Ultrasound Program

Vivek S. Tayal • Michael Blaivas • Troy R. Foster
Editors

Ultrasound Program Management

A Comprehensive Resource for
Administrating Point-of-Care, Emergency,
and Clinical Ultrasound

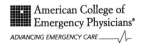 American College of
Emergency Physicians®
ADVANCING EMERGENCY CARE

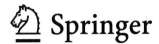 Springer

Editors
Vivek S. Tayal
Department of Emergency Medicine
Carolinas Medical Center
Charlotte, NC
USA

Troy R. Foster
Lutheran General Hospital
Park Ridge, IL
USA

Michael Blaivas
Department of Emergency Medicine
St. Francis Hospital
Columbus Georgia
University of South Carolina School
of Medicine
Columbia, SC
USA

ISBN 978-3-319-63141-7   ISBN 978-3-319-63143-1   (eBook)
https://doi.org/10.1007/978-3-319-63143-1

Library of Congress Control Number: 2018930883

Printed on acid-free paper

This Springer imprint is published by Springer Nature
The registered company is Springer International Publishing AG
The registered company address is: Gewerbestrasse 11, 6330 Cham, Switzerland

How to Use this Book

Clinicians face increasingly sicker and more complicated patients than ever before and physicians need access to life-saving technology. In the past two decades, ultrasound has become increasingly available at the bedside making tremendous impacts in patient care and patient safety. However, creating a successful ultrasound program that provides education, equipment management, and quality control is often the barrier that prevents this life-saving technology from reaching patients. Without a sound management program, point-of-care ultrasound (POC US) use is disorganized, unregulated, and unsafe.

As physicians, we hope to positively impact our patient's lives with innovative healthcare. As educators and administrators, our impact can be exponential, especially with a well-designed and a well-run ultrasound program providing our colleagues with ultrasound availability and future physicians with vibrant training.

Program directors confront many challenges when constructing their program starting with finding the right equipment to incorporating a successful workflow process. It is difficult to gather all the needed information and advice to make competent decisions without having to learn everything through trial and error. To overcome this burden, the editors enlisted an impressive legion of expert authors and compiled decades of cumulative experience. Now in one place, ultrasound directors have a comprehensive resource.

The Editors' goals are to provide all the tools necessary to make a program successful beginning with a conceptual framework and then providing specific templates and tools. The editors understand that program development and management is dynamic as national policies and available tools change. At the time of publication, this book is as current as possible. It also provides reference websites to keep you, the US program director, abreast of new developments.

In this first edition, we made some editing decisions that reflect the evolution in US practice and philosophy of the US management courses we have directed. First, the chapters in this book cover many subject areas, many of which overlap. We made a conscious decision to allow overlap, so that the reader did not have to move to another chapter for reference to a topic. However, individual topics are fully explored in their home chapter. Second, the topics are independent of experience level, so novice program directors may wish to follow our advice for the fundamental chapters. Third, as true in any area of knowledge, there will be practice, technical, regulatory, reimbursement, and legal changes that require you to correlate subject matter with current statutes.

Fourth, we have substitute POC US for the many terms for this field including clinical, clinician-performed, focused, emergency, critical, bedside, physician-performed, and others. Time will resolve the varying nomenclature. Finally, US is based on technology which changes at breakneck speed and alters practice and management.

Evolution of Program Management

POC US is relatively new and during its infancy it was a challenge for the program directors to manage. Traditional users have had a system set up with archiving, billing, and hospital policy. Bedside ultrasound used in the emergency department, intensive care units, and offices did not enjoy previously designed pathways for privileging, reimbursement, and archiving. As emergency physicians started to use this US technology, it became apparent that successful implementation of an ultrasound program required more than hands-on training and interpretation skills. Education on program management was needed to provide the key components to safe and effective diagnostic and procedural ultrasound.

In 2004, sponsored by a grant from the American College of Emergency Physicians, Dr. Vivek Tayal organized the first Emergency Ultrasound Management Course which had the mission to provide ultrasound program directors the tools to set up a well-functioning program. Now, several other courses offered around the United States also offer education regarding program management.

The course was the first recognized resource for emergency room ultrasound directors to learn the multifaceted components of program development. The faculty instructors were experts in their respective material including the core topic, the Ultrasound Director, given by Dr. Mike Blaivas.

Other specialties also recognize the need of program management and have included management education during their hands-on ultrasound courses, such as the American College of Chest Physicians Ultrasound Course at their national simulation center.

Although a few other small courses exist with a program management component and a few textbooks briefly introduce the basics of program management, there is no comprehensive guide to this topic. Thus, this book is relevant to the continued growth of POC US.

Starting Point and Section Organization

Dr. Tayal's introductory chapter is your first priority. It is a global perspective on clinician-performed bedside ultrasound. Be sure to digest this important chapter as your first task to becoming an informed ultrasound director.

The early chapters of this book focus on the leadership of your program whether in your department or institution.

The second section centers on education at all levels recognizing that smaller machines have made ultrasound available for medical students to advanced practitioners. It even includes a section on ultrasound simulation, a growing educational tool.

The third section provides detailed logistics on equipment, maintenance, and safety. This is, by far, the most practical section for useful information and advice immediately applicable to your program.

In the fourth section, we focus on the engine of a program, which is the quality improvement program. We devoted a chapter to workflow process which should get considerable attention of any new ultrasound director. For those with limited budgets we also offer a section on practical operating and educational solutions.

The fifth section offers insight into hospital level credentialing, quality assurance, national politics, and recent issues with accreditation. This is followed by reimbursement and coding, which hands you the monetary keys to pay for your program.

The last section covers topics in specialized communities. Chapters focus on ultrasound in pediatrics, critical care, community, and office-based practices. Finally, the book covers ultrasound programs in emergency medical services and the global health effort.

If the reader is starting a program from the ground floor, the editors recommend reading first the chapter titled: Ultrasound Director. The next steps are acquiring equipment, establishing a privileging pathway, providing education for the physician staff, and setting up quality assurance. A crucial component to easing the workload is a smooth functioning workflow solution. These are the priority chapters the editors recommend for fledgling programs.

Novel program recommended chapters
Chapter 2: Ultrasound Director
Chapter 12: Equipment Purchase
Chapter 5: Introductory Education
Chapter 16: Quality Assurance
Chapter 17: Workflow and Middleware

At whatever point your program is in its development, we make the promise to you that this book will give you the conceptual building blocks and ample specific details to take your program to the next level.

Park Ridge, IL   Troy R. Foster, MD

Contents

Section 6   US Special Communities

Contributors

Srikar Adhikari, MD, MS, FACEP Department of Emergency Medicine, University of Arizona, College of Medicine, Tucson, AZ, USA

David P. Bahner, MD, FACEP Department of Emergency Medicine, The Ohio State University Wexner Medical Center, Columbus, OH, USA

Michael Blaivas, MD, MBA, FACEP, FAIUM Department of Emergency Medicine, St. Francis Hospital, Columbus, GA, USA

University of South Carolina School of Medicine, Columbia, SC, USA

Christopher J. Bryczkowski, MD, FACEP Department of Emergency Medicine Robert Wood Johnson Medical School, New Brunswick, NJ, USA

Mark W. Byrne, MD Department of Emergency Medicine, Boston Medical Center, Boston University School of Medicine, Boston, MA, USA

Eric J. Chin, MD, FACEP Department of Emergency Medicine, San Antonio Military Medical Center, Fort Sam Houston, TX, USA

Gerardo Chiricolo, MD, FACEP Department of Emergency Medicine, NewYork-Presbyterian Brooklyn Methodist Hospital, Brooklyn, NY, USA

Haley Cochrane, MBBS Department of Emergency Medicine, Massachusetts General Hospital, Boston, MA, USA

Thomas Cook, MD Department of Emergency Medicine, Palmetto Health Richland, Columbia, SC, USA

Apostololos P. Dallas, MD, FACP, CHCP Department of Internal Medicine, Virginia Tech Carilion School of Medicine and Research Institute, Roanoke, VA, USA

Andreas Dewitz, MD, FACEP Department of Emergency Medicine, Boston University School of Medicine, Boston Medical Center, Boston, MA, USA

Petra E. Duran-Gehring, MD Department of Emergency Medicine, University of Florida College of Medicine-Jacksonville, Jacksonville, FL, USA

Robinson M. Ferre, MD, FACEP Department of Emergency Medicine, Vanderbilt University Medical Center, Nashville, TN, USA

Troy R. Foster, MD Lutheran General Hospital, Park Ridge, IL, USA

Rajesh N. Geria, MD, FACEP Department of Emergency Medicine, Robert Wood Johnson Medical School, New Brunswick, NJ, USA

Jessica R. Goldstein, MD, FACEP Department of Emergency Medicine, University Hospitals Ahuja Medical Center, Case Western Reserve University, Cleveland, OH, USA

Zachary T. Grambos, MD, FAAEM Emergency Department, Saint Thomas Rutherford/Midtown Hospital, Murfreesboro, TN, USA

Patrick S. Hunt, MD, MBA Department of Emergency Medicine, Palmetto Health Richland, Columbia, SC, USA

Robert Jones, DO, FACEP Department of Emergency Medicine, MetroHealth Medical Center, Case Western Reserve University, Cleveland, OH, USA

Dan Katz, MD, FACEP Department of Emergency Medicine, Cedars-Sinai Medical Center, Los Angeles, CA, USA

John L. Kendall, MD, FACEP Department of Emergency Medicine, CarePoint Healthcare, Denver, CO, USA

Department of Emergency Medicine, University of Colorado School of Medicine, Aurora, CO, USA

Heidi H. Kimberly, MD, FACEP Department of Emergency Medicine, Brigham and Women's Hospital, Boston, MA, USA

Resa E. Lewiss, MD Department of Emergency Medicine, Thomas Jefferson University Hospital, Philadelphia, PA, USA

Matthew Lipton, MD Department of Emergency Medicine, Vanderbilt University Medical Center, Nashville, TN, USA

Rachel Liu, MD, FACEP Department of Emergency Medicine, Yale School of Medicine, New Haven, CT, USA

Michael P. Mallin, MD, FACEP Division of Emergency Medicine, Department of Surgery, University of Utah School of Medicine, Salt Lake City, UT, USA

Jennifer R. Marin, MD, MSc Departments of Pediatrics and Emergency Medicine, Children's Hospital of Pittsburgh of UPMC, Pittsburgh, PA, USA

Christopher L. Moore, MD, FACEP Department of Emergency Medicine, Yale School of Medicine, New Haven, CT, USA

Brian B. Morgan, MD Department of Emergency Medicine, Denver Health Medical Center, Denver, CO, USA

Arun D. Nagdev, MD Department of Emergency Medicine, Highland General Hospital, Oakland, CA, USA

Bret P. Nelson, MD, FACEP Department of Emergency Medicine, Mount Sinai Hospital, New York, NY, USA

Vicki E. Noble, MD, FACEP Department of Emergency Medicine, University Hospitals, Cleveland Medical Center, Cleveland, OH, USA

Laura Nolting, MD, FACEP Department of Emergency Medicine, Palmetto Health Richland, Columbia, SC, USA

Jason T. Nomura, MD, FACEP, FACP, FAHA Department of Emergency Medicine, Neurosciences Service Line, Christiana Care Health System, Christiana Hospital, Newark, DE, USA

Laura Oh, MD, FACEP Department of Emergency Medicine, Emory University Grady Memorial Hospital, Atlanta VAMC ED, Atlanta, GA, USA

Aliaksei Pustavoitau, MD, MHS Department of Anesthesiology and Critical Care Medicine, Johns Hopkins Hospital, Baltimore, MD, USA

Christopher C. Raio, MD, MBA, FACEP Department of Emergency Medicine, Good Samaritan Hospital Medical Center, West Islip, NY, USA

Nelson A. Royall, MD Department of Surgery, The University of Oklahoma College of Medicine, Tulsa, OK, USA

Sachita P. Shah, MD, FACEP Department of Emergency Medicine, University of Washington, Harborview Medical Center, Seattle, WA, USA

Paul R. Sierzenski, MD, MS HQS, FACEP Acute Care Services, Renown Health, Reno, NV, USA

Erik Su, MD Department of Anesthesiology and Critical Care Medicine, Johns Hopkins Hospital, Baltimore, MD, USA

Shane M. Summers, MD, FACEP Department of Emergency Medicine, San Antonio Military Medical Center, Fort Sam Houston, TX, USA

Vivek S. Tayal, MD, FACEP Department of Emergency Medicine, Carolinas Medical Center, Charlotte, NC, USA

Molly E.W. Thiessen, MD, FACEP Department of Emergency Medicine, Denver Health Medical Center, Denver, CO, USA

Department of Emergency Medicine, University of Colorado School of Medicine, Aurora, CO, USA

Robert J. Tillotson, DO, FACEP Northwest Wisconsin Emergency Medicine, Mayo Clinic Health System, Eau Claire, WI, USA

Alfredo Tirado-Gonzalez, MD, FACEP Department of Emergency Medicine, Florida Hospital-East Orlando, Orlando, FL, USA

Christopher David Wilbert, MD Department of Emergency Medicine, St. Thomas Rutherford Hospital, Murfreesboro, TN, USA

Stanley Wu, MD, MBA, FACEP Department of Emergency Medicine, Baylor College of Medicine, Houston, TX, USA

Chapter 1
Initial Approach to Ultrasound Management: Making Ultrasound Meaningful from the Start

Vivek S. Tayal

Objectives

- Describe the clinical characteristics of clinical, point-of-care ultrasound
- Understand the importance of Ultrasound Management Goals
- Define the essential steps of Ultrasound program
- Understand the cycle of education, quality review, improvement, credentialing
- Recognize strategy and situational awareness in program design
- Define ultrasound program success

Perspective on Point-of-Care Ultrasound Evolution

Ultrasound is the ultimate application of engineering, computers, and medicine as a window into the human body. While there have been many technologies that utilize the application of physics to assess the human body, ultrasound is unique. Ultrasound is nonionizing, portable, rapid, economical, and synergistic with the clinical examination [1]. However, the most important development with this technology is the willingness of clinicians to perform and interpret ultrasound at the bedside for clinically occult conditions. This enthusiasm coupled with technological advances such as solid state chips, computerized engineering, man-made piezoelectric crystals, miniaturization, wireless and web-based communication, and digital storage has made ultrasound the practical diagnostic technology of this era.

V.S. Tayal, MD, FACEP
Department of Emergency Medicine, Carolinas Medical Center,
Charlotte, NC, USA
e-mail: vtayal@aol.com

© Springer International Publishing AG 2018
V. S. Tayal et al. (eds.), *Ultrasound Program Management*,
https://doi.org/10.1007/978-3-319-63143-1_1

1

Point-of-care ultrasonography (POC US), also known as "clinical ultrasonography," is the application of ultrasound technology to diagnose, resuscitate, monitor, and treat medical conditions in a focused manner relevant to the medical condition of the patient [1, 2]. Clinical point-of-care ultrasound programs are a natural evolution of the rapid adoption of ultrasonography into medicine throughout the world during the last 30 years. While ultrasonography was traditionally part of "imaging" or "radiology" or "cardiology" departments, adoption of powerful, portable, bedside ultrasound equipment has created the point-of-care revolution [3]. Not only can physicians of any specialty bring this technology to the bedside, it can be done with little infrastructure and resource need [4]. Ultrasound provides unique synergy of the bedside evaluation emphasizing safety of nonionizing radiation, value of an economical scientific test, and efficiency of the provider's time.

History of Point-of-Care, Clinical US

Clinical ultrasound programs historically began simply with machine acquisition, basic training, and initiation of scanning. As clinicians started to use ultrasound, there were unique historical characteristics to their use compared to traditional imaging. Specialties such as emergency medicine, family practice, surgery, urology, obstetrics/gynecology, critical care, and others started to use ultrasound in a focused manner to answer clinical questions like " is there fluid in the abdomen?" "is there an abdominal aortic aneurysm?" "is there urinary retention?" "what is the position of the fetus?" and many other clinical questions. Table 1.1 lists common ultrasound applications in clinical specialties.

Most of these ultrasound examinations were done to answer a specific clinical question, and not as a comprehensive imaging examination. Ultrasound machines used by clinicians were smaller, more portable, and simpler to use. The training for clinicians varied per specialty, but included physics, instrumentation, and the clinical area of ultrasonography [5]. Image production, if produced, was initially typically thermal printing or video, with movement to digital output only in the last decade. System software such as PACS (Picture Archiving Communication System) was not available for clinical ultrasound providers, and electronic medical records were not initially in existence. Politically, it became clear that there were issues at the hospital level in acceptance of clinical ultrasonography. In 1999, the AMA House of Delegate's resolution 802 provided guidance for hospital credentialing committees to accept specialty specific training guidelines [6]. From 1999 through the present, point-of-care ultrasound has grown both in applications and by specialty.

The greatest paradigm shift in the use of medical ultrasound technology was the concept that the clinician both performed and interpreted the ultrasound examination, in contrast to the traditional service of sonographer in a remote ultrasound laboratory followed by physician interpretation [7]. See Fig. 1.1. For all the reasons above, ultrasonography is considered a "disruptive innovation" in medicine [8, 9].

Table 1.1 Common examples of point-of-care ultrasound applications by clinical specialties

	EM	Surgery	Critical Care	FP	Ob/gyn	Urology	IM	Pediatrics	Orthopedics	Anesthesia
Free fluid in abdomen	X	X	X	X	X	X	X	X		
Pericardial effusion/cardiac function	X	X	X	X			X	X		X
Aortic aneurysm	X	X	X	X			X	X		
Pregnancy location or viability	X			X	X					
Pneumothorax/pleural effusion	X	X	X	X			X	X		X
Soft-tissue/musculoskeletal	X			X			X	X	X	
Procedural guidance	X	X	X	X	X	X	X	X	X	X
Deep vein thrombosis	X	X	X	X			X	X		
Urinary tract obstruction	X		X	X		X	X	X		

<u>Traditional Consultative US workflow</u>

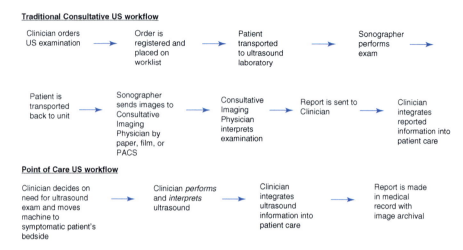

Fig. 1.1 Comparison of workflow in consultative US versus POC US

US Management

Picking up the ultrasound probe may be the easy part of an ultrasound program, but the hard part is delivering a safe, efficient, meaningful, transferable, and reimbursable service in modern medicine. Once a novice sonologist has moved on from exploring with the machine, they realize that there are significant ramifications to each part of the ultrasound service. The choice of machine and probes, the amount of education, the manual steps for image acquisition, acceptable cleaning protocols, availability of the machines, ultrasound supplies, written or digital transmission, reporting, coding, reimbursement, different clinical settings, and innovations are variables in the delivery of ultrasound services.

As point-of-care ultrasound started to gain acceptance and credibility throughout clinical medicine, it became clear that implementation had unique features that required guidance. Ultrasound program management is not intuitive to the clinicians or health systems where they work. The American College of Emergency Physicians (ACEP) Section on Emergency Ultrasound created a course to address these issues, the Emergency Ultrasound Management Course [10]. During the last 10 years, that course has been expanded and refined to a unique knowledge base for ultrasound program leaders. With the proliferation of the different specialties using ultrasound, it became clear that there was a shared basis to this information.

Ultrasound management describes the implementation and management of ultrasonography by clinicians in their unique setting. In this chapter, we will describe strategies and key concepts that should help any clinician initiate, grow, and manage an ultrasound program [10].

In Table 1.2 we define common terminology used in ultrasonography.

Table 1.2 Common terminology in clinical POC ultrasonography

Ultrasonography—use of high frequency sound waves in the diagnosis, monitoring, guidance or treatment in clinical care
Clinical, point-of-care, focused, bedside ultrasound—Physician or provider performing ultrasound to diagnose, monitor, resuscitate, and treat medical conditions
Consultative ultrasound—ultrasonography done in traditional manner with performance by sonographers and interpreted by a physician in a two component service
Sonographer—medical professional who performs ultrasonography. Most commonly refers to professional who has finished training in an ultrasound school or finished sonographer training in an undergraduate college degree. Often anyone who performs ultrasound may be given this name
Sonologist—a physician who performs, interprets, and integrates ultrasound into the clinical care of their patient
Ultrasound management—a program implementation, administration, and supervision of a program that makes ultrasound meaningful in clinical practice

Ultrasound Management Goals

Defining the goals of an ultrasound program is an important step in the implementation of a successful ultrasound program. The goals can vary depending on practice setting, economic model, quality goals, workflow, teaching, and research mission. Typically, clinicians perform ultrasound examinations because they are a test that gives more information than the history or physical, like soft-tissue ultrasound for occult cutaneous abscess. Ultrasound can be a standard test in the evaluation of certain patient types, such as in pregnancy. Ultrasound can be used to improve safety, such as the use of ultrasound guidance for internal jugular vascular access. Educational settings and programs are enhanced by using ultrasound to demonstrate the anatomic or pathophysiologic condition of a patient. Ultrasound can also be part of an investigational research question, by adding sonographic variables or outcomes. No matter the goal, ultrasound gives clinicians a powerful tool to improve care [11].

All programs should strive to make ultrasonography meaningful in the care of their patients and to the provider. While many ultrasound programs initially start out with educational ultrasound examinations that are supervised, confirmed, or overread, reliance on a "confirmatory test" should be temporary, as clinical competence is gained. But that process of reliance on a "confirmatory test" should be temporary, as clinical competence is gained. In addition, a common and erroneous description of point-of-care ultrasound is that it is an "extension of the physical examination." While ultrasound is complementary to the physical examination, ultrasound has separate science, technology, skills, interpretation, and value in clinical medicine [3, 12]. Meaningful use of ultrasound adds information to the patient's evaluation beyond the history or physical examination, and without the use of confirmatory testing.

Your priorities and sequence of steps in program design depends on many variables such as architecture of the health system, physician and provider training, machine availability, economic reimbursement model, practice setting, academic mission, medical specialty, and possibly cultural or national norms. For example, a

Table 1.3 Essential steps for your ultrasound program

1. Define your initial scope of ultrasound practice
2. Establish a leader
3. Get a machine that meets your needs
4. Get the training needed for practice
5. Get credentialing/certification in your system (if possible)
6. Integrate and invest in a system that integrates ultrasound images and reports into your medical record or medical system's method of communication
7. Appropriately bill for ultrasound services
8. Monitor and improve via quality improvement processes and cycles
9. Create a budget for your ultrasound program
10. Adopt new applications and technologies as your program matures

community hospital with a substantial amount of geriatric and non-trauma may want to start with a program that emphasizes procedural guidance for central lines, biliary, aortic renal, and cardiac scans for the middle aged and geriatric populations with a clear reporting and billing program. An academic center with the need to teach residents or students may wish to prioritize the resuscitative ultrasound applications of trauma, cardiac, obstetric, aorta, thoracic, and procedural guidance with substantial equipment investment. An office-based clinician may choose the applications that meet specific needs using existing billing codes with minimal equipment purchase.

The minimum requirements for an ultrasound program are an interested clinical physician, an ultrasound machine, ultrasound education, and clinical need for ultrasound evaluation. But there are more considerations than can make the implementation of your ultrasound program more complete, such as US leadership, provider credentialing, ultrasound examination reporting, quality improvement, clinical ultrasound protocols, coding and billing and incorporating new ultrasound applications. Table 1.3 outlines the essential steps for your ultrasound program (checklist).

Leadership

Ultrasound program management requires a dedicated physician who can understand the complexities and subtleties of an ultrasound program [2]. While most of the time this is usually one person (at least initially), it can be a cast of many, so long they are aligned to creating a successful program. Leadership in ultrasound management may start small in divisions or departments but also may grow into institutional or health system positions that span several departments, hospitals, clinics, and specialties (See Chaps. 2, 3, 4).

Ultrasound Equipment

As discussed later in the equipment chapter (Chap. 11) there is a vast availability of ultrasound equipment in various size and capability. In addition, a wide selection of ultrasound transducers may fit your clinical needs. Whether for a solo practice in an office, or large group practice in an urban emergency department, the usage models, education, maintenance, and continuing care models need to be considered carefully. Image quality is important but cost, ease of use, workflow, durability, reliability, and maintenance must be thought out.

US Training

Initial training may be implemented in variety of different pathways including undergraduate medical education, graduate medical education continuing medical education courses, departmental in-services, fellowships, or preceptorships (Chaps. 5 and 6). With the advent of new educational techniques such as free online education, downloadable digital courses that can be downloaded, and simulation products, you may find covering the didactic portion of education easier than in the past. However, nothing can be substituted for hands-on teaching for clinical ultrasound. The provider must be able to manipulate the probe and machine to the get the imaging required for sound decision-making. In addition, ultrasound education must be tailored to the educational level and goals of the providers.

Quality Improvement

The cycle (Fig. 1.2) of performance, assessment, feedback, and improvement is fundamental to the success of the ultrasound program. An assessment and feedback system should be considered as the program is developed. Images, reporting, and

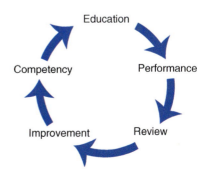

Fig. 1.2 Cycle of education—Performance—Review—Improvement—Competency

feedback can take considerable time and effort. Digital systems have helped but regardless of the hardware, software, and reporting systems, quality improvement programs must be in place to allow for appropriate training, credentialing, monitoring, improvement, and expansion of programs (Chap. 16).

Credentialing and Certification

Once physicians get trained to the level of acceptable competence, credentialing or certification within your health system can occur. Attention to the rules and requirements of the health system may be worthwhile as you design your program. Certification by third-party organizations such as sonographer or physician organizations may be obtained, but credentialing at hospital and hospital systems will still be required. Designing your credentialing plan with your national, state, healthcare system, and specialties guidelines in mind will create the architecture that makes your educational and training system successful, efficient, and accepted by your peers (Chaps. 19 and 20).

Clinical Protocols

Once education, equipment, and training are in place, ultrasound must be integrated into clinical scenarios, procedures, and algorithms. This aspect of management may be overlooked but is key to efficient, rational, and appropriate use of ultrasound. Examples of ultrasound in the undifferentiated hypotensive patient, procedural guidance of central lines, ultrasound for soft-tissue infection, monitoring of IVC diameter for the volume depleted patient, and US guidance of therapeutic injections. In each case, ultrasound has its place in the clinical sequence, practice algorithms, and expected results. Careful consideration of ultrasound's place in current clinical care will guarantee acceptance, performance, and success.

Information Management

Once an ultrasound examination is performed and interpreted, the information will need to be reported and documented in a medical record. The reporting may be minimal in the battlefield or a disaster, and very sophisticated in a tertiary care center with images and reports being integrated from the machine to the electronic medical record by wireless communication. You should have a thoughtful plan for rapid accurate, succinct, and reimbursable manner documentation (Chaps. 17 and 18).

Work Value and Reimbursement

Ultrasonography takes clinical time, which is the most important commodity to a physician. Ultrasonography must carry its own weight in regard to value. In the United States, there are codes for US services for both professional (interpretation) and technical elements (performance, equipment, supplies, and overhead), and this may help defray costs of equipment and supplies. Ultrasonography contributes to value in medical care in regard to sound medical-decision-making, more clinical efficiency, improved risk management, increased safety, and better outcomes. While the program's steps of education, machine acquisition, credentialing and integration usually precede the reimbursement phase, eventually a mature ultrasound program will want the appropriate recognition with value calculation and reimbursement for the ultrasonography examination (Chap. 22).

Ultrasound Strategy

Strategy depends on the practice environment and resources. Prioritizing education and machine purchase are obvious first steps, but thinking about your quality assurance, budget, archiving and reporting needs to be well thought out. See Fig. 1.1.

Are your needs at just one location? Are more than one user or specialist going to use that machine? How will the images and report get into medical record (paper or electronic). You may not be able to solve all these issues at once but keeping them in mind as you structure your program is wise.

Popular strategies for starting ultrasound programs include using quality, education, research, or practice needs as leverage. For those who are starting with initial resistance, emphasizing improving quality with the use of US with reference to national and specialty standards may be a good initial strategy. Research utilizing ultrasound as the diagnostic goal, monitor, or variable is certainly another strategy that can be employed and may provide data to start a program. Depending on the clinical specialty, your department may have to meet educational standards that require US at undergraduate, graduate, and postgraduate levels. Finally practice demands of patient care needs, such as obstetric patient waiting time, high rates of penetrating trauma, or lack of DVT US at off hours may be the initiating clinical requirement to start an US program.

Situational Awareness

We cannot overemphasize the importance of situational awareness (Table 1.4) in developing your ultrasound strategy. You understand resources in your health system, the rules and regulations of the institutions and jurisdictions in which you live,

Table 1.4 Situational awareness

Practice guidelines
Federal and state laws
Medical staff politics
Administrative health system politics and budget
Maintenance program and personnel
Departmental or group dynamics
Information technology policies and trends
Workload

and interaction of other providers with your adoption of ultrasound. A famous politician once said all politics is local, and we would say that the politics of ultrasound often are the application of more national and specialty politics to your local situation (Chap. 19). Knowing the atmosphere in your system, the credentialing or certification rules, budget structure, local politics, and temperaments of your institutional colleagues can help guide you overcome avoidable obstacles. These are the non-ultrasound issues that affect your US program.

Modern issues in American health system include the specialty specific ultrasound guidelines, evolution of the EMR, credentialing rules and regulations of the medical staff, budgets for equipment, information system platforms, provider workflow, payment models, infection control regulations, quality improvement systems, and other technologies and medical devices that are used or intervene in medical conditions where ultrasound is used.

Creating a US Network with Key System Personnel

Table 1.5 lists key personnel and departments that interface with your ultrasound program. This will depend on your setting and your healthcare system. It is important these key players understand the relevance, mission, and strategy of ultrasound in your clinical setting.

Timing

The timing of implementation can vary, but there should be some goals for implementation once a machine (machines) and initial education has been obtained. Credentialing plans and clinical protocols should be in place as soon as initial education is obtained. Administrative oversight will require reviewing intermittent review of individual and departmental goals throughout the year. A well-thought-out plan for a busy clinical group should allow completion within 1–2 years, but this depends on the size of group, individual clinical load, frequency of ultrasonographic abnormal scans, and credentialing plan requirements. See Table 1.6 for suggested grid of implementation.

Table 1.5 Key players in US program

Ultrasound Director or Lead Physician
Department Chair/leadership of group
Group/Department physician members
Equipment Manufacturers and Sales Representatives
Clinical engineering
Infection control
Materials management
Nursing
Traditional imaging specialties
Information services
Hospital or health system leadership/ CMO

Table 1.6 Timeline of management grid

	Suggested timeline of completion	Your timeline
Leadership	Months 0–3	
Machine	Months 0–3	
Initial education	Months 0–6	
Experiential training phase	Year 0–2	
Credentialing/certification	Year 0–2	
Archiving	Continuous	
Quality assessment	Continuous	
Reporting	Continuous after training	
Billing	After credentialing	

New Frontiers

Ultrasound is addictive, intriguing, and intellectually progressive. The anatomy and physiology learned in medical school can be seen within seconds of your initiation of placing the probe on the patient. Uses that go beyond the traditional boundaries are flourishing. One can expect to grow and expand your program as both new applications are created and your program naturally grows beyond its initial structure.

Definition of Success

A successful ultrasound program is defined by the performance, interpretation, and integration of ultrasonography by clinicians with accuracy, reliability, and consistency (Fig. 1.3). The ultrasound examination should stand on its own performance and interpretation separate from the clinical examination and other testing, especially other imaging. The ultrasound examination should have meaning to all in the medical system—patient, provider, peers, payers, and public.

Fig. 1.3 Maturation of ultrasound programs

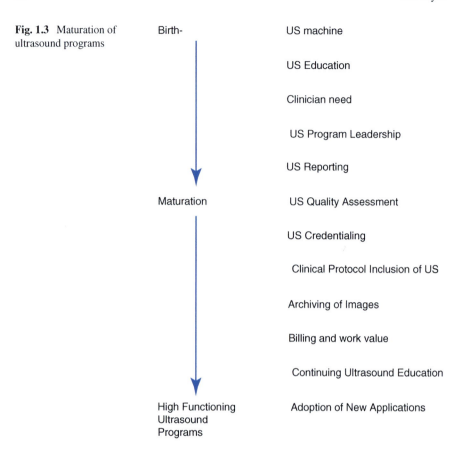

Birth-   US machine

US Education

Clinician need

US Program Leadership

US Reporting

Maturation   US Quality Assessment

US Credentialing

Clinical Protocol Inclusion of US

Archiving of Images

Billing and work value

Continuing Ultrasound Education

High Functioning Ultrasound Programs   Adoption of New Applications

Pitfalls

1. No leadership.
2. Lack of an ultrasound machine after education, and lack of education after obtaining a machine.
3. Imposing an ultrasound program without regard to clinical and provider workflow.
4. Lack of a quality improvement program that assesses technique and outcomes.
5. Not understanding that ultrasound program components are interdependent.
6. Clinicians not valuing ultrasound as reimbursed work or a skill separate from the physical examination.

Key Recommendations for US Program Management

1. Define your mission—why you want to use US in your setting.
2. Designate a leader to the ultrasound program.

3. Strategize with situational awareness of the opportunities and threats in your medical environment.
4. Get a machine that meets your practice's needs and integrates with your workflow.
5. Initiate the cycle of education, performance, improvement, competency.
6. Make decisions that align the components of your US program for maximum efficiency and effectiveness.
7. Make your ultrasound program meaningful to clinical care.

References

1. Moore CL, Copel JA. Point-of-care ultrasonography. N Engl J Med. 2011;364:749–57.
2. ACEP. Emergency ultrasound guidelines. Ann Emerg Med. 2009;53:550–70.
3. Greenbaum LD, Benson CB, Nelson LH, Bahner DP, Spitz JL, Platt LD. Proceedings of the compact ultrasound conference sponsored by the American Institute of ultrasound in medicine. J Ultrasound Med. 2004;23:1249–54.
4. Shah S, Noble VE, Umulisa I, et al. Development of an ultrasound training curriculum in a limited resource international setting: successes and challenges of ultrasound training in rural Rwanda. Int J Emerg Med. 2008;1:193–6.
5. Mateer J, Plummer D, Heller M, et al. Model curriculum for physician training in emergency ultrasonography. Ann Emerg Med. 1994;23:95–102.
6. H-230.960 Privileging for Ultrasound Imaging. http://www.ama-assn.org/apps/pf_online/pf_online?f_n=resultLink&doc=policyfiles/HOD/H-230.960.HTM&s_t=Ultrasound&catg=AMA/HOD&&nth=1&&st_p=0&nth=2&. Accessed 2001.
7. Physicians ACoE. American College of Emergency Physicians. ACEP emergency ultrasound guidelines-2001. Ann Emerg Med. 2001;38:470–81.
8. Lewiss R. How an old technology became a disruptive innovation. TEDMED2014.
9. Christensen C, Dann J. Sonosite: an insider's view. Boston: Harvard Business School; 2001.
10. ACEP. Emergency ultrasound management course. In: Tayal V, Foster T, editors. Emergency ultrasound management course. San Franscisco: ACEP; 2003.
11. FAST Consensus Conference Committee, RA STM, Chiu WC, et al. Focused assessment with sonography for trauma (FAST): results from an international consensus conference. J Trauma. 1999;46:466–72.
12. Geria RN, Raio CC, Tayal V. Point-of-care ultrasound: not a stethoscope-a separate clinical entity. J Ultrasound Med. 2015;34:172–3.

Chapter 2
Ultrasound Director

Michael Blaivas

Objectives

- Understanding the scope of an ultrasound director position
- Describe key components of organizing an ultrasound program as a director
- Describe incorporation of an ultrasound program into the wider system
- Understand strategic components critical to strengthening an ultrasound program

Introduction

The job of ultrasound director can take on many forms and differ based on setting. It also invariably changes throughout time. Given the nature of point-of-care ultrasound and its incredible growth over the last two decades, every ultrasound director should be prepared for and in fact push for growth in their program. One of the most frequently asked question is why does my institution, clinic, office, or department need an ultrasound director? The answer lies in the nature of point-of-care ultrasound itself and that it is different from most other things we do. This can be a particularly challenging concept to describe to seasoned providers. They have seen new applications come and go and are used to learning new methods in a short CME course or journal and adding it to their medical toolkit with a finite investment of time. A good example may be learning to inject joints, tendons or a new intubation technique. However, ultrasound is different from any of these individual applications.

M. Blaivas, MD, MBA, FACEP, FAIUM
Department of Emergency Medicine, Columbus, GA, USA

University of South Carolina School of Medicine, Columbia, SC, USA
e-mail: mike@blaivas.org

© Springer International Publishing AG 2018   15
V. S. Tayal et al. (eds.), *Ultrasound Program Management*,
https://doi.org/10.1007/978-3-319-63143-1_2

Many providers did not learn ultrasound in their training programs and as opposed to learning to use a video laryngoscope after using blind intubation for years, ultrasound has multiple components such as physics, machine optimization, multiple applications and providers have to learn ultrasound anatomy as well. Some providers may view the addition of ultrasound as a nuisance, especially if they are past the midpoint in their career. Many providers are simply struggling to keep up and adding one more thing leads to pushback, at least until those providers realize how point-of-care ultrasound can actually improve their practice. Fortunately this attitude has been changing, mostly because of the introduction of new practice guidelines.

In general, the ultrasound director is effectively a champion and cheerleader for ultrasound in the department or clinic and while this is the first duty, secondary duties like quality assurance and education are close behind. A common misstep would be to have someone take on the job who has lots of responsibilities in the department, such as the residency director, quality assurance director, or medical director.

Benefits to Having a Director or Coordinator

Much like the birth of a department or group itself, introduction of ultrasound is essentially a business venture. The benefits of introducing ultrasound should be outlined as well as the benefits of having an ultrasound director. Ideally the ultrasound director is appointed prior to starting an ultrasound program, but this may not be practical in many settings where the realization of a "need" only materializes after a disaster or sentinel event with ultrasound. Considerable management is required with ultrasound use, especially as it scales. While the benefits of ultrasound are numerous, so is the potential for missteps and conflict with traditional imagers. Lastly, many clinicians find it appropriate to be reimbursed for utilizing their new ultrasound skills and the benefits applications bring to their practice. Time and effort will have to be dedicated to streamlining the documentation, billing and negotiating processes that come naturally with the ultrasound. In fact, a centralized person with a fund of knowledge of ultrasound is mandatory for troubleshooting, education, billing, and liaison/political activities. These and other roles (Table 2.1) are part of the ultrasound director's job.

Table 2.1 US Director's typical interfaces with other healthcare system personnel	
	ED physicians
	Operations manager
	ED chair
	Residency director
	Nurse manager
	Hospital
	Credentialing committee
	Purchasing
	Clinical engineering
	Infection control
	Informatics

Things to Consider Ahead of Job Commitment

The clinician pondering taking on the job of ultrasound director should consider the commitment carefully, because it's such an important job and has to be taken seriously. The prospective ultrasound director should be well aware of the various components that will make up his or her job. Learning ultrasound from the ground up is simply not feasible at this stage in point-of-care ultrasound, so this is an important prerequisite. For the position to be sustainable and role successful, enough time and resources have to be dedicated by the clinic, department, or group to ultrasound.

Negotiations for protected time, staff support, moneys for equipment and meetings should be done upfront. Negotiating after the job has been accepted may be difficult in the current era of cost cutting and emphasis on clinical productivity. This is the case whether one is considering ultrasound directorship in an academic or private practice setting (See Chap. 3 – Job Search and Contract Negotiations).

Depending on the clinical setting and the relative power your specialty wields, resistance from traditional imagers may be expected. It is no longer accurate to blanket label radiologists as obstructionists to clinician use of ultrasound as it seemed to be years ago, but at the local level this is typically the most frequent point of conflict and friction. Other traditional imagers include cardiology, vascular surgery, and occasionally obstetric/gynecology. Before taking a new job it behooves the prospective director to survey the institutional imaging landscape and not depend on the departmental medical director or chairperson. They may not really be aware of how radiology and others will react or may have an incentive to underestimate possible challenges. Ideally, address your questions to the radiologists themselves or others, perhaps the vascular laboratory run by vascular surgery.

The great paradox is what to do when promises are broken, a machine is never purchased, protected time does not materialize, etc. While verbal agreements mean nothing, it is important to realize that a written contract may not offer you much more protection. Will you be willing to litigate to inforce your contract? Does state law give you a fighting chance of winning? How likely are you to keep your job if you push so hard? Will you get reference letters if you enforce your contract in a messy legal process? These are just a few things to consider and you may come to believe there is little you can do if agreements are broken. However, having agreements in writing is still a wise option. In some facilities such contracts will be enforced internally. It may be a good reminder to your supervisor what he/she promised to deliver. Alternatively if you do leave to another job, a letter showing the promised machine, protected time and staff support will give you a negotiation starting point and verify that you left for a credible reason. Even if you never plan to inforce or contest the promises broken, a written contract is good to have.

Prospective ultrasound directors often feel that being the first in a program or department is the ideal position and may be reluctant to be the second ultrasound director. While there may be merit to this line of thinking initially, many ultrasound directors, however, have found that it's best to be the second US director after the first one has initiated the departmental conversation. In the interim, the department or group may have realized more support is required, or you may simply be a better fit or more qualified. It is prudent to have an alternative plan. That plan B will differ from person to person, but if ultrasound is important enough to you, it is wise to know who else might be looking for ultrasound directors in the vicinity or are considering starting an ultrasound program. This is best performed on an ongoing basis. Business schools actually recommend this approach to executives. Always keep active in your network. Be aware of positions that are open and inquire with others in the industry about open position, plans, new programs, etc. This process can be couched as learning opportunities and continuous investigation into process improvement.

Taking on the New Job

When starting a new ultrasound directorship position, if you are coming in from the outside you will have disadvantages as well as advantages. Most directors experience a honeymoon period, while it may be short-lived, it should be taken advantage of. Coming in from the outside may allow you to be viewed as the "expert who is brought in." This can buy some instant credibility and ease your path to creating a program. Another time of opportunity which may not be evident on the surface is a time of upheaval or change in the practice, clinic, or department. As jobs shift, duties are expanded, increased flexibility may be available and shifting priorities may make it easier to get ultrasound off the ground with adequate support. There is a flip side to the opportunity which is broken promises, changes in direction, and sudden loss of funding as other projects come on line unexpectedly.

Established Patterns and Credentialing Pathways

Of particular interest should be any previously established practice patterns with ultrasound. Especially in newer specialties to point-of-care ultrasound, a credentialing pathway may be something that has not been discussed previously. As seen in this textbook, credentialing, if using ultrasound in the hospital setting, is of great importance (Chap. 20).

If the answer is yes, and a credentialing pathway exists, verify and obtain a copy. More often than not there will be unexpected surprises. While creating a credentialing pathway for your department or group at the hospital may be one of your first tasks, it is helpful to explore this process even before signing on. The same applies to a private office or clinic setting where the entire group may have to approve a plan and training outline for the group. Remember, just because the chairperson or medical director says they want ultrasound to happen, it is rarely a done deal. Look for landmines prior to stepping on them. If looking at a hospital setting, consider speaking with the credentialing committee or medical executive committee directors to get their sense for how receptive the committees may be to point-of-care ultrasound or if possible road blocks already exist. Keep in mind that roadblocks are just that and sometimes you simply have to drive off the road to get around them. The more you know about this ahead of time, the better you can plan.

Once you have a lay of the land you will need to consider your options. In some cases turning down an opportunity that seems fraught with too many obstacles or too good to be true is the best option. Groups often promise things they cannot deliver and it may be completely unintentional. If you start getting that sense, be honest with yourself, ask more questions, and decide how much risk you are willing to take. Always check to see if administration is on board and if they are, ask provocative questions such as "what if the radiology group threatens to leave if we start using ultrasound on the floors?" You may get a more honest answer at that point. Billing is a topic that often comes up, especially if radiology is involved. Make sure you are prepared to answer these questions. Also, read the chapter on reimbursement and be aware of your options. In some cases the revenue generated by billing can mean the difference between support for the program, administrative time or not. An US director's responsibilities and training is included in Table 2.2 (from CUAP website).

Table 2.2 Ultrasound director description

THIS IS A SAMPLE DOCUMENT ONLY
ACEPs policy statement, <u>Emergency Ultrasound Guidelines</u>, approved October 2008, states:
Emergency ultrasound director
The emergency ultrasound director or coordinator is a board-eligible or certified emergency physician who has been given administrative oversight of the emergency ultrasound program from the EM director or group. In addition to coordination of education, machine acquisition maintenance, the US director is responsible for developing, monitoring, and revising the QA process
Ultrasound director responsibilities (list all responsibilities pertaining to the ultrasound program)
For example, the Ultrasound Director's responsibilities might include:
– Developing and ensuring compliance to overall program goals: educational, clinical, financial, and academic.
– Designing and managing an appropriate credentialing and privileging program for physicians and/or residents within the group and/or academic facility.
– Designing and implementing in-house and/or out-sourced educational programs for all residents and attending physicians involved in the credentialing program.
– Monitoring and documenting physician privileges, educational experiences, ultrasound scans, and CME.
– Developing, maintaining, and improving an adequate QA process in which physician scans are reviewed for quality in a timely manner and from which feedback is generated.
– Developing and monitoring an ultrasound machine maintenance care plan to ensure quality and safety.
Ultrasound director training (include credentialing and length of time in position)
For example, it is recommended that the Emergency Ultrasound (EUS) Director meet the following requirements:
– Credentialed as an emergency physician
– Maintains privileges for EUS applications
– Designated as Ultrasound Director by the Medical Director of Emergency Medicine
– If less than 2 years in position as Ultrasound Director, directors are highly encouraged to have performed **one** of the **three** following tracks toward ultrasound management education:
1. Graduated from an EUS fellowship
2. Attended an EUS management course
3. Completed an EUS preceptorship or mini-fellowship

Who Else Is Using Ultrasound?

In the modern medical landscape there is almost certainly someone else in the hospital that is using ultrasound clinically. This may be other departments, specialties, or groups. In the majority of cases, unlike traditional imaging providers, these colleagues are likely to see your entry into ultrasound as a boost for them. The more clinicians use ultrasound, the more power they have to stave off pressure from contrarians, be they in the same specialty, a different one, or in administration. If you are able to find out, contact those individuals ahead of time, get some honest answers. If you are encouraged by their experience, start getting to know those clinicians early to make ties, even before taking on the role of ultrasound director.

If you cannot identify other users of ultrasound in the hospital or medical center other than cardiology and radiology, investigate deeper. Are there exclusive contracts? These may be illegal based on applicable laws, but may still be in place. Such contracts are often seen with radiology where the hospital has agreed that only the radiology group can provide imaging services. Such a contract may be used to stop your ultrasound program in its heels. However, upon a closer look, one often discovers that cardiology also uses ultrasound to image and possibly others as well. This may be your angle to get ultrasound into your practice.

The Ultrasound Director Job

Whether you are going to be running ultrasound in an emergency department, internal medicine clinic, intensive care unit, or any other location, it is important to realize just what this can entail. It is more than just checking where the machine is periodically and dusting it off. In fact, such ultrasound directors tend to make themselves and their colleagues miserable while stifling rather than promoting ultrasound use. It can be an all-encompassing job at the other extreme (See Table 2.1—Interactions with other health system). Depending on the setting, especially for emergency medicine, internal medicine, critical care, and other specialties where multiple ultrasound applications may be utilized, ultrasound may touch almost everything you do. For instance, there is little doubt that the physical examination will be forever altered in the future by ultrasound. Similarly, it is becoming too risky to insert a needle anywhere other than an obvious superficial vein without ultrasound.

Many ultrasound directors find that a flourishing ultrasound program is much like having your own department within a department. At least there is a possibility of growing the program to its full potential, with many examples around the country in critical care, emergency medicine, and internal medicine departments. Practically speaking, this means considerable power and influence for the ultrasound program as well as a real impact on patient care delivery in your facility.

At this point, ultrasound directors should you plan ahead. Time management is critical. Plan which initial topics to address, partition the approach to ultrasound adoption, and consider a staggered approach to ultrasound introduction. If your group or department is considering five ultrasound applications they would like to adopt, let's say DVT evaluation, central line placement, focused cardiac, joint injections, and lung ultrasound, it could be challenging to tackle all of these at once. While an ultrasound education course may be able to address all of these topics in 2 days, getting a number of clinicians up and running on all of these applications will be challenging, especially in a private practice setting where nonclinical time may be quite limited. It is important to communicate this to your employers so that they fully understand the pitfall of trying to tackle everything at once. If that is something they insist upon, then you will need much more protected time and colleagues will need real incentives to keep them motivated.

Ideally there will be general agreement to undertake just one ultrasound application at once. This does not mean an ultrasound course that teaches only how to stick a peripheral or central vein under ultrasound guidance. A full course that compasses several applications as well as physics, machine operations, etc. is very important. Indeed, if you are just going to put ultrasound-guided central lines, it makes sense to learn basic lung ultrasound to rule out pneumothorax and some soft tissue ultrasound to understand surprise findings on pre-scans. Yet, the ultrasound director's job will be more limited in such a setting than one where ten ultrasound applications will be practiced.

An inspiring ultrasound director never rests. One of my favorite statements about ultrasound was made by Dr. Alex Levitov, a successful critical care ultrasound pioneer: *"Ultrasound is the only infection I know of that cures."* Those who have been involved with point-of-care ultrasound over the years will recognize the accuracy of this statement. It reflects both the frustration of some with point-of-care ultrasound and the incredible utility of the technology. Once providers recognize how helpful it is in one clinical application, they start to wonder about using it elsewhere and start applying ultrasound more and more liberally.

A decade ago ultrasound directors were invariably in academic positions and training residents, faculty, fellows, and medical students was a large portion of their job. Currently, many ultrasound directors are needed in the private practice setting, but resident and medical students training is still very important. This will often fall under academic responsibilities expected from faculty and some specialties have found that starting fellowships is a great way to increase qualified future faculty for academic programs. Ultrasound in medical school education is an exploding topic. At the time of writing nearly a quarter of medical schools already have or are in the process of introducing 4 year integrated ultrasound education curricula (see undergraduate medical education chapter). This provides a great opportunity for ultrasound directors to become involved at the medical school and institutional level. While this may seem like simply additional work it also means additional leverage. Such leverage can be used to obtain needed equipment, protected time, and other resources. The larger the ultrasound program and the more widespread its impact on the department, clinic, hospital, or medical school, the less likely a chair or medical director can ignore requests for additional support (See Chap. 7 – Undergraduate US Education).

The planning of departmental ultrasound infrastructure is made additionally challenging when students and residents are added to the mix. It will become even more important to find allies in your group to help teach. This does not mean some-one who is already trained, although that would be ideal, but rather someone who is willing to learn. That one person can soon double your efficiency and show others that getting involved may be beneficial. Ideally, create several ultrasound colleagues to share work, training duties and discuss interesting cases and future goals.

Extramural Involvement

More and more frequently ultrasound directors in various specialties are being asked to help outside of their department or specialty. This may be working with nursing, EMTs, or other specialties to help introduce ultrasound. This is an oppor-tunity to attain additional allies and grow the influence your program has in the facility. Invariably that influence translates to better support and an increased degree of shielding from detractors or outright hostile forces. Time and resources should be considered as your time may be stretched thin.

Quality Assurance and Improvement

With all of these duties how can the ultrasound director do anything else? Yet one key function cannot be overlooked. This is quality assurance and improvement. It may be possible in a mature program to do little quality assurance, but even in such cases disaster will eventually strike. Quality assurance involves the review of all studies performed by providers who are not yet credentialed by the hospital or have not met clinic/practice goals for competency outside of a hospital setting. Such review is discussed later in the textbook but ideally is performed in person. The ideal is unreachable in most cases, so a good substitute is video, not just the cardiol-ogy habit of saving 1 s video clips, but longer digital videos such as 20–60 s. Such videos clips will tell the story of the path a novice took to find or miss the organ of interest or potential pathology. Even for procedures, one can gain incredible insight by reviewing video regarding improvements.

Making the Ultrasound Directors Job Easier

There are several general things which can make the ultrasound director's job easier and some have already been mentioned in this chapter. Carving out protected time is absolutely critical and the ultrasound director should be cautious in thinking that protected time will come after proof of concept. This may be the only approach and has definitely worked, but caution is warranted as many directors in this position have ultimately quit in frustration for lack of protected time. If you are getting push-back, it may simply be due to the novelty of ultrasound directorship for the group or specialty. Recall, those quality assurance directors, medical directors, and others will typically receive protected time. Document the hours spent per week if already in the position or project if simply considering. Looking at nearby groups, programs or even pulling information from the literature can be extremely helpful.

If you have never set up an ultrasound program, a text such as this is absolutely essential. The basics of setting up a program are fairly simple; avoiding the pitfalls that many of us fell into may be harder. Multiple medical societies have resources on line for providers that address documentation, quality assurance, education, billing, and other topics. Such a review is also a good idea to get a sense for what is happening in other specialties and what standards others may have. In fact, it is prudent to know what is happening in other specialties in terms of applications being used, policies and some higher profile studies or manuscripts which have been published. This will increase the potential for collaboration in research, patient care, and education, among others. The more you can partner with others in the clinical setting, the more leverage everyone will have to push ultrasound forward and stave off attacks from opponents.

Every ultrasound director learns that despite the rebellious nature of point-of-care ultrasound in the past, to be successful, one needs to align their ultrasound goals with that of the department or group. Once done, the path to winning over the department as a whole and especially individual providers will often be more obvious. To win over superiors and colleagues it is important to assume their view point first. How will ultrasound benefit them? Will it enhance the way the department or group is viewed because of cutting edge technology? Perhaps others in the area are using ultrasound or new providers are reluctant to join a group they perceive as not keeping up. For individuals it often means decreased risk of procedures. A harder concept to convince an experienced practitioner is that ultrasound will take their high level of competence and increase it further, often dramatically, whether this is placing a central line, injecting a shoulder, or assessing the heart during a physical examination.

Consider presenting your plan for ultrasound development and roadmap for the future to the group, after discussing it with leadership. Get input and be ready to explain your reasoning behind each step. This is where any standards, policy statements, or high profile research studies may be helpful in illustrating your assertions. You plan should reach several years in the future and does not have to be as complete as your master plan. Areas of immediate concern should be addressed first, such as a pneumothorax caused by a central line placement or frustration with time delays in getting DVT ultrasound studies or others which can be done rapidly at bedside.

Making a Service Plan

Creating a service plan is often helpful for the ultrasound director and chairperson or medical director. The service plan should not only include what ultrasound applications will be using but also how it will serve the department, clinic, or group. Additionally, do you offer the service outside of the department or clinic is an important question. Working with a nursing home, emergency medical services, local government or other in the medical center or clinic could potentially bring in additional funding.

The service plan should also include longer term plans, on the order of 3–5 years, for ultrasound equipment and any peripherals such as a workflow system, servers, and printers. Many programs find it beneficial to have a graded equipment response. They plan for increasing ultrasound use and resultant future purchases accordingly. If you start with placement of an occasional central line but will then adopt focused echo, then lung ultrasound and others you may need additional transducers and then even additional equipment as you grow from 1 user to 17. Obviously, budgeting is a very useful skill, even at a rudimentary level.

Compensation

Compensation is an important topic as in any case where you may be doing additional work or have expertise above their peers (Also see Chap. 3). This is no different from someone in the group or office that has IT expertise, a business expert, or the quality assurance guru. There is some psychological value to the additional recognition and compensation. It shows you and others that your work and expertise are valued and that they bring value to the group or department. There is an increasing amount of data being published regarding ultrasound director compensation, hours required to perform the job and impact ultrasound makes on the bottom lines of departments. Much of this is limited to emergency and critical care ultrasound at this time, but others will likely follow with similar publications. Regardless, parallels can be drawn even if from a different field to support your bid for compensation and salary support. Identifying someone in a similar situation and obtaining buy-down time information may further support your arguments, even if on a different scale or with a different payer mix. There is a significant time requirement for this role and Table 2.3 gives you some insight into the time requirements and the expertise level to complete tasks. It can be used when negotiating for protected time and salary, understanding that we did not attach actual hours in each task except QI, which is a little easier to quantify.

Table 2.3 US director's time commitment calculator (adopted from Troy Foster, MD)

Director task	Time	Skill requirement
Equipment		
Equipment purchase	1	2
Equipment maintenance	2	2
Accessory equipment logistics	1	1
Logistical help	−1	
Quality improvement		
Scans performed/month	3	2
Information technology work	4	5

Table 2.3 (continued)

Director task	Time	Skill requirement
Workflow solution	−3	
Education		
Attendings needing training	3	4
Residency training	4	3
Medical student training	4	2
Assistant directors/fellows	−2	
Politics		
Credentialing	1	5
Hospital politics/committee work	1	4
Reimbursement issues	2	5
Multiplication factors		
Patient volume	5	
Size of group/training level	4	
Number applications performed	4	
Number of machines	3	
Fellows to train	2	
Residents	3	
Medical students	2	
Growth	2	
QI time requirement formula		
[((Scans/day) × (1.5 minutes/scan))/60 min] × 7 days = Hours spent per week performing QI		

System Wide POC US Director

Somewhat of a new concept is the system wide ultrasound director. This will typically apply to a medical center, large clinic or a system of hospitals or clinics. In contrast to the typical siloed approach to point-of-care ultrasound, some systems realize that having too many different standards and no centralized quality improvement and educational approach can stifle growth and even lead to disasters. A leader overseeing all point-of-care ultrasound programs throughout a system leads to considerable efficiency improvements. Centralized education programs, across the board standards and coordination of resource utilization are all attractive to larger systems (Chap. 4).

Working with Industry/Consulting

This is a frequent question, probably not so much regarding do I say yes or no to a request, rather, how do I get involved. Why would someone consider consulting with industry or ultrasound vendors? The obvious is additional income, but there are other reasons. Consulting may be a way to affect healthcare on a much larger scale than you are able to in your clinic, office, or department. Additionally, it is often intellectually challenging. Most providers will never have a change in lifestyle from doing some consulting on the side, but it can be rewarding and also expand your horizons.

Medico-Legal Issues

Medico-legal concerns are both your friend and your enemy. Hospitals, medical systems, surgical centers, and others detest paying out litigation fees and awards and missed cases leading to law suits are a true motivating factor. Missed pulmonary emboli, abdominal aortic aneurysms, pneumonia, pneumothorax, DVT, and others are just a few of the long list of entities which can be diagnosed accurately at the bedside with point-of-care ultrasound. Never forget that risk management can be a great ally.

The converse may be a bigger fear for most providers and administrators. This fear is often stoked by contrarians who are protecting turf or hoping not to have to learn a new technology and applications. How often are point-of-care ultrasound providers being sued? The few data that have been published suggests that point-of-care ultrasound users are sued very infrequently and may be at more risk for being because they failed to utilize ultrasound rather than missing something on their scan [1, 2]. This may change in the future, as it is statistically an eventuality.

The best way to avoid successful litigation is having established policy and procedure. Fly by night scans with no trace of them in the medical record increase liability, not decease it. Invariably there is someone who recalls that the scan was performed just before the patient expired and a nurse may have even documented it. You may have done nothing wrong, but the mere failure to document and suggested impropriety from the plaintiffs that you were somehow hiding this fact can turn a jury against you or create suspicion and doubt. There are more and more guidelines available from clinical specialty societies regarding documentation, recording and reporting. Utilize these whenever possible. Fortunately, more and more workflow solutions now exist to make documenting ultrasound examinations in the electronic medical record easier and more seamless.

A proper credentialing process is also important to protect from litigation and in case of litigation. Some malpractice insurers may not cover you if you perform a procedure without credentialing for it. Similarly, if the credentialing process does not meet national guidelines, to the extent they are available, insurers may feel at risk during trial and force a settlement in an otherwise potentially defensible case. Recall that plaintiffs' attorneys are not too far behind us in reading policies and invariably have access to experts who might have an understanding of the lays of the land.

Defensive Planning

Defense planning is a critical component of the ultrasound director, at least a good ultrasound director that wants to protect their program and facility. It is important to be seen as valuable by the group, clinic, office, or medical facility. A valuable ultrasound program, one that improves patient care and hopefully generates revenue, either through savings or income, is much less likely to be shut down by administration than one which is not. As the cliché goes, the best defense is a good offense, please keep in mind this does not mean attacking anyone. However, think like your likely detractors might think? What are your programs weaknesses? Maybe you do not have published data to support the applications you are using? Find the data, it is likely out there or find something close. If you cannot, maybe you should not be using ultrasound in that fashion. At the very least, be able to show that others in your specialty or in a related setting are using ultrasound similarly. What are potential pitfalls of what you are doing based on common knowledge or published literature. If out of plane visualization for central venous cannulation has been shown to have a higher rate of complications, maybe you need to switch everyone to an in-plane cannulation approach. Be aware that some of the worst outcomes occur when administrators find out you have no written policy, procedure, and quality improvement process. These alone can back off risk management because you can show you are essentially operating safely and have a plan for improvement. Talk to others and anticipate mistakes which will be made by novice user, try to educate them out before they occur.

Having the facility vested in your program is critical to protect it from negative consequences. Perhaps in the case of a hospital a procedure service starts utilizing ultrasound and is offered to the hospital and to replace it would incur additional expense. Safety or risk reductions provided by your ultrasound program are also a benefit to the facility and will protect you. It is also helpful to keep a file of ultrasound issues even outside of you area. This may yield several benefits. First, it may give you a glimpse of potential pitfalls to avoid. Second, it levels the playing field when you realize that radiology misses things on ultrasound scans all the time as well, something that is not a sign of poor quality but reality. Third, if pressed you may need to produce this data at high level meetings if assertions are made that one department or service is perfect in its performance of ultrasound while you are inferior. Actual data in the form of multiple cases tend to bring out cooler heads among administrators, who will quickly realize you are being vilified due to turf reasons.

Lastly, know applicable federal and states laws and regulations and actively make sure you are adhering to them whether they deal with cleanliness of equipment, electrical safety or proper and secure documentation. These are simply obligations for you and your program to comply with but are also smart defensive moves to avoid potential complications downstream.

Key Recommendation

Taking on the role of ultrasound director should not cause anxiety, but approaching the job with an appropriate level of commitment, understanding, and skill is critical.

Relevant Literature

There is scant literature on directing an ultrasound program but several helpful tangential articles are available on billing, reimbursement, and administratively relevant issues.

References

1. Blaivas M, Pawl R. Analysis of lawsuits filed against emergency physicians for point-of-care emergency ultrasound examination performance and interpretation over a 20-year period. Am J Emerg Med. 2012 Feb;30(2):338–41.
2. Stolz L, O'Brien KM, Miller ML, Winters-Brown ND, Blaivas M, Adhikari S. A review of lawsuits related to point-of-care emergency ultrasound applications. West J Emerg Med. 2015 Jan;16(1):1–4.

Chapter 3
Job Search and Contract Negotiations

Laura Oh

Objectives

- Discuss the importance of clearly defined career, ultrasound-related, and personal goals prior to entering into a job search or contract negotiation
- Describe principled negotiation and how it differs from positional bargaining

Introduction

The transition from ultrasound training to a first-time ultrasound position represents a time of great excitement but also great uncertainty. In addition to defining more specific goals related to an ultrasound career and position, there is value in early identification of broader career and personal goals. For many applicants, the definition, alignment, and commitment to career, ultrasound, and personal goals is the most challenging part of the job search process.

L. Oh, MD, FACEP
Department of Emergency Medicine, Emory University Grady Memorial Hospital,
Atlanta VAMC ED, Atlanta, GA, USA
e-mail: laura.oh@emory.edu

© Springer International Publishing AG 2018
V. S. Tayal et al. (eds.), *Ultrasound Program Management*,
https://doi.org/10.1007/978-3-319-63143-1_3

Job Search

The traditional academic job application cycle begins in October, however, new opportunities can arise at any time. Although it may be tempting to start the job search as early as August or September, the downside of this strategy is that it may lead to an unnecessarily protracted search.

To prevent interview season fatigue, it is in the best interest of the applicant to cluster interviews within a few weeks of each other. An early and solo job offer may lead to unnecessary pressure for an applicant with an interview scheduled with a preferred employer later in the season, as most employers will want a reply to a job offer within 4 weeks. There are some advantages to applying very late in the season (i.e., spring), because of the relative lack of competition for late-breaking opportunities. However, the late season applicant runs the risk of an employment gap as the typical credentialing process can be lengthy, with some states taking 5 months to approve a medical license.

The peak of the community job interview season tends to be earlier than the peak of the academic job season. In addition, the typical time frame for a job offer in community practice differs from that in academics. It is not unusual to receive an offer from a community job on the day of interview. In contrast, most academic institutions receive federal funding and will use fair hiring practices; the industry standard is to post an academic position for 30 days before making an offer to any candidate. Academic job openings may involve the input of search committees balanced with respect to race, gender, and experience; the opinion of current faculty members may be sought at a division or department meeting. Applicants who are applying simultaneously to community and academic positions may find that because the community and academic job search seasons are asynchronous, it may not be possible to hold onto early community offers and fully explore academic job opportunities.

Peak Value

A pitfall common to fellows overwhelmed by the decision-making process is to procrastinate by taking a starter job with the assumption that life goals will become more clear a year later. The problem with procrastination, however, is that an applicant's peak value does not rise in linear fashion with experience and time. Paradoxically, an applicant who has just completed fellowship may be a more attractive applicant to an employer than a fellowship graduate with 1 year's clinical experience. This is due, in part, to the name recognition of the fellowship site and the importance of the place of last employment.

Where to Look; How to Write a Cover Letter and CV

Although ultrasound positions may be advertised in academic journals, job search websites, or on HR webpages, the most helpful way to obtain a position is to network and utilize personal contacts. Much of this networking happens by being involved at national meetings, particularly in ultrasound-related activities. If an applicant has exhausted personal contacts, they might use information available online to make an educated guess regarding the interest of potential employers in new ultrasound hires. If, for example, a 40 person department lists 8 physicians with specialized ultrasound training on their website, it is less likely they will require an additional ultrasound-trained provider vs. a department of similar size with only one ultrasound-trained provider.

A valuable resource for how to write a professional cover letter and CV is the Barb Katz series which is available for free online. Ms. Katz, who is an EM consultant, advises that cover letters be specific and sincere, detailing what is desired from a position and why the applicant is the right hire [1]. Krista Parkinson, adjunct professor at USC, gives more cheeky advice—a cover letter should be "like a mini skirt: long enough to cover the important parts, but short enough to be interesting!" [2]. Cover letters and CVs should be submitted in PDF format to potential employers to ensure that extraneous markings of grammar and spell check do not distract from an otherwise qualified candidate.

Typical responses for a job query include an offer to interview, a forwarding of materials to a search committee, or a response stating that there are no openings but the CV will be kept on file. The applicant should not be discouraged if the answer is not an immediate "yes" as applicants may be considered for unforeseen openings that arise in the near future. A response, however, should always be expected. Occasionally because of the red tape of the hiring process, a qualified application can get lost on an HR website. Applicants should follow up on all nonresponders to close out every job query if no response is given within a reasonable timeframe.

Evaluating an Ultrasound Position

When evaluating an ultrasound position, the applicant should make an effort to understand the ultrasound milieu and gauge the enthusiasm for point-of-care ultrasound by potential work colleagues and other stakeholders such as radiology, cardiology, and OB departments. The applicant should make sure there is adequate IT and biomed support.

The applicant should take into account the existing level of expertise of providers to anticipate the workload needed to credential all providers. Although an employer might be interested in having an ultrasound program, they might not fully realize what resources need to be budgeted to run an ultrasound program successfully.

If the applicant is tasked with building a program from ground zero, they should confirm that there are adequate resources for this endeavor. Some employers will anticipate the expenses for equipment needs such as ultrasound machines of sufficient quality with an appropriate number of probes, cleaning supplies, procedural supplies, training mannequins, and phantoms. Many employers, however, will neglect to fully budget for a workflow solution (which may entail initial licensing fee and yearly subscription fee), costs of maintenance (e.g., service contracts or 10% of the machine price per year for the service contract once a machine is out of warranty). Academic directors will also want to ask for administrative support, access to statisticians, and a research coordinator to aid in IRB applications. The employer should recognize that the creation of an ultrasound program is a long-term investment—equipment will need to be replaced as it wears out and program needs change with growth.

Just as the applicant should be able to clearly articulate what is desired out of an ultrasound position, the employer should also be able to clearly articulate a vision for ultrasound in their department. An employer may wish to limit the scope of ultrasound applications (e.g., no transvaginal ultrasound); the applicant should consider whether they would be satisfied to work in an environment that does not allow full utilization of skills. Also of note, some departments may or may not be interested in billing for ultrasound; since revenue from billing can be used to expand an ultrasound program, this decision has important consequences for future machine purchase and hiring of additional ultrasound-trained providers (See Chap. 2 – Ultrasound Director).

Contract Considerations

The contract should be read in its entirety, with special attention given to tail coverage, noncompete, and termination clauses. All significant elements of the compensation package should be detailed in writing (e.g., number of shifts, number of total yearly hours, number of vacation weeks, CME allowance). If protected time is expressed as a fraction, the applicant should also have in writing the expected total number of shifts or hours per year. When comparing contracts, benefits such as health care, retirement, long-term disability, life insurance, vacation, sick leave, and CME make up a significant portion of the offered package outside of salary. Some jobs may offer a pension, while others may offer educational debt forgiveness, assistance with purchasing a home, college tuition for the children of employees, or tuition support for additional degrees.

Some very desirable jobs may be "non-negotiable." However, many employers are open to negotiation with a desired candidate, especially for low-hanging fruit such as delayed start date, moving expenses, medical board/licensure fees, board review course and test fees, additional CME or funding for ultrasound education and meetings. Items such as an ultrasound job title (e.g., director or assistant director) may be cost-neutral to an employer, but have significant value to the applicant in terms of either promotion or as a platform for desired ultrasound resources. Office space can be a scarce commodity; if not immediately available the applicant may request future office space during the next ED renovation.

The savvy applicant will avoid mention of money or schedule until the very end of negotiation, when they are fairly certain that they are a desired candidate and that they desire the job in turn. The amount of protected time for an ultrasound position will vary depending on factors such as geographic region, maturity of the ultrasound program, and expectations of the position (a 25% reduction of clinical load may be a reasonable starting point for discussion). There may be an ultrasound stipend or a sign-on bonus for those that inquire.

As a rule of thumb, when annual exams exceed 3600 (>10 exams/day), additional support is needed, whether in the form of reduction of clinical hours or a second person to assist with QA. The contract might include a provision for funds for an assistant ultrasound director hire or additional protected time when this benchmark is met. Negotiations may revolve around absolute shift reduction or an administrative fee for ultrasound QA or some combination of the above. For example, if an applicant is asked to do QA at multiple community sites, they might first estimate how much time it will take to provide QA at each site (as a rough estimate, 3–5 min/scan) and then negotiate an admin hourly rate for QA at roughly 50% of the clinical hourly rate at each site in addition to a shift reduction (e.g., 1/8 reduction of clinical load as a starting point if also requesting an hourly admin compensation).

Most contracts will follow a generic template that will not be tailored to the specific items desired in a contract for an ultrasound position. If the contract itself cannot be altered, a written promise in an email is worth more than a verbal promise, but will not be enforceable.

Negotiation

A negotiation is an exploration of whether your interests can be best met through an agreement or by pursuing a better alternative [3]. For a negotiation to be good it must have the 5 E's (Table 3.1): it must be efficient, it must endure, it must be equitable, it must meet each side's needs, and it must maintain existing relationships [4].

A common way to negotiate with someone is to take a strong position and defend it. This positional bargaining, however, often leads to deadlock as neither side can back down from their position without appearing weak [4]. The Harvard Negotiation Project,

Table 3.1 Five E's of a good negotiation

1. Efficient
2. Enduring
3. Equitable
4. Each side's needs are met
5. Existing relationships are maintained

created in 1979, pioneered a new method of negotiation called "principled negotiation" which avoids positional bargaining and looks instead for mutual gain [4]. Where interests conflict, this method advocates the use of independent fair standards.

The principled negotiation method can be applied to the negotiation of an ultrasound contract. A key tenet of principled negotiation is to focus on shared interest. Rather than focusing on a hard position (e.g., 50% vs. 25% protected time), the prospective employee may approach the negotiation from the point of view of the prospective employer. Administrators value patient satisfaction, patient safety, quality of care, and the bottom line. If the hospital the applicant is interested in working for has had recent sentinel events that could have been averted by the use of ultrasound (e.g., accidental carotid artery cannulation in central line placement), he or she might approach the negotiation from a patient safety perspective. For example, the applicant might offer to train all providers on how to avoid future similar complications and request appropriate protected time for this endeavor.

The principled negotiation method recognizes that although "splitting the difference" is often the easiest solution, it is often not the best solution because it assumes a fixed pie; neither side is completely satisfied with their portion. Sometimes a negotiation can be reframed to make a bigger pie [4]. For example, if an applicant is not satisfied with offered compensation for an ultrasound position, he or she might inquire if they can take on additional responsibilities for additional compensation. This additional responsibility might mean taking over ultrasound direction for the entire hospital rather than for just one department, or ultrasound direction for multiple sites rather than a single site.

If negotiations stall there are a few strategies to move forward. If the applicant is at an impasse with someone who will not back down from a strong position, determine the reason behind the position and explore if the same goals can be accomplished in an alternative way [4]. A third party mediator can sometimes break a deadlock by aiding in reframing the conversation in terms of shared interest rather than divisive position.

An important component of the principled negotiation method is the referencing of objective criteria. If there is a disagreement about compensation or position expectations, both applicant and potential employer can look to institutional, regional, and national precedents. Sometimes this exploration of objective criteria may benefit the applicant, but other times it can benefit the employer. What matters is that both parties keep an open mind and are willing to acknowledge objective criteria that are brought into the discussion.

An important step in preinterview preparation is to try to determine the underlying interests of the prospective employer and to determine the interests of individual people who might be work colleagues. Not only does preparation lay the groundwork for smoother negotiation, it helps determine if a potential employer's core values are in alignment with the potential employee's. A major component of long-term job satisfaction for an employee is respect for the employer and belief in the group's mission (Table 3.2).

Table 3.2 Applicant checklist

1.	Articulate personal and professional goals.
	Know what you desire out of an ultrasound position
2.	Use personal contacts/network to move application forward
3.	Send out CV and cover letter as PDFs keeping in mind the "mini-skirt" approach
4.	Before the interview, research the underlying interests of the prospective employer and seek objective criteria for fair compensation
5.	Understand the milieu—are all stakeholders (radiology, cardiology, OB, etc.) amenable to POC US?
	Understand employer's vision (billing/no billing; scope of applications desired)
6.	Read contract in entirety, paying attention especially to tail coverage, noncompete, and termination clauses
7.	Ask that anything of significance be put in writing
8.	Negotiate money and schedule at the very end
	Ask for a sign-on bonus and/or US Director stipend
9.	Look ahead and negotiate future adjustments based on future successes
	Keep records to support future renegotiations
10.	Make sure your personal values are in line with the group's core values/mission

Renegotiating a Contract

As an ultrasound program matures, inevitably the workload for the ultrasound director increases as the volume of scans increases. Opportunities for renegotiating a contract arise at times of "great saves" or "great misses" or "great asks." The ultrasound director should keep a file of "great saves" where use of point-of-care ultrasound altered the clinical course of a patient in a life-saving way. Sometimes the excitement of a "great save," can generate goodwill and additional financial resources. In contrast, great misses also provide opportunity to ask for additional funds if the miss could have been averted by use of ultrasound by an ED provider.

Finally, an ultrasound director might renegotiate a contract when a large task is asked for by the administration (e.g., system-wide credentialing of providers in multiple core ultrasound applications within a short timeframe).

Good record-keeping of all the hours spent on ultrasound activities provides objective data for administrators who might underestimate how labor-intensive ultrasound direction can be. Extra efforts will sometimes go unnoticed by administration if not properly documented.

An ultrasound director might also renegotiate a contract by highlighting how much revenue is generated by ultrasound billing. One technique that has been employed successfully is to isolate how much income is generated for the department in an average month by sending a set of dual charts—one with all ultrasound charges included and one without, to department coders.

Discussion

The long-term success of an ultrasound program requires a sustained effort by a director who is passionate about ultrasound. It is often the case that the amount of protected time given by the employer will not fully account for all the extra hours than an ultrasound director invests.

Programs falter when ultrasound directors feel undervalued or when they do not receive the resources they need, or when the employer's expectations have not been met. Open communication between the ultrasound director and administration is essential for the well-being of both the ultrasound director and ultrasound program.

Pitfalls

1. Failure to pause prior to job search to define clear personal and professional goals.
2. Procrastination of job search beyond peak value immediate post-fellowship.
3. Failure to read and understand contract, and to ask for items of significance in writing.

Key Recommendations

1. Do not be afraid to negotiate.
2. Choose principled negotiation over positional negotiation.
3. Renegotiate as the ultrasound program matures and succeeds.

References

1. Katz B. Career source: truth or consequences. Emerg Med News. 2012;34(8):20. doi:10.1097/01. EEM.0000418682.02837.43.
2. Parkinson K.. The mini skirt method to getting your resume read. 2016 Aug 16. http://www.huffingtonpost.com/krista-parkinson/the-mini-skirt-method-to_b_11656976.html.
3. Ury W. Getting past NO: negotiating in difficult situations. New York: Bantam Deli; 2007.
4. Fisher R, Ury W. Getting to yes: negotiating agreement without giving in. New York: Penguin Group; 2011.

Chapter 4
Institutional Point of Care Ultrasound

Gerardo Chiricolo and Vicki E. Noble

Objectives

- Understand institutional point of care ultrasound leadership
- Review strategies for implementation of an institutional point of care ultrasound program
- Review a sample organizational structure for institutional point of care ultrasound
- Learn the administrative and operational responsibilities involved in an institutional program
- Highlight the importance of interdepartmental collaboration

Introduction

Over the last decade, as ultrasound machines have become more portable, easier to use, and more affordable, point of care ultrasound has diffused into the practice of almost every specialty in the house of medicine [1]. The ability to make rapid diagnoses and monitor response to therapy at the bedside encourages an ever broader user base. Moreover, the introduction of ultrasound imaging in medical school—as it is incorporated into early basic science curricula like gross anatomy and physiology—means that a generation of young physicians begin their careers with

G. Chiricolo, MD, FACEP (✉)
Department of Emergency Medicine,
NewYork-Presbyterian Brooklyn Methodist Hospital, Brooklyn, NY, USA
e-mail: j7chico@gmail.com

V.E. Noble, MD, FACEP
Department of Emergency Medicine, University Hospitals, Cleveland Medical Center, Cleveland, OH, USA

© Springer International Publishing AG 2018
V. S. Tayal et al. (eds.), *Ultrasound Program Management*,
https://doi.org/10.1007/978-3-319-63143-1_4

ultrasound experience and exposure [2]. As more physicians and more specialties start to use ultrasound in their practice, the need for governance and an institutional organizational structure grows. Universal oversight, leadership, and quality assurance become increasingly necessary. Most significantly, standardizing the workflow processes by which the use of ultrasound is operationalized throughout an institution will mean increased efficiency and performance and will lead to a safer practice and increased patient benefit.

Who should lead this effort? Consideration should be made for physicians of specialties that have successfully implemented POC programs, use POC in multiple, non-specialty-based applications, and perform and interpret US at the bedside in a clinical manner. While physicians from many specialties should be considered, there is a strong case to be made for having an emergency physician as the point person for an institutional clinician performed ultrasound program during this era. First, no other organization has done more to support the practice of clinician performed ultrasound than the American College of Emergency Physicians. ACEP is the primary organization that has experience establishing guidelines for training and credentialing, safety, and quality assurance in clinician performed ultrasound [3]. Emergency medicine is also the only residency training program that has a wide breadth of ultrasound examinations as part of the core competency for residency training [4]. This exposure and expertise is helpful in managing an institutional program as no other specialty will have training that includes cardiac, obstetrical, vascular, general abdominal, ophthalmologic, and musculoskeletal exams. Finally, to date emergency medicine has led the effort to train leaders and experts in all aspects of running a point of care ultrasound program with dedicated fellowships, although increasingly other specialties are seeking out this training [5].

Establishing the Need

The first step in setting up an institutional point of care ultrasound (POC US) program is getting buy-in from your department and chair. Running a hospital-wide ultrasound program will take time and money, and without the support of the chair for the initial startup investment, the effort will be stalled. The justification for a departmental chair to support the program are:

1. Standing within the hospital community. The acknowledgement of an area of expertise will lead to increased visibility and leadership within the hospital governance structure.
2. Academic productivity. Centralized training and quality assurance increases the ability for institution-wide research on outcomes, comparative effectiveness, and patient satisfaction. Indeed, this research is essential for demonstrating the effectiveness of an institutional POC US program and in maintaining the institution's commitment to such a program.
3. Budget support. The budget of any hospital is a zero sum game but by stepping into a void and providing a service that can demonstrate improved patient care

Table 4.1 Critical steps in program development

Phase I	Phase II	Phase III
Chair support	Presentation to board	Collect data
Demonstrate need	IT support	Celebrate successes
Baseline metrics	Budget	Long term planning
	Gather champions	

efficiency and decrease resource utilization the department can claim back some of the indirect financial gains and savings provided by the program. Some of these benefits may be shared back with the department as well as the program.

The second step is to demonstrate a need that is hospital-wide. Oftentimes this need becomes self-evident as the inefficiencies of individual archiving systems, training programs, and machine maintenance across departments are demonstrated. Gathering data on procedural complications or redundant imaging also can demonstrate a need for integrated training and documentation [6–8]. In the initial stages of program development it is essential to establish a relationship with the hospital's coding and billing personnel. Data driven evidence will make gathering and maintaining support for the program much easier (Table 4.1). In addition, obtaining the number of physicians and specialties who have requested privileges for ultrasound use by speaking with the chair of the credentialing committee or with the office of the medical board can also support the need for an institutional program. Demonstrating that widespread use is occurring without general oversight and standardization could have clinical implications, medicolegal ramifications, and most importantly patient safety concerns for the hospital. An institutional ultrasound program provides a solution to this problem. Finally, do not assume that the administrative leaders who will be approving the formation of an institutional point of care ultrasound program will even understand what point of care ultrasound is. It is essential in the initial presentations to overwhelm the administration with the evidence for how ultrasound has been shown to decrease length of stay [9], decrease redundant imaging in the intensive care unit [10], improve patient satisfaction [11], decrease procedural complications [12] and review any current literature demonstrating efficacy and comparative effectiveness.

Finally, before the initial presentation to the hospital administration, after garnering the support of your chair, gathering data as above and reviewing the literature, it is essential to know who the individuals are that you will need to convince on the merits of an institutional program. Do your homework prior to the meeting and find out if you have supporters or detractors. Try to anticipate what the sticking points will be. It never hurts to have the "meeting before the meeting" as well to feel out what the controversial points will be. This is just good politics. Early involvement of departmental leaders, i.e., chairmen and vice chairmen of the various specialties involved, is of critical importance and will foster the support you will need in moving forward with the program. Each department will have different needs and objectives. Acquiring this information so that your presentation will speak to their specific concerns and expectations will lead to success.

The Presentation

The presentation to the administration will be critical. This proposal should include a mission statement, an organized rollout plan, the various curricula for different departments, safety mechanisms, machine purchase and maintenance plans, and a quality assurance mechanism. If there are other cross-specialty institutions within the hospital, meet with them and model the program on their successes. One example often cited is a pain management program. It is important to include a solid return on investment analysis in your proposal. Although you may see the patient care benefits and the obvious indirect returns the program will provide, most administrators appreciate a neat, direct, and concise analysis of the return. Direct returns can be derived from an estimated volume of exams, the regional charges from the CMS fee schedule for the professional fees on inpatients and both professional fees and technical fees (or the global fee) for outpatients. In addition, include an estimate on decreased procedural complications as a potential for improved revenue capture. Indirect returns such as decreased length of stay because of more efficient diagnostic turnaround, point of care ultrasound use in bundled payment cases and value-based reimbursement, and physician retention and satisfaction can also be mentioned.

There is also a significant cost to the equipment and infrastructure including both hardware and software purchases. Electronic health record interfaces alone can costs tens of thousands of dollars. Make sure you include reasonable estimates as it will be hard to explain unplanned budgetary expenses later on. It is also important to be clear and specific as to how to fund the program. Solutions include grant support, philanthropy, institutional funding, or departmental budget contributions. Usually it is some combination of all of the above but you will want to have a clear outline of this up front. Finally, it is appropriate to negotiate a compensation structure for your time and effort. This may include a yearly stipend, an hourly rate, a reduced clinical load, or any combination of the above. Establishing a program requires a considerable time commitment and it is recommended that you do not underestimate the amount of work to be done. Many realize that much time will be spent with education, quality assurance, and competency assessment. But few initially note the time for the development of policies and procedures, delineation of privileges, assessment tools, and the myriad of other responsibilities associated with this role.

How to Structure a Program

Once the need for the program is established, the next step is determining the model of organization that best suits the needs of your institution and patient population. There are two differing ways to model the organization and administration of an institutional point of care ultrasound program. The first way is by having a single leader or director of the program. Ideally this physician should have POC (currently, emergency ultrasound) fellowship training or have significant administrative experience in an ultrasound program and be well versed in all exam types of point of care ultrasound. It is important that if going with a single leader approach, that expectations are managed and it is understood that this person will not be able to train the entire hospital in point of care ultrasound. Instead, a timeline for "train the trainers" should be presented and the institutional leader can gather champions in each department who can take active roles in the education, oversight, and quality assurance in a specialty-specific manner.

The second model of organization and administration is via governance by committee. In this model, key ultrasound leaders throughout the institution will all contribute to the management and oversight of the program. This model should include clinicians from various specialties and expertise that encompass all point of care exam types to be performed institution wide. In this case it is wise to develop a governance or committee charter with clearly defined structure, rules and regulations, and terms and conditions. In particular, the chair of the board position should have delineated qualifications and terms. As a committee structure, the work can be shared and regularly scheduled meetings and reassessments of that work can be accomplished. In this scenario, support for the program might be easier to obtain as more specialties—namely traditional imaging specialties of radiology, cardiology, and obstetrics and gynecology—are directly involved in the administration of the program.

The logistics of how the program should be housed will be institutional specific. It may be initiated as a pilot program, a division of an established department that offers cross credentialing, or maybe even a distinct department outright. However it is done, having a clear organizational plan is essential.

Programming

Once the program is established, it is reasonable to begin training and infrastructure development. Most programs will start with a training schedule and then move to roll out a workflow for clinical use. Remember that training needs will be guided by specialty-specific curricula. The education should include didactic modules accompanied with hands-on training that meets your a priori defined standards. As the training and individual physician privileging is beginning, workflow processes can be rolled out. Documentation, archiving, and quality assurance can be done uniformly across the hospital but will require significant support from the hospital's information technology department, so make sure to involve them early in any plan.

Capture Your Data

As with any new program, it will be important to make sure you capture any and all data especially with regard to the metrics that demonstrate increased efficiency. Track procedural complications, length of stay, and number of chest X-rays in the intensive care unit. Having this data at subsequent administration meetings will enable you to demonstrate the return on investment for the institutional program and will help solidify your position.

Synergy

Considerations of creating point of care institutional leadership should also be considered with interest in system-wide US educational, research, accreditation, and protocol-based pathways. For example, creation of an US curriculum in the medical school or the Graduate Medical Education program is a perfect time to create an institution-wide structure. Quality of care programs, like US-guided vascular access, that incorporate US are another natural initiators of an institutional POC program.

Finally, celebrate all successes. Having a "case of the month" or "save of the month" that can encourage ultrasound use by late adopters and advertise the potential of the program can really help to create goodwill as well as highlight the patient benefit we all know that clinician performed ultrasound confers.

Pitfalls

- Not discussing with key players before administration presentation.
- Not planning for deliverables—i.e., length of stay, decreased complications, decreased consultative testing—to demonstrate a return on investment and improved patient care.
- Not interacting with specialties interested in US to address their concerns.

Key Recommendations

- Be sure to get your chair's buy-in
- IT involvement early
- Do not promise revenue early

References

1. Moore CL, Copel JA. Point of care ultrasonography. N Engl J Med. 2011;364(8):749–57.
2. Day J, Davis J, Riesenberg LA, Heil D, Berg K, Davis R, Berg D. Integrating sonography training into undergraduate medical education: a study of the previous exposure of one institution's incoming residents. J Ultrasound Med. 2015;34(7):1253–7.

3. American College of Emergency Physicians. Emergency ultrasound guidelines. Ann Emerg Med. 2009;53(4):550–70.
4. Sakhtar S, Theodoro D, Gaspari R, Tayal V, Sierzenski P, LaMantia J, Stahmer S, Raio C. Resident training in emergency ultrasound: consensus recommendations from the 2008 Council of emergency Medicine Residency Directors Conference. Acad Emerg Med. 2009;16(12):S32–6.
5. Lewiss RE, Tayal VS, Hoffmann B, Kendall J, Liteplo AS, Moak JH, Panebianco N, Noble VE. The core content of clinical ultrasonography fellowship training. Acad Emerg Med. 2014;21(4):456–61.
6. Killu K, Coba V, Mendez M, Reddy S, Adrzejewski T, Huang Y, Ede J, Horst M. Model point-of-care ultrasound curriculum in an intensive care unit fellowship program and its impact on patient management. Crit Care Res Pract. 2014;2014:934796.
7. Andersen GN, Graven T, Skjetne K, Mjølstad OC, Kleinau JO, Olsen Ø, Haugen BO, Dalen H. Diagnostic influence of routine point-of-care pocket-size ultrasound examinations performed by medical residents. J Ultrasound Med. 2015;4:627–36.
8. Randolph AG, Cook DJ, Gonzales CA, Pribble CG. Ultrasound guidance for placement of central venous catheters: a meta-analysis of the literature. Crit Care Med. 1996;24:2053–8.
9. Howard ZD, Noble VE, Marill KA, Sajed D, Rodrigues M, Bertuzzi B, Liteplo AS. Bedside ultrasound maximizes patient satisfaction. J Emerg Med. 2014;46(1):46–53.
10. Blaivas M, Sierzenski P, Plecque D, Lambert M. Do emergency physicians save time when locating a live intrauterine pregnancy with bedside ultrasonography? Acad Emerg Med. 2000;7:988–93.
11. Barne TW, Morgenthaler TI, Olson EJ. Sonographically guided thoracentesis and rate of pneumothorax. J Clin Ultrasound. 2005;33:442–6.
12. Peris A, Tutino L, Zagli G, Batacchi S, Cianchi G, Spina R, Bonizzoli M, Migliaccio L, Perretta L, Bartolini M, Ban K, Balik M. The use of point of care bedside lung ultrasound significantly reduces the number of radiographs and computed tomography scans in the critically ill patients. Anesth Analg. 2010;111(3):687–92.

Chapter 5
Introductory Education

Brian B. Morgan and John L. Kendall

Objectives

- Provide introductory ultrasound education tailored to the learners' needs
- Distribute pre-course materials including text and multimedia
- Ensure ongoing education and continued support of trainees

Introduction

Fundamental to any clinical ultrasound program are defined education and training requirements appropriate to the ultrasound applications and techniques utilized by a variety of physician specialties. In each case, training requirements should be established that are in accordance with recommendations endorsed by the physician's specialty. The American College of Emergency Physicians 2008 Emergency Ultrasound Guidelines makes the following statement: [1]

> "Emergency ultrasound requires emergency physicians to become knowledgeable in the indications for ultrasound applications, competent in image acquisition and interpretation, and able to integrate the findings appropriately in the clinical management of his or her patients. These various aspects of the clinical use of emergency ultrasound all require

B.B. Morgan, MD (✉)
Department of Emergency Medicine, Denver Health Medical Center, Denver, CO, USA
e-mail: brian.b.morgan@gmail.com

J.L. Kendall, MD, FACEP
Department of Emergency Medicine, CarePoint Healthcare, Denver, CO, USA

Department of Emergency Medicine, University of Colorado School of Medicine,
Aurora, CO, USA
e-mail: John.Kendall@dhha.org

© Springer International Publishing AG 2018
V. S. Tayal et al. (eds.), *Ultrasound Program Management*,
https://doi.org/10.1007/978-3-319-63143-1_5

proper education and training. The ACGME mandates procedural competence for emergency medicine residents in emergency ultrasound as it is considered a 'skill integral to the practice of Emergency Medicine' as defined by the 2008 Model of Clinical Practice of Emergency Medicine…we recognize the new spectrum of training in emergency ultrasound from undergraduate medical education through post-graduate training, where skills are introduced, applications are learned, core concepts are reinforced and new applications and ideas are introduced in life-long practice of ultrasound in emergency medicine."

Ultrasound continues to be listed as a core skill on the 2013 update to the Model of Clinical Practice of Emergency Medicine [2].

In general there are two pathways for emergency physicians training in ultrasound. The first is securing training in an ACGME-approved residency that includes an ultrasound curriculum. The majority of emergency medicine residents are taught ultrasound and will meet emergency medicine training standards by the completion of their training [3]. Residency-trained physicians should be granted emergency ultrasound privileges when joining a medical staff that recognizes emergency ultrasound privileges. In many instances these privileges will simply be a part of emergency medicine core privileges. In other instances, additional evidence of competency may be required, such as confirmation by the physician's residency director of a sufficient number of cases with demonstrated quality. Candidates for recruitment who have been trained in ultrasound often view the use of ultrasound by a practice as an indicator of quality.

The second pathway includes practicing emergency physicians who did not receive ultrasound training during residency. Others were in training when ultrasound was being introduced and have had exposure without sufficient structured education to meet emergency ultrasound training guidelines. This situation is not unusual, as physicians practicing in all specialties add new skills on an ongoing basis. A 2006 survey reported that only 33% of nonacademic emergency departments had available an ultrasound device for use by physicians, yet 36% of those without a device planned to acquire one [4], signaling the expansion of point-of-care ultrasound. More recently, 56% of emergency physicians in a variety of practice settings reported using ultrasound at least sometimes when placing a central venous catheter [5]. Emergency physicians trained prior to the institution of emergency ultrasound in residency training must acquire the necessary instruction through continuing medical education in order to maintain a quality practice and meet evolving standards of care. ACEP's Ultrasound Guidelines recommend 16–24 h in introductory training consisting of both lecture and practical sessions. They also suggest 4–8 h CME courses for focused training in 1–2 core applications [1].

Ultrasound is a core skill among other specialties as well. The Accreditation Council for Graduate Medical Education (ACGME) published milestones that recommend educational goals for resident physicians in each specialty. They recommend ultrasound mastery for Obstetrics and Gynecology as a part of obstetrical technical skill [6]. The American College of Obstetrics and Gynecology (ACOG) released a practice bulletin that states "Physicians are responsible for the quality and accuracy of ultrasound examinations performed in their names, regardless of whether they personally produced the images" [7]. The American Society of Echocardiography (ASE) recommends "comprehensive, specialized education in the medical and technical aspects of diagnostic cardiac sonography" in order to be qualified to perform echocardiographic examinations [8]. The American College of Chest Physicians made this statement for Intensivists: "We suggest that critical care ultrasonography requires competence in modules in the following areas: pleural; vascular; thoracic; and cardiac (basic and advanced echocardiography)" [9].

This chapter is a guide for those seeking to provide or obtain initial ultrasound education. While the ultrasound trainee may very well be a physician or medical student, nonphysician care providers are also using bedside ultrasound. Perhaps the student is a Physician Assistant (PA) or Nurse Practitioner (NP) that will function as a clinician, with some or all of the same proficiencies as the physician they work with. Nurses and technicians increasingly utilize ultrasound to place intravenous catheters, or to assess a patient's bladder.

The best choice for training depends on the goals of the practitioner or the goals of the practice. Is this an individual wanting to explore the utility of ultrasound on behalf of his or her group, or is this a practitioner wanting to enhance specific skills, such as ultrasound-guided procedures? Is this an individual wanting special expertise in order to administer an ultrasound program? Or, is this a practice that has made the decision to train the entire group for the incorporation of bedside ultrasound? Each of these educational goals requires a different approach.

Pre-course Materials

Prior to the first educational session, pre-course materials should be distributed to the learner. This introduces content and provides the framework for the course. Pre-course materials accelerate learning, and let the student identify problem areas that may be more difficult for them to grasp. Learners will come to their first class with more pointed questions, having answered the more trivial ones at home. Offering pre-course materials primes the learners about the utility of ultrasound at the bedside, demonstrates its power, and engenders excitement for the learners' impending new skill.

There is a wealth of introductory texts available with focus on specialty-specific, population-specific, and even organ-specific topics. A reference textbook that covers the bulk of expected skills provides a structure for the students' progression toward competency. Consider purchasing textbooks for the practice, to encourage members to work together and pace each other and to have a universal reference.

A variety of multimedia training tools exist, which can add another dimension to pre-course education. This comes in the form of interactive computer software, tablet applications, websites, or documents embedded with videos and interactive elements. Multimedia combines text with images, videos, illustrations, and animations, and demonstrates probe handling and patient positioning techniques, and displays expected anatomic and pathologic findings. This format of presenting educational material can be more directed and illustrative, so abstract concepts such as the piezoelectric effect can be demonstrated with video, rather than described in text. Multimedia is an ideal medium to illustrate the dynamic and real-time nature of ultrasound. Additionally, some multimedia products offer assessments, which enable the learner to track progress and identify knowledge gaps.

Lastly, there are a number of websites that focus specifically on ultrasound education. Providing the student with web links for online tutorials, podcasts, blogs, or discussion boards may offer a palatable introduction for the uninitiated to the growing body of bedside ultrasound knowledge. On the other hand, these resources can be more experimental in nature, and many are not vetted for their accuracy or educational value. A recent survey of popular bloggers and podcasters in Emergency Medicine defined 31 quality measures to consider when assessing the educational value of podcasts and blogs [10]. A study of third year medical students showed that self-directed electronic modules are an effective method for teaching pattern recognition and image interpretation skills, however when compared with students who received expert-guided training, the students taught by electronic modules failed to demonstrate equivalent scanning technique [11]. While pre-course materials are vital, ultrasound training requires an expert educator to ensure students gain technical proficiency.

Ultrasound Courses

Course Setting

There are three basic setting options for an introductory ultrasound course. An *open course* is one where the location is set, complete with its facilities, equipment and educators. An *imported course* is one where the course travels to the participants. Lastly, *modular courses* are those that are presented as part of a larger conference or meeting. Each comes with its own benefits and drawbacks.

The benefit of an open course includes the sheer availability of many offerings from known established companies that stand by their quality, with reviews available to speak to their efficacy. Little planning is required by the participants. The downside involves an increased expense since it usually requires travel. Additionally, scanning is performed among strangers and with equipment that may not be the same installed in the home facility.

An imported course performed within the group's local facility offers the benefit of training the entire group at one time, using the group's own equipment. On-site training allows the group to address specific institutional political issues. It offers an opportunity for teambuilding. Participants of the training will be better rested, having no need to travel. This is often a more economical option, as well. One significant drawback to this model is occupying the entire group during a time where the facility needs staff. This can be abated by placing members experienced with ultrasound in the department for the particular period of time.

Table 5.1 Examples of courses for introductory education. Additional courses and up-to-date offerings can be found with a web search

Open courses
• Advanced Health Education Center (AHEC)
• Australian Institute of Ultrasound
• Emergency Ultrasound Course
• Essentials of Emergency Medicine
• Gulfcoast Ultrasound Institute
• Mediterranean Emergency Medicine Congress
• World Interactive Network Focused On Critical UltraSound (WINFOCUS)
Imported courses
• Advanced Health Education Center (AHEC)
• Emergency Ultrasound Course
• Emergency Ultrasound Services
• Insight Ultrasound
• GW Emergency Ultrasound
• Sonoran Ultrasound, LLC
• Rocky Mountain Ultrasound
Modular courses
• ACEP scientific assembly
– Trauma ultrasound
– Echocardiography
– Transvaginal ultrasound
– Venous ultrasound
• ACEP chapter/Regional meetings
• Other National/International conferences

Modular ultrasound education that is offered as part of a regional or national meeting is a relatively inexpensive option. Modules are directed toward specific diagnostic and procedural competencies, and offer an advanced curriculum. While this may be a good method to boost a handful of skills, it is not a replacement for a comprehensive introductory education. Topics are usually varied, and offerings are unpredictable. That being said, medical students, who were provided a 1-day ultrasound-focused course, reported a statistically significant increase in confidence with skills such as ultrasound-guided central venous catheter placement, foreign body removal, and the focused assessment with sonography for trauma (FAST) exam [12]. Table 5.1 summarizes examples of these course offerings.

Finding the Right Course

Finding the right course can be a difficult task. First, decide whether an open or imported course fits best with your practice setting. Ask around for recommendations, from members of the regional or national group. Request information regarding course content from educational organizations. Define the scope of initial education, i.e., one- versus two-day course.

Courses should include educators with expert knowledge in ultrasound. The course should contain a mix of didactic and hands-on training. Ninety-nine percent of medical students surveyed—with little to no experience using ultrasound—reported hands-on clinical skills stations and didactic sessions as the most helpful means of "solidifying understanding of point-of-care ultrasound" [12].

Scanning should be performed on machines expected to be used in practice. A 2-day course should contain laboratory sessions: ideally a minimum of 6–8 h during a 2-day course. Scanning stations should attempt to train no more than 5 students at a time. Models, phantoms, or simulators can demonstrate both normal and pathologic anatomy. For example, one study found that students trained with a paracentesis training model or a mannequin simulator attained similar proficiency in their ability to perform a focused assessment with sonography in trauma (FAST) exam and identify intra-abdominal fluid [13].

For those eligible, choosing a course that offers continuing medical education (CME) credits incentivizes participation. Apply for hospital-based CME through the CME department. Have ready to submit: a course syllabus, learning objectives, and curriculum vitae of course faculty. Expect about 4–6 weeks turnaround time. National CME may be available from the college of each specialty. A course with established AMA credit can apply for joint sponsorship with the national or regional chapter of the college of specialists.

Supplemental Education

Education does not need to end when the training course completes. Consider distributing helpful pocket cards, offering chart templates, and holding scanning shifts. Chart templates not only boost documentation, they can act as a reminder for views needed, indications, and image storage. Templates can serve as support for clinical decision-making.

Holding scanning shifts with the director, expert sonographer, or "ultrasound faculty" acts as an extended hands-on training session and buoys the number of scans toward credentialing. Ultrasound faculty can hold scanning "office hours" or educate during a clinical shift. Scanning shifts can be devoted to specific applications or be based on clinical care. While very effective, scanning shifts are labor intensive. When tested for knowledge-retention 6 months after attending a classroom-based ultrasound training course, emergency residents who were trained 1-on-1 by an experienced preceptor outperformed residents trained without the benefit of a preceptor [14].

That being said: when providing additional education, be sure to adapt to the needs and capabilities of the learners. Some benefit from more self-directed learning while others prefer a more interactive preceptorship. Some choose textbooks while others elect to use online text and multimedia tools. When polled, a pool of mostly emergency residents and nonphysician providers preferred education in a small-group format, with video-clips, and hands-on scanning sessions [15]. Coordinate across different efforts. Hold a case of the month, journal club, or offer an attending curriculum. Case simulation is proven as an effective means of reinforcing ultrasound skills, not only in terms of image acquisition and interpretation, but also to solidify the indications for use and integration into care-algorithms [16]. Adapting and providing a spectrum of educational tools allows for active and passive participation for all learners' needs.

Determining Competency

Testing of the trainees ensures the success of an introductory education session. Written exams, hands-on evaluation, or performance on simulation models gives an accurate assessment of learner progress. Outside of testing, learners can be evaluated and given feedback through over-reading of images during quality assurance sessions, video review, and even direct observation. Emergency Medicine residency programs are expected to teach ultrasound as a core skill. These programs use a variety of methods for assessing resident competency in ultrasound. Most often, objective structured clinical exams (OSCEs), standardized direct observation tools (SDOTs), standardized multiple choice testing, and practical examination are utilized [3].

The objective structured assessment of ultrasound skills (OSAUS) scale is a validated method of assessing a trainee's ability to function as a sonographer in practice (Table 5.2). Trainees' skills are assessed on a 5-point scale in the categories of applied knowledge of ultrasound equipment, image optimization, systematic examination, interpretation of images, and documentation of images [17, 18]. Physicians using ultrasound to examine four patients with known pathologic findings were evaluated both on their diagnostic accuracy and on their OSAUS scores. A group of physicians who were randomized in to a 4-h course in abdominal ultrasound scored significantly higher in the categories of systematic examination, interpretation, and documentation than a control group who was evaluated prior to training. The same study group also showed significantly improved diagnostic accuracy [19].

One method of determining competency involves using the Focused Professional Performance Evaluation (FPPE) model. In FPPE, an application is chosen, such as echocardiography or the FAST exam. The group is given an education strategy, using methods offered above, for example. Define specifically how the group's performance will be evaluated, i.e., number of exams performed or percent true positives. Finally, outline the duration of the monitoring over a period of time, like 6 months. Report back to the group on progress and use the data to define new goals for the next period [20]. Figure 5.1 demonstrates how the FPPE model can be used in practice.

Table 5.2 The objective structured assessment in ultrasound (OSAUS)

	1	2	3	4	5
1. Indication for the examination If applicable. Reviewing patient history and knowing why the examination is indicated.	Displays poor knowledge of the indication for the examination	2	Displays some knowledge of the indication for the examination	4	Displays ample knowledge of the indication for the examination
2. Applied knowledge of ultrasound equipment Familiarity with the equipment and its functions, i.e., selecting probe, using buttons and application of gel.	Unable to operate equipment	2	Operates the equipment with some experience	4	Familiar with operating the equipment
3. Image optimization Consistently ensuring optimal image quality by adjusting gain, depth, focus, frequency etc.	Fails to optimize images	2	Competent image optimization but not done consistently	4	Consistent optimization of images
4. Systematic examination Consistently displaying systematic approach to the examination and presentation of relevant structures according to guidelines.	Unsystematic approach	2	Displays some systematic approach	4	Consistently displays systematic approach
5. Interpretation of images Recognition of image pattern and interpretation of findings.	Unable to interpret any findings	2	Does not consistently interpret findings correctly	4	Consistently interprets findings correctly
6. Documentation of examination Image recording and focused verbal/written documentation.	Does not document any images	2	Documents most relevant images	4	Consistently documents relevant images
7. Medical decision-making If applicable. Ability to integrate scan results into the care of the patient and medical decision-making.	Unable to integrate findings into medical decision-making	2	Able to integrate findings into a clinical context	4	Consistent integration of findings into medical decision-making

doi:10.1371/journal.pone.00S76S7.t003
Reprinted with permission from: Todsen T, Tolsgaard MG, Olsen BH, et al. Reliable and valid assessment of point-of-care ultrasonography. Ann Surg. 2015;261(2):309–315

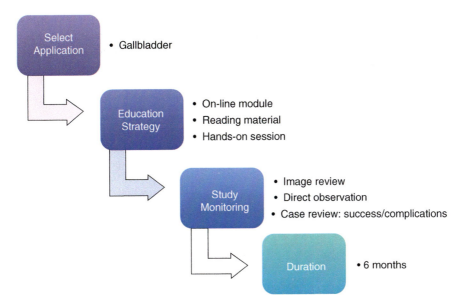

Fig. 5.1 Use of the Focused Professional Performance Evaluation (FFPE) as a framework to ensure continued competency in trained workers for an implemented ultrasound application. This example pertains to focused gallbladder ultrasound, but the FFPE framework can be applied to any application

Pitfalls

There are some pitfalls in navigating the provision of initial ultrasound education to a medical group. These can present in the course structure, from the source of training, or from within the group itself. Knowing about and preparing for these pitfalls can save time, money, and growing pains during this important introductory time.

Courses that pair too many students with an ultrasound preceptor will face challenges with too much "hands-off time." The practical component of training is invaluable, as skilled sonographers rely much on muscle memories. Courses that cover too much content over a miniscule time allotment will find diminished retention among students. The director who does their homework on courses and instructors will be rewarded with expediently trained staff, maximal retention, and minimal need for retraining.

Members of other specialties may offer ultrasound training to your practice. Relying on other specialties to conduct ultrasound education can detract from the perspective that a comember of your specialty can provide. Training provided solely by ultrasound technicians can lack the background or scientific expertise that a specialist could otherwise provide. Intra-specialty ultrasound experts make for the best educators.

Some groups may have no access to equipment or have no plans to purchase an ultrasound machine. Providing ultrasound education must be followed with implementation into clinical practice. Some learners in the group may dismiss the utility of ultrasound and may act as a barrier to broad implementation. Identifying these members early and offering focused time to demonstrate ultrasound's bedside efficacy can mitigate broader naysaying.

Key Recommendations

- Choose a course that fits your group and is conducted by experienced members of your specialty
- Provide pre-course materials to maximize classroom efficacy
- Set up ongoing training and provide support for practitioners

References

1. Physicians ACoE. Emergency ultrasound guidelines. Ann Emerg Med. 2009;53(4):550–70.
2. Counselman FL, Borenstein MA, Chisholm CD, et al. The 2013 model of the clinical practice of emergency medicine. Acad Emerg Med. 2014;21(5):574–98.
3. Amini R, Adhikari S, Fiorello A. Ultrasound competency assessment in emergency medicine residency programs. Acad Emerg Med. 2014;21(7):799–801.
4. Hamper UM, DeJong MR, Caskey CI, Sheth S. Power Doppler imaging: clinical experience and correlation with color Doppler US and other imaging modalities. Radiographics. 1997;17(2):499–513.
5. Buchanan MS, Backlund B, Liao MM, et al. Use of ultrasound guidance for central venous catheter placement: survey from the American Board of Emergency Medicine Longitudinal Study of Emergency Physicians. Acad Emerg Med. 2014;21(4):416–21.
6. Bienstock J, Adams K, Connolly A, Edgar L, Frishman G, Goepfert A. The obstetrics and gynecology milestone project. 2015. Accessed 14 Nov 2015.
7. Gynecologists ACoOa. ACOG Practice Bulletin No. 101: ultrasonography in pregnancy. Obstet Gynecol. 2009;113(2 Pt 1):451–61.
8. Quiñones MA, Douglas PS, Foster E, et al. American College of Cardiology/American Heart Association clinical competence statement on echocardiography: a report of the American College of Cardiology/American Heart Association/American College of Physicians—American Society of Internal Medicine Task Force on Clinical Competence. Circulation. 2003;107(7):1068–89.
9. Mayo PH, Beaulieu Y, Doelken P, et al. American College of Chest Physicians/La Société de Réanimation de Langue Française statement on competence in critical care ultrasonography. Chest. 2009;135(4):1050–60.
10. Thoma B, Chan TM, Paterson QS, Milne WK, Sanders JL, Lin M. Emergency medicine and critical care blogs and podcasts: establishing an international consensus on quality. Ann Emerg Med. 2015;66(4):396–402.e394.
11. Cawthorn TR, Nickel C, O'Reilly M, et al. Development and evaluation of methodologies for teaching focused cardiac ultrasound skills to medical students. J Am Soc Echocardiogr. 2014;27(3):302–9.
12. Amini R, Stolz LA, Gross A, et al. Theme-based teaching of point-of-care ultrasound in undergraduate medical education. Intern Emerg Med. 2015;10(5):613–8.

13. Salen P, O'Connor R, Passarello B, et al. Fast education: a comparison of teaching models for trauma sonography. J Emerg Med. 2001;20(4):421–5.
14. Noble VE, Nelson BP, Sutingco AN, Marill KA, Cranmer H. Assessment of knowledge retention and the value of proctored ultrasound exams after the introduction of an emergency ultrasound curriculum. BMC Med Educ. 2007;7:40.
15. Cartier RA, Skinner C, Laselle B. Perceived effectiveness of teaching methods for point of care ultrasound. J Emerg Med. 2014;47(1):86–91.
16. Bentley S, Mudan G, Strother C, Wong N. Are live ultrasound models replaceable? Traditional versus simulated education module for FAST exam. West J Emerg Med. 2015;16(6):818–22.
17. Todsen T, Tolsgaard MG, Olsen BH, et al. Reliable and valid assessment of point-of-care ultrasonography. Ann Surg. 2015;261(2):309–15.
18. Tolsgaard MG, Todsen T, Sorensen JL, et al. International multispecialty consensus on how to evaluate ultrasound competence: a Delphi consensus survey. PLoS One. 2013;8(2):e57687.
19. Todsen T, Jensen ML, Tolsgaard MG, et al. Transfer from point-of-care ultrasonography training to diagnostic performance on patients-a randomized controlled trial. Am J Surg. 2016;211(1):40–5.
20. Hunt JL. Assessing physician competency: an update on the joint commission requirement for ongoing and focused professional practice evaluation. Adv Anat Pathol. 2012;19(6):388–400.

Chapter 6
Continuing Education

Molly E.W. Thiessen and Resa E. Lewiss

Learning Objectives

- Describe the unique needs of practicing physicians for continuing education
- Describe Deliberate Practice theory and how it relates to continuing education
- Describe how to create a blended learning curriculum as a model for teaching point-of-care ultrasound
- State the uses, benefits, and limitations of web-based education
- State the uses, benefits, and limitations of simulation for learning and assessment

Introduction

In 2012, the Accreditation Council for Graduate Medical Education (ACGME) included point-of-care ultrasound (POC US) as one of 23 sub-comptencies that emergency medicine residents must master by residency completion [1]. The most recent consensus statement on resident training in POC US recommends that 50%

M.E.W. Thiessen, MD, FACEP
Department of Emergency Medicine, Denver Health Medical Center, Denver, CO, USA

Department of Emergency Medicine, University of Colorado School of Medicine, Aurora, CO, USA

R.E. Lewiss, MD (✉)
Department of Emergency Medicine, Thomas Jefferson University Hospital, Philadelphia, PA, USA
e-mail: resaelewiss@gmail.com

© Springer International Publishing AG 2018
V. S. Tayal et al. (eds.), *Ultrasound Program Management*,
https://doi.org/10.1007/978-3-319-63143-1_6

of core faculty be ultrasound credentialed [1]. Additionally, both General Surgery and Anesthesia critical care specialties have included POC US in their ACGME Milestones. Moreover, an international round table comprising 13 critical care organizations stated that POC US should be mandatory in critical care training [2–4]. At earlier stages of training, medical school educators have begun integrating POC US education into undergraduate medical curricula [5]. As such, continuing education in POC US for practicing physicians is essential.

The American College of Emergency Physicians and the American College of Cardiology have each set guidelines for continuing education [6, 7]. As these trends expand across specialties, quality continuing education for practicing clinicians will be essential.

Continuing education in POC US for practicing physicians is a unique endeavor. Experienced clinicians and adult learners have different needs and time constraints in the patient care environment in contrast to undergraduate or resident learners. Practicing physicians cite time constraints as the largest barrier to continuing education—the time needed to learn and master the skills, as well as the amount of time they have for each patient encounter to implement and utilize these skills [8]. Given the specific needs of practicing physicians as learners, incentivizing their participation in POC US educational activities is likely necessary. Educational activities must be user-friendly. The data on incentivizing physicians for continuing education is limited. The use of monetary incentive, academic advancement, actual CME credit, and other nonmonetary rewards has been studied. No one has stood out as a particularly helpful incentive [9]. A survey of physicians participating in a POC US continuing education course showed a preference for brief lectures and didactic materials combined with significantly more "hands-on" time [10]. A model of learning in which a variety of educational modalities are presented to learners, known as "blended learning" lends itself particularly well to POC US continuing education. Ideally, a framework of multimedia pre-course work and didactics are combined with rigorous hands-on scanning and simulation. The combination then entails specific, timely feedback and skills assessment in line with Deliberate Practice theory.

Deliberate Practice

The specific elements of Deliberate Practice are listed in Fig. 6.1 [11]. Essentially, the theory of Deliberate Practice emphasizes structured goal-oriented learning, with repetitive performance of skills, coupled with rigorous skills assessment rather than simply repeated practice of skills [12]. This method has specific applicability for

1.   Highly Motivated Learners

2.   Well-defined learning objectives that address knowledge or skills that matter clinically

3.   Appropriate level of difficulty for medical learners

4.   Focused, repetitive practice of the knowledge or skills

5.   Rigorous measurements that yield reliable data

6.   Informative feedback from educational sources (e.g., teachers, simulators)

7.   Frequent monitoring, error correction, and more deliberate practice

8.   Performance evaluation toward reaching a mastery standard

9.   Advancement toward the next clinical task or unit

Fig. 6.1 Elements of deliberate practice (Adapted from McGaghie et al. [16])

use after initial training, for practicing physicians and continuing education, and has been shown to be superior to traditional teaching methods, particularly when used in a simulation environment [13–15].

While web-based educational modules combined with simulation create a strong template for continuing education in a blended model, POC US education for practicing physicians requires special attention to the needs of advanced learners. Integration of blended learning with the Deliberate Practice theory creates an excellent framework for continuing education of POC US. In fact, improved performance has been found in learners who received simulator training using the elements of Deliberate Practice [17].

An essential element of deliberate practice, and education in general is competency assessment. Physicians must master image acquisition, interpretation, and be able to integrate these into their medical decision-making [18]. There are multiple methods available for POC US competency assessment, from the use of checklists (e.g., Council of Residency Directors peer reviewed standardized direct observational assessment tools [19]), to the use of management software, online quizzes, and direct observation. Methods for competency assessment are listed in Fig. 6.2.

Fig. 6.2 Methods for
competency assessment

- Checklists

    o   http://emmilestones.pbworks.com

- Quality Assurance Activities

    o   Software Supported Image Review

    o   In Person Image Review

- Written/Web Based Examinations

- Web-based online Examinations

    o   http://www.emsono.com/acep/exam.html

    o   http://www.ultrasoundninja.com

- Commercially Available Management Software

- Direct Observation

- Simulation

Educational Goals

The ideal educational outcome for any continuing education-based activity range is
a positive perception of the learning experience on the part of the physician. This
changes behavior, and eventually benefits patients. Kirkpatrick offers a way to
gauge effectiveness of an educational activity on the leaner. See Table 6.1 [20].

For reference, a 2007 Agency for Healthcare Research and Quality (AHRQ)
review found that in terms of the various possible educational modalities for continuing education, print media is less effective than live lectures. Multimedia educational tools are more effective than any single media alone. Interactive modalities
are more effective than noninteractive modalities, and multiple exposures over time
are more effective than single exposures. Simulation was shown to be effective in
improving psychomotor skills [9].

Table 6.1 Kirkpatrick's adapted hierarchy of evaluating educational outcomes [20]

Level 1	Reaction	Covers learners' views on the learning experience, its organization, presentation, content, teaching methods, and aspects of the instructional organization, materials, quality of instruction
Level 2a	Learning: change in attitudes/perception	Modification of attitudes/perceptions—outcomes here relate to changes in the reciprocal attitudes or perceptions between participant groups toward intervention/simulation
Level 2b	Learning: modification of knowledge or skills	Modification of knowledge/skills—for knowledge, this relates to the acquisition of concepts, procedures, and principles; for skills, this relates to the acquisition of thinking/problem-solving, psychomotor, and social skills
Level 3	Behavior	Documents the transfer of learning to the workplace or willingness of learners to apply new knowledge and skills
Level 4a	Results: change in the professional practice	Change in organizational practice—wider changes in the organizational delivery of care, attributable to an educational program
Level 4b	Benefits to patients	Any improvement in the health and well-being of patients/clients as a direct result of an educational program

Blended Learning

Based on the findings of the AHRQ, web-based instruction, simulation, and elements of Deliberate Practice in a blended learning format create an ideal framework for POC US education. Blended learning has been shown to be an effective educational format and lends itself well to POC US [21, 22]. Blended learning integrates multiple educational modalities to maximize knowledge acquisition and skill mastery on the part of the learner [18]. Modalities can include in-person lectures, online educational modules or recorded lectures, hands-on scanning with live models or simulators, and simulation time. The importance of integrating simulation and hands-on teaching with faculty present cannot be overemphasized. Particularly for POC US, the psychomotor skill of image acquisition and real-time interpretation are essential. Learners who receive only web-based education do not perform as well with hands-on skills [23, 24]. Additionally, blended learning provides skill retention [25].

Web-Based Instruction

Web-based learning appeals specifically to the continuing education audience because it allows for individualized learning, flexible scheduling, novel instructional methods, and distance learning. It also insures consistent content, and means of assessment [26]. It is an effective tool for POC US as part of a blended educational experience [27, 28].

Web-based learning may consist of online modules to read, lectures to view, interactive scenarios, social media communication, online discussion groups, multiple choice examinations, and others. Online discussions and novel ideas are especially appealing to engage experienced learners [29]. Figure 6.3 lists examples of online education tools. One paper has suggested that the financial cost of a web-based or blended curriculum may be similar to that of a traditional ultrasound course. Arguably, the number of hours dedicated to preparation is significantly less for web-based education [27]. Even when used as adjunct educational tools, web-based educational resources have improved outcomes over the traditional method for teaching ultrasound skills [30].

Studies demonstrate that web-based learning for continuing education improves knowledge, attitude, and even skills, albeit to a lesser extent. For POC US specifically, web-based education is best utilized in a blended curriculum that includes a hands-on scanning and/or simulation component to assist in motor skill acquisition [31–33]. Web-based education, in which participants complete multiple online modules over time, benefits learners with repeated exposure [34].

A completely web-based curriculum has limitations: social isolation, de-individualized instruction, lack of timely or in-person feedback. However, there is

Fig. 6.3 Web-based online educational tools

- Blogs

- Competency Lists

- Google Hangout Discussions

- Narrated lectures

- Videos including YouTube and Vimeo

- Organizational Websites

- Podcasts

- Question Banks

- Text Documents

- Social media including Twitter

1. Match Instruction Difficulty to Your Learners' Developmental Level

2. Minimize Extraneoues Features that Inhibit Learning

3. Balance Interactivity with Cognitive Load

4. Provide Rich Feedback and Guidance

5. Maximize Learner Control

6. Use Web-Based Instruction to Enhance Learning Around and Within It

7. Clearly Define and Communicate the Reasons for Using Web-Based Instruction

8. Integrate Space and Time for the Web-Based Instruction into the Curriculum

9. Be Explicit About How Using Web-Based Instruction Relates to Assessment

10. Address Faculty Motives and Perceptions

11. Identify and Mitigate Issues that may Diminish the Effectiveness of Web-Based Instruction

12. Engage in Quality Monitoring and Improvement

Fig. 6.4 Twelve tips for effective web-based instruction (adapted from Yavner et al. [35])

evidence to support that when utilized wisely and appropriately, a blended curriculum including web-based elements leads to education success [26].

There are several essential steps to ensure an effective learning experience for POC US web-based education as part of a blended curriculum. First and foremost, the educator must assess the learners in order to tailor the content appropriately. Additional tips for creating effective web-based educational tools can be seen in Fig. 6.4 [35]. Web-based instruction should contain a minimum of extraneous material. It should be interactive enough to maintain the attention of the learner, but not so interactive that it is distracting. Ideally, the program would allow the learner to tailor the educational module or curriculum to their preferred style of learning. This is particularly important for POC US education as studies have shown that simulation and hands-on education are necessary to improve psychomotor skills. If a schedule and curriculum are utilized, time to work on the web-based content should be allotted. Educators should elucidate the purpose of the web-based instruction is being used, as well as how it will be used for assessment. Finally, educators should solicit feedback from stakeholders and learners to continue to improve the web-based instruction content and effectiveness [35].

Simulation and Hands-On Education

Simulation entails the use of low- or high-fidelity US trainers either in a simulated clinical environment. Live human models can be used. Table 6.2 describes characteristics of high- and low-fidelity ultrasound simulators [18]. Simulation allows for reproducible clinical scenarios, ease of performance evaluation, and the ability to learn outside of the patient care environment [36, 37]. Simulation has been widely used in graduate medical education [37–39], and more recently in continuing education (See Chap. 11 – Simulation) [20].

Use of simulation and hands-on training for POC US skills has met with great success, usually as a part of a blended educational experience [11, 25, 40–44]. With respect to continuing education, simulation has been shown to be positively received by learners, as well as impart a perceived improvement in confidence and clinical preparedness. It has also been shown to improve knowledge and long-term retention of skills. Most educators feel that while current evidence supporting the implementation of simulation education in POC US is limited, use of this educational format is necessary as the evidence moves forward [20].

Critics of simulation-based POC US education question if certain skills transfer from the simulated to the patient care environment [45]. Simulation provided with faculty presence has been found to be superior to self-guided simulation [46]. Others worry that learned skills will decay without continued practice [47]. While the literature on simulation for continuing medical education and POC US is still limited, most educators agree it is an essential element of training [18].

The features of effective simulation education are listed in Fig. 6.5 [13–15]. Feedback has been found to be the most important element of simulation education. Additional important factors include repetetive practice, the ability to tailor the simulation to the learner in a high-fidelity, reproducible scenario and active participation. As with any educational activity, clearly stated learning objectives and learner expectations result in better learning [48]. Simulation has the benefit of providing the opportunity for practice and competency evaluations. Checklists can be utilized for this element [49]. CORD recommends that competency assessment on POC US technique, image acquisition, and image interpretation be demonstrated by practicing clinicians [50].

Table 6.2 Characteristics of ultrasound simulators (from Lewiss et al. [18])

Characteristic	Low-fidelity simulators	High-fidelity simulators
Condition	Static	Static or dynamic
Availability	Handmade or commercial	Commercial
Skill tested	1 Skill	1 Skill or multiple skills
Separate ultrasound machine required	Yes	No
Tissue motion	No	Yes
Ultrasound transducer	Required and needs to be connected to actual machine	Mock probe with position sensor or patient dummy with position sensor
Real-time 2-dimensional images	Yes	Yes
Real-time haptic feedback	Possible	Yes
Cost	Inexpensive	Expensive

1.   Provide feedback during the learning experience with the simulator.

2.   Learners should repetitively practice skills on the simulator.

3.   Integrate simulators into the overall curriculum.

4.   Learners should practice with increasing levels of difficulty.

5.   Adapt the simulator to complement multiple learning strategies.

6.   Ensure the simulator provides for clinical variation.

7.   Learning on the simulator should occur in a controlled environment.

8.   Provide individualized (in addition to team) learning on the simulator.

9.   Clearly define outcomes and benchmarks for the learners to achieve using the simulator.

10. Ensure the simulator is a valid learning tool.

Fig. 6.5   Features of effective simulation education (Adapted from Issenberg [48])

Pitfalls

1. Failure to assess the learner prior to the educational activity.
2. Not providing specific goals and objectives for the learning activity.
3. Lack of preparation prior to the activity will detract from the educational value.
4. Inadequate assessment of the learners and the educational activity will limit improvement.

Key Recommendations

1. Utilize a blended approach to continuing education
2. Utilize an ideal education workflow (Figure 5.1)
3. Know your learner

References

1. ACGME [Internet]. www.acgme.org/acWebsite/RRC-110/110_guidelines.asp.
2. Cohen N. The critical care anesthesiology milestone project [Internet]. 2014. https://www.acgme.org/acgmeweb/Portals/0/PDFs/Milestones/CriticalCareMedicine.pdf.
3. Malangoni M. The surgical critical care milestone project [Internet]. http://www.acgme.org/acgmeweb/portals/0/pdfs/milestones/surgicalcriticalcaremilestones.pdf.

4. Expert Round Table on Ultrasound in ICU. International expert statement on training standards for critical care ultrasonography. Intensive Care Med. 2011;37(7):1077–83.
5. Hoppmann RA, Rao VV, Poston MB, Howe DB, Hunt PS, Fowler SD, et al. An integrated ultrasound curriculum (iUSC) for medical students: 4-year experience. Crit Ultrasound J. 2011;3(1):1–12.
6. American College of Emergency Physicians. Emergency ultrasound guidelines. Ann Emerg Med. 2009;53(4):550–70.
7. Quinones MA, et al. American College of Cardiology/American Heart Association Clinical Competence Statement on Echocardiography: a report of the American College of Cardiology/American Heart Association/American College of Physicians—American Society of Internal Medicine Task Force on Clinical Competence. Circulation. 2003;107(7):1068–89.
8. Price DW, Miller EK, Rahm AK, Brace NE, Larson RS. Assessment of barriers to changing practice as CME outcomes. J Contin Educ Heal Prof. 2010;30(4):237–45.
9. Marinopoulos SS, Dorman T, Ratanawongsa N, Wilson LM, Ashar BH, Magaziner JL, et al. Effectiveness of continuing medical education. Evid Rep Technol Assess. 2007;149:1–69.
10. Hofer M, Kamper L, Miese F, Kröpil P, Naujoks C, Handschel J, et al. Quality indicators for the development and didactics of ultrasound courses in continuing medical education. Ultraschall Med. 2012;33(1):68–75.
11. McGaghie WC, Issenberg SB, Cohen ER, Barsuk JH, Wayne DB. Does simulation-based medical education with deliberate practice yield better results than traditional clinical education? A meta-analytic comparative review of the evidence. Acad Med. 2011;86(6):706–11.
12. Duvivier RJ, van Dalen J, Muijtjens AM, Moulaert VRMP, van der Vleuten CPM, Scherpbier AJJA. The role of deliberate practice in the acquisition of clinical skills. BMC Med Educ. 2011;11:101.
13. Ericsson KA. Deliberate practice and the acquisition and maintenance of expert performance in medicine and related domains. Acad Med. 2004;79(10 Suppl):S70–81.
14. Ericsson KA. Deliberate practice and acquisition of expert performance: a general overview. Acad Emerg Med. 2008;15(11):988–94.
15. Cook DA, Hatala R, Brydges R, Zendejas B, Szostek JH, Wang AT, et al. Technology-enhanced simulation for health professions education: a systematic review and meta-analysis. JAMA. 2011;306(9):978–88.
16. McGaghie WC, Issenberg SB, Cohen ER, Barsuk JH, Wayne DB. Medical education featuring mastery learning with deliberate practice can lead to better health for individuals and populations. Acad Med. 2011;86(11):e8–9.
17. Ericsson KA. An expert-performance perspective of research on medical expertise: the study of clinical performance. Med Educ. 2007;41(12):1124–30.
18. Lewiss RE, Hoffmann B, Beaulieu Y, Phelan MB. Point-of-care ultrasound education: the increasing role of simulation and multimedia resources. J Ultrasound Med. 2014;33(1):27–32.
19. Lewiss RE, Pearl M, Nomura JT, Baty G, Bengiamin R, Duprey K, et al. CORD-AEUS: consensus document for the emergency ultrasound milestone project. 2013.
20. Khanduja PK, Bould MD, Naik VN, Hladkowicz E, Boet S. The role of simulation in continuing medical education for acute care physicians: a systematic review. Crit Care Med. 2015;43(1):186–93.
21. Kempinska AY, Bhanji F, Larouche S, Dubrovsky AS. A novel simulation-based program for ultrasound-guided fracture reductions: program evaluation. Am J Emerg Med. 2014;32(12):1547–9.
22. Mitchell JD, Mahmood F, Wong V, Bose R, Nicolai DA, Wang A, et al. Teaching concepts of transesophageal echocardiography via web-based modules. J Cardiothorac Vasc Anesth. 2015;29(2):402–9.
23. Filippucci E, Meenagh G, Ciapetti A, Iagnocco A, Taggart A, Grassi W. E-learning in ultrasonography: a web-based approach. Ann Rheum Dis. 2007;66(7):962–5.
24. Woodworth GE, Chen EM, Horn J-LE, Aziz MF. Efficacy of computer-based video and simulation in ultrasound-guided regional anesthesia training. J Clin Anesth. 2014;26(3):212–21.

25. Laack TA, Dong Y, Goyal DG, Sadosty AT, Suri HS, Dunn WF. Short-term and long-term impact of the central line workshop on resident clinical performance during simulated central line placement. Simul Healthc. 2014;9(4):228–33.
26. Cook DA. Web-based learning: pros, cons and controversies. Clin Med (Lond). 2007;7(1):37–42.
27. Kang TL, Berona K, Elkhunovich MA, Medero-Colon R, Seif D, Chilstrom ML, et al. Web-based teaching in point-of-care ultrasound: an alternative to the classroom? Adv Med Educ Pract. 2015;6:171–5.
28. Chenkin J, Lee S, Huynh T, Bandiera G. Procedures can be learned on the web: a randomized study of ultrasound-guided vascular access training. Acad Emerg Med. 2008;15(10):949–54.
29. Chan TM, Thoma B, Lin M. Creating, curating, and sharing online faculty development resources: the medical education in cases series experience. Acad Med. 2015;90(6):785–9.
30. Arroyo-Morales M, Cantarero-Villanueva I, Fernández-Lao C, Guirao-Piñeyro M, Castro-Martín E, Díaz-Rodríguez L. A blended learning approach to palpation and ultrasound imaging skills through supplementation of traditional classroom teaching with an e-learning package. Man Ther. 2012;17(5):474–8.
31. Curran VR, Fleet L. A review of evaluation outcomes of web-based continuing medical education. Med Educ. 2005;39(6):561–7.
32. Fordis M, King JE, Ballantyne CM, Jones PH, Schneider KH, Spann SJ, et al. Comparison of the instructional efficacy of internet-based CME with live interactive CME workshops: a randomized controlled trial. JAMA. 2005;294(9):1043–51.
33. Wutoh R, Boren SA, Balas EA. eLearning: a review of internet-based continuing medical education. J Contin Educ Heal Prof. 2004;24(1):20–30.
34. Shaw T, Long A, Chopra S, Kerfoot BP. Impact on clinical behavior of face-to-face continuing medical education blended with online spaced education: a randomized controlled trial. J Contin Educ Heal Prof. 2011;31(2):103–8.
35. Yavner SD, Pusic MV, Kalet AL, Song HS, Hopkins MA, Nick MW, et al. Twelve tips for improving the effectiveness of web-based multimedia instruction for clinical learners. Med Teach. 2015;37(3):239–44.
36. Gordon JA. As accessible as a book on a library shelf: the imperative of routine simulation in modern health care. Chest. 2012;141(1):12–6.
37. McLaughlin S, Fitch MT, Goyal DG, Hayden E, Kauh CY, Laack TA, et al. Simulation in graduate medical education 2008: a review for emergency medicine. Acad Emerg Med. 2008;15(11):1117–29.
38. Schroedl CJ, Corbridge TC, Cohen ER, Fakhran SS, Schimmel D, McGaghie WC, et al. Use of simulation-based education to improve resident learning and patient care in the medical intensive care unit: a randomized trial. J Crit Care. 2012;27(2):219.e7–13.
39. Okuda Y, Bond W, Bonfante G, McLaughlin S, Spillane L, Wang E, et al. National growth in simulation training within emergency medicine residency programs, 2003–2008. Acad Emerg Med. 2008;15(11):1113–6.
40. Mendiratta-Lala M, Williams T, de Quadros N, Bonnett J, Mendiratta V. The use of a simulation center to improve resident proficiency in performing ultrasound-guided procedures. Acad Radiol. 2010;17(4):535–40.
41. Ahmad R, Alhashmi G, Ajlan A, Eldeek B. Impact of high-fidelity transvaginal ultrasound simulation for radiology on residents' performance and satisfaction. Acad Radiol. 2015;22(2):234–9.
42. Girzadas DVJ, Antonis MS, Zerth H, Lambert M, Clay L, Bose S, et al. Hybrid simulation combining a high fidelity scenario with a pelvic ultrasound task trainer enhances the training and evaluation of endovaginal ultrasound skills. Acad Emerg Med. 2009;16(5):429–35.
43. Knudson MM, Sisley AC. Training residents using simulation technology: experience with ultrasound for trauma. J Trauma. 2000;48(4):659–65.
44. Evans LV, Dodge KL, Shah TD, Kaplan LJ, Siegel MD, Moore CL, et al. Simulation training in central venous catheter insertion: improved performance in clinical practice. Acad Med. 2010;85(9):1462–9.
45. Sidhu HS, Olubaniyi BO, Bhatnagar G, Shuen V, Dubbins P. Role of simulation-based education in ultrasound practice training. J Ultrasound Med. 2012;31(5):785–91.

46. Alba GA, Kelmenson DA, Noble VE, Murray AF, Currier PF. Faculty staff-guided versus self-guided ultrasound training for internal medicine residents. Med Educ. 2013;47(11):1099–108.
47. Wang EE, Quinones J, Fitch MT, Dooley-Hash S, Griswold-Theodorson S, Medzon R, et al. Developing technical expertise in emergency medicine—the role of simulation in procedural skill acquisition. Acad Emerg Med. 2008;15(11):1046–57.
48. Issenberg SB. The scope of simulation-based healthcare education. Simul Healthc. 2006;1(4):203–8.
49. Dong Y, Suri HS, Cook DA, Kashani KB, Mullon JJ, Enders FT, et al. Simulation-based objective assessment discerns clinical proficiency in central line placement: a construct validation. Chest. 2010;137(5):1050–6.
50. Akhtar S, Theodoro D, Gaspari R, Tayal V, Sierzenski P, Lamantia J, et al. Resident training in emergency ultrasound: consensus recommendations from the 2008 Council of Emergency Medicine Residency Directors Conference. Acad Emerg Med. 2009;16(Suppl 2):S32–6.

Chapter 7
Undergraduate Ultrasound Education

David P. Bahner and Nelson A. Royall

Objectives

1. Understand the current state of ultrasound in medical schools, as a first step in an educational competency path.
2. Hypothesize a clear educational ultrasound outcome for the proficient and safe practice of point of care ultrasound in clinical medicine.
3. Distinguish the necessary steps to initiate and maintain an ultrasound program for undergraduate medical education.
4. Perform a needs assessment for an ultrasound program and include those elements essential in creating a curriculum for preclinical and clinical medical students.
5. Address the management issues associated with the initiation, maintenance, and growth of undergraduate ultrasound education and personalizing the approach to each institution's mission, vision, and values.

Introduction

Point of care (POC) focused ultrasound has become ubiquitous across most medical specialties without a corresponding emergence of consistent training pathways for physicians. Physician demand for ultrasound competency has drastically increased

D.P. Bahner, MD, FACEP
Department of Emergency Medicine,
The Ohio State University Wexner Medical Center, Columbus, OH, USA
e-mail: David.Bahner@osumc.edu

N.A. Royall, MD (✉)
Department of Surgery, The University of Oklahoma College of Medicine,
Tulsa, OK, USA

© Springer International Publishing AG 2018
V. S. Tayal et al. (eds.), *Ultrasound Program Management*,
https://doi.org/10.1007/978-3-319-63143-1_7

since "To Err is Human: Building a Safer Health System" and the Agency for Healthcare Research Quality (AHRQ) identified ultrasound-guided vascular access as a practice which should be adopted by all physicians [1, 2]. Since that time, focused ultrasound as part of the bedside patient evaluation across different body systems has been shown to improve patient experience and decrease healthcare expenditures.

Yet a significant gap remains for physician training in undergraduate medical education. In a 2012 survey of U.S. medical schools, only 51 of the 134 MD-granting medical schools reported having ultrasound training at any point in their curriculum [3]. The survey showed most medical school deans agree ultrasound should be a component of the medical school curriculum, but only a minority of schools have placed emphasis on integrating this into their curricula citing such reasons as financial cost of equipment and limited space within existing curricula. Despite these perceptions, many early adopters have developed robust training experiences while utilizing existing equipment and without the removal of existing curricular content [4–7].

This chapter will seek to codify the development and integration of ultrasound into undergraduate medical education. The objective of undergraduate ultrasound education must fit within the larger medical education paradigm. This chapter will demonstrate the pathway for developing a novice medical student into a graduate prepared to utilize ultrasound upon entering residency.

Main Ideas

Curriculum Development

The process of training an individual within a course, rotation, or longitudinal curriculum requires administrative coordination and efficiency. Progression of a functional skill such as focused sonography can be understood by applying the principles of Miller's pyramid to the training paradigm (Fig. 7.1) [8]. In this model, the trainee progresses from the "knows" (knowledge), "knows how" (competence), "shows how" (performance), and finally "does" (action) steps of the pyramid. An undergraduate ultrasound curriculum which follows these progression steps will train physicians capable of performing focused ultrasound safely and efficiently. An example of an integrated vertical ultrasound curriculum in the undergraduate medical curriculum can be found in Appendix 7.1.

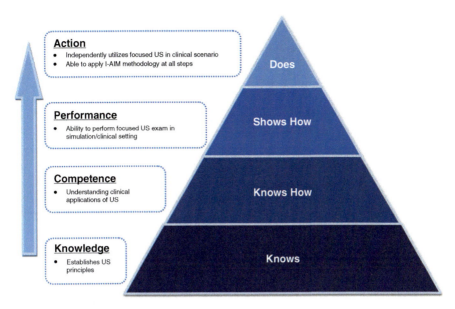

Fig. 7.1 Miller's pyramid of clinical assessment applied to focused ultrasound follows the "Knows," "Knows How," "Shows How," and "Does" progression of a learners' development of clinical competency. A learner must establish the knowledge base (Knows) of how ultrasound works and basic principles of scanning before they can create a competency (Knows How) of focused ultrasonography at the patient's bedside. The learner then establishes ability to perform (Shows How) focused ultrasound exams in either clinical or simulated settings before reaching the ability to independently utilize focused ultrasound through the complete I-AIM process for point of care ultrasound exams (Does). I-AIM: Indications, Acquisition, Interpretation, and Medical Decision-Making [23]

Designing an undergraduate curriculum is a significant task, with multiple pathways for potential tangents that have little benefit to the student or the institution. A top-down approach to curriculum development is critical in focused ultrasound integration at the undergraduate medical education level. The Kern 6-step process is an accepted model for medical curricula development that provides a framework for creating an undergraduate ultrasound curriculum [9]. The Kern process relies upon six steps for curriculum development: problem identification and general needs assessment, targeted needs assessment of learners, measurable goals and objectives, educational strategies, implementation, and evaluation and feedback (Fig. 7.2).

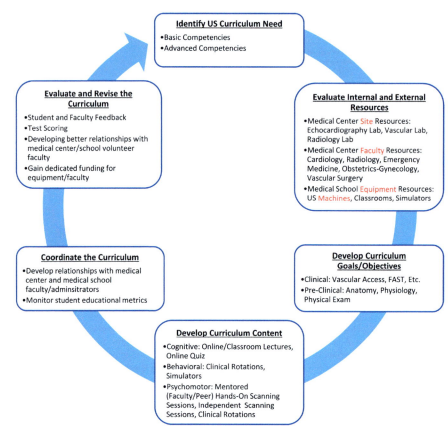

Fig. 7.2 An overview of the process for developing an undergraduate ultrasound curriculum. The cycle follows the 6-step process outlined by Kern for development of undergraduate ultrasound curriculum [9]. As the curriculum is developed and integrated, the institution should review the initial steps of the process to develop subsequent components of the curriculum

Problem Identification and General Needs Assessment

Questions medical schools face in implementing ultrasound include: when should training begin, where should it be placed in the curriculum, which skills should be taught, and what techniques should be used to teach the skills? Confounding the development of ultrasound training programs is the lack of any unifying body at each medical education level to direct the differentiation of learners along the course. The final product of any ultrasound training curriculum should be the creation of physician Sonologists, those who are capable of utilizing basic and advanced ultrasound in a clinical setting.

Focused ultrasound literacy improved dramatically over the past few decades, although remains highly variable, even within the same institution. Although early ultrasound training was described in Germany during the late twentieth century, the experience with ultrasound education in U.S. medical schools decades later remains among the early adopters and innovators [3]. Exemplifying the problem was a study of entering emergency medicine interns in 2012–2013 at one U.S. residency program which found 25% of their residents had not been exposed to ultrasound during medical school at any point and approximately 55% had never used ultrasound in a simulated setting in their medical education [10]. What the expectation and ideal implementation of an ultrasound program in the medical education pedagogy remains to be determined [11]. Regardless of the eventual strategies used at each institution and training level, focused ultrasound training must be a requisite component in the medical education for *all* future physicians given evidence supporting focused ultrasound in most specialties.

Significant fragmentation of ultrasound training programs exists in U.S. medical schools. One major factor is the lack of central leadership in defining ultrasound training expectations of physicians. Ultrasound training is poorly defined along the undergraduate (AAMC-LCME), graduate (ACGME-RRC), and professional societies (ABMS-MOC) governing training requirements [12, 13]. This uncertainty has led to variation not only in the quantity of practitioners electing to utilize ultrasound, but more importantly the quality and consistency with which they apply it to patient care. An additional factor in the fragmentation is the lack of understanding in both what focused ultrasound is and how one reaches a relative competency in the skill.

Implementing an undergraduate ultrasound program is surely feasible, and embraced by a variety of current professionals. Healthcare providers involved in training includes: sonographers, radiologists, gynecologists, intensivists, cardiologists, hospitalists, primary care physicians, and prehospital personnel. Emergency medicine, however, has the most expansive, organized, and engaged ultrasound scope of practice among physicians, which lends this group to become the stewards for the house of medicine to develop focused ultrasound programs.

An additional challenge for medical schools is to ensure graduates are not only exposed to ultrasound, but progress along the training model to fulfill the satisfactory performance phase of using bedside ultrasound. Clinicians will have a multitude of uses and need to be trained to become comfortable with ultrasound as a clinical tool. The successful curriculum engages the learner and leads the novice through the enlightenment of knowledge and skill to perform focused ultrasound examinations.

Beyond medical school ultrasound education, the healthcare institution has the responsibility for ultrasound education. Training overconfident practitioners with limited skills risks the misdiagnosis from inappropriately applying ultrasound to medical decision-making. Each institution with existing GME programs is likely to have already implemented some form of ultrasound education. However, the current implementation of ultrasound education lacks a centralized pathway between the UGME and GME programs even at a single institution. This problem of fractured ultrasound training components is a major point which must be addressed from an institutional perspective as ultrasound programs continue to develop [14].

General Needs Assessment

At an institutional level, the goal of a general needs assessment is to identify available resources and potential barriers for an ultrasound curriculum. Determining the scope will help identify available resources, such as existing mature ultrasound resources, and significance of the potential barriers, such as administrative support from physicians that have not learned the benefits of focused ultrasound in practice. The scope may be limited to the medical school or expanded to an entire medical center (medical school, residency and fellowship programs, nursing school, etc.). A coordinated pathway for the entire medical center almost certainly will reduce curricular redundancy and improve resource utilization, although this will require significant administrative coordination.

Faculty resistance is a common barrier since focused ultrasound integration is not defined throughout the different fields. A successful program will lead to perceptual changes, trust among faculty, and enhance faculty interest as the program demonstrates improved outcomes. These changes eventually lead to a greater willingness of faculty to donate teaching time to the program.

Within any institution, there will be existing ultrasound equipment and physical spaces in use for other educational or clinical purposes. The program champion can develop relationships with departmental staff and faculty to ask to share these resources. This requires fostering relationships with these professionals as well as significant coordination and cooperation. Ideally, dedicated equipment in a simulation lab and/or cadaver lab entails a capital expenditure and investment. Finally, curricular space for any added programs must be accounted for in understanding the impedance of an ultrasound program. With the limited curricular space for all medical education at the medical school and residency level, a program must work within the space of a curriculum rather than add to the bulk of the existing curriculum load.

The sonographic footprint is the conglomeration of ultrasound equipment, trained faculty, and ultrasound utilization at each institution, which may be nonexistent or well developed. A survey of an institutional footprint should attempt to differentiate those resources which are comprehensive or focused [15]. A comprehensive ultrasound application requires the sonographer, physician, equipment, and examination spaces, whereas focused ultrasonography traditionally is limited to the physician and the ultrasound equipment. Faculty from Emergency Medicine, Critical Care, or Radiology or sonographers (Vascular or Echocardiography Labs) are generally asked to contribute to ultrasound programs without compensation. Eventually an undergraduate ultrasound program will expand and the addition of funded faculty time and dedicated ultrasound equipment lessens the burden on these existing institutional resources. A bridge between the volunteer faculty and the addition of funded resources is the use of prior learners within the program. Senior medical students that have developed the appropriate proficiency can serve as valuable mentors for junior students [16–18].

Targeted Needs Assessment

What is required of the medical school for a graduate to be prepared for residency training and eventual practice as it relates to ultrasound? The targeted needs assessment of learners focuses on the learner and their planned educational journey with specific milestones along this path. After graduation, virtually all medical students will enter into one of 24 specialties that utilize focused ultrasound for diagnostic or therapeutic purposes [19]. However, undergraduate medical education does not need to develop graduates competent in all the forms of focused ultrasound. Rather the medical student will need the foundation in focused ultrasound that allows the learner to differentiate and advance their skills towards specific practices within their specialty.

Defining competencies provides the foundation for the ultrasound curriculum. To better stratify medical school curricular competencies, most institutes categorize a competency as "Core" versus "Enriched" or "Basic" versus "Advanced". Basic (Core) competencies are those that must be achieved by all medical students and they must also demonstrate their proficiency before graduating within the curriculum at a specific timeframe. In contrast, Advanced (Enriched) competencies are optional achievements that allow learners to become exposed to certain skills expected of only certain specialties.

Basic Competencies

Evaluating the needs for all medical school students at an institute should be based upon established evidence-based practices that coordinate well with existing curricula. Although there are different perspectives among existing focused ultrasound educators at the undergraduate level, there is general agreement among physicians and healthcare authorities as to specific applications that constitute a core competency [11, 20].

Ultrasound safety and basic science principles are the most critical basic competencies. These principles are nonphysical in nature and can be developed predominately separate from ultrasound equipment. Specific basic science components include wave development and propagation, image generation, Doppler shift, and artifact generation. With respect to ultrasound safety, a student must demonstrate techniques to limit thermal tissue damage using the ALARA principle [21]. Additionally, students must be able to safely utilize ultrasound equipment without increasing the spread of communicable disease [22]. Regardless of the scope or breadth of an ultrasound program, these basic competencies are expected to be accomplished by all focused ultrasound users. Ultrasound knobology, the use of machine controls to acquire and optimize imaging, is an additional basic competency [23]. This is distinct from isolating techniques to acquire ultrasound images as a competency.

The overwhelming body of evidence supporting ultrasound-guided vascular access for both central and peripheral vascular structures necessitates developing a competency for all students in the medical school setting. Given the national guidance from government and societal organizations which have set the standard of care for central venous access using ultrasound-guidance students must therefore be trained in this skill [24, 25]. Basic competencies beyond ultrasound principles and vascular access must be chosen carefully for an early ultrasound program. Creating a large volume of mandatory ultrasound competencies can cause a program to fail because of the resources required to support such broad programs. Basic competencies should be added to a curriculum in stepwise fashion to allow necessary adjustments to the entire curriculum based upon resource strain or changes in the needs assessment.

Advanced Competencies

Advanced competencies support specific subpopulations in a medical education system, which if applied to all learners would distract students. Advanced competencies also help assess the feasibility of potential curricular components. Mature ultrasound programs will integrate advanced competencies in a serial fashion to ensure there are adequate resources and need for each competency. A frequent failure is a program which instates multiple advanced competencies into their program which leads to resource fatigue and high variability in learner outcomes.

The practical determination of which focused ultrasound competencies should be implemented as advanced competencies is unique to a program. Maturing ultrasound programs should initially develop advanced competencies in their program which address common focused ultrasound needs in medical education that are not currently met in their existing basic competencies. In fact, many current undergraduate ultrasound programs have developed their curriculum through serial additions of advanced competencies [26]. After a period of program assessment and revisions, many of these advanced competencies are later added to the curriculum as basic competencies. This is the method for developing a robust list of basic competencies in an ultrasound curriculum. Examples at these programs are: transthoracic echocardiography to determine pericardial effusion and estimated left ventricular ejection fraction, pulmonary survey to evaluate for pleural effusion or pneumothorax and differentiation of pulmonary edema from pneumonia and atelectasis, musculoskeletal joint survey for joint effusion and ligament disruption, and abdominal survey for appendicitis and cholecystitis [4, 11].

Measurable Goals and Objectives

The overarching goal for an undergraduate ultrasound program is to develop the skills to lead to a sonologist through undergraduate and graduate medical training to a practicing physician; a practitioner who can determine the appropriateness for a specific exam, perform the technical skill of obtaining video and images, interpret those findings, and integrate those findings into the care of a patient. Sonologists follow the I-AIM (Indication, Acquisition, Integration, and Medical Decision-Making) methodology to utilize focused ultrasound, whereas sonographers are those that only have the technical skill of performing ultrasound examinations without the clinical component [23]. Measurable goals and objectives are created to develop the physician Sonologist. The difference between goals and objectives, while both being measurable outcomes, is that goals represent the student population and are a reflection of the curriculum as a whole while the objectives represent student performance which can be tracked to assess an individual's competency.

Although this component of the program development relies upon an understanding of the general and targeted needs, goals and objectives ultimately must match institutional resources. Educational goals for the program are developed by identifying each basic or advanced competency and creating a set of goals to be met by the eventual curriculum implementation. Examples of educational goals for a basic competency such as ultrasound equipment utilization would be: (1) students can utilize an ultrasound machine to perform and record an ultrasound examination, (2) students can optimize examination results for subsequent review and documentation, and (3) students can demonstrate ultrasound Doppler principles in utilizing Doppler functions in an examination. In contrast, the learners' objectives for a basic competency more closely mirror the tasks a student will be expected to become proficient at during the curriculum. Examples of learner objectives for a basic competency such as ultrasound equipment utilization would be for the learner to be able to: (1) turn a portable ultrasound machine on and off, (2) identify an appropriate probe for a specific intended examination and ensure it is connected to the machine, (3) acquire a 2D image and record both still images and video to the storage drive, (4) utilize the screen markup features to label an image or video for later review, and (5) obtain a Doppler waveform using the Doppler mode and identify specific measurements.

In addition to specific educational goals, a specific goal for coordination and acquisition of resources for the curriculum must be established. This goal ultimately drives future growth of an undergraduate ultrasound program as well as maintenance of existing curricular components. Establishing a specific goal for the program to develop and maintain resources such as teaching faculty, ultrasound equipment, simulation models, and didactic resources emphasizes the significant effort required to coordinate ultrasound medical school programs. Other specific goals may be set at this point for an ultrasound program including: advanced competency development, medical center faculty training and adoption, and planned contributions to educational literature.

Educational Strategies

POC focused ultrasound learning occurs through three main components: cognitive, behavioral, and psychomotor. Each skill within focused ultrasound can be taught in isolation; however this approach ignores the constant crossing over between the components. An ultrasound curriculum should ensure to accomplish the three components across each objective. Although certain objectives may rely more on one component than another, each objective should have all three components from a teaching standpoint.

Current training models for both basic and advanced competencies in undergraduate ultrasound curricula utilize a multimodal approach to achieving cognitive, behavioral, and psychomotor training. Cognitive components are traditionally based in didactic lectures given either in a classroom setting or online video. An advantage of combining the two approaches is the obvious ability for the learner to review the topic at their freedom and personalize their education towards their learning weakness and strengths. There are numerous lecture series already in existence through an internet search both available for general use or a subscription basis (Appendix 7.2). An institute can benefit from the development of a series of lectures developed by their own faculty to ensure all desired content is covered.

Behavioral components emphasize the hands-on experience associated with patient encounters. Oftentimes, the behavioral aspect is least emphasized because of the need to develop psychomotor skills and the cognitive ability to utilize ultrasound. However, the ability to integrate focused ultrasound within the clinical setting is highly tied to a learner's ability to know when and how to utilize ultrasound. The hands-on sessions should emphasize learners applying the findings to a clinical scenario. For example, while performing a neck ultrasound a learner should be able to interact with the patient to coordinate patient positioning, arrange equipment, and differentiate the internal jugular vein from carotid artery based upon B-mode and Doppler. Additionally, emotional intelligence and situational awareness can be scripted [27, 28].

Psychomotor components requires the greatest resource allocation, similar to any physical skill development. Psychomotor skills can be developed through the hands-on sessions where experienced users demonstrate proper probe scanning and examination techniques. Peer-based teaching also provides learners the ability as a student model to appreciate the impact of various psychomotor techniques on exam efficiency (i.e., probe pressure, gel application) [16, 18, 29]. Independent hands-on experiences will drive a large portion of a learner's development of the psychomotor skills necessary for focused ultrasound. As the most variable skill to acquire of the main components, psychomotor skills may develop rapidly for those accustomed to hand-eye coordination whereas those who have less experience may require a significant amount of practice.

Equipment selection for the undergraduate curriculum can rapidly outpace the available resources allocated to the program. Faculty-developed simulation equipment can yield equivalent educational value for programs without the resources to afford advanced feedback simulators. For example, gel models can be developed at minimal cost and replaced easily depending on the desired application such as venous cannulation or demonstration of specific artifacts [30, 31]. High fidelity ultrasound simulators which can provide feedback have also been shown to aid in the development of competency among trainees as discussed further in Chap. 25. Institutes must avoid sole reliance upon these simulator and online resources given the inferior results seen with this methodology when performed without coaching-based models [32].

Proficiency Assessment

Evaluation is the final component to be addressed in the development of an ultrasound program. As documented in a series of studies, simply completing a volume of examinations does not demonstrate competency in focused ultrasound. Rather, the program should utilize a type of checkout that has at least a psychomotor and cognitive component to evaluate the learners. A cognitive checkout examination is traditionally a written or online examination where users must demonstrate the knowledge necessary for each objective. Inclusion of image review and evaluation in the examination can satisfy the need to demonstrate some of the behavioral skills learners must gain during the curriculum. Similarly, standardized ultrasound examination templates are available through an internet search designed to meet specific program objectives (Appendix 7.2). In the psychomotor checkout, trainees demonstrate procedural competency on a simulator in addition to maintaining a log of completed examinations. An advantage of this digital portfolio is the use as a longitudinal log other institutions can review to satisfy future training requirements, obviating the need for repetitive training as a resident [33].

In longitudinal or vertical ultrasound curricula, there remains a need for a method to monitor individual learner progression. Although there is no universally accepted method for this currently, milestones are a commonly accepted form for tracking graduate medical education competencies and can be easily adapted to undergraduate ultrasound curricula. Depending upon the period of time an institution is following learners across, these milestones may be narrow or broad in scope. For example, a program with specific objectives of developing basic ultrasound procedural competency should develop milestones which focus on the tasks their learners should aim to progress along (Table 7.1). In contrast, a more mature ultrasound program with undergraduate and graduates in training can utilize milestones which track leaner development towards that expected of an independently functioning physician (Table 7.2). Universally accepted methods to track learner development across

Table 7.1 A milestone consists of progressive levels of competency a learner demonstrates through time. Learners are provided the subjective feedback of their progression relative to the anticipated final level of competency in the skill. A narrow scope for milestones are appropriate for ultrasound programs with limited time to develop competency

Level 1	Level 2	Level 3	Level 4	Level 5
Knows indication and safety principles for US procedures	Able to differentiate US anatomy	Able to demonstrate psychomotor skills for US procedure	Able to perform US procedure independently	Completes 100 US procedures

Table 7.2 A potential milestone for focused ultrasound which accounts for the continuum of an ultrasound curriculum across the undergraduate and graduate medical system. This milestone should be blinded to the specialty and delineate the levels of progressive competency in professional and technical utilization of focused ultrasound. A medical student should achieve at least a level 2 competency prior to graduation, whereas a graduating resident must be at the level 4 competency in order to utilize focused ultrasound after training completion. Level 5 recognizes advanced applications yet the core ability is to generate a billable report and document an exam

Level 1	Level 2	Level 3	Level 4	Level 5
Knows indication for US	Able to perform US scans in simulated setting	Able to perform multiple scans in clinical setting	Completes 150 exams	Able to save images, document and bill for US

the ultrasound competency spectrum are clearly needed with increasing adoption of focused ultrasound in medical education.

Implementation

A common starting point for undergraduate ultrasound programs will be in the clinical years of the curriculum utilizing specialties with high-volume ultrasound exposure such as Emergency Medicine, Cardiology, Obstetrics-Gynecology, Critical Care, and Radiology. The program can be directed to develop objectives and goals that align with certain specialties that are being supported by a medical center. For example, if an institution has substantial resources dedicated to Interventional Cardiology, the availability of faculty for teaching focused echocardiography will likely allow for early integration and maturation of focused cardiac ultrasound education. Echocardiography labs in this setting can serve as sites for healthy volunteer hands-on sessions for students to learn about ultrasound knobology and basic science principles while reviewing cardiac anatomy and physiology.

A critical transformation of an undergraduate ultrasound program is the progression of ultrasound training into preclinical training. Coordination with anatomy or physiology staff can allow for scanning sessions with volunteer faculty to demonstrate relevant concepts through volunteer scanning sessions. During cadaver lab sessions, a separate room may be used for healthy volunteer scanning under supervision of the anatomy faculty to demonstrate the functional anatomy of the heart and great vessels during the period used to dissect the cardiothoracic anatomy [34]. A similar type of integration can be used during physical examination courses to combine focused echocardiography with pulsed wave Doppler and overlying cardiac audiograms. One study demonstrated that this method markedly improved medical students' ability to recognize cardiac pathology with auscultation during physical exam courses in preclinical years [35]. These examples of ultrasound integration in preclinical coursework can serve to solidify support for undergraduate ultrasound curriculum and develop support for eventual dedicated resources.

Of the potential applications of focused ultrasound within the preclinical curriculum, anatomy curricula is the most commonly favored site currently [34, 36, 37]. Gross Anatomy courses follow a similar process to the early training required for understanding focused ultrasonography, the first level of developing competency. Students in this setting are able to perform focused ultrasound examinations of the anatomical structures on either cadaver or volunteers to better understand the location and function of each structure. Furthermore, integration of focused ultrasound in this manner allows students to familiarize themselves with nonphysical principles of ultrasound basics including knobology, ultrasound wave principles, and artifact generation in an active fashion [34]. Integration at this level can allow students to develop and demonstrate competencies in multiple basic competencies including ultrasound safety, scanning techniques, and anatomy identification.

Ultrasound Champion

An integrated undergraduate ultrasound curriculum requires a coordinated approach led through an ultrasound champion. The champion ensures that learner experiences align with the needs assessments and goals of the program. As the ultrasound program matures, the ultrasound champion must delegate responsibilities, based upon available resources such as additional sponsored faculty, institutional resources, or experienced student peers. An example of the various duties an ultrasound champion may be expected to complete depending on the institute can be seen in Fig. 7.3.

The ultrasound champion must have protected time to perform the duties of equipment allocation and volunteer coordination/recruitment. Because of the significant time required for this position, a medical school dean may not have the time available to commit to the position. Faculty from within a high-volume ultrasound specialty is where the ultrasound champion should be called upon to implement initial ultrasound programs at the undergraduate level.

Funding Considerations

The reality of the undergraduate medical education landscape is the absence of necessary funding for novel educational projects. Without administrative support, the role of the Ultrasound Champion can be difficult to create. Dedicated time for an Ultrasound Champion is based upon the amount of ultrasound experiences expected to be established. For a 1 month rotation with 2–4 students in clinical ultrasound exposure there will be approximately 20–40 h of administrative work to develop the course materials and experiences in addition to the 80–120 h required to operate the course each month. Although many of these hours can be divided among administrative leadership often, without support from institutional leaders these hours will be solely the responsibility of the Ultrasound Champion. Dedicated time is clearly a necessity for an Ultrasound Champion to develop a longitudinal or vertical curricula at this level.

In a more common setting, motivated personnel may seek to develop ultrasound programs at the undergraduate level prior to securing program funding. This path has inherent risk to the individuals as without funding, the institutional leadership has not demonstrated any value of the significant effort to be accomplished. Without a large population of physicians trained in the use of ultrasound, the field of Emergency Medicine has an opportunity to be the primary source for ultrasound education. Other specialties such as Cardiology and Obstetrics-Gynecology may not have the breadth of skills Emergency Medicine physicians have in evaluating the entirety of the anatomy performed in emergency ultrasound.

In establishing administrative funding for the Ultrasound Champion, the emphasis must be on the specialty and the amount of dedicated time for faculty. As mentioned, Emergency Medicine faculty have the greatest ability to provide the scope of curricular initiatives in focused ultrasound and this needs to be emphasized to the leadership early in the decision-making process. Support for the Ultrasound Champion is based

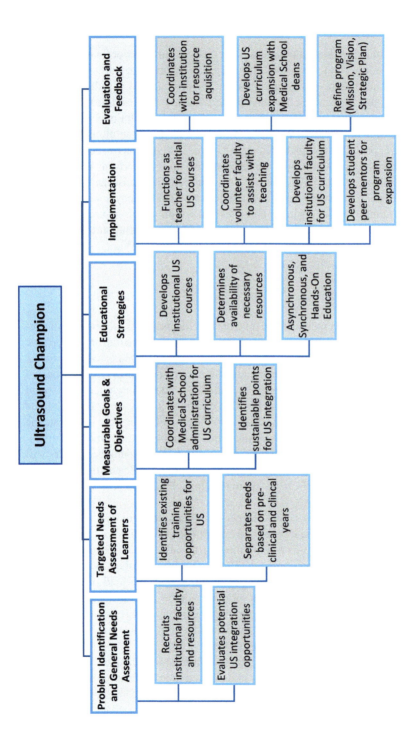

Fig. 7.3 Overview of the responsibilities of an institutional Ultrasound Champion. The Ultrasound Champion is intricately involved in the teaching component of the early ultrasound curriculum, however with the development of additional ultrasound resources there is a shift towards coordination and administrative responsibilities. A robust undergraduate ultrasound curriculum requires an Ultrasound Champion to develop teaching faculty and student peer mentors to assist with teaching roles

upon the percentage of a full time equivalent (FTE), where a 5 day 8 h week equates to 2080 h. Ideally a 1.0 FTE position is created as part of the ultrasound initiative, although the reality is this is rarely the case. Practically, funding can be appropriated from the Dean's budget for education as a separate line item of ultrasound education. More frequently, the funding is coupled into Radiology or other specialty electives. A shared appropriation of the FTE percentage from these budgets should then be used to develop a singular Ultrasound Champion position with the ability to coordinate the tasks of the ultrasound program across the multiple specialties.

Other interesting concepts do exist for the funding of an Ultrasound Champion position and the ultrasound program. Educational grants do exist and are more commonly found when collaborating with other healthcare practitioners such as nursing. Additional sources of grants can be those appropriated for safety initiatives, an area which focused ultrasound has been used such as for improving safety for central venous cannulation. Other options include activity fees from student tuition or the development of an institutional endowment for community donations.

Evaluation and Feedback

A study of the effectiveness of an ultrasound program is derived from both the administrative faculty and students. Institutional leadership will expect proof of goals and objectives from the program being accomplished within a certain period of time. Failure to accomplish goals regardless of how broad or narrow the program's scope will jeopardize future administrative support. This fact supports the restraint ultrasound faculty must have in the development and expansion of ultrasound opportunities until adequate resources and institutional experience exists.

Student evaluations at the completion of each component of the curriculum drives further expansion of the program into preclinical years. Students have traditionally demonstrated strong support for ultrasound training in clinical and preclinical years across most institutions [6, 7]. Demonstration of student engagement and improved performance across other components of the curriculum will drive institutional support if it was lacking. Therefore the charge of the ultrasound champion at an institution will be to design evaluation studies of students and faculty that can be used to not only lead to program revisions, but also support for acquisition of resources. For example, an ongoing log of student utilization of dedicated ultrasound equipment or simulator equipment must be kept to ensure replacement of these resources.

The ultrasound champion will encounter a variable amount of ease for program expansion depending on the institutional support. A top-down approach through deans allows the champion to recruit faculty, coordinate experiences, and schedule hands-on sessions with greater ease. If the institutional support is lacking, the champion must have significant perseverance to change institutional perceptions. This approach requires significant time and travel requirements and may not be feasible for faculty with other significant institutional duties.

Discussion

The state of ultrasound training drastically changed with the advent of emergency ultrasound. As practitioners have gained incremental experience largely from emergency ultrasound applications, the practice of medicine developed more applications for focused ultrasound [19]. The education of future physicians however needs to be formalized to ensure safe performance and continued growth of the field. As there is a significant emphasis on anatomy and physiology within a medical school curriculum, there is an equal opportunity for ultrasound to play a role in learning.

There is a growing preponderance of evidence for ultrasound education in the undergraduate medical education system. Blended curricula are becoming more prevalent as the advent of online content, FOAMed and other resources help augment resource limited efforts within the medical school mission. The fact that investing in this tool can help programs with teaching preclinical topics and improve retention rates while simultaneously preparing future clinicians for practical skills needed in residency further supports its adoption.

Unfortunately, the robust nature of medical school ultrasound also has led to significant fragmentation in its implementation until a more central direction is applied from our governing bodies. Emergency Medicine has been shown to be the most common site for training ultrasound in U.S. medical schools, although the faculty from this specialty have not yet adopted a consensus on the best method to train medical students [38]. In contrast, the American College of Emergency Physicians (ACEP) has been a leader in the realm of graduate medical education by adopting specific guidelines for ultrasound education for Emergency Medicine residents which have since been incorporated into clear milestones by the ACGME [39]. Similar approaches are necessary at an undergraduate level to assist in coordinating ultrasound adoption and standardization within medical schools.

Until this unification of focused ultrasound education occurs, each institution must determine their development of ultrasound training at the undergraduate level based upon their mission and values. Clearly basic competencies, which must be taught at this level, include ultrasound basic science principles, safety, equipment utilization, and standard examination techniques. In addition, all medical students should be expected to have developed ultrasound-guided vascular access competency given the ubiquitous nature of the skill in the field of medicine. Beyond these clear basic competencies, significant resources become requisite which many institutions may not be willing to devote initially. An emphasis on training medical students in the core components of cognitive, behavioral, and psychomotor skills will establish graduates with the best ability to utilize ultrasound in their eventual practice regardless of the competencies covered in the curriculum.

The final product from undergraduate medical education should be a physician prepared to succeed in a graduate medical education program. Development of new undergraduate curricula is an ongoing process that requires coordination from each field to ensure modern approaches are integrated. Focused ultrasound has clearly shown its role within the practice of medicine and warrants an increased role within the undergraduate medical education curriculum.

Pitfalls

- Doing too much too soon, not well, and underperforming.
- Trying to train students to perform comprehensive exams.
- Stating ultrasound is an aid to the physical exam (it can aid in teaching the physical exam yet has no specified role as such in the completion of a physical exam in clinical practice).
- Having students perform unsupervised exams in the clinical setting (patients can confuse the educational exam and findings for a more comprehensive exam).
- Failing to get internal support from administration and institutional faculty early.

Key Recommendations

- Utilize the six-step approach to undergraduate ultrasound curriculum development.
- A general needs assessment at an institution will determine the scope of resources available to initiate an ultrasound curriculum.
- Distinguish basic and advanced ultrasound competencies to compartmentalize competencies for all physicians versus specialty-based training.
- Ultrasound-guided vascular access should be a component of every undergraduate ultrasound curriculum.
- Specialty selection will often determine the needs of learners for advanced ultrasound competencies.
- Ultrasound curricula must seek to develop competencies in all components of focused ultrasonology (cognitive, behavioral, and psychomotor). Overemphasis of the cognitive component is common among early programs seeking to match the needs assessment.
- Online resources exist for undergraduate ultrasound curriculum and lessen the challenge of program content development.
- A modern digital portfolio demonstrates the training of a sonologist. Included components may include labeled images and video of performed examinations, case reports of clinical performance, written works within the field, social media and other samples of applied ultrasound education.
- Identify an Ultrasound Champion early to coordinate program development.
- Since a majority of practicing physicians may not have been trained in focused ultrasound, institutional administration must be shown the benefits of ultrasound to form internal support.
- Establishment and growth of an ultrasound curriculum requires maintaining evaluations from students and faculty demonstrating program success. The ultrasound program may positively impact other areas of the curriculum and can serve as a method to gain program support.

Appendix 7.1 Sample Undergraduate Medical Education (UME) Integrated Vertical Ultrasound Curriculum

Medical School Year 1

3 Months			7 Months	2 Months
Gross Anatomy and Laboratory			Basic Science Curriculum	Vacation
Musculoskeletal anatomy US	*Thorax, abdomen and pelvis anatomy US*	*Head and neck anatomy US*	*Introduction to focused US*	

Medical School Year 2

8 Months	2 Weeks	2 Months
Basic science curriculum	Introduction to clinical medicine	Vacation
Basic focused US protocols	*US-guided vascular access*	

Ultrasound model pool elective

Medical School Year 3

8 Weeks	8 Weeks	8 Weeks	8 Weeks	8 Weeks	6 Weeks	2 Weeks
Internal medicine	Pediatrics	Family medicine	General surgery	Neurology/psychiatry	Obstetrics-gynecology	Clinical topics
Integrated specialty-based hands-on US experience						*Core focused US protocols*

Medical School Year 4

1 Month	1 Month	1 Month	1 Month	7 Months
Emergency medicine rotation	Ambulatory medicine rotation	Chronic care rotation	Sub-internship rotation	Elective rotations
Emergency US	*Integrated specialty-based hands-on US experience*			

Advanced course in focused US elective

Medical School Year 1

US in Anatomy

- 12 h (four 3-h) Lectures: Basic physics, knobology, scanning techniques, and image acquisition in cadaver lab
- 12 h (four 3-h) Hands-On Sessions: Practical scanning on cadavers and student models

Introduction to Focused US

- 10 h (five 2-h) Lectures: Basic science principles, I-AIM introduction, common focused US protocols
- 12 h (six 2-h) Hands-On Sessions: Practical scanning on student models and simulators

Total: 46 h

Medical School Year 2

Basic Focused US Protocols

- 12 h (six 2-h) Lectures and Hands-On Sessions: Focused US protocols and US procedural guidance

US Vascular-Guided Access

- 2 h Lecture and Hands-On Session: US-guided vascular access and simulator use

US Model Pool Elective

- 12 h (six 2-h) Volunteer Student Modeling for Hands-On Sessions

Total: 14 h (26 h with Elective)

Medical School Year 3

Integrated Specialty-Based Hands-On US Experience

- 12 h (six 2-h) Lectures and Hands-On Session: Focused US for each specialty rotation with student models/simulators
- Variable Hours Hands-On Clinical Sessions: Rotation-specific hands-on experience with patients

Core Focused US Protocols

- 8 h (four 2-h) Lectures and Hands-On Session: Focused US protocol review and student model/simulators

Total: 20 h

Medical School Year 4

Emergency US Rotation

- 2 h Lectures and Hands-On Session: Emergency US protocols with student models/simulators
- Variable Hours Hands-On Clinical Sessions: Emergency Department patient hands-on experience

Integrated Specialty-Based Hands-On US Experience

- Variable Hours Hands-On Clinical Sessions: Rotation-specific patient hands-on experience

Advanced Course in Focused US Elective

- 20 h (ten 2-h) Lectures: Advanced topics in focused US
- 20 h (ten 2-h) Hands-On Sessions: Proctored hands-on sessions with student models/simulators
- 20 h (ten 2-h) Journal Club Sessions: Literature review of focused US topics
- 15 h Independent Hands-On Sessions: Student-directed hands-on experience with student models/simulators
- 4 h (two 2-h) Hands-On Clinical Sessions: Intensive Care and Emergency Department proctored patient hands-on experiences

Total: ~2–5 h (≥81 h with Elective)

Appendix 7.2 Summary of Free Open Access Medical Education (FOAMed) Ultrasound Resources

Curriculum design
• AIUM ultrasound in medical education portal (http://meded.aium.org/home)
Reading materials
• Ultrasound guide for emergency physicians (www.sonoguide.om)
Video lectures
• Academy of emergency ultrasound (http://vimeo.com/channels/aeus/videos)
• Emergency bedside ultrasound training series (http://learn-us.vanderbiltem.com)
• Emergency ultrasound teaching (http://emergencyultrasoundteaching.com)
• Mount Sinai emergency ultrasound (www.youtube.com/user/SinaiEMultrasound)
• University of California-Irvine critical care ultrasound (https//itunes.apple.com/us/itunes-u/ucimc-ultrasound-education/id452550953)
• University of South Carolina School of Medicine Ultrasound Institute (http://ultrasoundinstitute.med.sc.du)
Proficiency assessments
• Emergency ultrasound exam (www.emsono.com/acep/exam.html)
• Emergency ultrasound teaching (http://emergencyultrasoundteaching.com)

References

1. Shojania KG, Duncan BW, McDonald KM, Wachter RM, Markowitz AJ. Making health care safer: a critical analysis of patient safety practices. Rockville: Agency for Healthcare Research and Quality; 2001.
2. Kohn LT, Corrigan JM, Donaldson MS. To err is human: building a Safer health system, vol. 6. Washington, DC: National Academies Press; 2000.
3. Bahner DP, Goldman E, Way D, Royall NA, Liu YT. The state of ultrasound education in U.S. medical schools: results of a national survey. Acad Med. 2014;89(12):1681–6.
4. Bahner DP, Adkins EJ, Hughes D, Barrie M, Boulger CT, Royall NA. Integrated medical school ultrasound: development of an ultrasound vertical curriculum. Crit Ultrasound J. 2013;5(1):6.
5. Fox JC, Schlang JR, Maldonado G, Lotfipour S, Clayman RV. Proactive medicine: the "UCI 30," an ultrasound-based clinical initiative from the University of California, Irvine. Acad Med. 2014;89(7):984–9.
6. Hoppmann RA, Rao VV, Poston MB, et al. An integrated ultrasound curriculum (iUSC) for medical students: 4-year experience. Crit Ultrasound J. 2011;3(1):1–12.
7. Rao S, van Holsbeeck L, Musial JL, et al. A pilot study of comprehensive ultrasound education at the Wayne State University School of Medicine: a pioneer year review. J Ultrasound Med. 2008;27(5):745–9.
8. Miller GE. The assessment of clinical skills/competence/performance. Acad Med. 1990;65(9):S63–7.
9. Kern DE, Thomas PA, Hughes MT. Curriculum development for medical education: a six-step approach. Baltimore: JHU Press; 2010.
10. Day J, Davis J, Riesenberg LA, et al. Integrating sonography training into undergraduate medical education: a study of the previous exposure of one institution's incoming residents. J Ultrasound Med. 2015;34(7):1253–7.
11. Lane N, Lahham S, Joseph L, Bahner D, Fox J. Ultrasound in medical education: listening to the echoes of the past to shape a vision for the future. Eur J Trauma Emerg Surg. 2015;41(5):461–7.
12. Goldstein SR. Accreditation, certification: why all the confusion? Obstet Gynecol. 2007;110(6):1396–8.
13. Watanabe H. Accreditation for ultrasound in the world. Ultrasound Med Biol. 2004;30(9):1251–4.
14. Ahern M, Mallin MP, Weitzel S, Madsen T, Hunt P. Variability in ultrasound education among emergency medicine residencies. West J Emerg Med. 2010;11(4):314–8.
15. Greenbaum LD, Benson CB, Nelson LH 3rd, Bahner DP, Spitz JL, Platt LD. Proceedings of the Compact Ultrasound Conference sponsored by the American Institute of ultrasound in medicine. J Ultrasound Med. 2004;23(10):1249–54.
16. Jeppesen KM, Bahner DP. Teaching bedside sonography using peer mentoring: a prospective randomized trial. J Ultrasound Med. 2012;31(3):455–9.
17. Kühl M, Wagner R, Bauder M, et al. Student tutors for hands-on training in focused emergency echocardiography–a randomized controlled trial. BMC Med Educ. 2012;12(1):101.
18. Ahn JS, French AJ, Thiessen ME, Kendall JL. Training peer instructors for a combined ultrasound/physical exam curriculum. Teach Learn Med. 2014;26(3):292–5.
19. Moore CL, Copel JA. Point-of-care ultrasonography. N Engl J Med. 2011;364(8):749–57.
20. Baltarowich OH, Di Salvo DN, Scoutt LM, et al. National ultrasound curriculum for medical students. Ultrasound Q. 2014;30(1):13–9.
21. Medicine AIoUi. Prudent use and clinical safety. American Institute of Ultrasound in Medicine; 2012. www.aium.org.
22. Medicine AIoUi. Guidelines for cleaning and preparing external- and internal-use ultrasound probes between patients. American Institute of Ultrasound in Medicine; 2012. www.aium.org.
23. Bahner DP, Hughes D, Royall NA. I-AIM: a novel model for teaching and performing focused ultrasound. J Ultrasound Med. 2012;31(2):295–300.

24. Revised statement on recommendations for use of real-time ultrasound guidance for placement of central venous catheters, ST-60 (2010).
25. Shekelle PG, Wachter RM, Pronovost PJ, et al. Making health care safer II: an updated critical analysis of the evidence for patient safety practices. Evid Rep Technol Assess (Full Rep). 2013;211:1–945.
26. Bahner DP, Royall NA. Advanced ultrasound training for fourth-year medical students: a novel training program at The Ohio State University College of Medicine. Acad Med. 2013;88(2):206–13.
27. Gorgas DL, Greenberger S, Bahner DP, Way DP. Teaching emotional intelligence: a control group study of a brief educational intervention for emergency medicine residents. West J Emerg Med. 2015;16(6):899–906.
28. Dugan JW, Weatherly RA, Girod DA, Barber CE, Tsue TT. A longitudinal study of emotional intelligence training for otolaryngology residents and faculty. JAMA Otolaryngol Head Neck Surg. 2014;140(8):720–6.
29. Knobe M, Munker R, Sellei RM, et al. Peer teaching: a randomised controlled trial using student-teachers to teach musculoskeletal ultrasound. Med Educ. 2010;44(2):148–55.
30. Kingstone LL, Castonguay M, Torres C, Currie G. Carotid artery disease imaging: a home-produced, easily made phantom for two-and three-dimensional ultrasound simulation. J Vasc Ultrasound. 2013;37(2):76–80.
31. Kendall JL, Faragher JP. Ultrasound-guided central venous access: a homemade phantom for simulation. CJEM. 2007;9(05):371–3.
32. Cawthorn TR, Nickel C, O'Reilly M, et al. Development and evaluation of methodologies for teaching focused cardiac ultrasound skills to medical students. J Am Soc Echocardiogr. 2014;27(3):302–9.
33. Hughes DR, Kube E, Gable BD, Madore FE, Bahner DP. The sonographic digital portfolio: a longitudinal ultrasound image tracking program. Crit Ultrasound J. 2012;4(1):15.
34. Dreher SM, Dephilip R, Bahner D. Ultrasound exposure during gross anatomy. J Emerg Med. 2014;46(2):231–40.
35. Wittich CM, Montgomery SC, Neben MA, et al. Teaching cardiovascular anatomy to medical students by using a handheld ultrasound device. JAMA. 2002;288(9):1062–3.
36. Teichgräber U, Meyer J, Nautrup CP, Rautenfeld DB. Ultrasound anatomy: a practical teaching system in human gross anatomy. Med Educ. 1996;30(4):296–8.
37. Tshibwabwa ET, Groves HM. Integration of ultrasound in the education programme in anatomy. Med Educ. 2005;39(11):1148.
38. Cook T, Hunt P, Hoppman R. Emergency medicine leads the way for training medical students in clinician-based ultrasound: a radical paradigm shift in patient imaging. Acad Emerg Med. 2007;14(6):558–61.
39. American College of Emergency Physicians. Emergency ultrasound guidelines. Ann Emerg Med. 2009;53(4):550–70. www.osuultrasound.edu

Chapter 8
Residency Ultrasound Education

Laura Nolting and Thomas Cook

Objectives

- Discuss ACGME Requirements for point of care ultrasound training.
- Highlight ultrasound training recommendations by the American College of Emergency Physicians.
- Discuss development of a residency ultrasound training program in emergency medicine.
- Compare different specialty residency training guidelines.

Introduction

In the 1990s, ultrasound began to evolve as a key diagnostic tool for a number of clinical specialties. The disseminated use of this technology caused established organizations of medical imaging to discourage ultrasound training outside historical boundaries. However, it also stimulated the formation of groups composed of passionate clinical physicians dedicated to expand ultrasound utilization into nearly every clinical environment short of psychiatry. By the turn of the twenty-first century many US universities had taken notice and had begun to include ultrasound training as a fixed component of the education for all of their medical students.

This chapter reviews the requirements for point of care (POC) ultrasound education in residency training in the United States and includes recommendations to

L. Nolting, MD, FACEP (✉) • T. Cook, MD
Department of Emergency Medicine, Palmetto Health Richland, Columbia, SC, USA
e-mail: tpcookmd@hotmail.com

© Springer International Publishing AG 2018   91
V. S. Tayal et al. (eds.), *Ultrasound Program Management*,
https://doi.org/10.1007/978-3-319-63143-1_8

integrate ultrasound education into an existing residency program. The authors' perspective is from residency training in emergency medicine, but many recommendations can be applied to residency training in other specialties.

ACGME Requirements for Clinical Ultrasound Training

Utilization of diagnostic ultrasound by clinical specialists began in the 1960s with cardiology and obstetrics-gynecology. However, it was not until the beginning of the twenty-first century that the Accreditation Council for Graduate Medical Education (ACGME) began to formulate training requirements for CUS. These new requirements were initially included in the ACGME Program Requirements for emergency medicine in 2001 [1].

Revised in 2013, the emergency medicine program requirements for ultrasound training is as follows:

> "Residents must use ultrasound for the bedside diagnostic evaluation of emergency medical conditions and diagnoses, resuscitation of the acutely ill or injured patient, and procedural guidance [1]."

The use of the word "must" specifically requires programs to provide ultrasound training, but the statement is relatively general compared to other ultrasound policy statements for professional organizations (e.g., ACEP). There are no requirements for the competence of emergency medicine faculty in bedside ultrasound or the presence of an adequate number of ultrasound systems capable of providing quality imaging in the emergency departments that serve as teaching sites for emergency medicine residents.

In 2013, ACGME also rolled out "The Next Step in the Outcomes-Based Accreditation Project [2]" (often referred to as "Next Accreditation System" or "NAS") as a joint effort by the ACGME and medical specialty boards. For emergency medicine this collaboration included the American Board of Emergency Medicine (ABEM). The goal of NAS was to overhaul the evaluation system for postgraduate medical education in the United States, clearly define observable skills expected at particular stages of training within a given specialty, and recommend competency assessment tools [2]. The cornerstone of this process was the development of "Milestones" for each specialty to act as a framework for the assessment of resident physician competencies [2].

For emergency medicine there are 23 milestones [2] (Table 8.1). Of these, five are clinical procedures:

- Airway Management
- Anesthesia and Acute Pain Management
- Goal-Directed Focused Ultrasound
- Vascular Access
- Wound Management

The inclusion of POC US as a milestone firmly established the importance of this skill from the viewpoint of ABEM and the ACGME.

Emergency medicine programs are now required to assess and regularly report directly to ACGME a given resident's progress at utilizing POC US over the course of their training (Table 8.2). This includes a requirement that each resident perform 150 "focused ultrasound examinations," and it is still used as the primary benchmark for the ACGME milestone for POC US in emergency medicine residency training.

Table 8.1 ACGME milestones for emergency medicine [2]

Emergency Stabilization	Performance of Focused History and Physical Exam
Diagnostic Studies	Diagnosis
Pharmacotherapy	Observation and Reassessment
Disposition	Multi-Tasking
General Approach to Procedures	Airway Management
Anesthesia and Acute Pain Management	Goal-directed Focused Ultrasound
Wound Management	Vascular Access
Medical Knowledge	Professional Values
Accountability	Patient Centered Communication
Team Management	Practice-based Performance Improvement
Patient Safety	Systems-based Management
Technology	

Table 8.2 Other diagnostic and therapeutic procedures: goal-directed focused ultrasound (diagnostic/procedural) (PC12)

Level 1	• Describes relevant anatomy to basic goal-directed clinical ultrasound
	• Describes the indications for goal-directed clinical ultrasound and how it differs from consultative ultrasound
	• Demonstrates the hand motions of scanning with proper transducer manipulation
	• Performs an eFAST with direct supervision
Level 2	• Identifies the proper probe, settings, and protocols to obtain and optimize images for goal-directed clinical ultrasound
	• Correctly acquires images for goal-direct clinical ultrasound
	• Visualizes and identifies relevant anatomy for goal-directed clinical ultrasound
	• Performs goal-directed clinical ultrasound in critical situations, e.g., eFAST, Echo, Aorta
Level 3	• Correctly interprets acquired images and completes goal-directed clinical ultrasound protocols
	• Describes limitations of bedside goal-directed clinical ultrasound exams and protocols
	• Describes clinical algorithms incorporating goal-directed clinical ultrasound
	• Performs a minimum of 150 adequate and reviewed goal-directed clinical ultrasound examinations with scans in each core application
	• Uses ultrasound for dynamic guidance of procedures
Level 4	• Demonstrates competency of documentation of clinical ultrasound in the medical record
	• Consistently utilizes and integrates appropriate ultrasound applications in clinical management
	• Utilizes ultrasound to identify procedural success and anticipate complications

(continued)

Table 8.2 (continued)

Level 5	• Teaches other providers goal-direct clinical ultrasound
	• Expands ultrasonography skills to advanced applications
	• Understands the key components to developing and maintaining a successful emergency ultrasound program
	• Participates in ultrasound-related research
	• Contributes to advancing the field of goal-directed clinical ultrasound

Uses goal-directed focused ultrasound for the bedside diagnostic evaluation of emergency medical conditions and diagnoses, resuscitation of the acutely ill or injured patient, and procedural guidance [3]

Suggested assessment tools for the POC US milestone include:

- Standardized Direct Observation Tool (SDOT)
- Observation of Resuscitations
- Simulation
- Video Review

Ultrasound Training Recommendations by the American College of Emergency Physicians

There are many professional medical colleges, societies, and associations that have developed policies and position statements on POC US. Many of these have undergone revisions as POC US implementation has matured in various specialties, and negotiations between the leaders of organizations for different specialties have searched for common ground to safely increase POC US utilization.

The American College of Emergency Physicians (ACEP) is the largest organization of this type in emergency medicine. In the 1990s, ACEP convened a group of experts in POC US to produce a consensus document for emergency physicians interested in using POC US.

This document described two pathways for emergency physicians to competently use POC US (Table 8.3).

This became the first document sanctioned by ACEP to include a specific number of examinations to acquire competence (150 studies) [5]. Although it has been criticized, it became the standard for most policies in emergency ultrasound as well as credentialing standards for hospital privileges. Even as ACEP broadened its recommendations to achieve competence in subsequent revisions of its policy, the required number of examinations has remained constant.

In 2008, ACEP significantly expanded its policy to include recommendations that physicians should perform 25–50 reviewed examinations for all common applications of POC US in the emergency department [6]. In addition, the document provided guidelines for ultrasound education in residency training that are discussed below.

Table 8.3 ACEP pathways for emergency physicians to proficiency in ultrasound [4]

Pathway	Residency training	Practicing physician
Didactics	Receives ultrasound training in residency	Attends introductory CUS Course
Experiential	Performs US examinations with experienced residency program faculty members	Performs US examinations under supervision or using Gold Standards, confirmatory testing, or patient outcome review within departmental US plan
Proficiency	Residency Director and/or US Director certifies US training	Ultrasounds are obtained with documentation and review to meet ACEP proficiency guidelines.
Credentialing	Acquired at local hospital settings within departmental privileges	
Continuing medical proficiency and education	Quality review of ultrasound performed continuously, CME attended in accordance with specialty guidelines	
New applications	New applications adopted after CME, research or other training	

Development of a Residency Ultrasound Training Program

The development and implementation of an ultrasound training program for a residency is a complicated and time-consuming process. It requires dedicated and skilled faculty members and has significant expenses. It takes several years to reach maturity at which point residents can utilize the technology to simultaneously evaluate and manage patients in the emergency department.

There are four assets required for the successful deployment of such a program:

- Curriculum
- Faculty
- Equipment
- Competency Assessment

Curriculum

Residents should be exposed to an introductory course at the beginning of their training. All residents attend a variety of courses during the first weeks of their PGY 1 year (e.g., Advanced Trauma Life Support and Advanced Cardiac Life Support). POC US training courses should also be included at this time. The course should provide residents with important basic information:

- Machine operation and maintenance
- Exam setup
- Screen orientation
- Logging exams for technical and interpretive review by faculty
- How to access additional educational resources

A dedicated rotation to POC US should be a component of the first year of residency training as well. In general, the length of the rotation should not be less than 2 weeks in duration and should be composed of dedicated shifts to perform POC US without the burden of patient management. Shifts dedicated to ultrasound scanning should be designed to spend some time examining patients directly with faculty that possess expertise in POC US.

In addition, ACEP recommends that the rotation include:

- Didactic sessions covering basic and advanced POC US applications
- Scheduled reading assignments in texts and journals
- Access to other digital educational resources including question banks on POC US applications

Beyond the PGY 1 ultrasound rotation the program should have longitudinal educational tools aimed specifically at teaching residents to integrate ultrasound into their daily practice. Examples include case presentation series during conference, continued online training modules, and simulation medicine training emphasizing the use of ultrasound in resuscitation and procedural guidance.

Faculty

ACEP recommends that all emergency residency programs should identify a full-time faculty member as its emergency ultrasound director. It is not required that the ultrasound director be fellowship trained. However, it is paramount for programs to recognize the substantial time commitment to developing and managing a successful program. In the past this position has often been relegated to junior faculty with little compensation in terms of protected time to accomplish a colossal task. Since there may be no older faculty mentors within the program to advise them, it is imperative that new directors are supported to attend outside conferences to encourage networking with directors at other institutions.

Per ACEP guidelines, a minimum of 50% of the "Core Faculty" members of a program should also be designated as core ultrasound faculty and credentialed by the host institution in the use of ultrasound. The ultrasound faculty should be responsible for direct and indirect review of the majority of the resident examinations and be able to provide feedback on scanning technique and interpretation. Ultrasound fellows may be delegated ultrasound faculty responsibilities.

Equipment

There are an increasing number of choices for ultrasound equipment for CUS. System capabilities continue to expand while cost has remained constant and in some cases decreased. Computer miniaturization has allowed for the production of small systems that can even fit into the lab coat of a physician.

The choice of equipment depends on many factors:

- Number of residents
- Patient census
- Physical size of the emergency department
- Budgetary issues

The number and type of ultrasound probes should be chosen based on the applications performed in each program's clinical environment, but generally includes linear, curved linear, phased array, and endocavitary transducers.

Other important factors to consider include the mundane issues of durability, product warrantees, and regular maintenance. Product information should not only be obtained through sales representatives, but also through consultation with ultrasound program directors at other institutions.

Both new and experienced ultrasound program directors will benefit from routinely sampling a large number of systems to keep abreast of technology advances and to determine the best fit for their current and future needs.

Competency Assessment

The goal of competency assessment is to assure that each resident can integrate ultrasound into daily clinical practice. Two parameters are used to make this assessment:

- Number of exams performed
- Evaluation of technique and interpretation

Many organizations including the ACGME recognize that at least 150 ultrasound examinations in "critical" or "life-saving" scenarios promote a minimum acceptable level of exposure. However, completion of these exams does not establish competency, and the residency program must also qualitatively assess each resident's ability to perform studies routinely conducted in an emergency department setting. This process should include assessment of the following parameters:

- Proper machine settings
- Probe positions
- Image acquisition and documentation
- Image quality
- Identification of landmarks
- Completeness of imaging protocol
- Interpretation of findings

The majority of these experiences should be conducted while working with patients in an emergency department setting, but can also be performed in simulated settings using standardized patients or ultrasound simulators. Assessment methods include:

- Standard Direct Observations Tool (SDOT)
- Objective Structured Clinical Examination

The program should provide a system for residents to log their ultrasound exam experiences during training. This system should include a method to store images for each exam that can be reviewed by faculty with POC US expertise. Commercial systems are also available with annual fee structures based on the number of residents and the number of submitted exams (e.g., Q-path at http://www.telexy.com).

Medical knowledge of POC US can be assessed using a standardized multiple-choice examination. Emsono (http://www.emsono.com/acep/exam.html) provides a free interactive modular exam covering all of the core applications of emergency ultrasound. This test includes video, still image, and case-based questions.

Other Residency Experiences

ACGME utilizes two documents to establish requirements for postgraduate medical training:

- ACGME Program Requirements
- The Milestones Project

The only specialty other than emergency medicine with written requirements for ultrasound education in both the ACGME Program Requirements and Milestones is anesthesiology (Table 8.4). Other clinical specialties that can utilize POC US have very limited written requirements that pertain specifically to ultrasound education. Cardiology is the only specialty other than emergency medicine to require the performance of a specific number of studies during postgraduate training (ironically also 150 examinations), but there are no milestones for ultrasound competence. Although obstetrics and gynecology (OB-GYN) is historically an early adopter of clinical ultrasound, OB-GYN does not have specific language in the ACGME program requirements for POC US education. However, there is a reference to ultrasound competence within one of the OB-GYN milestones. There are no ACGME specific requirements or milestones for POC US education in family medicine, internal medicine, pediatrics, or surgery.

Only a handful of the nation's internal medicine programs incorporate bedside ultrasound training into their curriculum. A survey of internal medicine training programs found that while there is substantial interest in point of care ultrasound among internal medicine educators, only 25% indicated their program has a formal curriculum [25].

Although ACGME does not require POC US training in family medicine, the American Academy of Family Physicians (AAFP) Practice Profile Survey from 2008 reported that 18% of AAFP members offer obstetric ultrasound in their practices, 15% offer non-OB ultrasound, and 14% offer echocardiography [26]. The Society of Teachers of Family Medicine (STFM) and the American Academy of Family Physicians (AAFP) commission on education state that family medicine residents should learn basic and advanced obstetric ultrasound and be exposed to ultrasound-guided procedures including central vascular access, paracentesis, and thoracentesis [26].

Table 8.4 Comparison between specialties regarding ACGME program requirements and NAS milestones on ultrasound education [1–3, 7–24]

Specialty	ACGME program requirements	NAS milestones
Anesthesia	**Section IV.A.5.a).(2). (l).(ii)**	**Acute, chronic, and cancer-related pain consultations and management** with regard to nerve location and regional anesthesia.
	… central vein and pulmonary artery catheter placement, and the use of transesophageal echocardiography and evoked potentials…	**Technical skills: Use and Interpretation of Monitoring and Equipment** related to central line placement and transesophageal ultrasound for advanced monitoring techniques
Cardiology	**Section IV.A.5.a).(2). (a).(ii)**	None (from The Internal Medicine Subspecialty Milestones Project)
	… must demonstrate competence in the performance of … echocardiography; Each fellow must perform a minimum and interpret a minimum of 150 studies, and observe the performance and interpretation of transesophageal cardiac studies	
Emergency medicine	**Section IV.A.5.a).(2). (c). (viii). (a)**	**Other Diagnostic and Therapeutic Procedures: Goal-directed Focused Ultrasound (Diagnostic/Procedural).** Uses goal-directed focused ultrasound for the bedside diagnostic evaluation of emergency medical conditions and diagnoses, resuscitation of the acutely ill or injured patient, and procedural guidance
	Residents must use ultrasound for the bedside diagnostic evaluation of emergency medical conditions and diagnoses, resuscitation of the acutely ill or injured patient, and procedural guidance	
Family medicine	None	None
Internal medicine	None	None
Obstetrics and gynecology	None	Mentions ultrasound competence briefly in the **Obstetrical Technical Skills—Patient Care** milestone
Pediatrics	None	None
Pulmonary critical care	**Section IV.A.5.a).(2). (b). (xiii)**	None
	… use of ultrasound techniques to perform thoracentesis and place intravascular and intracavitary tubes and catheters	
Surgical critical care	None	Mentions as "Advanced Monitoring Technique" in the **Patient Care Shock/ Resuscitation** milestone
Surgery	None	None

ACGME program requirements for pulmonary critical care includes POC US training to *"perform thoracentesis and place intravascular and intracavitary tubes and catheters,"* but there are no milestones for ultrasound competence. The Surgical Critical Care Milestones document mentions ultrasound as an *"advanced monitoring technique"* for shock and resuscitation, but it is not discussed in the ACGME program requirements.

Pitfall for Ultrasound Training in Residency

1. **Not introducing POC US early in residency training**

   - Many programs fail to introduce residents to POC US until after their PGY 1 year of training.
   - By this point many residents become resistant to new techniques and skills.
   - Setting expectations on the first day of residency is critical to developing the habit of POC US utilization.

2. **Depending on training venues or specialties outside your department to teach your residents**

   - Depending on other specialties for POC US training often allows your program faculty to avoid learning how to utilize POC US.
   - This creates a clinical environment where residents are not actively encouraged to use POC US in their regular patient care.

3. **Recreating the "educational wheel" of didactics, training, and testing rather than utilizing previously developed education resources**

   - Curriculum development is a tremendous burden for a dynamic topic like POC US.
   - There is an enormous amount of previously developed educational content that can be used to assist in resident POC US education.

4. **Not having faculty that are trained and supportive of POC US**

   - Require minimum standards for your faculty regarding POC US competence.
   - Provide educational support through didactic training as well as hiring new faculty with POC US skills.

Key Recommendations

- Development and implementation of a residency ultrasound training program requires significant planning and resources.
- The ultrasound program director must be compensated to dedicate adequate time and effort to the process.

- ACGME now requires the evaluation of clinical ultrasound skills for residents training in emergency medicine with evolving standards in other specialties.
- There are four assets required for the successful deployment of a POC US program: curriculum, trained faculty, adequate equipment, and competency assessment tools.

References

1. Accreditation Council for Graduate Medical Education Program Requirements for Graduate Medical Education in Emergency Medicine. http://www.acgme.org/acgmeweb/portals/0/pfassets/2013-pr-faq-pif/110_emergency_medicine_07012013.pdf.
2. Beeson MS, Carter WA, Christopher TA, et al. Emergency medicine milestones. J Grad Med Educ. 2013;5(1S):5–13.
3. Nelson M, Abdi A, Adhikari S, et al. Goal-directed focused ultrasound milestones revised: a multiorganizational consensus. Acad Emerg Med. 2016;23(11):1274–9. doi:10.1111/acem.13069.
4. Kelly B, Sicilia J, Forman S, Ellert W, Nothnagle M. Family medicine residency education advanced procedural training in family medicine: a group consensus statement. http://www.aafp.org/dam/AAFP/documents/medical_education_residency/fmig/FMAdvancedProceduralTraining.pdf.
5. American College of Emergency Physicians. ACEP emergency ultrasound guidelines—2001. Ann Emerg Med. 2001;38:470–81.
6. ACEP policy guidelines. http://www.acep.org/workarea/downloadasset.aspx?id=32878.
7. American College of Emergency Physicians. American College of Emergency Physicians. Use of ultrasound imaging by emergency by emergency physicians [policy statement]. Ann Emerg Med. 2001;38:469–70.
8. Accreditation Council for Graduate Medical Education Program Requirements for Graduate Medical Education in Anesthesiology: https://www.acgme.org/Portals/0/PFAssets/ProgramRequirements/040_anesthesiology_2016.pdf.
9. The Anesthesiology Milestones Project. Accreditation Council for Graduate Medical Education and the American Board of Anesthesiology. https://www.acgme.org/Portals/0/PDFs/Milestones/AnesthesiologyMilestones.pdf.
10. Accreditation Council for Graduate Medical Education Program Requirements for Graduate Medical Education in Cardiovascular Disease: http://www.acgme.org/Portals/0/PFAssets/ProgramRequirements/141_cardiovascular_disease_int_med_2016.pdf.
11. The Internal Medicine Subspecialty Milestones Project. Accreditation Council for Graduate Medical Education and the American Board of Internal Medicine, Alliance for Academic Internal Medicine, and Association of Specialty Professors. http://www.acgme.org/portals/0/pdfs/milestones/internalmedicinesubspecialtymilestones.pdf.
12. Accreditation Council for Graduate Medical Education Program Requirements for Graduate Medical Education in Family Medicine. http://www.acgme.org/Portals/0/PFAssets/ProgramRequirements/120_family_medicine_2016.pdf.
13. The Family Medicine Milestones Project. Accreditation Council for Graduate Medical Education and the American Board of Family Medicine. http://www.acgme.org/portals/0/pdfs/milestones/familymedicinemilestones.pdf.
14. Accreditation Council for Graduate Medical Education Program Requirements for Graduate Medical Education in Internal Medicine. http://www.acgme.org/portals/0/pfassets/programrequirements/140_internal_medicine_2016.pdf.
15. The Internal Medicine Milestones Project. Accreditation Council for Graduate Medical Education and the American Board of Internal Medicine. http://www.acgme.org/portals/0/pdfs/milestones/internalmedicinemilestones.pdf.

16. Accreditation Council for Graduate Medical Education Program Requirements for Graduate Medical Education in Obstetrics and Gynecology. https://www.acgme.org/Portals/0/PFAssets/ProgramRequirements/220_obstetrics_and_gynecology_2016.pdf.
17. The Obstetrics and Gynecology Milestones Project. Accreditation Council for Graduate Medical Education, American College of Obstetrics and Gynecology, American Board of Obstetrics and Gynecology. https://www.acgme.org/Portals/0/PDFs/Milestones/Obstetricsand GynecologyMilestones.pdf.
18. Accreditation Council for Graduate Medical Education Program Requirements for Graduate Medical Education in Pediatrics. https://www.acgme.org/Portals/0/PFAssets/ProgramRequirements/320_pediatrics_2016.pdf.
19. The Pediatrics Milestones Project. Accreditation Council for Graduate Medical Education and the American Board of Pediatrics. https://www.acgme.org/Portals/0/PDFs/Milestones/PediatricsMilestones.pdf.
20. Accreditation Council for Graduate Medical Education Program Requirements for Graduate Medical Education in Pulmonary Critical Care.
21. Accreditation Council for Graduate Medical Education Program Requirements for Graduate Medical Education in Surgical Critical Care. https://www.acgme.org/Portals/0/PFAssets/ProgramRequirements/442_surgical_critical_care_2016_1-YR.pdf.
22. The Surgical Critical Care Milestones Project. Accreditation Council for Graduate Medical Education and the American Board of Surgery. http://www.acgme.org/portals/0/pdfs/milestones/surgicalcriticalcaremilestones.pdf.
23. Accreditation Council for Graduate Medical Education Program Requirements for Graduate Medical Education in General Surgery. http://www.acgme.org/portals/0/pfassets/programrequirements/440_general_surgery_2016.pdf.
24. The General Surgery Milestones Project. Accreditation Council for Graduate Medical Education and the American Board of Surgery. http://www.acgme.org/portals/0/pdfs/milestones/surgerymilestones.pdf.
25. Schnobrich D, Gladding S, Olson A, Duran-Nelson A. Point-of-care ultrasound in internal medicine: a national survey of educational leadership. J Grad Med Educ. 2013;5(3):498–502.
26. American Academy of Family Physicians. Practice profile II. Leawood: American Academy of Family Physicians; 2009.

Chapter 9
Ultrasound Fellowship Programs

Christopher C. Raio and Srikar Adhikari

Objectives

- Describe the importance and role of ultrasound management, administrative and leadership education in clinical ultrasound fellowship programs.
- Provide an overview of core topics integral to an ultrasound fellow's education in the area of ultrasound management, administration, and leadership.
- Provide a framework for educating fellows in ultrasound management, administration, and leadership topics.
- Describe the challenges in integrating nonclinical ultrasound education into clinical ultrasound fellowship programs.

Introduction

Over the past three decades clinical ultrasound use by non-traditional users has skyrocketed and Emergency Medicine specialists have pioneered this development. As point-of-care ultrasound (POC US) has evolved, the breadth of applications has also greatly expanded for users at the POC US, and this growth has triggered a need to train future experts and leaders in the field. Ultrasound fellowship training programs, and in particular Emergency Ultrasound (EUS) fellowship

C.C. Raio, MD, MBA, FACEP (✉)
Department of Emergency Medicine, Good Samaritan Hospital Medical Center,
West Islip, NY, USA
e-mail: craio7@gmail.com

S. Adhikari, MD, MS, FACEP
Department of Emergency Medicine, University of Arizona,
College of Medicine, Tucson, AZ, USA

© Springer International Publishing AG 2018   103
V. S. Tayal et al. (eds.), *Ultrasound Program Management*,
https://doi.org/10.1007/978-3-319-63143-1_9

programs, have filled this void. There now exist approximately 96 programs nationwide (http://www.eusfellowships.com/). Initially concentrated in the northeast, programs have been introduced in 30 states and Canada. The goal of these programs is not solely to graduate clinical ultrasound experts, but also to mentor and develop the future administrative and academic leaders in the field.

The importance of ultrasound management, administration, and leadership has increased as clinical ultrasound training has penetrated earlier into physician education. Competency in the core applications is now a requirement for completion of an Emergency Medicine ACGME (Accreditation Council for Graduate Medical Education)-approved residency program [1]. Some physicians are even obtaining extensive training in their undergraduate medical training [2]. Fellowships are geared towards mastery of not only "advanced" clinical applications, but also focus on the nonclinical aspects of ultrasound program development.

Fellows generally gain expertise in image acquisition and interpretation in all basic and advanced point-of-care EUS applications. Fellows are required to be active in EUS research and are responsible for teaching faculty, residents, and medical students. In addition, fellows should become proficient in the critical components required to establish and run a EUS program. The importance of involvement in regional and national organizations is also of critical importance and must be stressed during fellowship training (See Chap. 12 – Equipment, Chap. 15 – US Safety and Infection Control).

The Need for Fellowship Training in EUS

EUS is one of the most coveted fellowships in Emergency Medicine. Training is typically 1 year in length, though there are a few programs that offer multi-year positions in combination with alternative degrees, research experience, or specified focus areas such as international medicine and ultrasound integration. Fellowship training aims to elevate the level of clinical expertise far beyond that of "well-trained residents in EUS." Fellows receive higher level, focused training and mentoring by his or her fellowship director and other EUS-trained faculty members. Scanning technique, limitations, pearls and pitfalls and advanced applications are all integrated into the various programs. However, pursuing an ultrasound fellowship will not only increase the fellow's proficiency in the technical aspects of performing bedside ultrasound, but also help acquire administrative skills that are essential to develop a point-of-care ultrasound program. In our era of medicine where reimbursement is a constant challenge and moving target, ultrasound can produce an alternative source of revenue via both direct and indirect mechanisms. This will benefit not only the individual clinician, but also the emergency medicine group or practice and institution. The expertise gained over the course of fellowship can open opportunities whether it be in an academic institution, community hospital, or global healthcare. Choosing a niche such as ultrasound will also increase professional satisfaction and also provide opportunities to reduce clinical workload and prevent burnout.

EUS Fellowship Guidelines/Core Content

Over the past decade, EUS fellowships have rapidly proliferated and currently 96 such fellowships are offered in the United States (http://www.eusfellowships.com/programs.php). Despite guidelines and educational recommendations proposed by national emergency medicine organizations, variability still exists in exposure that the fellows receive during the course of their programs.

In an attempt to provide uniformity and minimum standards, in 2011, the "Emergency Ultrasound Fellowship Guidelines" were released [3]. This consensus document published by the American College of Emergency Physicians (ACEP) Emergency Ultrasound Section outlines site qualification requirements, minimum criteria to be an EUS fellowship director, and minimum criteria for fellows to graduate. These guidelines recommend participation in various administrative and quality assurance activities including reimbursement audits, interdepartmental meetings, and monitoring the credentialing process of colleagues. Subsequently in 2014, Lewiss et al. published "The Core Content of Clinical Ultrasonography Fellowship Training" to provide a framework to standardize the clinical scope of fellowship training [4]. The EUS fellow is expected to master the core content listed in the document, and potential applications that may be used for future board certification examinations are outlined. The proposed curriculum is broadly divided into Image Acquisition and Interpretation Skills, Education Skills, Research Skills, and Administration Skills. The administration skills listed in this document include Quality improvement principles and program, Leadership, Program systems, Relationships and networks, Coding and billing, and Economics.

Fellowship Training Models and Methods

As mentioned above, there are over 96 EUS fellowship programs in the United States and Canada. Even though there are the ACEP guidelines and published core content, there is significant variability in the training across programs and currently there is no standardized method to train EUS fellows in ultrasound management skills. A team-based approach to train EUS fellows in the management skills has been successfully implemented in some programs [5]. Other programs distribute administrative responsibilities on a rotating basis where fellows spend a designated period of time responsible for a specified aspect of the ultrasound program, i.e., resident education/rotation, quality assurance and feedback, credentialing, etc. There are also several national and regional course offerings, such as the hugely popular ACEP Ultrasound Management course, which deliver focused education covering the key administrative and leadership topics. Many programs still teach these skills via "on the job" training where fellows are thrown into the processes on a daily basis and learn on-the-go. Typically as programs advance, this type of training gives way to a more formalized approach, which we recommend. Regardless of the training model, fellows should be actively involved in various aspects of ultrasound program management. Fellows must be integrated into all aspects of ultrasound program development and maintenance of that program. It is critical for fellows to not only understand the policies, procedures, and processes but also to realize the time, effort, and dedication required to sustain high level ultrasound programs.

Below, we discuss various components of EUS management fellows need to master during their fellowship training.

Education Skills

Part of the fellow's training is to learn how to become an effective ultrasound educator. This is a key component of any point-of-care ultrasound program since ultrasound management is closely tied to training physician colleagues in the clinical skill. It is crucial to have a strong ongoing education program. Fellows should receive instruction in both content development and presentation. This should include curricular development, creating a portfolio of didactic lectures, image bank development, critical literature review and coordinating journal clubs, utilization of social media resources, visual presentation and public speaking skills [4]. Typically fellows receive training in bedside teaching of residents and medical students. Focus should be not only teaching residents and medical students, but also faculty and experienced physicians. Fellowship directors should focus on training fellows how to teach learners at different levels and different settings and assist with faculty development at their institution. Challenges in training faculty members should be stressed as this is often the most difficult aspect of any educational program.

Additionally, clinicians from other specialties and practice environments will request ultrasound training and education, and the fellow should learn how to set up outreach education and online educational programs. An interesting dilemma that needs to be taught is how to negotiate time and resources as they relate to these educational objectives. "When to say no" is often a difficult question, but it must be answered. Online forums and social media are valuable assets to any educational portfolio and ways to engage with these tools also needs to be included in the fellows' education.

Fellows should be specifically trained in bedside hands-on instruction and organizing courses workshops, such as SonoCamp/Ultrasound Challenge, Ultrafest, etc. Fellows should actively send out weekly cases and host cadaver and or procedural labs. They should also receive instruction in competency assessment, both for overall knowledge and hands-on skills. Various methods of competency assessment including Objective Structured Clinical Examinations and Standardized Direct Observation Tools should be reviewed, and question writing skills also must be described. They should be familiar with ACGME milestones for residents as well as practice-based pathways for nonresident physicians. Fellows should be trained in evaluation of knowledge through written or online examinations, clinical image and video review, formal ultrasound report review and evaluation of psychomotor skills either on live patients, standardized patients or simulation exercises. They should also gain experience in assessment of teaching skills including direct observation, lectures, and written evaluations.

Quality Assurance

A quality assurance program is crucial to maintain a successful point-of-care ultrasound program. Quality assurance generally includes image review for technical quality of image acquisition, image interpretation, documentation, and clinical integration leading to patient outcomes. A majority of programs review all ultrasound examinations performed at their institutions for quality assurance via video and still images at "tape review sessions." This type of review can be performed on a daily or weekly basis and is best practice. Fellows should be integrally involved in this process. Alternatively, reviews can cover a percentage of departmental examinations performed. Fellows should be specifically trained how to give feedback to the sonographer as a part of this process, address missed critical and incidental findings, and ensure physician compliance with documentation of ultrasound examinations.

Unfortunately, every active ultrasound program will eventually encounter a troubling case, missed findings, or complications related to ultrasound use. Dealing with these issues and integrating them into a valuable performance improvement program is an essential skill that must be learned. Often this involves interacting with leadership from other departments or the hospital. Handling these issues from the quality perspective again must be stressed, as well as appropriate documentation of these issues.

Leadership

During the fellowship year, fellows must acquire leadership skills essential to lead point-of-care ultrasound program. Effective leadership skills are often difficult to obtain, however, the overriding principle is effective communication. Communication skills can be taught in a variety of ways, and this will vary from program to program. An overview of varying leadership styles can also be reviewed during the course of fellowship year. And finally the differences between managing and taking the next step to leading should be discussed. After global leadership skills are incorporated into a fellows training the integration of those skills to oversight of education, equipment, workflow, research, administration, and risk management will ensue.

Equipment

Fellows should receive instruction in purchasing and maintaining the equipment required to operate a program including ultrasound machines, middleware solutions, transducers, and disinfection equipment. Fellows should learn how to assess equipment from different vendors and how to interact and negotiate with those vendors. Working with hospital administration in submitting capital requests and purchasing new equipment and service contracts is also a learned knowledge. The purchasing process is often difficult to navigate. Installing new equipment, setting up presets, labels, protocols, worksheets, working with biomedical engineers and information technologists all must be part of their formalized training.

Fellows should be equipped with knowledge and skills to troubleshoot both hardware and software problems, Digital Imaging and Communications in Medicine (DICOM) and wireless connectivity issues. The fellowship training should also include items such as Health Insurance Portability and Accountability Act (HIPAA) compliance and social media institutional policies. Ensuring accessibility and adequate stocking of ultrasound supplies in the emergency department is also critical. Because of the large number of users and the harsh environment these systems are used in, emergency department (ED) ultrasound equipment frequently sustain hardware damage or encounter software errors. Fellows should learn how to solve these issues, contacting Biomedical Engineering department or vendors directly. Additionally, fellows should be trained in solving issues related to interfaces with middleware or Picture Archiving and Communication System (PACS).

Policies and procedures related to cleaning of the systems themselves, transducers, and overall infection control must be developed and fellows should become knowledgeable in this process. Safety principles as they relate to point-of-care ultrasound including As Low As Reasonably Achievable (ALARA) must also be delivered.

Workflow

As fellows go on to take leadership positions, they should be equipped with tools and skills to set up POC ultrasound workflow. Fellows should be trained in different components of workflow including order entry, modality worklists, entering demographic identifiers on ultrasound systems, distinguishing educational vs. patient care examinations, wireless image management including archiving in PACS, web-based archival system or middleware for documentation and electronic signature, Electronic Medical Record (EMR) documentation, ED coder notification and electronic and digital interfaces. All front-end and back-end workflow processes must be understood. Fellows should be able to develop sophisticated wireless and workflow solutions, develop policies and procedures with regard to ED POC ultrasound workflow after their training. Fellows should be taught not only how to set up the workflow but also how to train physician colleagues and coders to adopt the workflow.

Physician compliance with documentation and workflow process is crucial for generating ultrasound billing revenue. Fellows should be trained how to address the barriers and motivate colleagues to be compliant with workflow processes and also increase ultrasound use. It is also important to comprehend the oversight of these processes, and any metrics to track to ensure the workflow system is supporting the clinical ultrasound program (See Chap. 17 – Workflow).

Networking

Fellows should actively participate in all ultrasound-related meetings including performance improvement, operations, credentialing, information technology, biomedical engineering, infection control, risk management, and revenue stream. They should attend departmental faculty meetings to provide ultrasound updates and interdepartmental meetings to discuss issues and developments related to point-of-care ultrasound. In addition to meetings directly related to ultrasound, fellows should also participate in meetings and discussions regarding budget, ED policy and procedure, clinical guidelines, and institutional POC ultrasound development.

Besides intramural meetings, they should be encouraged to network and meet others in the EUS field at national meetings such as ACEP, Society of Academic Emergency Medicine (SAEM), and American Institute of Ultrasound in medicine (AIUM). They should also be encouraged to attend the annual Society for Ultrasound Fellowships (SCUF) meeting. Any exposure to regional, national, or international ultrasound specialty groups must be encouraged. Committee engagement at this level is critical to advancing fellow expertise. Fellows are expected to develop professional working relationships with other specialties as well. There are multiple venues to encourage these interactions including social media and online webinars and blogs.

Another aspect of networking that cannot be overlooked is the ability to recruit individuals to join ones group or practice. In most regions of the country there exist emergency physician shortages and the ability to recruit colleagues is a key skill that involves networking and must be stressed.

Coding/Billing/Reimbursement

Understanding the financial piece of ultrasound is a key fellowship educational objective. At the end of fellowship training, fellows should be equipped with all tools necessary to initiate a reimbursement program. Successful implementation of a point-of-care ultrasound program requires financial integration of ultrasound into existing departmental reimbursement strategies. Fellows should be familiar with International Classification of Diseases (ICD) codes/Current Procedural Terminology (CPT) codes of limited ultrasound examinations, documentation requirements and the importance of payer mix and contracting with private insurers. Fellows should be trained in how to integrate reimbursement into POC ultrasound workflow including EMR documentation, electronic signature, physician training, timely billing reminders to physicians, and ED coder training and communication.

Physician compliance with documentation is crucial for generating ultrasound billing revenue, and fellows should be trained to address the barriers with documentation and motivate physicians to improve documentation. Fellows should be familiar with strategies to improve physician documentation and participate in ongoing education of these strategies (middleware navigation, indications for POC ultrasound, required images, required components of documentation including medical necessity, description of organs studied and study findings).

Efficiency of ED coders is the key to increase the ultrasound billing revenue. Fellows should learn how to work closely with ED coders, ensure ongoing education of ED coders, and address billing issues that are critical for reimbursement. Fellows should be trained in regularly reviewing metrics including billing volume, reimbursement rates, denials, and collections with the ED coders consistently. Fellows should also be knowledgeable about ongoing reimbursement changes regionally and nationally (Medicare vs. Private insurance). They should also learn how to address billing errors and denials. They should learn strategies to motivate physicians to use ultrasound including integration of ultrasound into relative value units Relative Value Units, incentive packages for using ultrasound and providing productivity reports (See Chap. 22 – Reimbursement and Coding).

Budget/Economics

It is crucial for fellows to learn how to allocate resources available to maintain and grow their respective programs. Resources will vary from institution to institution. Understanding return on investment strategies for point-of-care ultrasound is critical to gaining these resources. There is not only direct return through revenue generation from CPT codes on the professional and technical side, but also potential Evaluation & Management coding uplift on cases where ultrasound exams are performed. In addition, indirect return on investment is likely far greater including improved patient flow, reduced length of stay, patient and provider satisfaction, reduced complications and expenses related, and reduced malpractice costs.

They should understand the principles of department and division budgeting and develop negotiation skills to better their positions. Fellows should learn how to submit budget requests and justify costs for expenditures such as equipment and service contracts. They should learn how to negotiate and manage ultrasound section funds, ultrasound faculty salary support, equipment, facilities and support for performing quality assurance review. Effective negotiation skills is a topic that should be formally taught during fellowship training.

Credentialing/Privileges

Fellows must learn to distinguish certification, credentialing, and accreditation. These terms are often inappropriately interchanged and misunderstood. They should understand that no standardized method exists for POC ultrasound credentialing, and the process is institution-specific. The process of developing delineation of privileges specific to POC ultrasound housed either within the department or at the level of a hospital's credentialing committee is critical. Most experts agree that global ultrasound credentialing at the hospital credentialing committee level combined with application specific privileges tracked within the Department of Emergency Medicine is best practice. A recent survey indicates that hiring physicians with additional training in emergency ultrasonography assists with credentialing other staff in POC ultrasound [6].

Fellows should be assigned the task of facilitating the credentialing of other faculty within their departments during the fellowship year. They should be required to send comprehensive reports on a regular basis to faculty and residents tracking volume of application specific examinations, quality (appropriate probe/preset selection, appropriate gain/depth adjustments, and acquisition of required views), documentation, accuracy of interpretation, and frequency of billing. This will ensure active participation and understanding of the credentialing process. Assigning an individual fellow to a specific small group of residents or attendings to help expedite their credentialing may be useful. Understanding strategies to motivate physician colleagues to obtain ultrasound credentials and continue to expand their skills is important. These strategies include periodic reminders and monitoring of metrics, monthly workshops, and continuous feedback.

Fellows should also become familiar with different credentialing pathways and the criteria for credentialing and recredentialing. They should be equipped with the skills to navigate this process at the intra-, interdepartmental, hospital, and health system levels.

As part of the formalized fellowship education Focused Professional Practice Evaluations (FPPE) and Ongoing Professional Practice Evaluations (OPPE) must be learned and understood. FPPE is a process whereby the organization evaluates the privilege-specific competence of a practitioner who does not have documented evidence of competently performing the requested privilege at the organization, or encounters an issue while performing the requested privilege. OPPE is the ongoing assessment of an existing medical staff member's performance. These are Joint Commission standards for the medical staff. The development and of these policies and procedures and carrying them out should be incorporated into the role the fellow plays within their ultrasound program (See Chap. 20 – Credentialing and Privileging).

Point-of-Care Ultrasound Program Accreditation

Fellows should become familiar with the ACEP-governed Clinical Ultrasound Accreditation Program standards in the areas of administration of ultrasound programs, education and training of healthcare providers, performing and interpreting ultrasound examinations, equipment management, transducer disinfection, image acquisition and retention, and confidentiality and privacy. This will ensure quality, patient safety, communication, responsibility, and clarity regarding the use of clinical ultrasound in their future endeavors (See Chap. 21 – Accreditation).

Problem Solving

Fellows should also be trained to address complaints related to use of POC ultrasound, from either within the Emergency Medicine group or other departments or patients. They should gain experience how to handle medicolegal issues related to POC ultrasound. They also need to develop expertise to resolve issues related to billing, documentation, and of course patient care. Negotiating through these issues and appropriately documenting the process and any corrective actions is critical.

Politics/Institutional POC US/Negotiation Skills

Fellows should have good understanding of departmental, institutional, regional, and national politics related to ultrasound. They should learn how to negotiate support for the Ultrasound Director position and additional ultrasound faculty. They should be mentored to effectively communicate and negotiate with ED and hospital leadership to help determine the position of their respective faculty, group, or division.

Discussion

Ultrasound management, administration, and leadership is complex and multi-faceted. Every aspect of an EUS fellowship requires some element, from educating faculty to optimizing workflow. Increasingly, many specialties have an interest in utilizing ultrasound in their clinical practice across diverse patient care settings. Consequently, there is a need for direction, leadership and administrative oversight for hospital systems to efficiently deliver this technology in an organized and coordinated manner. Emergency physicians by nature have a broad scope of practice and interact with essentially all specialties and are thus uniquely positioned to take this role. It is crucial to train fellows in these skills to meet the growing needs of ultrasound users. To lead an EUS program efficiently in the future, fellows must have rigorous experience in the various components of POC ultrasound management, administration, and leadership. This is even more vital as clinical ultrasound skills training penetrates deeper into undergraduate and graduate medical education, giving fellowships the perfect time and opportunity to teach the nonclinical core expertise.

Pitfalls

1. Primary challenges in delivering this experience and education is that not every fellow has equal interest is these nonclinical topics, and not all fellowship-directors were exposed themselves to every administrative and leadership skill.

2. In addition, there is no empowered oversight for these non-ACGME accredited clinical ultrasound fellowships which leads to lack of uniformity in training, and potentially lack of resources and expertise at some institutions.

Key Recommendations

1. Fellows must be actively involved in all aspects of ultrasound management, administration, and leadership in order to receive the most well-rounded fellowship experience.
2. Assigning administrative responsibilities during fellowship training will ensure depth of exposure for fellows to understand and learn all aspects of running a successful EUS program.

References

1. Lewiss RE, Pearl M, Nomura JT, Baty G, Bengiamin R, Duprey K, Stone M, Theodoro D, Akhtar S. CORD-AEUS: consensus document for the emergency ultrasound milestone project. Acad Emerg Med. 2013;20(7):740–5.
2. Bahner DP, Goldman E, Way D, Royall NA, Liu YT. The state of ultrasound education in U.S. medical schools: results of a national survey. Acad Med. 2014;89(12):1681–6.
3. American College of Emergency Physicians. Emergency ultrasound guidelines. Ann Emerg Med. 2009;53(4):550–70.
4. Lewiss RE, et al. The core content of clinical ultrasonography fellowship training. Acad Emerg Med. 2014;21(4):456–61.
5. Adhikari S, Fiorello A. Emergency ultrasound fellowship training: a novel team-based approach. J Ultrasound Med. 2014;33(10):1821–6.
6. Das D, Kapoor M, Brown C, Ndubuisi A, Gupta S. Current status of emergency department attending physician ultrasound credentialing and quality assurance in the United States. Crit Ultrasound J. 2016;8(1):6.

Chapter 10
Point of Care Ultrasound Issues for Advanced Practice Providers and Nursing Programs

Eric J. Chin and Shane M. Summers

Objectives

1. Perspective on US use by APPs
2. US Educational Pathways for APPs
3. Credentialing and Supervision issues for the APP
4. Nursing use of US
5. Pitfalls and Controversies for the APP's use of US

Introduction

Early use of point of care ultrasonography (POC US) by advanced practice providers (APPs) and nursing programs can be traced back to the early 2000s for percutaneous liver biopsies, abscess localization, and peripheral intravenous catheter insertion [1–3]. Notably, there is a paucity of published examples of formal curricula designed to train and evaluate APPs in the discipline of POC US, with the earliest one dating as far back as 2007, specifically for emergency medicine-trained physician assistants [4].

E.J. Chin, MD, FACEP (✉) • S.M. Summers, MD, FACEP
Department of Emergency Medicine, San Antonio Military Medical Center,
Fort Sam Houston, TX, USA
e-mail: sammc@thechinfamily.com

© Springer International Publishing AG 2018
V. S. Tayal et al. (eds.), *Ultrasound Program Management*,
https://doi.org/10.1007/978-3-319-63143-1_10

Over the past decade, utilization of POC US applications has continued to increase across many different disciplines and types of clinicians [5–7]. APPs are as diverse and varied as there are medical and surgical specialties in medicine. This includes a wide range of training experiences, training levels, and practice environments upon which POC US can be utilized—such as in the operating room by a nurse anesthetist performing regional anesthesia; in the intensive care unit by a physician assistant assessing volume status in a hypotensive patient; in a primary care clinic by a nurse practitioner evaluating an ankle joint for an effusion; or in the emergency department by a nurse placing a peripheral intravenous (IV) catheter in a chronic IV drug abuser. With these wide ranging factors in mind, this chapter will discuss a practical approach to implementing initial POC US education, equipment considerations, supervision, credentialing, and documentation for APPs and nursing programs.

Initial Education

There are many types of APPs (e.g., nurse practitioners, physician assistants, nurse anesthetists) and nursing programs training in POC US across a wide variety of settings. The training platform will mostly depend upon the skill level necessary for the practice setting and the educational status of the learner (e.g., currently in primary medical schooling as opposed to being in active clinical practice) (Chaps. 5, 6 and 7).

A reasonable approach to ensuring competency in POC US should follow one of two pathways, analogous to those described by some medical specialty organizations [8, 9]: a trainee-based pathway and a practice-based pathway (see Fig. 10.1). Both of these pathways should include didactics, practical clinical skills sessions, and a skills validation assessment. Beyond the initial POC US education, it is imperative that POC US Directors maintain a quality assurance program and users mitigate skill decay through continuing medical education and regular practice with POC US.

Trainee-Based Pathway

This pathway is intended for novice POC US users who are still in a formal educational setting (e.g., nursing school, physician assistant medical school, midwifery school). It is an optimal setting for acquiring POC US skills, since a formalized curriculum including an introductory didactic course, hand-on skills training, and competency assessment can be coordinated from start to finish.

An introductory course with didactic content and an experiential hands-on component will typically require several hours for a single modality, and up to 24 h for a more comprehensive training program (see Fig. 10.2 for sample curriculum). This introductory content does not need to occur all at once; however, this may prove to be the most efficient and effective way of covering the material for logistical reasons. Many training

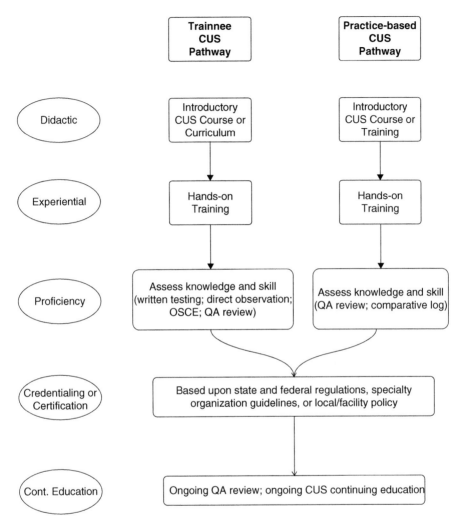

Fig. 10.1 Recommended clinical ultrasound (POC US) training pathways. *OSCE* objective structured clinical examination, *QA* quality assurance. Adapted from: [10]

programs may not have enough faculty experienced in POC US to instruct a course; therefore, it may be necessary to augment POC US course faculty from other areas of medicine (ultrasonographers, emergency physicians, radiologists, etc.).

Minimum competency can be assessed through written testing, online educational modules, direct observation, objective structured clinical examinations (OSCEs), and quality assurance review of completed POC US studies. Many programs utilize scoring systems for image quality, such as the American College of Emergency Physicians Ultrasound Reporting Guidelines [12]. Training programs desiring more advanced expertise may consider POC US-specific rotations that provide dedicated scanning sessions and direct feedback (such as a POC US block or elective).

1. Define limited POC US as compared to comprehensive radiology-performed exams.

2. Discuss POC US operation and optimization of ultrasound systems, equipment handling, and infection control.

3. Identify and describe specialty-specific POC US applications.

4. Describe physics principles of image formation, instrumentation and artifacts in image acquisition.

5. Describe the indications, contraindications, limitations and safety for each POC US applications.

6. Define the relevant sonographic windows, anatomical landmarks and potential pitfalls.

7. Describe normal and abnormal findings and their clinical implications.

8. Describe the techniques used to perform a particular POC US.

9. Describe required elements and components of image acquisition, data storage and documentation.

10. Provide experiential hands-on skills training for each POC US application.

Fig. 10.2 Sample curriculum for introductory clinical ultrasound (POC US) course. Adapted from: [9, 10]; Pustavoitau A, Blaivas M, Brown SM, et al. From the Ultrasound Certification Task Force on behalf of the Society of Critical Care Medicine [11]

A more synergistic approach is to integrate the POC US curriculum into the overall APP or nurse training program. In this model, a POC US application (e.g., biliary ultrasound) can be inserted into a related anatomy or pathology portion of the medical curriculum. The benefit of formulating a comprehensive and integrated approach is that adding POC US can facilitate and enhance medical learning, while also developing a valuable clinical skill. There are several examples of medical schools that have successfully integrated just such a curriculum into their medical training program [13–15].

Practice-Based Pathway

This practice-based pathway is ideal for POC US users who are already in clinical practice. In this pathway, the learner should complete an introductory or refresher course, depending on prior POC US exposure, followed by an experiential hands-on component. The learner's knowledge and skill should be assessed through review of POC US studies performed or through a "cumulative log comparing training ultrasound examinations to other imaging tests, surgical findings, or patient outcome(s)" [10]. Protected time in the schedule to practice POC US examinations is ideal to ensure procedural competency, but this is not always feasible.

There are several reasonable avenues for obtaining introductory POC US content. Listed below, from most basic to advanced, they are:

(a) *Asynchronous*. There are numerous traditional textbooks, electronic textbooks, and online learning modules and programs that can provide a basic foundation for learning POC US [16–18]. This approach is not recommended without a defined experiential hands-on component, since POC US requires the development of cognitive *and* psychomotor skills not available otherwise. There are some commercially available educational ultrasound simulation systems ([19–22]), which may provide some component of psychomotor development, however, their efficacy as a stand-alone curriculum has not been widely validated.

(b) *Course-based*. This educational format is a concise option for acquiring introductory POC US content and hands-on skills training in a discrete period of time. There are many commercially organized POC US courses scheduled throughout the country, as well as courses affiliated with professional organizations' conferences and meetings. Depending on the skill level and content desired, these courses typically consist of didactics and small-group hands-on sessions held over several hours to days.

(c) *Preceptorship*. This model consists of a POC US expert providing direct mentoring and/or supervision in a clinical environment (e.g., radiology department, emergency department, surgical setting). This approach may be limited by preceptor expertise, time, and volume of pathology. In addition, if a preceptor does not establish a formalized curriculum, it is recommended that a supplemental asynchronous platform is utilized to provide structured didactics that covers core POC US content.

(d) *Residencies and Fellowships*. In addition to primary schooling, there is an increasing interest in residencies and fellowships for the APP. Many APP residencies, such as emergency medicine and critical care programs, have integrated POC US into their training curriculum to facilitate the development of this valuable skill [23, 24].

For APPs interested in the most comprehensive approach to acquiring and mastering POC US skills, and potentially establishing and administering a POC US training program, there are at least six physician POC US fellowships that offer training to nonphysicians [8, 25]. Alternatively, there are online/distance-learning fellowships, which may provide an alternative platform for developing this expertise [26].

Experiential Component

POC US requires a combination of cognitive *and* psychomotor skills. Therefore, it is essential that regardless of the educational pathway an experiential component is included in POC US training. At a minimum, a clinician proficient in the desired application(s) should supervise or review the quality of the POC US exams being performed. This may be not be possible in all clinical settings and alternative arrangements should be considered—such as a "cumulative log comparing training POC US exams to other imaging tests, surgical findings, or patient outcome" [10]. The primary goal is providing enough repetition, preferably with direct feedback, to develop an overall proficiency or minimum competency when performing a POC US.

The ideal number of POC US exams to obtain a minimum competency is unclear, and published guidelines vary by specialty organization (see Table 10.1). A reasonable number of examinations performed per application appears to be 25–100, depending on the complexity of the study [10, 29, 30].

Table 10.1 Comparison of minimum number of recommended ultrasound exams for competency by specialty organization

Organization	Per application	Overall	Notes
American College of Emergency Physicians[a]	25–50	150–300	
American Registry for Diagnostic Medical Sonography[b]		Up to 800	Requirements vary based on ARDMS certification.
American Society of Echocardiography[c]		240–480	Varies based on duration of training.
International Expert Statement on Critical Care Ultrasonography/Echocardiography[d]	30–100	150	No firmly defined standards.

[a] American College of Emergency Physicians [10]
[b]ARDMS [27]
[c]Ehler et al. [28]
[d]Expert Round Table on Ultrasound in ICU [29]; Expert Round Table on Echocardiography in ICU [30]

Credentialing

Credentialing is the process of gathering and verifying clinician qualifications to establish a scope of practice for a particular clinical environment. These are typically determined by individual facilities or healthcare systems and can be influenced by state and federal regulations, specialty-specific training guidelines, and certifications (Chap. 20). For APPs and nurses, there are few detailed guidelines available regarding the credentialing or certification in POC US.

In the rare instance that specialty-specific guidelines or certifications are available, it is recommended that credentialing bodies utilize these as a framework for defining a scope of privileges. However, guidelines and certifications, or the lack thereof, should not be the sole determinant of delineating POC US privileges for APPs. POC US is a rapidly expanding area of medicine and novel applications will likely outpace the publication of specific guidelines; therefore, POC US guidelines from other medical specialties may be used as a foundation for credentialing depending on the practice setting. These may include the American College of Emergency Physicians Ultrasound Guidelines [31]; Midwives' Performance of Ultrasound in Clinical Practice Position Statement [5]; and the Society of Critical Care Recommendations for Achieving and Maintaining Competence and Credentialing in Critical Care Ultrasound with Focused Cardiac Ultrasound and Advanced Critical Care Echocardiography [11].

Supervision

Supervision of APPs and nurses performing POC US will vary based on the clinical environment, specialty-specific guidelines [32], as well as dictated by state and federal regulations [33, 34]. Although state regulations vary widely regarding supervision of APPs and nurses, most can be categorized as either allowing licensing as an independent practitioner or as a non-independent practitioner (i.e., requires some form of supervisory oversight). In both instances, it is highly recommend that medical practices and healthcare entities develop and adhere to well-defined policies for POC US oversight. This will help define the scope of practice for APPs working in environments with other clinicians, facilitate collaboration with other healthcare team members, and potentially reduce vicarious liability.

Independently Practicing APPs

Supervision of POC US should be specifically tailored to the level of clinician and their work environment. For APPs in a group practice or larger healthcare entity, the level of supervision should be based on the local scope of practice, which is defined by the credentialing process and the medical or facility director. A designated supervisor should be any clinician appropriately trained in POC US, which may sometimes include APPs or nurses as permitted by state and federal regulations.

Non-independently Practicing APPs

Models for supervision will vary based on the needs and capabilities of the APP's or nurse's practice setting. There are many factors to consider when defining the type and details of a supervision policy (see Figs. 10.3 and 10.4). Additional considerations may include geography, availability of supervisors, patient population, practice setting type, and training and experience level of the APP or nurse.

1. Are there state or federal regulatory requirements? Billing and reimbursement requirements?

2. How will the supervisor be designated (e.g., by case, shift, location, etc.)?

3. What is the maximum numbers of APPs that can be supervised at a time?

4. What form of supervision is desired?

5. Are review and feedback of POC US exams required? What proportion? What timeframe? How is it documented?

6. Are there specific scenarios or cases that require more or less supervision (e.g., complex cases; abnormal findings; life-threatening emergencies, etc)?

7. Is there a process for resolving diagnostic discrepancies (e.g., obtain a radiology-performed comprehensive ultrasound)?

Fig. 10.3 Factors to consider when supervising non-independently practicing APPs performing POC US

1. Direct - the supervisor is physically present during POC US exam
2. Indirect with direct supervision immediately available - the supervisor is physically in the same facility or practice location, and immediately available for direct supervision
3. Indirect with direct supervision available - the supervisor may not be in the same facility or practice location, and is available telephonically or electronically
4. Oversight - the supervisor provides a review of POC US exams after it is performed

Fig. 10.4 Types of supervision. Adapted from: Accreditation Council for Graduate Medical Education [35]

When supervision is not possible (e.g., due to geography, lack of adequate training, lack of experience), we recommend establishing a POC US quality assurance system (QA) or process. Some examples of QA processes may include:

1. Peer review and feedback for a proportion of POC US examinations performed.
2. Comparison of POC US examinations to other imaging studies, surgical pathology, and/or patient outcomes.
3. Establishing an agreement or affiliation with an outside POC US program to review a proportion of POC US examinations.

Documentation and Reimbursement

POC US is complementary to the physical examination but should be considered a separate and discrete diagnostic procedure in the evaluation and management of a patient. Appropriate documentation is an important component of providing quality patient care, conveying key information to other members of a healthcare team, and for optimizing healthcare reimbursement. Documentation and reimbursement of POC US exams performed by APPs should be similar to studies performed by physicians. The specific requirements for reimbursement will depend upon the applicable payor (e.g., private insurer, Medicare) (Chap. 22). At a minimum, the following elements should be included when documenting a POC US exam:

1. An indication of medical necessity documented in a patient's medical record.
2. A description of the views obtained, and the organs or structures studied.
3. An interpretation of the findings of the study.
4. Archiving of relevant images should be stored as part of the medical record.

Pitfalls and Controversies

The scope of practice of APPs and nurses varies greatly across the United States, which reflects the broad difference of opinions on the role of APPs and nurses in the U.S. healthcare system. Similarly, POC US utilization by APPs and nurses is likely to result in some areas of controversy and potential pitfalls regarding its use in clinical settings. Below are a few issues and recommended solutions.

- *Failure to provide an adequate experiential component to POC US education.* Proficiency with POC US is directly proportional to the number of exams performed. Developing and adhering to a standardized number of supervised or reviewed POC US exams per modality will help ensure a minimum competency is obtained.
- *Failure to clearly define the scope of practice for APPs and nurses.* Despite its rapid growth in medicine, the integration of POC US across medical specialties is unevenly distributed. On occasion, this has led to the situation where an APP or nurse may be the only clinician trained in POC US. Therefore, it is important to delineate the POC US scope of practice for non-independently practicing APPs to establish the POC US applications that are permitted in a particular clinical setting.
- *Failure to establish a clear supervision policy.* A POC US supervision policy should outline a process for when a more senior clinician does not agree with the utilization or interpretation of a POC US examination. Without establishing an explicit POC US policy or guideline for APPs and nurses, a provider or healthcare entity may have increased exposure to vicarious liability associated with POC US exams.
- *Failure to document POC US exams.* Appropriate documentation of POC US will ensure continuity of care among healthcare providers, permit quality assurance review, and enable reimbursement for professional services rendered.

Key Recommendations

- Establish a structured training pathway for POC US based on the educational status and anticipated practice environment of the POC US learner.
- All POC US training should include a didactic component, experiential component, competency or proficiency assessment, an ongoing quality assurance system, and continuing medical education requirements.
- Credentialing and certification in POC US should be based upon state and federal regulations and specialty-specific guidelines or policies, if available. However, the lack of these elements should not be the sole basis for restricting the privileging of POC US for APPs and nurses.
- Supervision policies for POC US should be established in writing and tailored to local circumstances.
- Appropriate documentation should be a key component of all POC US exams.

References

1. Blaivas M, Lyon M. The effect of ultrasound guidance on the perceived difficulty of emergency nurse-obtained peripheral IV access. J Emerg Med. 2006;31(4):407–10.

2. Gunneson TJ, et al. Ultrasound-assisted percutaneous liver biopsy performed by a physician assistant. Am J Gastroenterol. 2002;97(6):1472–5.
3. Roppolo LP, et al. Can midlevel providers perform ultrasonography on superficial abscesses? Ann Emerg Med. 2004;44(4):S83–4.
4. Daymude ML, Sumeru M, Gruppo L. Use of emergency bedside ultrasound by emergency medicine physician assistants: a new training concept. J Physician Assist Educ. 2007;18(1):29–33.
5. American College of Nurse-Midwives. Midwives' performance of ultrasound in clinical practice. 2012. http://www.midwife.org/ACNM/files/ACNMLibraryData/UPLOADFILENAME/000000000228/Ultrasound-Position-Statement-June-2012.pdf. [Accessed June 23, 2016].
6. Shaw-Battista J. et al. Interprofessional Obstetric Ultrasound Education: Successful Development of Online Learning Modules; Case-Based Seminars; and Skills Labs for Registered and Advanced Practice Nurses, Midwives, Physicians, and Trainees. J Midwifery & Women's Health. 2015;60(6):727–34.
7. Bellamkonda VR. et al. Ultrasound credentialing in North American emergency department systems with ultrasound fellowships: a cross-sectional survey. Emerg Med J. 2015;32:804–8.
8. American College of Emergency Physicians, American College of Emergency Physicians Ultrasound Section. American College of Emergency Physicians. https://www.acep.org/Membership-top-banner/Education-and-Training-2147459189/. Accessed 1 July 2016.
9. American College of Nurse-Midwives. ACNM Ultrasound Education Task Force. ACNM. 2013. http://www.midwife.org/ACNM-Ultrasound-Education-Task-Force. Accessed 24 June 2016.
10. American College of Emergency Physicians. Emergency ultrasound guidelines. Ann Emerg Med. 2009;53(4):550–70.
11. Pustavoitau A, Blaivas M, Brown SM, et al. From the ultrasound certification task force on behalf of the society of critical care medicine. Recommendations for achieving and maintaining competence and credentialing in critical care ultrasound with focused cardiac ultrasound and advanced critical care echocardiography. 2013. http://journals.lww.com/ccmjournal/Documents/Critical%20Care%20Ultrasound.pdf. Accessed 26 June 2016.
12. American College of Emergency Physicians. Emergency Ultrasound Standard Reporting Guidelines. 2011. https://www.acep.org/workarea/DownloadAsset.aspx?id=104378. Accessed 1 July 2016.
13. Chiem AT, et al. Integration of ultrasound in Undergraduate Medical Education at the California Medical Schools: a discussion of common challenges and strategies from the UMeCali experience. J Ultrasound Med. 2016;35(2):221–33.
14. Fox JC, et al. Proactive medicine: the "UCI 30," an ultrasound-based clinical initiative from the University of California, Irvine. Acad Med. 2014;89(7):984–9.
15. Hoppmann RA, et al. An integrated ultrasound curriculum (iUSC) for medical students: 4-year experience. Crit Ultrasound J. 2011;3(1):1–12.
16. EMSono, Online Emergency Medicine Ultrasound Education by Emsono. http://www.emsono.com/. Accessed 26 June 2016.
17. Mallin M, Dawson M. (2013) Introduction to bedside ultrasound. Volume 1 & 2. Ultrasound Podcast. http://www.ultrasoundpodcast.com/portfolio-item/ebooks/. Accessed 26 June 2016.
18. Noble VE, Nelson BP. Manual of emergency and critical care ultrasound. New York: Cambridge University Press; 2011.
19. CAE Healthcare. CAE Healthcare—Product & Services: Vimedix. http://www.caehealthcare.com/ultrasound-simulators/vimedix. Accessed 26 June 2016.
20. MedSim, MedSim I Advanced Ultrasound Simulation. http://www.medsim.com/. Accessed 26 June 2016.
21. SonoSim, SonoSim—Ultrasound Training Solution. SonoSim—The easiest way to learn ultrasonography®. http://sonosim.com/. Accessed 26 June 2016.

22. Simulab Corporation. SonoMan Diagnostic Ultrasound Simulator | Simulab Corporation. https://www.simulab.com/products/sonoman-diagnostic-ultrasound-simulator. Accessed 26 June 2016.
23. American Academy of Emergency Nurse Practitioners, American Academy of Emergency Nurse Practitioners—Fellowship Programs. http://aaenp-natl.org/content.php?page=Fellowship_Programs. Accessed 26 June 2016.
24. Society for Emergency Medicine Physician Assistants, SEMPA. https://www.sempa.org/Default.aspx. Accessed 26 June 2016.
25. Emergency Ultrasound Fellowships. Emergency Ultrasound Fellowship. http://www.eusfellowships.com/index.php. Accessed 1 July 2016.
26. Ultrasound Leadership Academy, Ultrasound Leadership Academy. Ultrasound Leadership Academy. http://www.ultrasoundleadershipacademy.com/. Accessed 26 June 2016.
27. ARDMS. Spi requirement and general prerequisites. 2014. http://www.ardms.org/Prerequisite%20Charts/generalprerequisites_-_2014-2.pdf. Accessed 26 June 2016.
28. Ehler D, et al. Guidelines for cardiac sonographer education: recommendations of the American Society of Echocardiography Sonographer Training and Education Committee. J Am Soc Echocardiogr. 2001;14(1):77–84.
29. Expert Round Table on Ultrasound in ICU. International expert statement on training standards for critical care ultrasonography. Intensive Care Med. 2011;37(7):1077–83.
30. Expert Round Table on Echocardiography in ICU. International consensus statement on training standards for advanced critical care echocardiography. Intensive Care Med. 2014;40(5):654–66.
31. Ultrasound guidelines: emergency, point-of-care and clinical ultrasound guidelines in medicine. Ann Emerg Med. 2017;69(5):e27–54.
32. American Academy of Physician Assistants. Guidelines for State Regulation of Physician Assistants. 2011. https://www.aapa.org/Workarea/DownloadAsset.aspx?id=795. Accessed 27 June 2016.
33. American Association of Nurse Practitioners, AANP—State Practice Environment. https://www.aanp.org/legislation-regulation/state-legislation/state-practice-environment. Accessed 27 June 2016.
34. Department of Health and Human Services—Centers for Medicare & Medicaid Services. Medicare Information for Advanced Practice Registered Nurses, Anesthesiologist Assistants, and Physician Assistants. 2015. https://www.cms.gov/Outreach-and-Education/Medicare-Learning-Network-MLN/MLNProducts/Downloads/Medicare-Information-for-APRNs-AAs-PAs-Booklet-ICN-901623.pdf. Accessed 27 June 2016.
35. Accreditation Council for Graduate Medical Education. ACGME Common Program Requirements. 2011. https://www.acgme.org/Portals/0/PDFs/Common_Program_Requirements_07012011[2].pdf. Accessed 28 June 2016.

Chapter 11
Simulation Medicine

Bret P. Nelson and Dan Katz

Objectives

- Discuss the role of simulation in ultrasound training, competency assessment
- Describe use of models for simulation to facilitate deliberate practice
- Highlight major types of simulators currently available

Introduction

Like many critical skills in emergency medicine, point-of-care ultrasound is a combination of cognitive and psychomotor skills. Once an ideal image is acquired and interpreted, the information needs to be correctly applied to patient care. Although traditional didactic lectures, readings, videos, and other sources of knowledge transfer have long been used to improve cognitive knowledge, psychomotor skill training requires different techniques. A challenge faced by medical educators is the inherent inefficiency of procedural training, which generally mandates significant resources including qualified instructors, standardized educational objectives, ultrasound equipment, and unpredictable access to patient pathology in a clinical setting. Ultrasound image acquisition and interpretation is operator-dependent and it is critical to allow learners to build knowledge and confidence in a safe

B.P. Nelson, MD, FACEP (✉)
Emergency Ultrasound Division, Department of Emergency Medicine,
Mount Sinai Hospital, New York, NY, USA
e-mail: bret.nelson@mountsinai.org

D. Katz, MD, FACEP
Department of Emergency Medicine, Cedars-Sinai Medical Center,
Los Angeles, CA, USA

© Springer International Publishing AG 2018
V. S. Tayal et al. (eds.), *Ultrasound Program Management*,
https://doi.org/10.1007/978-3-319-63143-1_11

environment. Ideally, this learning environment should mimic the clinical environment to the greatest extent possible. It may take learners months to years before they are able to scan a sufficient number of patients to develop competence, especially in recognizing rarely encountered pathology. Thus, over the past decade simulation in medical education has grown to become a standard component of undergraduate and graduate medical curricula [1–3]. A variety of medical simulators are available and relevant to point-of-care ultrasound training. The purpose of this chapter is to review the rationale and evidence for the use of medical simulation in ultrasound training, discuss the types of simulators available, and outline best practices for their use.

Training and Deliberate Practice

A typical ultrasound curriculum includes both didactic and hands-on instruction. Didactic training presents instruction on the principles of ultrasonography, an introduction to ultrasound mechanics or knobology, and a discussion of the purpose, method, and interpretation of the ultrasound examination. The hands-on training component is the practical application of instruction and also the most constrained due to limitations of practicing with model patients [4, 5]. In general, ultrasound training should develop trainees' speed of image acquisition, target structure (image window) acquisition, and diagnostic interpretation. The outcomes of training should be linked to a performance review and improvement process.

The American College of Emergency Physicians Emergency Ultrasound Guidelines list simulation among the range of tools to be considered for training and assessment of ultrasound skill [6]. These guidelines are echoed by an international expert statement on training standards for critical care ultrasound, and the recommendations of the American Thoracic Society Education Committee [7, 8]. One end goal of medical education is mastery of clinical skill, and deliberate practice is often employed as the primary technique in attaining mastery. Deliberate practice requires intense repetition of a skill, rigorous assessment of performance, specific informative feedback, and improved performance in a controlled setting [9, 10]. Simulation facilitates deliberate practice by allowing educators to consistently reproduce learning conditions for students, in a safe environment.

A conceptual framework for evaluating clinical simulation used for learning procedure skills was described by Kneebone, who proposed four key areas critical to simulation-based learning [11]:

1. Simulations should allow for sustained, deliberate practice within a safe environment, ensuring that recently acquired skills are consolidated within a defined curriculum that assures regular reinforcement.
2. Simulations should provide access to expert tutors, ensuring that such support fades when it is no longer needed.

Table 11.1 Characteristics of high-fidelity medical simulations that lead to effective learning

1. Mechanism for repetitive practice
2. Ability to integrate into a curriculum
3. Ability to alter the degree of difficulty
4. Ability to capture clinical variation
5. Ability to practice in a controlled environment
6. Individualized, active learning
7. Adaptability to multiple learning strategies
8. Existence of tangible/measurable outcomes
9. Use of intra-experience feedback
10. Validity of simulation as an approximation of clinical practice

Adapted from Okuda et al. [2, 3], Issenberg et al. [12] and McGaghie et al. [13]

3. Simulations should map onto real-life clinical experience, ensuring that learning supports the experience gained within communities of actual practice.
4. Simulation-based learning environments should provide a supportive, motivational, and learner-centered milieu that is conducive to learning.

When considering which types of simulators to employ, and which components of the curriculum they should augment or replace, it is helpful to consider which simulator features best facilitate learning. These features, described by Issenberg et al. and McGaghie et al., are summarized in Table 11.1, [12, 13] and can serve as a starting point in assessing any particular tool or curricular model.

Efficacy of Simulation

Studies assessing point-of-care ultrasound training frequently utilize simulation in one form or another. Ultrasound training courses across a variety of medical specialties provide hands-on training using live patient models and instructors to facilitate real-time feedback. Though sometimes overlooked, standardized patients can be categorized as simulation tools. ACEP recommends simulation to augment real-time patient-based learning for residency and post-residency training in ultrasound, as do critical care societies [6, 7]. A study using an ultrasound simulator demonstrated improved test performance and hands-on skills with human models compared to traditional didactics [14]. Even after both groups were trained on human models, the benefits to the simulator group persisted.

Multi-organ system assessments are commonly employed in emergency and critical care environments, and numerous studies have demonstrated the utility of simulation-based training. Surgical residents randomized to simulation versus hands-on patient formats showed improved test scores and image interpretation in the Focused Assessment with Sonography for Trauma (FAST); both teaching modalities showed similar efficacy [15]. Similar results were found in a study of fourth-year medical students learning the FAST exam [16]. No difference in image acquisition, interpretation, or confidence was found between students using the multimedia simulator or normal human models. A study of mixed-provider disaster response teams comprised of nurses, physicians, and paramedic/EMTs suggested that a portable ultrasound simulator may provide equivalent skills training in comparison to traditional live instructor and model training [17]. A high-fidelity simulation curriculum on the Abdominal and Cardiothoracic Evaluation by Sonography (ACES) protocol created a high degree of competency in image acquisition and interpretation among clerks and residents as well [18].

Endovaginal ultrasound education can be enhanced using simulation, and this in one area where the expense and logistics of obtaining live models for skill practice can be particularly challenging. A combination of high-fidelity simulation and a task trainer improved self-reported learner educational experience and faculty found the addition of the ultrasound task trainer was better for evaluating residents' skills in interpreting endovaginal ultrasound images [19]. Another study demonstrated Radiology residents' ability to perform adequate transvaginal examinations improved with high-fidelity simulation, as did their confidence in performing these studies [20].

Transesophageal echocardiography is an emerging application for both critical care and emergency medicine point of care ultrasound. A single-center study of anesthesia residents demonstrated that simulation led to improved TEE image acquisition on anesthetized patients compared to training with traditional didactics [21]. Another study of a curriculum for emergency physicians incorporating high-fidelity TEE simulation used a 4-h didactic and hands-on training session. Fourteen learners were assessed at course completion and again 6 weeks after the course. Good competency and retention were demonstrated; all learners assessed were able to demonstrate adequate midesophageal 4-chamber views at both time intervals. Adequate views for the remaining windows ranged from 71.4 to 78.6% upon course completion and 91.7–100% at 6 weeks [22]. A study of anesthesia residents and faculty found that a high-fidelity simulator was not inferior to the use of human models when competency was assessed using written and practical examinations [23].

Many studies have attempted to assess the utility of simulation in training and assessment of venous catheter placement. Study designs vary widely, and generally the simulation training itself rather than the ultrasound component specifically was the tool being assessed. In one metanalysis of 20 studies on simulation in central venous catheter placement, improvement in operator performance on simulators, knowledge and confidence were improved after training, as did patient outcomes such as fewer needle passes and decreased rate of pneumothorax [24, 25].

Simulation training for ultrasound-guided thoracentesis has been demonstrated to reduce the rate of pneumothorax from 8.6 to 1.1% [26]. A validated tool to assess thoracic ultrasound training on simulators, Ultrasound-Guided Thoracentesis Skills and Tasks Assessment Test (UGSTAT) has been described [27]. This tool could potentially be used to assess ongoing competency as well as initial training prior to clinical practice.

Simulator Considerations

A general consensus is emerging on the broad set of knowledge, skills, and abilities comprising competent sonography. For example, Tolsgaard et al. [28] identified seven ultrasound competencies agreed to by an international sample of experts from specialties that use sonography: (a) indication for the examination, (b) applied knowledge of ultrasound equipment, (c) image optimization, (d) systematic examination, (e) interpretation of images, (f) documentation of examination, and (g) medical decision-making. Skilled sonography is based on a complex interaction between gross and fine probe manipulation in light of the sonographer's knowledge of patient anatomy, optimal views, diagnostic interpretation, disease states, artifacts, machine settings, and individual differences.

As noted, simulations seek to approximate reality, requiring students to react to problems or conditions faced in actual real-life patient care. A wide variety of simulation types exist, and most can be categorized into one of the following [1]:

- Standardized patients
- Partial-task trainers
- Mannequins (specifically, high-fidelity patient simulators)
- Screen-based computer simulators
- Virtual-reality simulators

Simulators can also be classified as high-fidelity or low-fidelity, based on how closely they replicate actual scanning in terms of real-time image display, image quality, and haptic feedback [29]. There are inherent advantages and disadvantages to each simulator, and the decision regarding which type(s) to incorporate into a holistic curriculum or assessment tool must take into account many factors.

Wider adoption of point-of-care ultrasound has been hindered by the high opportunity cost of training users using traditional live instructor and model training. Although not conceptually a primary consideration, cost is an important factor when deciding what type of simulator to integrate into a teaching session or curriculum, and must be weighed against the cost of traditional live instructor and model training.

Volunteer models by definition are free, though there are often opportunity costs to finding willing models, and addressing secondary gains such as the desire to be taught, pressure to please course instructors, and obtaining a free medical ultrasound scan. These are important factors that can result in unforeseen costs in real money, instructor time, favors used, and risk management. At times, simulator operation may require skilled technicians who understand the mechanical aspects of the product, and a fee may be assessed by the simulation center that employs these technicians upon the learners. Clinical faculty are often relied upon to facilitate simulation sessions and ensure learning objectives are achieved. Unfortunately, academic time is infrequently valued as a commodity, and clinicians are asked to volunteer their time at the expense of other academic or clinical responsibilities. This, too, is an opportunity cost that must be taken into consideration.

On the low end of the cost scale are "homemade" task trainers such as soft tissue phantoms made from gelatin, candle wax, tofu, or meats. Paid models, often used to teach pelvic or testicular examinations, can be inexpensive or quite costly, depending on whether a formal hiring service is used, if they are being employed to demonstrate known stable pathology, or other factors. Commercially purchased task trainers and scanning phantoms are more expensive, but offer the benefit of multiple uses and decreased logistical overhead compared to those manufactured for a specific course. High-fidelity simulators are generally at the upper end of the cost scale, ranging from several hundred dollars to over one hundred thousand dollars. A wide array of benefits is offered with such products, including expansive case banks with real or simulated pathology, real-time feedback on probe placement or image acquisition, built-in tutorials, course management software to track learner progress, and a host of other features depending on the model selected.

Finances aside, perhaps the most important consideration when selecting a simulation tool is the curricular goal. Simulation can augment didactics and allow for asynchronous learning of core content. Some medical schools have described peer-to-peer ultrasound instruction programs that decrease faculty involvement for each learner [30–32]. Simulators with built-in tracking and learning content management systems can act as immersive interactive textbooks of anatomy, physiology, pathology, and technique. These systems allow learners to access didactic content and explore hands-on training cases in a self-directed fashion. Simulators can also facilitate hands-on learning as part of a larger course curriculum. Used in conjunction with standardized patients and high-fidelity mannequins, or in a stand-alone fashion, simulators can augment the pathology offered in nonclinical learning environments. Within a simulated environment (e.g., trauma or critical care scenario), simulators can portray vital ultrasound pathology and allow for controlled practice in a safe environment, with immediate feedback on performance and medical decision-making. Given the steep skill decay curves for sonography, simulation can be used in a spaced-learning model for independent refresher training that follows group sessions.

Simulation can be used to evaluate the effectiveness of a curriculum, and for competency assessments at various time intervals of a training course, as continued performance improvement, or as remediation for clinicians demonstrating a proficiency gap. Current student competency assessment is hindered by a variety of logistical constraints, such as lack of access to standardized patient pathology, ill-defined competency metrics, and the time and resources required to assess a multitude of variables defining competency. While commercial virtual training systems for ultrasound provide can provide effective training, there is a growing demand to further develop the capability to rapidly and efficiently assess ultrasound competency across large number of users. In 2010, Frank et al. reported that "adopting competency-based medical education on a larger scale would require new teaching techniques, new modules, and new assessment tools to be practical and effective" [33]. This was reinforced by the recent IOM report, which restated the need for new educational technologies to support performance-based teaching initiatives (IOM). Diligently designed and executed academic and private industry partnerships that leverage the guidance and expertise of medical educators and the private sector's ability to deliver scalable performance-based training solutions will be required to implement large-scale, robust performance-based medical education solutions that are responsive to stakeholder needs.

Commercially Available Simulators

In the context of the previously outlined simulator classification, some key questions surrounding educational objectives should be asked prior to making a decision on which type of simulator to include in a training session:

1. Does the simulator reliably replicate the hand movements required to acquire an image in real-time?
2. Does the displayed image reflect a real or simulated ultrasound image?
3. Does the simulator offer a broad range of ultrasound applications (e.g., cardiac, obstetric, musculoskeletal, e-FAST) and pathology?
4. Can the simulator be used for ultrasound-guided procedural skills training?
5. Can the simulator be used as part of a more comprehensive simulated patient care scenario?
6. Can learners operate the simulator independently prior to or following a course for the purpose of asynchronous learning or refresher training?
7. Can the simulator be used to help with medical decision-making training?
8. Can the simulator track student progress and provide metrics and feedback?

With these questions in mind, it is helpful to consider ultrasound simulators currently available in terms of the previously discussed categories of simulators.

Partial-Task Trainers: Phantoms

Hands-on training models are purpose-built for a single procedural task, such as central venous access, nerve blocks, thoracentesis, and lumbar puncture. Used in conjunction with any real ultrasound machine, these phantoms render simulated ultrasound images. Because this group of products is often punctured with needles, they are generally made from sturdy materials that necessitate some trade-offs in image realism in comparison to real human tissue. Many low-cost, homemade alternatives to these task trainers have been described, and may be worth considering if cost is an issue or when many simultaneous simulators are required for an educational activity [34–40] (Figs. 11.1, 11.2, and 11.3).

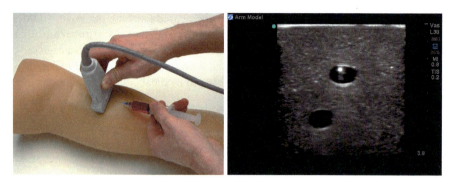

Fig. 11.1 Blue Phantom (CAE Healthcare, Quebec, Canada) vascular access simulators use real ultrasound equipment for real-time dynamic scanning through simulated patient anatomy

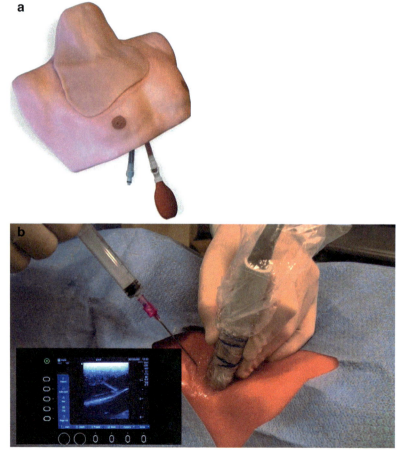

Fig. 11.2 (**a**, **b**) Simulab (Seattle, WA) vascular access simulators use real ultrasound equipment for real-time dynamic scanning through simulated patient anatomy

Fig. 11.3 Limbs & Things
(Savannah, GA) vascular
access simulators use real
ultrasound equipment for
real-time dynamic
scanning through
simulated patient anatomy

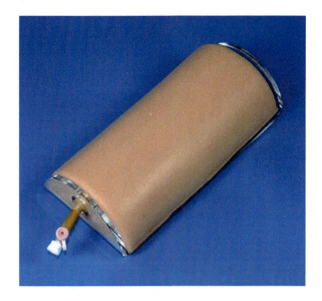

Anatomic Simulator: Live Model

Simulation-based training utilizing live models has been the standard for ultrasound training courses. Standardized patients (SPs) can be utilized to evaluate a
learners' global understanding of ultrasonography, examining their ability to
interpret and image and apply it to medical decision-making in the context of a
clinical scenario. They can also be used to evaluate a learner's interaction with a
patient, including attentiveness to patient comfort (e.g., amount of pressure used
with probe manipulation). Volunteers can be sought among medical students, residents, or learners who take turns scanning each other. With the exception of incidental findings or patients with previously identified abnormalities, the use of SPs
has been somewhat limited by their ability to depict pathology. Recently, however, radiofrequency communications technologies have been used to overcome
this barrier. Using a motion-sensing probe connected to an ultrasound graphic
user interface and anatomically labeled radiofrequency markers, simulated pathology can be projected into a healthy patient for a variety of applications, and
scanned in real-time (Figs. 11.4 and 11.5).

Anatomic Simulator: Phantom

Similar to the partial-task training phantoms described above, this group includes
durable hands-on training models for a variety of applications, including thorax,
abdomen, pelvis, and soft tissue. Once again, used in conjunction with any real

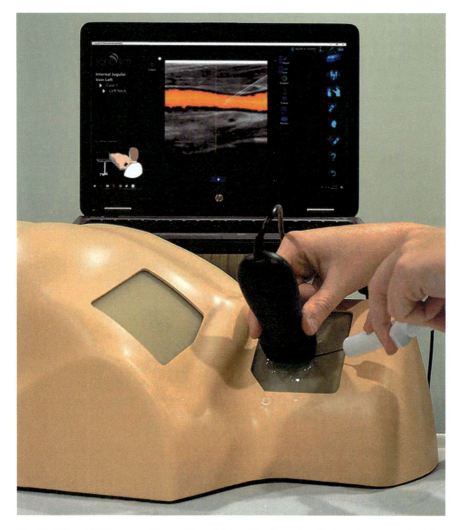

Fig. 11.4 Laerdal (Stavenger, Norway) Laerdal-SonoSim Procedure Trainer - first release includes a vascular access simulator using real patient anatomy that features color, power, and spectral Doppler tracings, automated real-time performance assessment, and virtual instruction. Anatomic Simulator: Live Model

ultrasound machine, these phantoms render simulated ultrasound images with variable realism in image quality compared to real human tissue. In addition, these models are static, limiting assessment of cardiac activity, lung movement, fetal heart tones, and other dynamic images (Figs. 11.6 and 11.7).

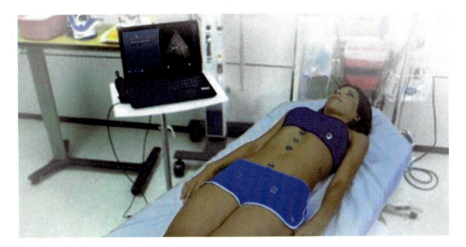

Fig. 11.5 The SonoSim® LiveScan (SonoSim, Santa Monica, CA) anatomic simulator uses simulated ultrasound equipment, real and simulated patient anatomy, and real-time dynamic scanning through the imaging data set which is localized to the proper anatomic location using ID tags placed on the model

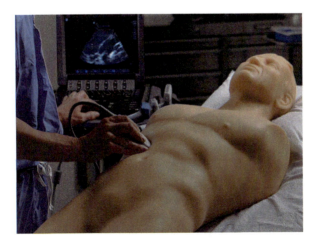

Fig. 11.6 Blue Phantom anatomic simulators use real ultrasound equipment for real-time dynamic scanning through simulated patient anatomy

Fig. 11.7 Kyoto Kagaku
(Kyoto, Japan) anatomic
simulators use real
ultrasound equipment for
real-time dynamic
scanning through
simulated patient anatomy

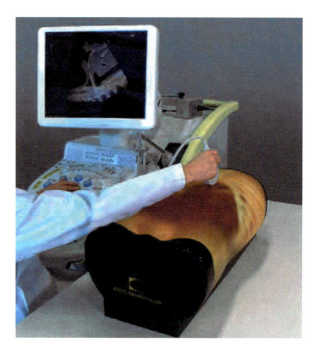

Anatomic Simulator: Computer-Based

Multiple computer-based ultrasound simulators are available with variable degrees
of image and scanning fidelity. Some simulators display looped videos or static
images when a simulated probe makes contact with a scanning surface (Fig. 11.8).
The opposite side of this spectrum includes simulators that offer ultrasound images
that can be manipulated in real-time through the movement of a hand-held probe.
An important distinction in computer-based ultrasound simulators surrounds the
ultrasound image itself. Some render computer graphic images (Figs. 11.9 and
11.10) while others use images and video from actual patient scans (Figs. 11.11,
11.12, and 11.13). Although the use of computer graphic imagery renders visually
appealing images, this method often omits fundamental image artifacts and pathologic findings critical to interpreting an ultrasound image. Breadth of content and
access to pathology are important considerations, as some simulators focus on core
applications such as thoracic, abdominal, and pelvic ultrasound, while others
include wider applications of point of care ultrasound such as ocular, soft tissue, or
musculoskeletal imaging. A host of other features is available among computer-
based simulators, including interfaces that display the trajectory of the beam as it
penetrates the underlying anatomy, on-screen probe positioning guidance, advanced
imaging modes such as Doppler, "reel feel" haptic feedback, side-by-side CT/MRI
to ultrasound comparisons, metrics-based assessment, and robust tracking of performance using learning management systems.

Fig. 11.8 Simulab
anatomic simulators use
simulated ultrasound
equipment, real patient
anatomy, and static,
landmark-based scanning
through the imaging
data set

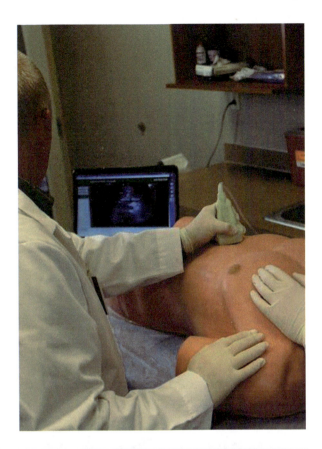

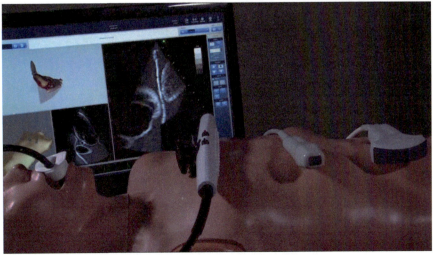

Fig. 11.9 The Vimedix system (CAE Healthcare) uses simulated ultrasound equipment, simulated
patient anatomy, and real-time dynamic scanning through the imaging data set

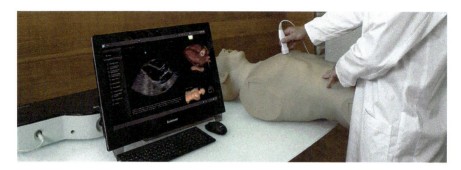

Fig. 11.10 The U/S Mentor (Simbionix, Airport City, Israel) anatomic simulator uses simulated ultrasound equipment, simulated patient anatomy, and real-time dynamic scanning through the imaging data set

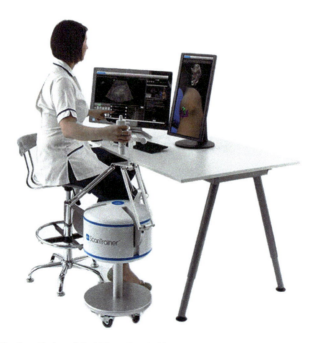

Fig. 11.11 The ScanTrainer (MedaPhor, South Glamorgan, United Kingdom) anatomic simulator uses simulated ultrasound equipment, real patient anatomy, and real-time dynamic scanning through the imaging data set with haptic feedback

Fig. 11.12 The SonoSim Ultrasound Training Solution® anatomic simulator uses simulated ultrasound equipment, real and simulated patient anatomy, and real-time dynamic scanning through the imaging data set

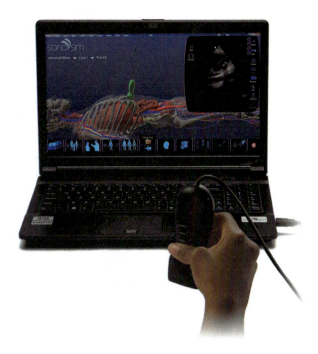

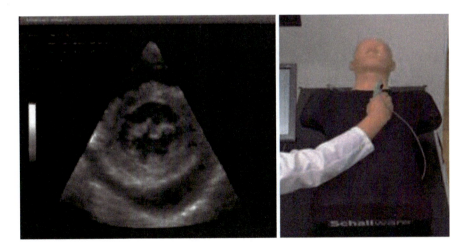

Fig. 11.13 The Schallware (Berlin, Germany) anatomic simulator uses simulated ultrasound equipment, real patient anatomy, and real-time dynamic scanning through the imaging data set

Discussion

Pressure for efficient and effective training comes from all sides—learners, educators, patients, hospital administrators, regulatory groups, and others. There is growing evidence that simulation enhances ultrasound education, but incorporating this technology remains a challenge at many levels. Funding for resources can be found through educational grants, from administrators or malpractice insurers interested in risk management solutions, or offset from revenue generated through billing for clinical ultrasound studies performed in the department. In some institutions simulation equipment is a shared interdepartmental resource, so costs are spread through multiple departments or built into institutional overhead.

Simulation is scalable in ways traditional hands-on training is not. Simulators can recreate the same clinical scenario for every learner indefinitely, allowing for large-scale consistent training. It can demonstrate a high volume of pathology in a short time compared to the unreliable flow of pathology in the clinical environment. Over time, the upfront cost of a high-fidelity simulator purchase is often less expensive than the repeated use of faculty time and hiring models, and either purchasing educational ultrasound machines or taking clinical machines out of service for education.

Thus, simulation can augment ultrasound education for every level of learner, including students, trainees, and faculty. It can provide an ongoing platform for deliberate practice, competency assessment, and remediation. And simulation can play a large role in standardizing assessment metrics which can be validated across specialties or institutions.

Pitfalls

1. Failure to connect micro-tasks back to overall skill
2. Use cases to highlight how to incorporate ultrasound into overall care plan
3. Use each simulator appropriately—some teach proprioception, some image recognition, etc.

Key Recommendations

1. Use simulation to augment cognitive and skills-based learning, creating a safe environment for deliberate practice
2. Incorporate task simulators, case-based learning, and self-direction in a multimodal educational approach
3. Collaborate with other departments for funding, expert faculty, and administrative support.

References

1. Chakravarthy B, ter Haar E, Bhat SS, et al. Simulation in medical school education: review for emergency medicine. West J Emerg Med. 2011;12(4):461–6.
2. Okuda Y, Bond W, Bonfante G, et al. National growth in simulation training within emergency medicine residency programs, 2003–2008. Acad Emerg Med. 2008;15:1113–6.
3. Okuda Y, Bryson EO, DeMaria S, et al. The utility of simulation in medical education: what is the evidence? Mt Sinai J Med. 2009;76:330–43.
4. Salen PN, Melanson SW, Heller MB. The focused abdominal sonography for trauma (FAST) examination: considerations and recommendations for training physicians in the use of a new clinical tool. Acad Emerg Med. 2000;7(2):162–8.
5. Shackford SR, Rogers FB, Osler TM, et al. Focused abdominal sonogram for trauma: the learning curve of nonradiologist clinicians in detecting hemoperitoneum. J Trauma. 1999;46(4):553–62.
6. American College of Emergency Physicians. Emergency ultrasound guidelines. Ann Emerg Med. 2009 Apr;53(4):550–70.
7. Expert round table on ultrasound in ICU. International expert statement on training standards for critical care ultrasonography. Intensive Care Med. 2011;37:1077–83.
8. McSparron JI, Michaud GC, Gordan PL, et al. Simulation for skills-based education in pulmonary and critical care medicine. Ann Am Thorac Soc. 2015;12(4):579–86.
9. Ericsson KA. Deliberate practice and the acquisition and maintenance of expert performance in medicine and related domains. Acad Med. 2004;79(suppl):S70–81.
10. Duvivier RJ, van Dalen J, Muijtjens AM, et al. The role of deliberate practice in the acquisition of clinical skills. BMC Med Educ. 2011;11:101.
11. Kneebone R. Evaluating clinical simulations for learning procedural skills: a theory-based approach. Acad Med. 2005;80:549–53.
12. Issenberg SB, McGaghie WC, Petrusa ER, et al. Features and uses of high-fidelity medical simulations that lead to effective learning: a BEME systematic review. Med Teach. 2005;27:10–28.
13. McGaghie WC, Issenberg SB, Petrusa ER, et al. Effect of practice on standardized learning outcomes in simulation-based medical education. Med Educ. 2006;40:792–7.
14. Neelankavil J, Howard-Quijano K, Hsieh TC, et al. Transthoracic echocardiography simulation is an efficient method to train anesthesiologists in basic transthoracic echocardiography skills. Anesth Analg. 2012;115:1042–51.
15. Knudson MM, Sisley AC. Training residents using simulation technology: experience with ultrasound for trauma. J Trauma. 2000;48:659–65.
16. Damewood S, Jeanmonod D, Cadigan B. Comparison of a multimedia simulator to a human model for teaching FAST exam image interpretation and image acquisition. Acad Emerg Med. 2011;18:413–9.
17. Paddock MT, Bailitz J, Howowitz R, et al. Disaster response team FAST skills training with a portable ultrasound simulator compared to traditional training: pilot study. West J Emerg Med. 2015;26(2):325–30.
18. Parks AR, Atkinson P, Verheul G, et al. Can medical learners achieve point-of-care ultrasound competency using a high-fidelity ultrasound simulator? A pilot study. Crit Ultrasound J. 2013;5:9.
19. Girzadas DV Jr, Antonis MS, Zerth H, et al. Hybrid simulation combining high fidelity scenario with a pelvic ultrasound task trainer enhances the training and evaluation of endovaginal ultrasound skills. Acad Emerg Med. 2009;16:429–35.
20. Ahmad R, Alhashmi G, Ajlan A, et al. Impact of high-fidelity transvaginal ultrasound simulation for radiology on residents' performance and satisfaction. Acad Radiol. 2015;22:234–9.

21. Ferrero NA, Bortsov AV, Arora H, et al. Simulator training enhances resident performance in transesophageal echocardiography. Anesthesiology. 2014;120:149–59.
22. Arntfield R, Pace J, McLeod S, et al. Focused transesophageal echocardiography for emergency physicians-description and results from simulation training of a structured four-view examination. Crit Ultrasound J. 2015;7(1):27.
23. Edrich T, Seethala RR, Olenchock BA, et al. Providing initial transthoracic echocardiography training for anesthesiologists: simulator training is not inferior to live training. J Cardiothorac Vasc Anesth. 2014;28:49–53.
24. Ma IW, Brindle ME, Ronksley PE, et al. Use of simulation-based education to improve outcomes of central venous catheterization: a systematic review and meta-analysis. Acad Med. 2011;86(9):1137–47.
25. Ma IW, Sharma N, Brindle ME, et al. Measuring competence in central venous catheterization: a systematic-review. Springerplus. 2014;3:33.
26. Duncan DR, Morgenthaler TI, Ryu JH, Daniels CE. Reducing iatrogenic risk in thoracentesis: establishing best practice via experiential training in a zero-risk environment. Chest. 2009;135:1315–20.
27. Salamonsen M, McGrath D, Steiler G, Ware R, Colt H, Fielding D. A new instrument to assess physician skill at thoracic ultrasound, including pleural effusion markup. Chest. 2013;144:930–4.
28. Tolsgaard MG, Todsen T, Sorensen JL, et al. International multispecialty consensus on how to evaluate ultrasound competence: a Delphi consensus survey. PLoS One. 2013;8(2):e57687.
29. Lewiss RE, Hoffmann B, Beaulieu Y, et al. Point-of-care ultrasound education: the increasing role of simulation and multimedia resources. J Ultrasound Med. 2014;33:27–32.
30. Fox JC, Chiem AT, Rooney KP, et al. Web-based lectures, peer instruction and ultrasound-integrated medical education. Med Educ. 2012 Nov;46(11):1109–10.
31. Ahn JS, French AJ, Thiessen ME, et al. Training peer instructors for a combined ultrasound/physical exam curriculum. Teach Learn Med. 2014;26(3):292–5.
32. Jeppesen KM, Bahner DP. Teaching bedside sonography using peer mentoring: a prospective randomized trial. J Ultrasound Med. 2012 Mar;31(3):455–9.
33. Frank JR, Snell LS, Cate OT, et al. Competency-based medical education: theory to practice. Med Teach. 2010;32:638–45.
34. Morrow DS, Broder J. Cost-effective, reusable, leak-resistant ultrasound-guided vascular access trainer. J Emerg Med. 2015;49(3):313–7.
35. Wojtczak JA, Pyne S. Teaching ultrasound procedural skills-low cost phantoms and animal models. Middle East J Anaesthesiol. 2014 Oct;22(6):603–8.
36. Sparks S, Evans D, Byars D. A low cost, high fidelity nerve block model. Crit Ultrasound J. 2014;6(1):12.
37. Campo Dell'orto M, Hempel D, Starzetz A, et al. Assessment of a low-cost ultrasound pericardiocentesis model. Emerg Med Int. 2013;2013:1–7.
38. Cheruparambath V, Sampath S, Deshikar LN, et al. A low-cost reusable phantom for ultrasound-guided subclavian vein cannulation. Indian J Crit Care Med. 2012;16(3):163–5.
39. Bude RO, Adler RS. An easily made, low-cost, tissue-like ultrasound phantom material. J Clin Ultrasound. 1995 May;23(4):271–3.
40. Di Domenico S, Santori G, Porcile E, et al. Inexpensive homemade models for ultrasound-guided vein cannulation training. J Clin Anesth. 2007;19:491–6.

Chapter 12
Ultrasound Equipment and Purchase

Rachel Liu, Christopher L. Moore, and Vivek S. Tayal

Objectives

1. Review machine types in the point-of-care community
2. Review most common probe types in the point-of-care community
3. Discuss advantages and disadvantages of different equipment choices
4. Review currently available features that influence machine selection
5. Outline costs

In many ways, the development of ultrasound equipment has facilitated the expansion of point-of-care ultrasound (POC US). As machines have become more compact, durable, and less expensive while maintaining high image quality, they have spread to diverse practice environments. In the last decade, POC US has been recognized as the fastest growing sector of the ultrasonography market, and now nearly all major manufacturers have equipment that is targeted to this market [1]. Machines that "handle the rigors of the multi-user, multi-location practice environment" [2] have been driven by user needs with each year bringing new models for consideration.

Purchase of a machine requires thoughtful deliberation, aided by knowledge of machine hardware, intended operator skill set, site infrastructure, IT capabilities, and workflow logistics of the clinical practice environment. In emergency care settings where a diverse range of applications are required, considerations related to machine portability, transducers, image quality, adaptability, ease of use, durability,

R. Liu, MD, FACEP • C.L. Moore, MD, FACEP (✉)
Department of Emergency Medicine, Yale School of Medicine, New Haven, CT, USA
e-mail: chris.moore@yale.edu

V.S. Tayal, MD, FACEP
Department of Emergency Medicine, Carolinas Medical Center,
Charlotte, NC, USA

© Springer International Publishing AG 2018   145
V. S. Tayal et al. (eds.), *Ultrasound Program Management*,
https://doi.org/10.1007/978-3-319-63143-1_12

image archival, interface with quality assurance systems, workflow, and connectivity are continuously being addressed with industry [3]. The purpose of this chapter is to review basic considerations regarding machine form factors, probes, and other features that are important for use in the point-of-care setting, as well as provide guidance on the process of selecting, purchasing, and maintaining equipment.

Machine Selection

Point-of-care ultrasound machines are by definition more compact than standard cart-based machines, as they are intended to move (Fig. 12.1) to the patient as opposed to remaining in a fixed location. Within the field of point-of-care ultrasound, machines are manufactured using different form factors. These are typically classified as: "compact cart-based" (Fig. 12.2), "hand-carried" (laptop size) (Fig. 12.3), and "pocket-carried" (Fig. 12.4); some interchangeability between different classifications are made possible by accessories or machine modifications. For example, several companies offer setups where laptop-sized machines may function as compact cart-based systems by mounting them on attached wheeled carts (Fig. 12.5). This gives the option to remove the laptop portion for independent use, transport, and service. In addition, companies are now adding monitor-size machines that can be set on a moveable pole or on a monitor arm (Fig. 12.6 Monitor/arm mounted—S series and TE7).

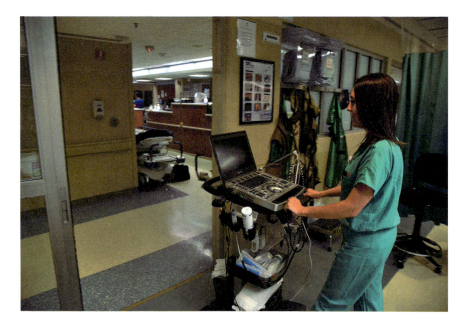

Fig. 12.1 Mobile Ultrasound

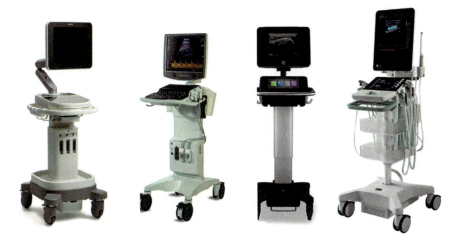

Fig. 12.2 Cart-based systems

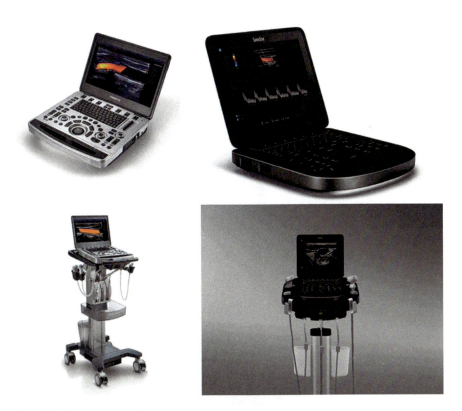

Fig. 12.3 Hand-carried machines on cart

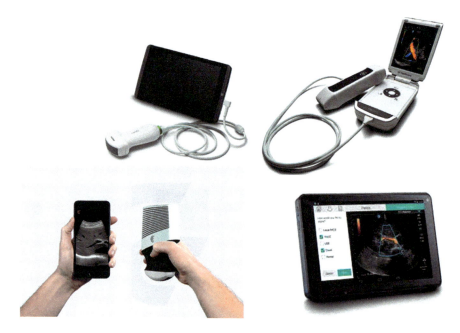

Fig. 12.4 Pocket-size ultrasound machines

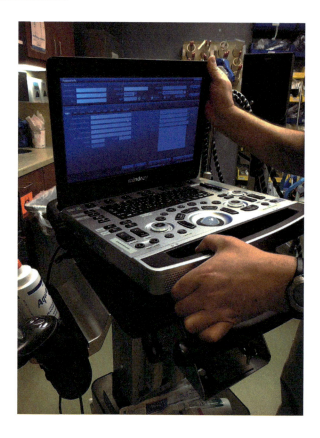

Fig. 12.5 Laptop machine
off cart

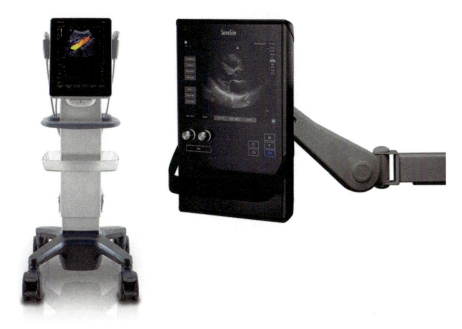

Fig. 12.6 Pole and arm mounted machine

The type of machine chosen for purchase depends mainly upon the practice environment of machine use. Wheeled cart-based machines are often the best form factor for emergency department or ICU settings, but would not be suitable for nonhospital field work. Likewise, smaller tablet and phone-sized machines may not provide features robust enough for certain in-hospital scenarios. Different classifications of machines have variations in mobility, durability, ease of use, image quality, access to advanced features, and adaptability to IT infrastructure. Most companies offer a trade-in price for older machines, and recycling machines may offset purchase costs.

Compact Cart-Based Ultrasound Machines

Compact cart-based machines are designed to be wheeled to the patient bedside (Fig. 12.2). They are termed "compact" as they are smaller than the nonmobile systems that reside in radiology or cardiology suites. Ideally their widths and depths are minimized, but they often have a large screen (Fig. 12.7), space for storage of equipment (Fig. 12.8), and more functionality than ultrasound equipment with smaller form factors. Based on the additional features and parts required, they are typically more expensive than other point-of-care machines (2017 price range approximately $30,000–$80,000). They consist of central processing units housed in casing that accommodate multiple transducers (Fig. 12.9), internet connectivity transmitter ("wireless dongle" (Fig. 12.10)), video output ports (Fig. 12.11), a keyboard (Fig. 12.12), and storage bins. They are often

Fig. 12.7 Large screen

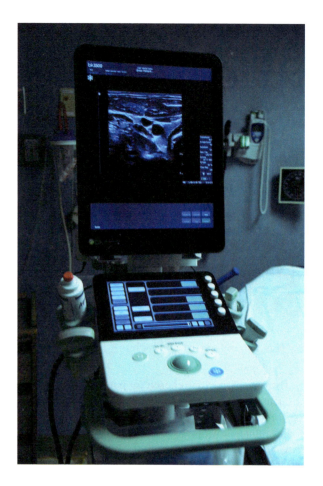

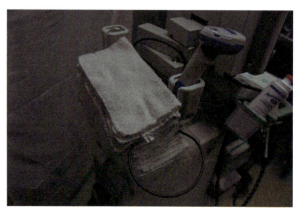

Fig. 12.8 Storage towels

Fig. 12.9 Probe ports

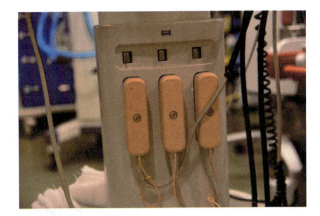

Fig. 12.10 Wireless
connectivity, external
wireless dongle

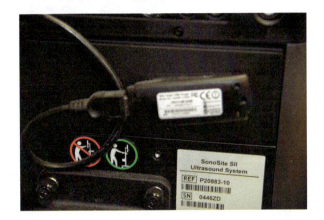

Fig. 12.11 Video input and
output digital connections

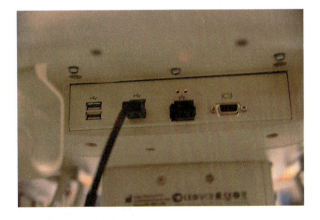

Fig. 12.12 Built-in keyboard

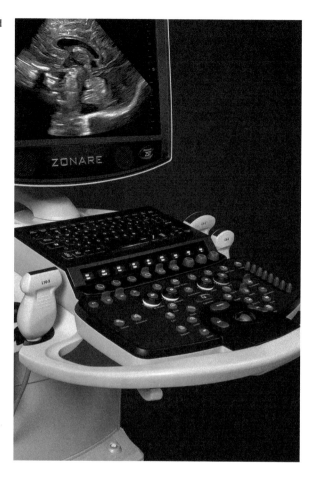

height adjustable with an articulating monitor (Fig. 12.13), allowing viewing from multiple angles. Some machines have separate touchscreens (Fig. 12.14), sealed control panels (Fig. 12.15), or retractable keyboards (Fig. 12.16) that offer more versatility in machine interactions than smaller form factors. The computers are robust enough to offer software packages that allow the most advanced functions (e.g. advanced cardiac imaging, transesophageal echocardiography, 3-D ultrasound). In general, their hardware performs at the highest levels and their processors are capable of producing the best image quality. They are wheeled from room to room, with modern designs structured to fit next to the patient's stretcher. They require adequate space surrounding the patient as well as dedicated storage space for the machine when not in use. Most modern compact cart-based machines have battery packs (Fig. 12.17) that allow use in the patient room without being plugged in, though they will need to be charged between use. Battery life typically lasts 1–2 h before requiring recharge. These machines will have onboard storage of digital clips, with Ethernet or wireless transfer to PACS and middleware programs available. Other options such as thermal printing, VHS, DVD, and USB image transfer are also available. Warranties for these machines are typically 3–5 years.

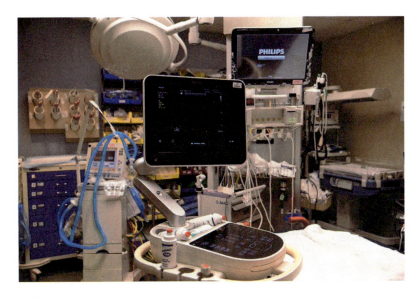

Fig. 12.13 Angled monitor arm

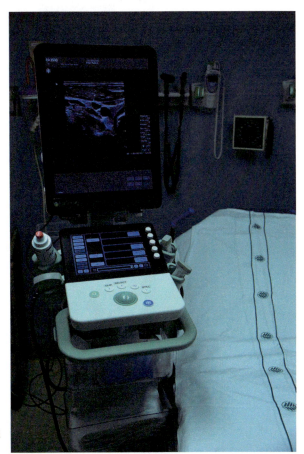

Fig. 12.14 Touchscreen and hard controls

Fig. 12.15 Glass panel

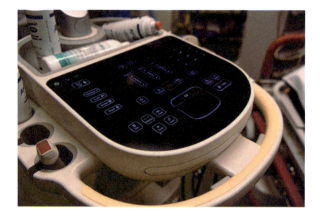

Fig. 12.16 Keyboard

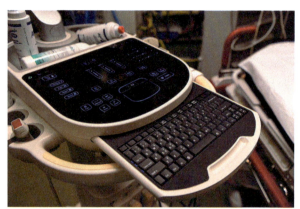

Fig. 12.17 Compact battery

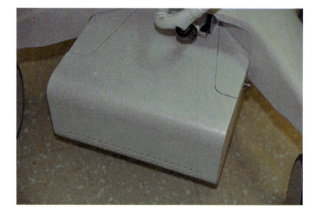

Hand-Carried Ultrasound Machines

These machines use a clamshell laptop or small television design (Fig. 12.3), and newer machines have touchscreen monitors contained in durable plastic housing. They usually have handles that allow the machine to be carried like a briefcase, and some can fit into a backpack. These systems may also be mounted on wheeled carts with cups to hold transducers and gel. They have the advantage of being detachable from the cart and carried if field portability is needed. They usually have one connection port for one transducer to be attached, and do not have the ability to add multiple probes simultaneously unless connected to a multiport adapter. Some companies are exploring Bluetooth cable-free transducers for this level of machine to free users from cable entanglement while changing probes. Hand-carried machines require less storage space than larger cart-based systems, but still require designated housing areas. Many of them can handle advanced applications, but software packages and certain capabilities may not be offered for all machines. They may provide less video output options, and may not possess inbuilt internet solutions like a wi-fi card, thus requiring external Ethernet adaptors or USB/SD card storage and retrieval. In 2017, these machines typically cost between $20,000 and $50,000 USD depending on the probes, cart, and software packages purchased with it. They also carry warranties lasting about a 3–5 year span.

Pocket-Carried Ultrasound Machines

With advancements in technology, the size of machines has become much smaller—small enough to fit inside a white coat pocket (Fig. 12.4). Some companies have created their own proprietary tablet-like devices, and may incorporate secured transducers that are not interchangeable. Others have placed hardware into their probes that connect with existing market tablets or smartphones with control of features through a downloadable app. The first of these pocket-carried ultrasounds were the GE Vscan and the Siemens Acuson P10. In 2015, tablet and smartphone android-based ultrasounds like the Philips Lumify and Sonosite iViz were introduced, with a transducer drawing power through the tablet micro-USB port. Now, other companies like Clarius and Healcerion are offering similar tablet-based machines that are compatible with both iOS and android, as well as wireless or Bluetooth transmission capabilities. This market is still relatively new and expanding quickly; newer models may not be ready for prime time marketing, but highlight promising features of future designs. They are much better for field use, but there may be issues with connectivity. They use various techniques to create sound waves, depending on the design of their device. Upfront costs are less than cart-based or hand-carried machines but warranties may be shorter and features are not robust. Some companies propose monthly or annual subscription models that may cumulatively equal the cost of larger machines.

The newest models employ touchscreens, with other models using Blackberry-like qwerty buttons or dials. "Older" generation machines available in the early 2000s do not have wireless connectivity options and require docking to a computer to transfer images. The latest devices support USB or micro-SD card image storage and transfer of images via wireless internet (cloud or email). Some of these machines may not offer video output connection, and, in general, are not designed for intermediate-advanced features. Image quality is not as good as cart-based or hand-carried machines, but as technology advances, this is improving. They are easily storable, but theft may be a problem. They are also prone to issues that affect current tablets: screen glare, difficulty obtaining optimum viewing angle, fingerprint smudges, freezes or forced reboots, and "buggy" image export. However, interest is increasing as their accessibility, relative low cost, easy storage, and decent image quality caters to populations (primary care, international work, EMS field use, education, etc.) that have been hindered in the past. As of 2015, these machines typically cost $7500–$15,000 USD. Their warranties last 1–5 years, though shorter warranties are more typical with this type of equipment. As of late 2017, new pocket-size machines based on non-piezoelectric technology called CMUT (capacitive micromachined ultrasound transducer) were announced for shipping in 2018. These machines use silicon chips to create voltage sent across a membrane to generate a sound wave. They have the ability to create a wide beam-width and enable one transducer to perform across a variety of US probe formats, from linear to curved to phased array, which then can be utilized for multiple applications. They use algorithms and signal processing to create optimal images. With the ability to plug into a smartphone, and the advertised price of near $2000, the new CMUT technology may have a large effect on portable US use with POC US, remote, prehospital, and even home use.

Pole or Arm Mounted US Machines

These machines are mobile, either by mounting on a rolling pole or a monitor arm, with the monitor containing touch controls (Fig. 12.6). Many pocket-sized US machines can be made "less pocket" and more mounted, rendering them multifunctional as a cross between a hand-carried machine on a cart and a true pocket, machine. In the past, most of these machines had small monitors and raised knobs or buttons, but most recently the trend has been to use touchscreen and controls similar to mobile phones to facilitate ease of use. While most have some advanced features, these machines are meant for particular purposes like intravenous line placement guidance, trauma assessment or resuscitation US in the resuscitation rooms, nerve blocks in the preoperative area, vascular guidance in the angiography suites, or other uses. Most can hold one to three transducers, similar to other transducers from the same vendor. All have battery capacity, and moderate screen size. While functionality is similar to hand-carried machines, touchscreens, footprint and visual access is often felt to superior. Disadvantages may include lack of keyboards, easy access to secondary controls, and buried advanced features.

Table 12.1 provides a comparison of the types of POC US machine types.

Table 12.1 Summary of advantages and disadvantages regarding machine types

	Cart-based machines	Hand-carried machines	Pocket-sized machines	Pole/arm mounted machines
Pros	• Most advanced features	• Fits into a briefcase	• Most portable	• Portable on moveable pole or arm
	• Robust processors	• Can be carried	• Lightest weight	• Monitor and controls usually n one screen or face
	• Largest hard drive/ memory	• Relatively lightweight	• Needs least holding space	• Can adapt pocket size onto moveable pole or arm
	• Large screen size	• Wheeled cart option	• Some offer both wifi and 3 g/4 g connectivity	• Not carried
	• Multidirectional mobile screen	• Less holding space needed	• Longer battery life (2–9 h depending on use)	• Wifi connectivity
	• Typically has best image quality	• Can be wall mounted	• Least expensive, although expensive for size	• Battery life similar to hand carried (2 h)
	• Holds 3 or more probes	• Good image quality		• Often dedicated to particular clinical purpose (procedural guidance, resuscitation)
	• Storage for accessories	• Rugged and durable		
	• Wheeled	• Some designed for field use		
	• Integrates best with electronic workflow solutions/processes	• Longer battery life (about 2 h)		

(continued)

Table 12.1 (continued)

	Cart-based machines	Hand-carried machines	Pocket-sized machines	Pole/arm mounted machines
Cons	• Larger size	• May not offer advanced features	• Typically not good image quality (although newest models are impressive)	• Limited features
	• Requires dedicated holding space for storage and charging	• Not as much storage space	• Older models with cumbersome connectivity	• Limited storage space
	• Less maneuverable	• May not accommodate multiple probe attachment	• Screen glare	• Keyboard on monitor or mobile
	• Heavier	• Screens not as adjustable	• May not simultaneously charge and be useable	• External wifi adapters
	• For indoor use only	• Some offer only external wifi adapters	• Less video output options	• Workflow solutions may be limited in function
	• Too big to mount to a wall		• May not interface with workflow processes	• Screen unidirectional
	• Short battery life (1 h) before requiring wall charge		• Security issues with wireless image handling	• Controls are menu-designed
	• Highest cost			

Probe Selection

Choosing which probe(s) to purchase depends on cost, ultrasound applications desired, probe frequency ranges, and patient population. A probe (also called a "transducer") is defined by the size and shape of its "footprint," which is the face of the probe (Fig. 12.18) that contacts the patient and encases the crystals that transmit and receive sound waves. Probe footprint will determine where a probe can best be used: wide footprint probes (Fig. 12.19) are best for the abdomen, where ribs do not obscure the view. Small footprint probes (microconvex or phased array) (Fig. 12.20) will be best for evaluations of the chest, as they can image between the ribs without interference.

Fig. 12.18 Footprint
enhanced phased array face

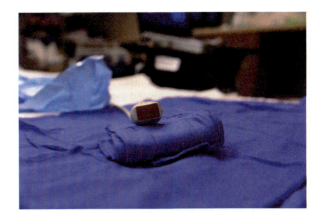

Fig. 12.19 Wide footprint
curvilinear face

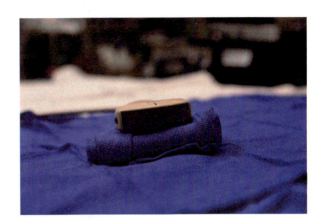

Fig. 12.20 Small curvilinear
face

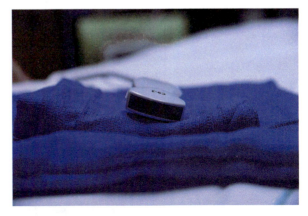

Probe footprint is often associated with probe frequency. Probes transmitting lower frequency waves are able to penetrate deeper into body cavities while higher frequency probes produce greater image resolution of superficial structures. Linear and endocavitary probes tend to be higher frequency, while abdominal and cardiac probes (curvilinear and phased array) are lower frequency. However, there may be frequency range options available for these standard probes. For example, practitioners imaging pediatric patients may want to look at higher frequency abdominal probes. Of note, most probes today are "broadband," utilizing multiple frequencies within a certain range to optimize the image based on depth.

There are four main types of probes that are used in clinician-performed ultrasound: curvilinear (Fig. 12.21), linear (Fig. 12.22), phased array (Fig. 12.23), and endocavitary (Fig. 12.24) (Table 12.2) [4]. These will allow performance of nearly every application for point-of-care ultrasound. Recently, there have been some publications about performing transesophageal echocardiography (TEE) in the point-of-care setting. This would require a separate special probe (Fig. 12.25), but this practice

Fig. 12.21 Curvilinear transducer

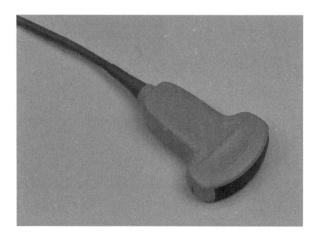

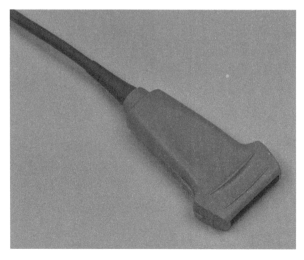

Fig. 12.22 Linear transducer

is not currently widespread. Probes on compact cart-based machines typically attach to the ultrasound machine through a set of ports (Fig. 12.26) that allow switching of probes without physically changing the port. Laptop-sized machines usually require the probe to be physically interchanged (Fig. 12.27). Pocket-carried machines often have a fixed probe that cannot be changed, although recent models have combined more than one probe type in a single transducer (Fig. 12.28). Innovative wireless probes have been developed by some companies, with control functions on the probe itself to allow one-handed operation (Fig. 12.29) or use of Bluetooth and wifi to transmit images to smartphones or tablets (Fig. 12.30). All transducers have raised color-marked lines or dots called "indicators" which correspond to a marker on the screen for assisting operators' spatial orientation. Probes generally cost between $7000 and $12,000 USD each, with warranties lasting 1–5 years [5]. Vendors manufacture their probes differently, influencing their durability and degradation time. It is worth asking companies about their manner of probe construction.

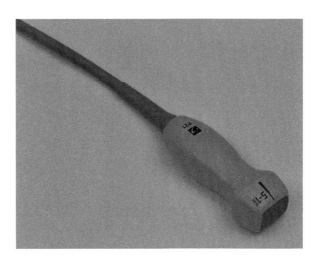

Fig. 12.23 Phased array transducer

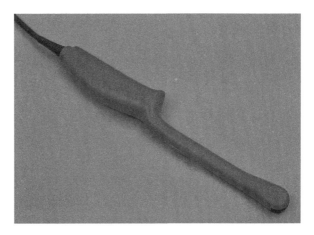

Fig. 12.24 Endocavity transducer

Table 12.2 Summary of the advantages of disadvantages of different probe types

	Phased array	Curvilinear	Linear	Endocavitary	TEE
Pros	• Best for cardiac scanning • Lower frequency with small footprint • Contains ideal tissue harmonic imaging for echo • May be used for thoracic & abdominal imaging too • May be used for transcranial applications	• Best for abdominal and OB imaging • May be used for thoracic and MSK imaging, particularly of deeper structures	• Best for vascular, MSK, ocular applications • Essential for the most common procedures (peripheral IV, central access) • May be used for transabdominal OB, bowel evaluations in thin patients • Variations exist that offer better ergonomic form factors like the "hockey stick" probe • New technologies offer very high-frequency imaging	• Best for transvaginal imaging • May be used for intra-oral peritonsillar abscess evaluation • May be used for suprasternal notch aortic arch assessment	• Exclusively for cardiac imaging • Potential POC US applications in cardiac resuscitation
Limits	• Image quality may be limited in obese patients • Image quality may be limited in non-cardiac presets • Depending on vendor, crystals and image quality may degrade relatively quickly • Not good for superficial imaging	• Larger footprint • Due to heavy use, especially for eFAST exams, rone to being dropped or mistreated	• Depth of field typically does not extend past 4 cm	• Applications are relatively specialist • Needs specific consideration of operator use/ proficiency in the clinical environment	• Requires training beyond normal current • POC US training Probes are expensive • Unclear definitive role in current resuscitation care

Fig. 12.25 TEE probe

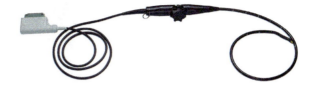

Fig. 12.26 Probe ports

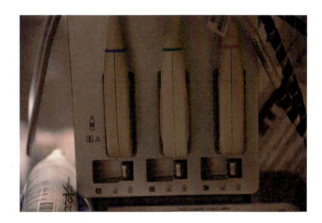

Fig. 12.27 Probe connection
into laptop

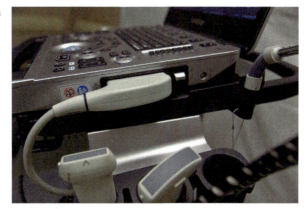

Fig. 12.28 Plug in probe—pocket size

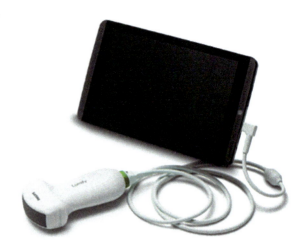

Fig. 12.29 Freestyle hand image

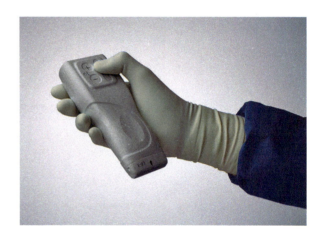

Fig. 12.30 Smart phone controlled portable ultrasound

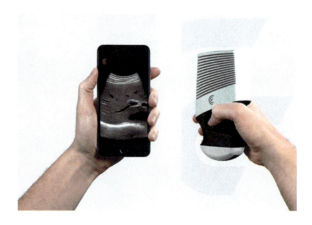

Linear transducers (also known as straight linear array probes) have a flat, oblong rectangular surface (Fig. 12.22). They are sometimes referred to as "vascular" probes as they are often used for this indication, although they have more diverse applications. The crystals are aligned parallel to each other in a straight line, and therefore produce sound waves that travel in straight lines. The field of the image on screen is rectangular, like a box. This probe has a high-frequency range (5–13 MHz) and so provides good resolution of images but less penetration into body cavities. Therefore, it is ideal for imaging superficial structures involved in soft tissue, musculoskeletal, vascular, pleural, and ocular imaging. Of note, it is commonly used for procedural guidance.

Variations of the linear probe exist, like the "hockey stick" probe (Fig. 12.31) that allows the probe to be gripped like a pencil. This can afford a more stable grip when performing procedures or applications that need fine motor action. In addition, since 2016 vendors have developed ultrasound high-frequency probes with capabilities up to 70 MHz (e.g., Sonosite Vevo MD transducers) that offer advancements in neonatal, vascular, and MSK examinations. The advantage of this in the point-of-care community has yet to be seen.

Curvilinear probes (Fig. 12.21) (also called convex) have crystals arranged along a large curved surface and produce sound waves traveling in a fan-shaped arcing beam. This allows a field of view that is wider than the probe's footprint, so images appear narrower on top of the screen and wider at the bottom. This configuration is often referred to as a "sector" probe, which also refers to phased array and endocavitary probes, as distinct from linear. The frequency of a curvilinear abdominal probe typically ranges between 2 and 6 MHz, allowing sound waves to penetrate

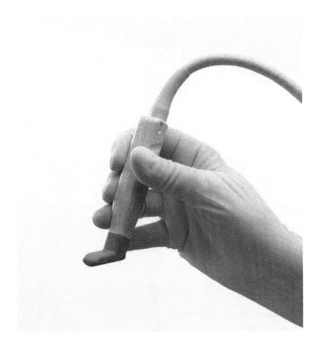

Fig. 12.31 Hockey stick probe

deeper into the body but providing less resolution. Curvilinear probes are commonly used to ultrasound the abdominal cavity, perform transabdominal fetal evaluation, evaluate the pelvis and bladder transabdominally, assess the pleural cavity, and perform certain musculoskeletal procedures (e.g. intra-articular shoulder injection and reduction, lumbar puncture). Highly curved small curvilinear probes with mid-level frequencies (4–8 MHz) are available for pediatric scanning (Fig. 12.32— small short radius mid-frequency range curvilinear probe).

Phased array probes have a flat, square surface shape and its crystals are grouped closely together in a point (Fig. 12.23). Sound waves originate from this single point and spread outward, creating a triangular or sector image. The probe frequency is between 2 and 8 MHz. As the footprint is smaller and flatter than the curvilinear probe, it is easier to maneuver between rib spaces and use in smaller areas. It is ideal for cardiac imaging as well as abdominal evaluation of thinner, smaller patients. Users should be aware that when selecting the phased array probe the machine may default to a cardiology convention, which may reverse the indicator-to-screen orientation from other indications.

The *endocavitary* probe (Fig. 12.24) has a small circular curved face that is narrower than the curvilinear probe and produces higher frequencies (8–13MHz). Because of its small size, it is ideal for placement into smaller cavities (intra-oral or intra-vaginal) for evaluation of peritonsillar abscess and most commonly, for OBGYN applications [4]. It can also be used for central line placement and assessment of the aortic arch at the sternal notch.

A *transesophageal* probe (Fig. 12.25) has the ultrasound face at the end of a flexible apparatus designed to be inserted and manipulated to visualize the heart adjacent to the esophagus. These probes are uncommonly used in the emergency department setting, but have been adopted by intensivists particularly in Europe. The transesophageal probe is more expensive than other probes (typically about $20–30 K), but provides unparalleled visualization of the heart.

In addition to TEE probes, there are many other probes that may be useful in POC imaging, such as biplanar probes and 3D probes (Fig. 12.33—biplanar probe, and Fig. 12.34 xplane 3D probe).

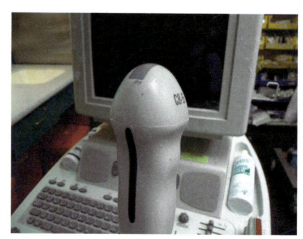

Fig. 12.32 Middle frequency curvilinear probe

Fig. 12.33 Biplane probe

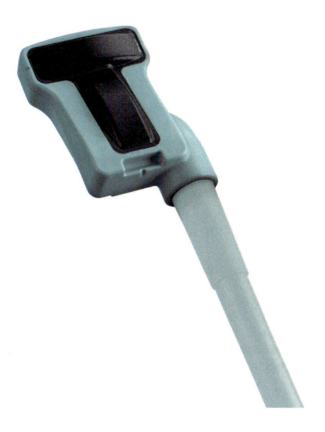

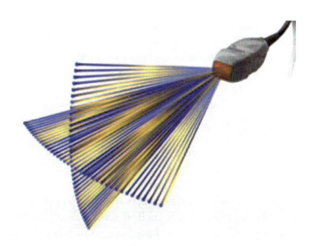

Fig. 12.34 Xplane 3D probe

In an ideal situation, a clinical ultrasonographer will have access to all available types of probes. However, due to budgetary constraints it may be necessary to prioritize which probes are obtained. Transabdominal imaging can often be reasonably performed with a phased array probe. However, cardiac imaging is difficult with a large footprint curvilinear probe. Thus when programs are trying to economize, they may choose a phased array or microconvex probe instead of both a phased array and large footprint curvilinear. This will work, although the quality of abdominal imaging will be improved if a high quality curvilinear probe is available. A linear probe is required for vascular, ocular, and musculoskeletal imaging, and an endocavitary probe is required for transvaginal imaging. Most point-of-care ultrasound machines will require at least phased array and linear probes, with probe selection tailored to the uses intended.

Equipment Purchase Considerations

The uniqueness of clinical ultrasonography is that it brings imaging to the patient bedside and so the practice environment is frequently changing. An operator can work in a hospital, detach a machine, and bring it to an international site. Or, the provider may choose to work primarily with smaller machines for personal use at multiple sites. Whether in a hospital, the back of an ambulance, helicopter, cruise ship, campsite, on top of a mountain, or in space, all environments of practice can be harsh. Machines need adaptability to keep pace with growing demands while withstanding the elements.

Portability and Durability

Sizing of machines have been addressed above, and it would benefit the buyer to physically measure the dimensions of patient care space and docking areas to ensure a machine fits.

While all buyers wish their units to be easily maneuverable and indestructible these characteristics will vary by manufacturer and model. Cart systems and hand-carried machines mounted on carts should be lightweight and easily turned. Wheels and wheel casings need to consist of durable material and perform multidirectional functions to enable movement. The composition of machine housing and articulating joints (e.g., height adjustment levers, monitor arms) need to be rugged, as machines run into walls during transport and are splashed by corrosive substances. Laptop-sized and smaller machines should have casing and screens that withstand being dropped.

Similarly, crystals within transducer footprints and seams in the probe casing need to be resilient if dropped accidentally. Cable management solutions that prevent cord entanglement and trampling are essential for transducer protection. If probe cables are run over by the machine, cables should withstand wear and tear to protect the wires inside. Wireless transducers are a way to combat this issue, but lead to concerns of probe misplacement or theft. Retractable cords have been proposed, but sterility, cleaning, and functionality have been problematic and to our knowledge there are no commercially available retractable probe connectors. Some companies have employed power stations to prevent power cord trampling, alleviate ergonomic issues associated with machine charging, and avoid handling of dirty cords that have dragged on the floor. Machines should contain storage options for transducers, gel, cleaning solution, and accessories to provide further protection. All surfaces associated with a machine have to be easily accessible and cleaned with readily available solutions.

Ease of Use

In critical care situations, quick machine boot-up time is a must and this can be facilitated by a power sleep mode. Comparing "cold boot" and "awakening from sleep" times should be done prior to purchase. Battery life is also an important feature, as situations arise where usage for 2–3 h or more is needed away from a wall socket. Quick battery charge time or ability for battery replacement during transport is ideal. Critical features (e.g., power, gain, depth, measure, freeze, save image, change transducer) must be easy to find and intuitively located. Keyboard and knobs should be backlit to accommodate imaging in darkened rooms. The machine's features and controls need appeal to users of differing skill levels, easily upgraded when new software and advanced packages are desired. Machines using touchscreen keypads need to be responsive, without lag or oversensitivity.

Integration of particular equipment into current or future department workflow should be considered. Some manufacturers and models will integrate better with particular electronic health records and image management systems (including both "middleware" or a more traditional picture archival and communication service—PACS). It may be very helpful to discuss machine integration with someone who uses a similar workflow, and vendors are often able to provide prospective customers with these references. Patient demographics should be available for selection from a work list and convenient to enter manually if needed. Some companies have enabled automatic transfer of patient information to their machines using a patient identity band barcode reader. The ability to select a patient without manual entry facilitates correct documentation for electronic medical record transfer and quality assurance [3]. Likewise, "ending an exam" facilitates image storage and the ability to create a new patient. Most systems will do this automatically, but a cumbersome process will hinder workflow. The prospective buyer should think carefully about how images will be stored and transferred from the machine and if possible discuss with someone using a similar configuration. Some ultrasound companies are now interfacing with middleware documentation companies to allow the completion of interpretation worksheets on their machines. This enhances operator compliance with documentation and speeds workflow.

Image Storage and Transfer

Definitive image archival is required for ultrasound reimbursement, and effective image management can enhance quality assurance and communication with other practitioners. While thermal printing, VHS cassette, and even DVD recording of images are still performed in some places, current equipment is designed for digital transfer of still and moving images or "cineloops," which are preferred by many users. Export of images in general formats such as jpeg or mp4 is typically available from the machine if desired, but most modern units will utilize the DICOM image storage format (a standard format that stands for Digital Imaging and Communication in Medicine). If manual export is anticipated, efficient export will prevent long download times and file corruption. Contemporary file storage options (USB drives, SD cards, wireless or cloud transfer) should be available. Wireless transfer of images is much more suited to the point-of-care environment if it can be configured. While most machines can have an external wi-fi adapter added, ideally this should be housed internally to ensure durability and functionality. Machines using plug-in ethernet connectors need to secure them to protect against accidental dislodgement when attaching or removing ethernet cables. Ethernet standards offered on the machines need to follow hospital security protocols, and it is beneficial to involve hospital IT during purchase discussions to ensure a machine is compatible with the hospital intranet system. Like computers, internal components and storage should be upgradeable and replaceable if needed (See Chap. 17 – Workflow and Middleware).

Service

Warranties or service contracts should be carefully reviewed prior to purchase, as they are essential for the maintenance of machines and probes. While some manufacturers include a full 5-year warranty as part of the initial purchase price, most vendors will offer a 1-year warranty with a service plan to be purchased after the initial warranty period. Service plans should typically be budgeted at about 10% of the machine cost per year, and spending more money for higher service packages is often a wise decision [5]. They should include replacement of broken parts and loan of either parts or full machine support during repair, ideally with pickup and shipping included. The warranty coverage of probes should be explicitly addressed, as these are often the most vulnerable parts of the machine. Warranties may not cover a probe repair or replacement if there is evidence of "excessive wear and tear" (something that unfortunately may be difficult to avoid in the point-of-care setting), while other companies will do this once but not subsequently.

Company replies to service calls need to be prompt, since delay of service could impact patient care. As many clinical ultrasonography practitioners are in emergency settings that are open 24/7, repair services need to be available past typical business hours. It is worth questioning representatives on service technicians' response times, methods of communication, location, and hours of service. This should ideally be verified by speaking with someone in your area who is working with similar equipment. The most convenient plans involve technicians investigating defects at the hospital site itself. System software upgrades should be quickly performed via USB drive, CD, or remote internet connection without requiring full hardware replacement (See Chap. 14 – Equipment Maintenance).

Image Quality

Image quality overall has improved markedly over the last decade in the point-of-care market. Having good image quality across the spectrum of patients (thin and

obese) and across examination types (abdominal and cardiac) will be a huge con-
tributor to success of a point-of-care ultrasound program. While images will often
look excellent on the healthy model recruited for a trade show, they may not be as
good on the 300 lb patient that arrives in the ED. It is recommended that a purchaser
invites more than one vendor to do side-by-side comparisons of image quality (as
well as workflow and other features) prior to purchase, and to speak with other
practitioners who are using similar equipment.

Considerations for Budgeting, Shopping, and Buying Equipment

For most purchasers, the first step in considering point-of-care ultrasound equipment will be budgeting, and many practice environments will require a business
plan for purchase. Those driving the purchasing are often physicians, and their
focus will be on patient care as well as reimbursement of professional fees. In some
cases, particularly when privileging is not yet in place, it may be necessary for the
physician group to buy a machine. However, it is typically more optimal for the
hospital to purchase the equipment. If reimbursement for point-of-care ultrasound is
already in place or anticipated, the hospital should be receiving a technical fee for
ultrasound performance. The purpose of this fee is to provide for equipment and
resources that support the ultrasound performance, separate from the professional
fee (See Chap. 22 – Reimbursement). While this information is sometimes challenging to obtain, someone from hospital accounting should be involved in the budgeting and business plan if possible. It is essential that the budget be comprehensive,
including the full cost of the equipment and probes as well as the anticipated service
contract (see Table 12.3).

Table 12.3 Basic checklist for budget considerations

	Budget considerations	Approximate costs
Equipment	• Machine type and form factor	• $30,000–$60,000 depending on features
	• Number of machines	• $7000–$18,000 for tablet machines
	• Purchase of refurbished machines or trade-in of old machines	• About $6000–$8000 per probe
	• Number of probes desired	• $30,000 for a TEE probe
	• Any specialist probes desired (TEE, TCD, TVUS)	
	• Extra warranty coverage and maintenance contracts	
	• Desired accessories (power packs, carts, wall mounting, etc.)	
Other IT needs	• Wifi routers and amplifiers	• Server may cost $20,000
	• Dedicated hospital server if desired	
Workflow solutions	• Middleware interface between machines, interpretation, EMR and QA (like Telexy Healthcare Qpath, Ultrasonix SonixHub)	• About $10,000–$15,000

Once a budget has been obtained, it is recommended that the purchaser look at multiple vendors to understand the options available and compare costs. A list of ideal US machine features has been included from the Emergency US section of the American College of Emergency Physicians (Table 12.4).

A good place to compare machines and speak to vendors is at a professional meeting such as the American College of Emergency Physicians or the American Institute of Ultrasound in Medicine, where most point-of-care ultrasound vendors will showcase equipment. Once potential equipment is narrowed down to a few machines, it is usually worthwhile to test them in your environment of care through vendor visits. As mentioned previously, arranging for a "side-by-side" with two or more vendors at once will both economize your time and allow you to compare such things as image quality in similar subjects. Price will obviously be an issue, but keep in mind that the actual price of ultrasound equipment may be widely variable, and will likely be negotiated by your hospital, as noted below. Most companies offer a trade-in price for older machines, and recycling machines may offset purchase costs.

Table 12.4 ACEP emergency US section essential machine features checklist

ACEP emergency ultrasound: essential machine features checklist (adapted with permission)
1. Compact and easily mobile
• Fits into patient rooms, limited spaces
• Width and depth kept to a minimum
• Wheels are high quality, multidirectional
• Light weight, easy maneuverability
• Most ED applications best served by a compact cart-based system
• Storage options (e.g., for extra gel, cleaning agents, probe covers, angiocaths)
2. Image quality and versatility
• 2-D image quality is essential
• Maximize in difficult/obese patients
• Capabilities for multiple applications
– General/abdominal (wide footprint curvilinear probe)
– Cardiac (phased array probe)
– Vascular, soft tissue, procedural (high-frequency linear probe)
– Pelvic, obstetrical (endocavitary/transvaginal probe)
• Midline mark on linear, curvilinear probes to facilitate procedural applications
• Multiple probe ports (minimum 3, preferably 4), easy switching between transducers
• Multiple holders to accommodate 3–4 probes, gel bottle(s), and barcode scanner
• Large, bright screen, broad viewing angles
• Monitor easily articulates in all directions
• Needle localization/guidance technologies highly desirable

Table 12.4 (continued)

ACEP emergency ultrasound: essential machine features checklist (adapted with permission)

3. Ease-of-use and simplification

• Quick boot-up time (including "cold boot")

• Battery powered sleep mode

• Maximal battery life (at least 2–3 h battery powered scanning)

• Rapid battery recharging

• Reminders (visual and auditory) when battery level low

• Simplified control panel, essential functions highlighted

– On/Off	– Zoom
– Start/End exam	– Freeze
– Exam type	– Measure
– Depth	– Calculations
– Gain	– Still image
– Optimize	– Video

• Control panel should be backlit, with large buttons and large print

• Physical knobs/dials preferable for functions such as depth, gain

• Sealed control panel surface for easy cleaning

• Keyboard best if sealed (not easily penetrated by liquids) or pull-out

• Should be as intuitive as possible (users of varying skill levels)

• Retain ability to pull up more advanced features

• Touchscreen panel on cart (not monitor) well-suited for this purpose

  – Allow for maximal customization (i.e., which functions to include/exclude)

  – Default to basic functions, with option to access more advanced modes

• Touch panels must be responsive (do not lag) and reliable, functions despite exposure to gel or bodily fluids

• Start exam screen fields

  – Patient name

  – Medical record number

  – Accession number

  – Examiner name(s) (two fields to allow for trainee/supervisor)

  – Probe selection

  – Exam type preset

4. Durability and service

• ED is a harsh environment, demands 24/7 upkeep

• Machine, probes, cords need to be rugged

  – Probes may be dropped onto the ground

  – Probe cords, power cords may be run over by the machine wheels

  – Probes, machine may be exposed to bodily fluids (blood, pus, etc.)

• Machine cord management commonly under-appreciated

• Probe cords must be durable (protected), cart designed to minimize cords tangling or being run over by machine wheels

• Probe holders should be stable, strong, easily cleaned

(continued)

Table 12.4 (continued)

ACEP emergency ultrasound: essential machine features checklist (adapted with permission)
• Power cord ideally retractable, otherwise easily stowed and should not originate from bottom of cart, which promotes tangling in cart wheels
• Service needs to be prompt and accessible 24/7
– Need availability beyond Monday–Friday 9 am–5 pm business hours
– ED required to be in full operation nights, weekends, and holidays
• Affordable service plan options, either included plan (5 years) or contract paid yearly
• Commonly broken parts should be separate (modular) and easily replaceable
• Ability to export and import machine system settings (i.e., for loaner machines in case primary machine is out of service for repairs)
• Software failures (freezes, reboots) unacceptable
5. Image archival and workflow
• Record as still images and cine loops to internal storage
• Internal storage capacity upgradeable (not fixed in size)
• DICOM capabilities should be standard on all machines
• Widely used export formats for still images (JPEG) and cine loops (MOV, AVI, MP4)
• Export options should include USB, CD/DVD, and (less commonly) thermal print
• Integrated Wi-Fi capabilities essential for all future machines models
• Wi-Fi adapter housed within a secured location on machine cart (not attached externally)
• Support for all IEEE 802.11 standards, security protocols used in healthcare IT
• Workflow should be designed using standardized, non-proprietary formats
• Front-end workflow: getting information into the machine (i.e., patient information, sonographer name(s), exam type, indication for scan)
• Optimize front-end workflow via barcode scanners, DICOM modality worklists
• Separate diagnostic studies from those performed for educational purposes
• Ultrasound interpretation ("worksheets") filled out directly on machines
• Worksheets should include indication, views, findings, interpretation based on ACEP Standard Reporting Guidelines, but essential that they are fully user customizable
• Back-end workflow: getting information out of the machine (i.e., transfer ultrasound images and interpretations to the PACS and EMR)
• Ideal workflow to obtain images and document findings directly on the machine, then wireless transfer of ultrasound images and report from machine to the PACS and EMR
6. Future innovations
• Wireless probe technologies highly desirable for the ED setting
• Consider incorporation of basic controls (e.g., image capture, depth, gain) onto the ultrasound probe
• Ability to pull up teaching images (standard views, probe placement, pathologic images)
• Directly on machines

Once a vendor and machine model is selected, purchase will need to be negotiated. While this may be done by individual physicians, often there is a hospital or institutional infrastructure in place for negotiating this. This process should be sought well ahead of making any commitments to a purchase. Even if there is a preferred vendor or model, the institution will often require two or more proposals, with rationale for purchase of the preferred machine.

Machine Companies

Excellent POC US products are now being offered that include Sonosite, General Electric, Philips Healthcare, Mindray (which acquired Zonare Medical Systems), Terason, Siemens Healthcare, Toshiba, Hitachi, Aloka, BK Ultrasound (which incorporated Ultrasonix), and others. Emergency Medicine comprises the largest share of the emerging markets, with rapid growth exhibited by anesthesiology, critical care, and musculoskeletal medicine [2].

Summary

The lifespan of a machine is about 3–7 years which can be prolonged by regular maintenance via service contracts and gentle care. General pricing for cart-based systems including 3–4 probes is $30,000–$70,000 USD. Hand-carried machines are priced less than that, but costs vary depending on additions like wheeled carts or the types of transducers purchased. Pocket-carried devices generally run from $7500 to $15,000 and may have subscription-based purchasing models. Some companies offer group pricing, education pricing, and leasing options. Purchasing decisions should not be rushed—involvement with hospital IT, asking for other practice's references, arranging company demonstrations for side-by-side comparison, and asking about each company's financing plans will help decision-making. Before meeting with companies, it can be helpful to create a checklist containing a starting budget, the desired probes, equipment crucial to the site's practice environment, maintenance needs, clinical workflow solutions, and image documentation requirements before engaging a prioritized wish list.

Pitfalls

1. Not understanding that US machine selection is a key and decisive action in US Program Management
2. Not comparing US machines on real-life models side-by-side
3. Lack of attention to key machine features and probe use for POC applications
4. Not understanding the service needs and replacement costs of equipment
5. Not understanding workflow integration of image capture, examination reporting, and communication to system networks in your health system
6. Not preparing for service life and replacement of US machines

Key Recommendations

1. Compare and contrast US machines in your environment prior to purchase
2. Make a checklist of key features that you require for your purchase

3. Buy probes that meet your application needs across age, location, and volume considerations.
4. Understand that POC US is done in a harsh, demanding, and constrained environment with respect to US machine
5. Decide on machines with provider workflow, communication, and documentation requirement in mind; involve departmental IT, biomedical engineering, and departmental budget personnel.
6. Integrate US machine into the mission and practice of your site with continual attention to the needs of your department or unit

Acknowledgments We gratefully acknowledge images from the following US manufacturers: BK Ultrasound, Philips Ultrasound, Fuji-Sonosite, Mindray, GE Ultrasound, Ultrasound, and Clarius Ultrasound.

References

1. "Versatile Point of Care Ultrasound Technology Quickly Gaining Market Share in the United States." prweb. 15 Apr 2015. Web. 8 Aug 2015. http://www.prweb.com/releases/2015/04/prweb12653454.htm.
2. American College of Emergency Physicians Policy Statement: Emergency Ultrasound Guidelines. Ann Emerg Med. 2009;53(4): 557.
3. Byrne M. Emergency ultrasound: essential machine features. American College of Emergency Physicians. 2014. Web. 8 Aug 2015. http://www.acep.org/uploadedFiles/ACEP/member-Center/SectionsofMembership/ultra/Essential%20Machine%20Features%202014.pdf.
4. Markowitz J. Probe selection, machine controls and equipment. In: Carmody K, Moore C, Feller-Kopman D, editors. Handbook of critical care and emergency ultrasound. New York: McGraw-Hill; 2011. p. 25–8.
5. Moore, C. "Ultrasound Equipment Purchase." American College of Emergency Physicians Emergency Ultrasound Management Course. San Francisco. 14 Oct 2011.

Chapter 13
Ultrasound Equipment Maintenance

Andreas Dewitz

Objectives

- Understand the daily operational issues associated with US machine maintenance in the point-of-care environment
- Understand the supply issues with US practice
- Development of a plan for US machine service

Introduction

Anyone involved in the creation or administration of a point-of-care ultrasound program will soon recognize that there are many moving parts to oversee and there are many hats that you will be required to wear. Knowing how to keep your ultrasound fleet shipshape and clean and making sure the requisite supplies for your ultrasound program's day-to-day operation are flowing smoothly is as essential a part of the job description as ultrasound education and QA. What follows in this chapter are many practical operational guidelines and a broad collection of tips and tricks—gleaned from several decades of practice—on how to keep the equipment and logistical aspects of your ultrasound program running smoothly.

The scenario typically begins with jubilation. Someone in your hospital's finance department signs off on a large purchase order, and sometime not long thereafter a large crate arrives. After a bit of assembly, your spotless new

A. Dewitz, MD, FACEP
Department of Emergency Medicine, Boston University School of Medicine,
Boston Medical Center, Boston, MA, USA
e-mail: dewitz@bu.edu

© Springer International Publishing AG 2018   177
V. S. Tayal et al. (eds.), *Ultrasound Program Management*,
https://doi.org/10.1007/978-3-319-63143-1_13

ultrasound machine emerges, looking just like the glossy photo in the brochure and you are now most eager to launch your new arrival on its maiden voyage. Your goals are simple: 100% operational uptime, ready access to equipment and supplies, and a clean and professional looking machine. In its new home, however, your new machine will face a wide variety of inevitable physical insults. A busy ED is not an inherently clean place. Look closely at your keyboards, the phones, the ubiquitous dust bunnies, your communal ED lounge refrigerator, or your trauma room after a messy clinical case for a preview of things to come. Your pristine machine will be used by multiple providers, most of whom will <u>not</u> take care of your equipment as you would. Your machine will be exposed to all manner of assaults (dust, blood, dried ultrasound gel, adhesive glue, and on occasion, vomit, charcoal, urine, hematemesis, plaster, coffee, sputum-yes, I have encountered them all!) and your machine will soon no longer resemble what you initially saw in the brochure. Your baby (or babies), will age in dog years. With multiple machines to care for you may wonder how you can possibly manage to stay on course? The information that follows will hopefully serve as a useful guide for you on this journey (Figs. 13.1, 13.2, 13.3, and 13.4).

First, some practical ultrasound fleet management guidelines should help you start your journey on an auspicious note. Then, a discussion of the many ultrasound equipment maintenance issues you are likely to encounter and will need to address, and how you can easily customize your ultrasound equipment to best suit your

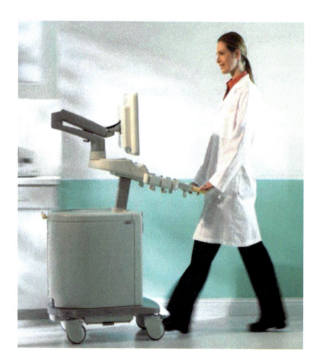

Fig. 13.1 A clean new US machine as it appeared in the brochure. Note the complete absence of any messy power cords, transducers, transducer cords, gel, and cleaning sprays in the photo!

Fig. 13.2 An ED Nursing lounge refrigerator, your first clue that communal cleanup responsibility may not be a successful strategy for cleaning your machine

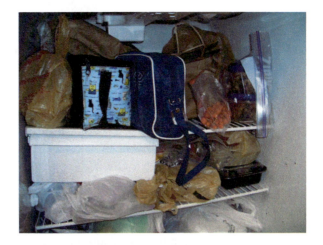

Fig. 13.3 ED desktop computer keyboard close-up: the shape of things to come for your new US machine

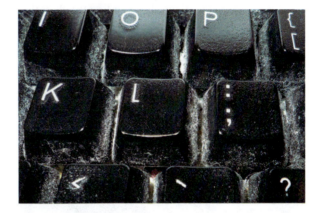

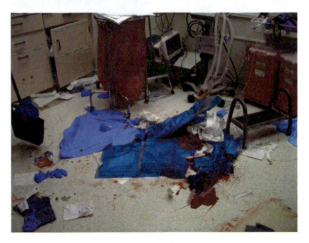

Fig. 13.4 ED Trauma Room after a messy case: how does the US machine look now?

practice needs. Finally, a review of various service contract options follows. Sprinkled throughout will be many photos of tips and tricks that should make the maintenance and logistics part of the job easier and more fun.

So, what important operational guidelines should you follow from the outset?

Choose Well-Designed Equipment and Purchase Your Equipment Carefully

Make note of the cart size, footprint, and how it will function in your practice setting. Examine the keyboard layout and ease of use of the user interface. Pay attention to ergonomics: are the handles conveniently located for ease of use? How easily the cart is moved about? How easy is the keyboard adjusted for various user heights? Look very carefully at how ultrasound probes, gel, and cleaning spray are stored, where other supplies can be placed on the cart, how transducer cords are managed (more in this later), and the solidity of the machine's overall construction. Sealed control surfaces are a must. A flat control surface will facilitate speedier and more successful disinfection. A standard laptop keyboard surface provides many nooks and crannies for hospital pathogens to reside in and will be harder to clean properly. Visit ultrasound equipment vendors at the national conventions and make sure you try out a piece of equipment before you buy it. Confer with your colleagues, road test a loaner unit in your practice setting. Fortunately, ever more attention is being paid to the design and construction of point-of-care ultrasound machines with better designs forthcoming every few years (Figs. 13.5 and 13.6) (See Chap. 12 – US Equipment and Purchase).

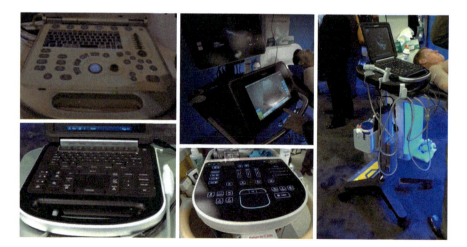

Fig. 13.5 Choosing your equipment: assess control surface layouts, user interfaces, and overall ease of use. Look at how transducer cords are managed, how easy the control surfaces are to clean, ease of cart mobility, are there locations for supplies that you will want on the cart?

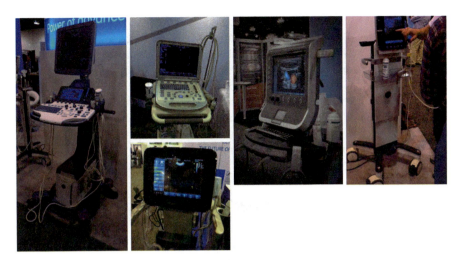

Fig. 13.6 Choosing your equipment: assess control surface layouts, user interfaces, and overall ease of use. Look at how transducer cords are managed, how easy the control surfaces are to clean, ease of cart mobility, are there locations for supplies that you will want on the cart?

User Education and Orientation Is Essential

A new ultrasound machine can cost as much as a small used plane or boat. No one should use the machine until they can demonstrate an understanding of proper start-up and shut down procedures, transducer selection, and image optimization. Most importantly, prospective users must be trained in the proper handling and storage of transducers (the most expensive part of the machine that is most likely to get broken). Education in proper care of your transducers is key. "In your hand, in the cup holder, or on your VISA" can be a useful mantra to instill appropriate user respect for transducer care and it will simultaneously remind your users to never leave an unsecured probe on a bed or tray table surface. Finally, all users need to demonstrate an understanding of proper cleanup procedures for transducers, cords, and control surfaces after use. Users should know where to return the ultrasound equipment after patient use, with all cords tidied and equipment plugged in for recharging. Education in equipment orientation and machine care should be included in all introductory US lectures.

Find a Safe Harbor

You will need to designate safe storage areas for your ultrasound machines when they are not in clinical use. Your equipment should be easy to locate by the clinician when needed and should be parked in a safe location where it can be plugged in for recharging and avoid getting prematurely dinged and broken. Lobby for front and center space that is convenient for the providers who will be using this equipment many times a day. Do not allow your equipment to be relegated to a back corner of your ED or other clinical care setting. Make sure you obtain appropriate signage to mark the storage areas and train your users and medical workers to return the ultrasound equipment to its designated home port when not in use. If you have multiple storage areas, label your machines with directions as to where the machine should be returned when done. Make sure to have your hospital electricians install the charging outlets at waist height for ease of use for the many providers who will be plugging the machines in and out many times a day.

Provision for the Journey Ahead

Streamline and automate the supply and distribution process as much as possible. Regular stocking and distribution of numerous ultrasound supplies will be required for smooth program operation. Enlist the support of your ED/ICU or clinic manager, and get your nursing staff and medical workers involved. Typical ultrasound supplies needed for a busy ED ultrasound program will include: a gel warmer in each patient care area, LOTS of US gel (this can add up to many hundreds of bottles a year), probe disinfection solutions or wipes, thermal print paper, squeezable gel-proof skin markers that will facilitate your many map-and-mark US procedures (Fig. 13.7). Since you will most likely also be using your machines for placing ultrasound-guided peripheral IVs in your difficult access patients, you will need a steady supply of sterile adhesive dressings, sterile probe covers, appropriate length needles for US-guided PIV access, chlorhexidine skin wipes, tourniquets, sterile surgical lubricant, catheter securing systems, and benzoin swabs, ideally all stocked and stored on your ultrasound cart for ease of use (Figs. 13.8 and 13.9).

Equipment cleaning and routine equipment maintenance is an unglamorous but essential component of your US program operation that cannot be overlooked. Day-to-day equipment care and oversight, as well as a host of preventive maintenance issues will need to be regularly attended to, some weekly, some monthly, some biannually. Day-to-day care includes routine cleaning of control

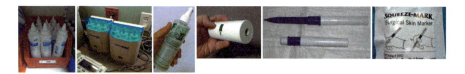

Fig. 13.7 Typical supply needs include US gel, gel warmers, low level disinfection sprays or wipes, thermal print paper, gel-proof markers for your "map and mark" procedures

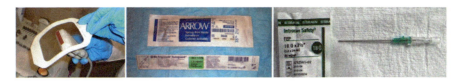

Fig. 13.8 US-guided PIV access supplies: sterile adhesive dressings, 48 mm and 64 mm needle options

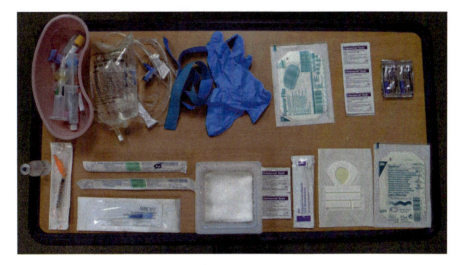

Fig. 13.9 Tray table layout of all the supplies needed for USG PIV line insertion: blood draw setup and tubes, spiked IV setup, tourniquets, non-sterile gloves, sterile adhesive dressing for probe cover, Chloraprep skin wipes, sterile surgical lubricant for US gel, (lidocaine and TB syringe optional for skin anesthesia, if needed), correct length US PIV needles, 48 and 64 mm, (NO standard 30 mm Angiocaths), gauze for skin cleanup after the line is placed, Chloraprep to remove any remaining gel/blood that may impede adhesion of the dressing, Benzoin swabs for added dressing adhesion success, sticky foam IV securing device or equivalent, final sterile adhesive dressing placed over the foam dressing to help prevent accidental line dislodgement

surfaces, inspection of transducers, transducer cords and power cords, cart cleanup after unanticipated exposures, as well as gel distribution and inspection of what needs restocking on the carts. Routine maintenance and cleaning seems to fall disproportionately onto US section staff unless you plan wisely. Enlist your ultrasound rotators, medical students, residents, and your faculty to help you, but above all, advocate for dedicated medical worker or ED manager time for these essential tasks. A maintenance checklist can be useful if you have many machines to care for and can provide an organized system for keeping track of which items will need attention or repair on which machines (Fig. 13.10).

ED Ultrasound Equipment Checklist				
Service Contact Name:				
Phone:		**Email:**		
Make/Model:				
Serial number:				
Transducers on cart: Serial numbers:				
Ancillary cart equipment:				
Maintenance Schedule:				
Control deck, transducer cup holders and cart clean?				
Transducers checked and clean? Midline marked?				
Trackball/trackpad clean and working?				
Transducer bungees correctly positioned?				
Control knobs damaged?				
Wiring and plugs checked?				
Any parts/attachments loose?				
Control deck labels intact?				
Filters and fans cleaned?				
Supply baskets stocked?				
Cart wheel lubrication/cleaning needed?				
Endocavitary probe cleaning station functioning?				
Gel warmers stocked?				
Printer with paper and functioning?				
Group e-mail reminder?				
Anything else?				

Fig. 13.10 US equipment checklist

What follows are some of the ultrasound equipment maintenance issues that you are likely encounter and will need to attend to.

Most day-to-day disinfection will be accomplished with a topical disinfectant spray such as T-Spray, Pi-Spray, or chlorhexidine disinfectant wipes on the probes and control surfaces. Isopropyl alcohol soaked gauze can be used on the cart body (A more detailed review of probe disinfection is discussed in another chapter) (Fig. 13.11). Transducer storage cups will inevitably become a repository for dust and dried adherent ultrasound gel and they will need regular (at least weekly) cleaning. A short bottlebrush purchased in any hardware store comes in handy for cleaning these transducer cup holders very efficiently, and will be particularly useful if

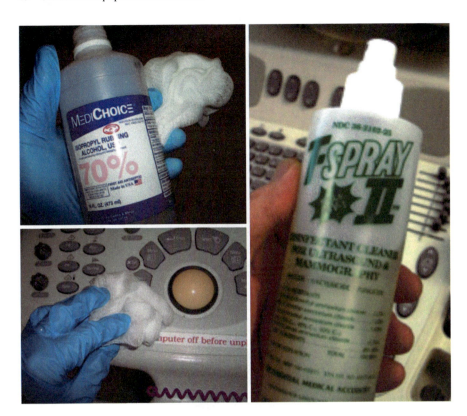

Fig. 13.11 Products for daily cleaning of the US machine

you have a lot of machines to maintain. The large Q-tips that you might carry on your OB/GYN cart may also be used for this purpose (Fig. 13.12).

Inspect your transducers and transducer cords for defects and cracks. You should not be using transducers with cracks on the scan head or splits in the housing or cord cover. If you find such defects you need to make arrangements to have the transducer replaced (Fig. 13.13).

Set up an equipment maintenance supply bucket and stock it with products you will need for tackling the various mystery fluids and adhesive assaults your machine will inevitably encounter. Useful agents include hydrogen peroxide for dried blood, isopropyl alcohol, bleach wipes, or general-purpose spray surface cleaners for cart body cleaning (Fig. 13.14). Do not use isopropyl alcohol to clean your transducer cords. You will additionally need to purchase a non-acetone based adhesive-removal solvent like Goo Gone or Goof Off. There isn't much else that will safely remove the adhesive goo that will inevitably mar your control surfaces, cart body and cart wheels. Adhesive foam EKG electrodes, foam IV securing devices, remnants of patient labels,

Fig. 13.12 A short bottle brush or GYN Q-tips work well for cleaning out dust and gel from transducer cup holders

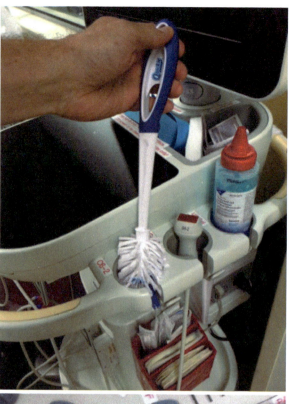

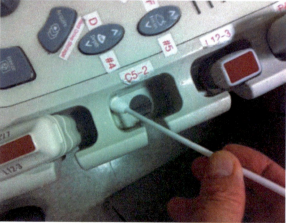

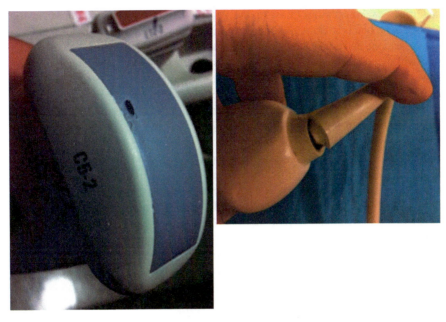

Fig. 13.13 Transducers with visible defects such as these will need to be replaced

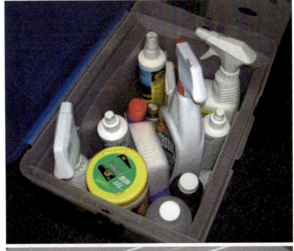

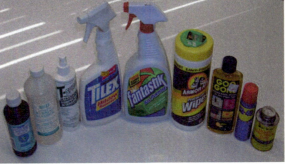

Fig. 13.14 The US fleet cleaning and maintenance supply bucket, ready for any eventuality

and dried benzoin splashes (most vexing!) appear to be the most common offenders; hopefully no one is sticking used bubble gum under your deck! Do <u>not</u> be tempted to use the acetone nail polish wipes you might have in your ED for this purpose. Although they will successfully remove adherent adhesive items or residue, they might also dissolve and irrevocably mar the plastic surfaces of your cart or control panel in the process! (Fig. 13.15). Periodically oiling the wheels of your US cart can help keep them gliding smoothly, and a can of compressed air comes in handy for cleaning out dust in any fan openings and in the TGC nooks and crannies if you have an older machine with button-based TGC controls (Figs. 13.16 and 13.17).

What should you do when you show up to a shift and find a blood-spattered machine, blood on the transducers and cords, or if you frequently encounter dirty transducer probe covers that have not been removed after use? (Fig. 13.18). Repetitive maladaptive behaviors need to be addressed and should merit the occasional group e-mail and photo reminding your staff members of their equipment cleanup obligations after any ultrasound-guided procedure or after the evaluation of a bloody trauma patient. Periodic "public service announcement" reminders during your US conferences can also be helpful to inculcate good equipment cleanup habits and establish a culture of shared responsibility for US equipment cleanliness. You will additionally need to periodically remind your staff that the ultrasound control panel is NOT to be

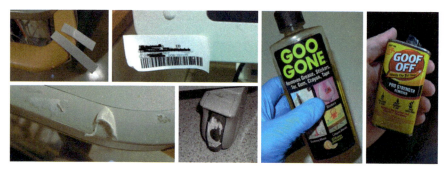

Fig. 13.15 Essential adhesive-removal solvents that will be needed for equipment cleaning; no acetone!

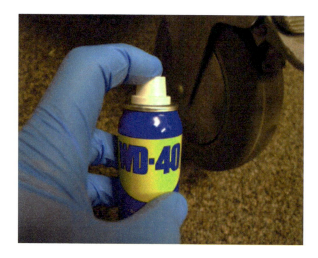

Fig. 13.16 Caster wheels will roll more smoothly with occasional oiling

used as a storage surface for coffee, used intubation blades, and random supplies being distributed about the ED or ICU (Fig. 13.19). A spilled cup of coffee on an unsealed ultrasound control panel can turn into a very costly misadventure. Start your group e-mail with the gentle subject line "It takes a village…."

If you have an active ultrasound training program and multiple ultrasound machines in use, you will likely find yourself using prodigious amounts of ultrasound gel (Fig. 13.20). Outsource this stocking and distribution task if you can, as it can add up to many hundreds of bottles to distribute each year. Although buying your ultrasound gel in 5 L bulk containers is cheaper, it is safer to stick with prefilled bottles since bacterial contamination with Pseudomonas and Klebsiella and Staph species has been reported to occur from refilling used ultrasound gel bottles. Other

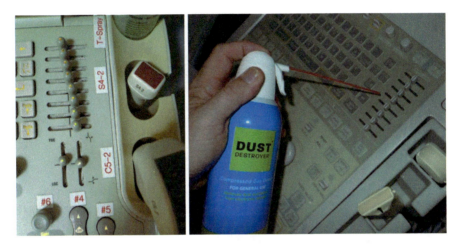

Fig. 13.17 A can of compressed air will help clean out dusty TGC buttons on older machines

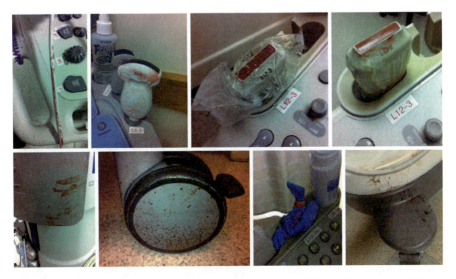

Fig. 13.18 The wall of shame: your staff will need periodic reminders of their responsibility to remove used probe covers and clean the machine after a messy trauma room encounter

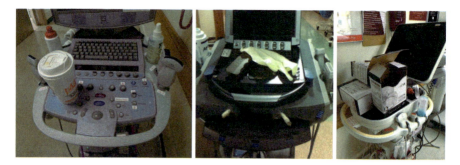

Fig. 13.19 The US control panel should not be used as a storage surface; strongly discourage such behaviors

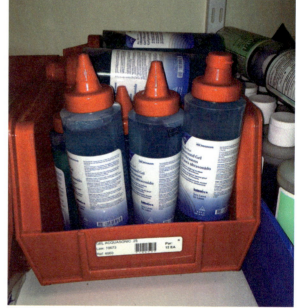

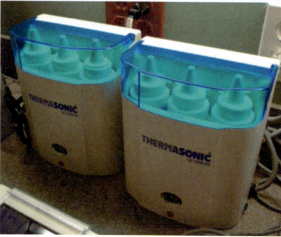

Fig. 13.20 Place a gel warmer in each patient care area and make sure you have easy access to extra gel for restocking

ultrasound coupling agents have been touted to be equally effective and less messy; in the future, we may be using small amounts of a residue-free ultrasound coupling liquid applied with a cloth just prior to scanning.

US Machine Cleaning

(See Chap. 15 – Safety and Infection Control for probe cleaning)

Preventive Maintenance

This is somewhat machine dependent but may include any or all of the following:

Basic Toolkit

Invest in a basic multipurpose toolkit that includes slotted and Phillips screwdrivers, and an adjustable wrench so you can tighten up some of the common trouble spots on your carts. Many ultrasound machines will use Torx type screws, so a folding Torx wrench may come in handy. Common cart trouble spots include cart housing screws, power cord attachment sites, and wheel assemblies. Having a few basic tools available will allow you to attend to some of these machine specific problems yourself (Fig. 13.21).

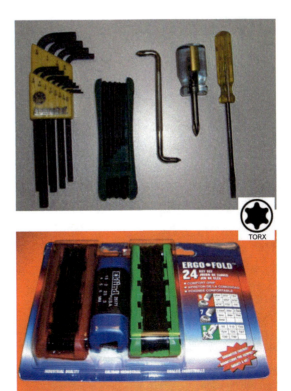

Fig. 13.21 It is helpful to have a basic equipment repair toolkit for some of the cart items that you will periodically want to adjust or tighten up yourself. Many carts use a Torx based system

Cleaning the Track Ball

You can learn how to do it yourself or have it done during semiannual preventive maintenance visits. Why bother? The internal trackball mechanism gets coated with US gel over time impairing its function. A track pad or touch screen panel avoids this problem altogether (Fig. 13.22).

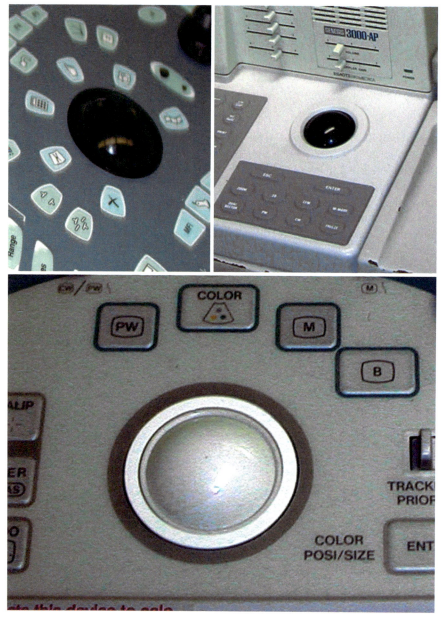

Fig. 13.22 Trackballs need periodic cleaning to remove ultrasound gel that can impede smooth trackball function

Filter and Fan Care

The ED is a VERY dusty place. Many ultrasound units have dedicated power supplies with cooling fans and filters to keep the electronics from overheating. Ideally these filters should be cleaned every few months. Waiting for a biannual or annual preventive maintenance visit is often inadequate and the filters may be clogged up by then. The filters need to be removed, washed with soap and water, then dried and replaced. If you don't clean them, the fans will no longer function efficiently, and your electronics can overheat, give you error messages or crash your equipment software. Any piece of equipment in your clinical care setting that has an onboard cooling fan running will inevitably vacuum up lots of ever-present dust. This is yet another reason why we should not leave our ultrasound machines running when not in use (Fig. 13.23).

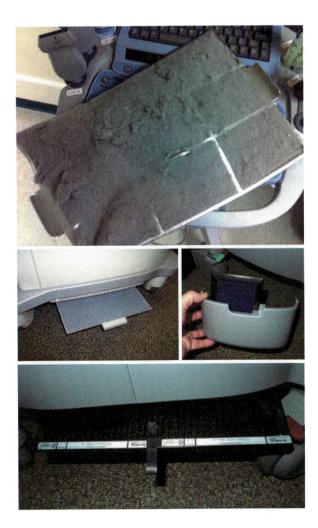

Fig. 13.23 The ER is a very dusty place. Onboard filters should be cleaned every several months to avoid overheated electronics. Once a year cleaning is inadequate

Fig. 13.24 A VCR head cleaner will help maintain good quality video images if you are still using this type of image storage medium

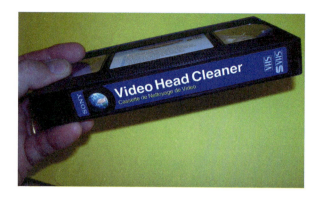

VCRs/CD Recorders

Not a lot of people are still recording ultrasound images with videotape, but if you still use this medium for image review, your VCR's image quality can be improved by using a $5–$10 tape head cleaner every few months (Fig. 13.24). Digital image capture devices like CD recorders simply need a periodic cleaning of the control surfaces and a periodic check of their plugs and connectors.

Tighten the Loose Stuff

Problem spots are machine specific. Your biomedical engineering folks or your equipment repair tech can point out what gets attended to on a routine preventive maintenance visit. Power cord holders on some older machines need monthly attention to keep them from loosening and falling off due to the heavy forces placed on them.

Broken Control Surface Buttons

Older machines often have plastic buttons that dry out and crack after having been T-Sprayed a few thousand times; TGC control buttons seem to be the first to break down. You can order a bag of replacement buttons and knobs from your ultrasound equipment vendor and with a bag of replacements handy you can address these small annoyances yourself (Fig. 13.25).

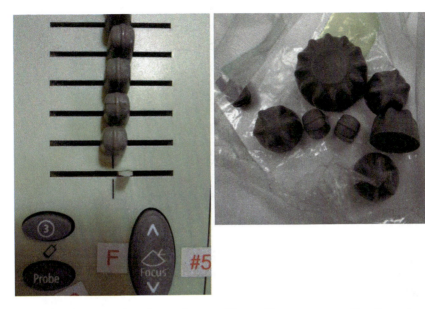

Fig. 13.25 Buy a bag of new buttons for your older machines so you can replace them when they break

Ultrasound Cart Wheel Assemblies

The plastic wheel housings on some ultrasound carts are poorly designed for the rigors of clinical use and will predictably loosen and fall off. This is mostly a cosmetic issue. The plastic housing simply hides the fact that the wheels get mightily gunked up over time, usually with a combination of dried blood, EKG electrode stickies, foam IV securing devices, tape of various sorts, and unbelievable amounts of hair! (Fig. 13.26). When your cart starts to shimmy or be noticeably difficult to roll around, it is time to give the wheels some attention. Ultrasound cart wheel assemblies need periodic cleaning and oiling, removal of the many adherent adhesive items with a solvent like Goo Gone or Goof Off, and the occasional haircut (forceps and scissors work best, high and tight!). The foot controlled wheel locking switches get very dirty over time but can be easily cleaned with any general-purpose spray cleaner and a bristle brush or old toothbrush. Seriously unglamorous stuff (Fig. 13.27).

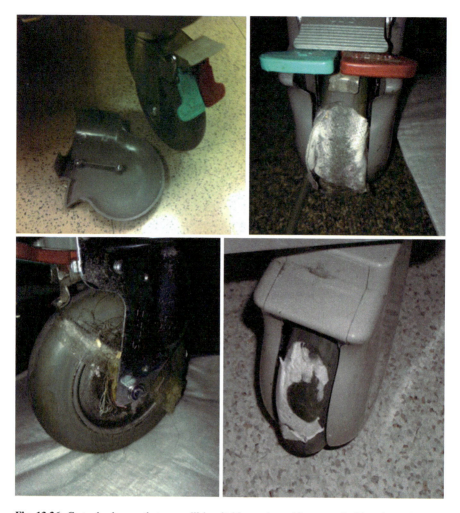

Fig. 13.26 Cart wheel woes that you will inevitably need to address: cracked housings, glued on EKG electrodes, dressing materials, foam IV securing devices, and more hair than you can imagine

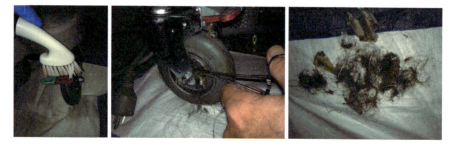

Fig. 13.27 Cart wheel cleaning: soak and brush off the foot pedals, forceps and scissors for the haircuts. Wear gloves!

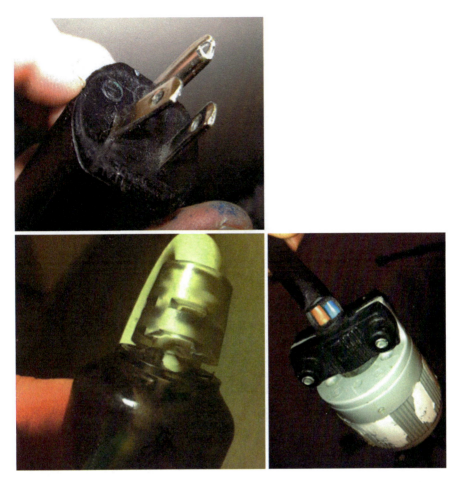

Fig. 13.28 Power cord plug end woes: bent pins, a cracked housing, exposed wires: all bad, time for replacement

Wiring Check

Power cord plug ends take lots of abuse. The machines get plugged in and out many times a day, 365 days a year, and occasionally the cord will take an extra whack when people move the ultrasound machine having forgotten that it is still plugged in. When the plug pins get bent, if the plug end housing is cracked and has wires peeking through anywhere, or if the power cord has nicks in it from being run over a few too many times it is time for repair or replacement (Fig. 13.28). It can be helpful to have a backup power cord on hand. If you just need to replace a bent plug pin that you can no longer straighten, you can have your hospital electrician install a new hospital grade plug end (Fig. 13.29). Periodically you should also visually inspect the power cord for nicks and defects in the housing.

Fig. 13.29 The famed
"Hospital Grade" plug

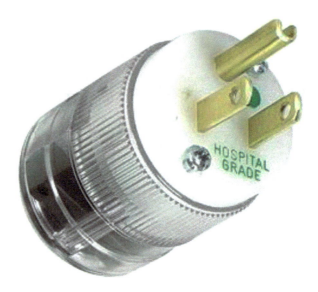

Ideally, a well-designed machine should have all important wiring hidden and protected within the cart or housing. This is rare with older machines in particular. Important but exposed wiring can get disconnected. Velcro cable ties (1/2 × 6 in., purchased at any hardware store) can be used to help neaten up this clutter and can help keep your equipment wiring tidy and out of harm's way.

Customizing

Customizing your new ultrasound equipment to suit your specific practice needs is an essential and fun part of the process of getting your machine ready for use in your clinical setting. Even after many years in the business and many (14!) machine purchases later, I have yet to see an ultrasound machine that didn't benefit from customization and modifications to make it more user friendly and better suited to our ED practice setting. All our ultrasound machines start out their lives in the Ultrasound Section "Chop Shop" (our Ultrasound Section office) before they get launched into the ED. If you buy several machines at a time you can do them up in bulk.

Essential Supplies

So what are the essentials? You're going to need some 4″ × 2″ industrial Velcro strips, ¾″ Velcro sticky-back tape, ¾″ × 8″ Velcro cable ties, plastic cable ties, metal extension springs or Kevlar/polycarbonate retractable key fobs, coiled plastic key rings and clips, and some metal key rings (Fig. 13.30).

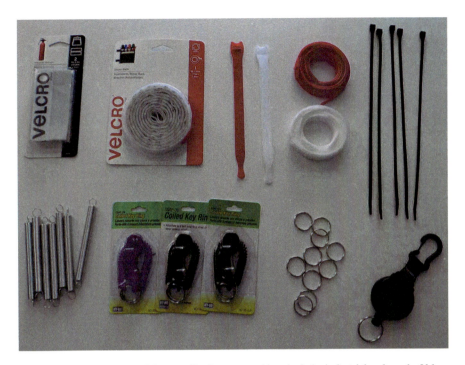

Fig. 13.30 Essential customizing supplies for new machines include: industrial and regular Velcro sticky-back tape, Velcro cable ties, plastic cable ties, piano wire extension springs, coiled key, metal key rings, and robust key fobs

Transducers and Transducer Cords

Implementing a system to protect your transducers and transducer cords will be your number one customizing task. Surprisingly little attention has been paid to this issue by ultrasound vendors, likely due to the fact that historically, ultrasound carts were mostly parked in one location and the patient was brought to that location for imaging. Most older ultrasound machines were very poorly designed for high mobility applications. Newer point-of-care machines and carts are much better designed in terms of footprint, wheel assemblies and simplified keyboards, but they are still mostly lacking in good transducer cord management solutions. At 4000 to over 10,000 dollars each times three to four transducers on each machine, you have a big incentive to protect these most essential and pricy parts of your ultrasound fleet. If your transducer cords are not properly secured it is almost guaranteed that you will at some point in time find a transducer cord snugly wrapped around one of your ultrasound cart's caster wheels (Fig. 13.31). While this will predictably cause you severe agita and might even bring the occasional tear to an ultrasound director's eye, it is an entirely avoidable event.

Transducer trauma can be likened to neuro trauma. For the transducer head, the closed head injury model applies. You drop it, your crystals get damaged, and things

Fig. 13.31 A transducer cord wrapped around a cart caster wheel; guaranteed agitation

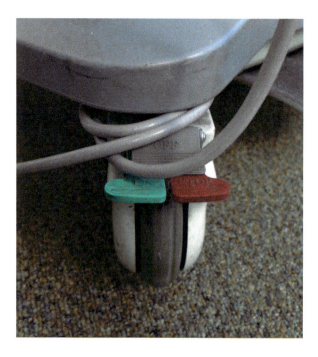

are never quite the same thereafter. User education on proper transducer care is the best preventive medicine to keep this type of trauma from occurring. Users should be taught from the outset that the transducer is very expensive, somewhat fragile, and should always be protected. There should be zero tolerance for laying the probe on a stretcher, a tray table, or on top of the ultrasound machine. "In your hand, in the cup holder, or on your VISA" is a useful mantra for inculcating good transducer care behaviors.

For the transducer cord, the spinal cord injury model applies. An unsecured transducer cord will drape onto the floor, and will at some point inevitably get run over and caught in the cart's wheel assembly. As a result, the cord housing may be violated, some essential wiring may have been severed, and the transducer rendered less than optimal, possibly useless. For this issue there is a simple fix: don't let the cord ever hit the floor.

Transducer and transducer cord protection can take on many forms. Years ago I had our hospital welder build a stainless steel cage for cord storage on a "mobile" 285 lb machine that was probably originally designed to just sit it one location and not be moved around a lot. (But what a good workout we got every shift!) The idea of a transducer cord bungee system began many years ago when Dr. Anthony Dean sent me pictures demonstrating how he used a bicycle cable, some coiled key rings and carabiners to improvise a system to keep his transducer cords from draping onto the floor, getting run over and traumatized (Fig. 13.32). I used the coiled key

Fig. 13.32 Early
transducer cord bungee
system: 2004, thanks to Dr.
Anthony Dean

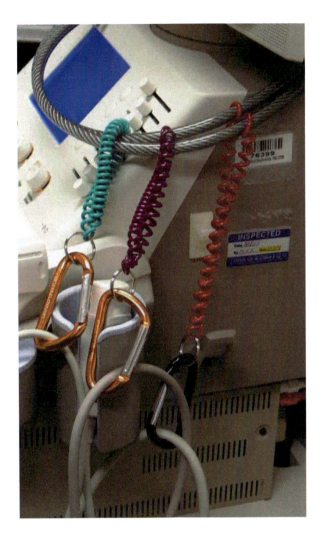

rings he suggested but modified the system by adding ¾ in. × 8 in. Velcro cable ties to the key ring bungees, so there would be a firm but still adjustable point of attachment to the transducer cord. Total cost for the system was about $2.50 per cord (Fig. 13.33).

So what is the process? Attach the Velcro cable tie snug around the transducer cord, and then wrap it through the key ring several times, adjusting the Velcro attachment to a location along the mid length of the cord such that the cord can never hit the floor. Depending on the machine and number of transducer cords and attachment sites, you can either bundle several transducer cords together or wrap them individually (Fig. 13.34). Some machines may end up with four individual

Fig. 13.33 Transducer cord bungee parts, next version: coiled key rings and ¾″ × 8″ Velcro cable ties

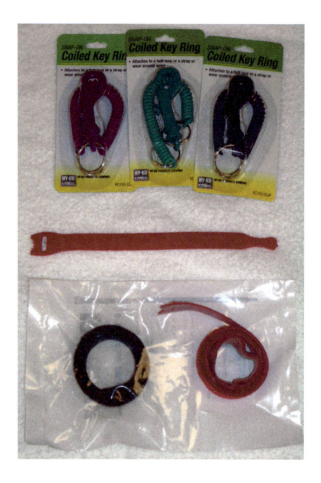

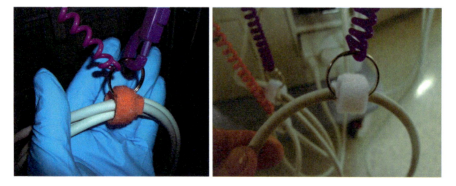

Fig. 13.34 Transducer cords can be bundled together or attached individually, depending on the machine.

Fig. 13.35 A four-transducer ultrasound machine with cord bungees in place; note that the cords never touch the floor

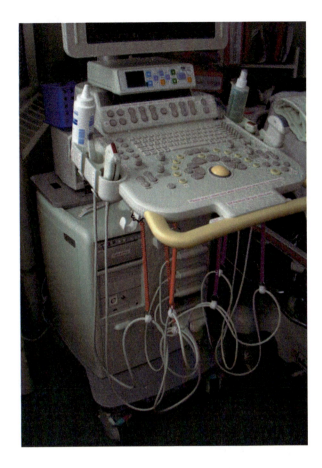

transducer cord bungees (Fig. 13.35) Points of attachment are going to be dictated by what you have available to work with on the underside of the machine in question. You can use plastic cable ties to provide an attachment site to the underside of the frame if no other suitable locations can be found.

The return on your investment is fantastic! $30 in supplies can provide protection for about $30,000 worth of transducers. The only down side with the coiled key ring bungee system is that over time, the coiled plastic will stretch out and lose some of it springiness, so they will need periodic replacement.

After digging around in my local hardware store's spring section, my more recent iteration of this bungee system replaces the coiled key rings with a 4.5 in. stainless steel extension spring (rated maximum load 1.61 lbs., part number 304, Jones Spring Company, about $1.50 apiece). After 3 years of use on multiple ED ultrasound machines these piano wire extension springs have worked very well and are much more robust than the coiled plastic key ring bungees used previously (Fig. 13.36a).

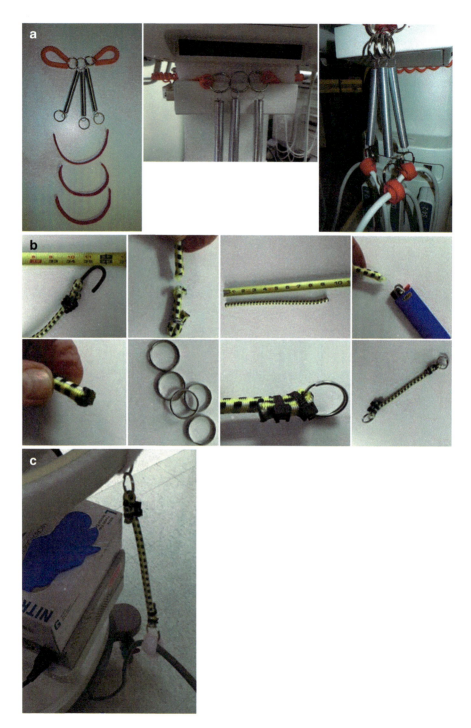

Fig. 13.36 (**a**) Newer transducer cord bungee system using coiled key rings, extension springs, metal key rings and Velcro cable ties. Close-ups of setup technique. (**b**) Technique for fashioning a custom power cord bungee. (**c**) Intalled custom power cord bungee

A similar cord bungee solution can also be used to keep your power cords from getting run over. One option is to use a metal extension spring that has a higher maximum load rating (Jones Spring company, part number 306, rated maximum load 2.61 lbs.) as a bungee device suitable for use on the ultrasound machine's heavier power cord. Most recently I have found that a short piece of actual bungee cord can be easily customized and very successfully employed for this purpose (Figs. 13.36b, c).

One final transducer cord bungee option uses a retractable key ring system with an extraordinarily robust polycarbonate and Kevlar retractable key fob (KEY-BAK #488B—about $13 apiece) that serves as a stellar cord bungee device (thank you Dr. Mike Stone for finding this!). If you chose this option and have lots of machines to outfit, your initial outlay for supplies may be several hundred dollars, but this is still cheap when compared to the price of the equipment being protected. The key fobs can be attached with a Velcro cable tie similar to the extension spring based system, one retractable fob for each cord (Fig. 13.37).

Once the Velcro cable ties are attached to the transducer cord and adjusted to the optimal location that keeps the cord off the floor, you can mark the cord's "sweet spot" with a gentian violet skin marker to make this location readily visually apparent. (Tape off the edges of this designated "sweet spot" about 1.5 in. apart, and make sure you wear gloves when applying the marker ink! Remove the tape when dry.) If added transducer cord length is needed for a procedure such as a central line placement, you can simply slide the transducer cord through its snug (but not immobile) Velcro cable tie attachment in order to lengthen the amount of transducer cord available. When the procedure is done, you simply slide the cord bungee back to its visually prominent "sweet spot" ensuring once again, that your transducer cords will not hit the floor and get run over (Fig. 13.38).

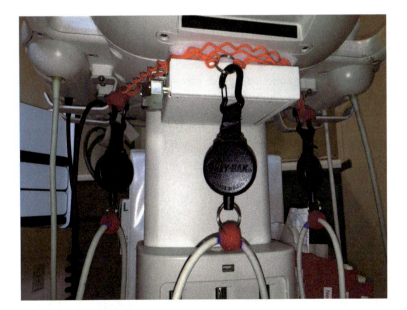

Fig. 13.37 Key fob bungee set up, same idea, key fobs used instead of extension springs

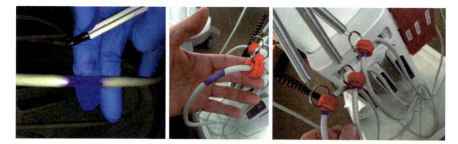

Fig. 13.38 Mark the sweet spot along the cord where the Velcro cable tie keeps the transducer cord off the floor. Tape off the area first, wear gloves, and remove tape when dry. The transducer cord can slide out from its usual attachment site if a longer length is needed for a procedure. Return the cable tie and cord bungee back to the easily visible "sweet spot" when done

Fig. 13.39 Spiral loom—another transducer cord protection strategy

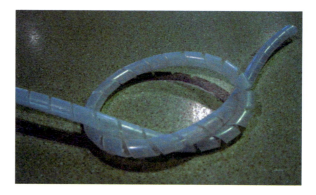

Another suggested transducer cord protection approach forwarded to me by Dr. Hal Minnigan is to armor coat the proximal transducer cord with a thick spiral plastic material (spiral loom) (Fig. 13.39). The transducer cord near the floor is thereby protected with a much more rigid exterior coating.

After many years of requests for more robust transducer cords, one vendor now offers armored cable technology with an armored cable jacket surrounding the electrical conductors of their transducer cords.

There are many other ultrasound equipment modifications that can make our machines more user friendly and fun and I will briefly run through some of these additional modifications below.

Power Cords

Power cords can present any one of a number of challenges. An overly stiff power cord can be difficult to coil up when the machine is stored, plug end pins will inevitably get broken or bent, power cord storage sites on the cart are often placed in ergonomically challenging locations, and these attachment sites may break from overuse/excessive force. I have yet to see an ultrasound machine with a

Fig. 13.40 A low power cord attachment site: a poor design feature for any mobile US machine that needs to be backed into a patient care area, and a guarantee that the power cord will be run over

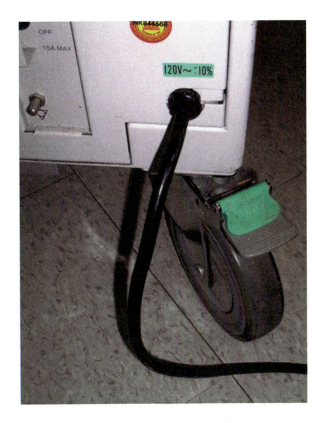

well-designed power cord storage solution. A low power cord attachment site on the back of the ultrasound cart is a poor design feature for a machine that is typically rolled into a corner of a patient examining room (Fig. 13.40). Inevitably, the power cord will get run over and impede cart movement in the process. A simple work-around involves creating a higher power cord tether point so that the cord will not contact the caster wheels when the machine is pushed into the corner of a room. Tethering options include using coiled key rings (they will stretch out with time, however), using the heavier gauge wire extension springs mentioned above (part #306) to create a power cord bungee (attach with metal key rings and Velcro cable ties), or using a small piece of actual bungee cord customized for the job. Alternatively you can just tether the power cord with Velcro sticky-back tape to a higher location on the back of the cart handle or frame if such a space is available; make sure you do this at maximal cart height so you don't limit the cart's potential for vertical adjustment (Fig. 13.41).

What about other power cord solutions? Retractable cord systems are already found on many portable X-ray machines. My 10⁺-year-old vacuum cleaner has a trouble-free retractable power cord system, so why haven't we yet seen something like this on an ultrasound machine to help provide us with a convenient cord man-agement solution? Or at the very minimum, a robust, well-designed, and

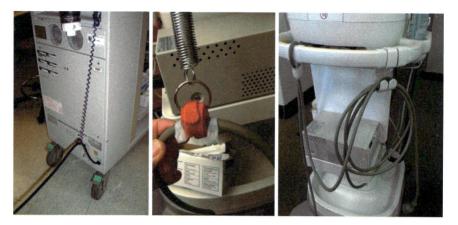

Fig. 13.41 Three power cord tethering solutions: use a coiled key ring bungee, or a more robust extension spring, or tether the power cord to the back handle of the cart if this option is available. See Fig. 13.36c for the custom power cord bungee option

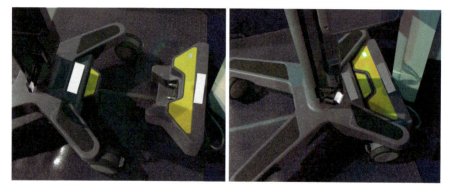

Fig. 13.42 A docking station system for recharging the ultrasound machine. No power cord issues here

ergonomically located cord storage area integral to the cart, not a cheaply made, plastic, and poorly located afterthought destined for an early demise. After many years of requests, one vendor now offers a retractable power cord system on their US cart; hopefully, more will follow. Another appealing option would be to avoid having a power cord altogether. One ultrasound equipment vendor offers a no-cord option with a power docking station on the cart base. The machine slides onto a fixed charging port when it is placed in its storage area to recharge its battery (Fig. 13.42).

In our search for electrons to feed our point-of-care buddy, it is not uncommon to find that the only available outlet in the patient care booth is located in a poorly accessible and ergonomically challenging location. With advancements in battery

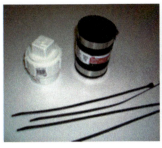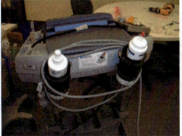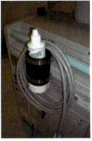

Fig. 13.43 Supply holders for your US gel and disinfectant sprays made from common hardware store plumbing supplies and plastic cable ties. Plastic cable ties were used to attach them to the cart body or the cart handle. Here they do double duty as power cord holders

technology and induction-based battery charging systems we can hope for a time in the not too distant future when we can move away from the tether of a power cord on our ultrasound equipment altogether.

Gel and Cleaning Spay Holders

Some of our older machines were designed without much thought as to where ultrasound gel and cleaning spray were to be stored. Common hardware store supplies such as PVC pipe ends and rubber plumbing parts can be easily fashioned into US gel and cleaning spray holders. These storage cups can then do double duty and serve as a convenient place to store your power cord as well (Fig. 13.43).

Small Parts Transducer Holder

Shortly after purchase of a brand new $10,000 small parts transducer, I attached it and placed it in the cup holder of a $100,000+ US machine for storage, whereupon it slipped right through the opening and onto the floor! There was no mention from the vendor that the built-in cup holders would not work for this transducer, and no vendor work-around or remedy was offered or suggested. So, another invitation to customize. Our hospital plumbers happened to be working in the ED that week installing some thick but flexible adhesive plastic bathroom baseboard. A small piece of this product was easily trimmed to size with scissors and a scalpel, with just the right size opening for the transducer cord but too small for the hockey stick transducer to fall through. Make sure to place it sticky side down to glue it firmly into the base of the cup holder. Another problem successfully MacGuyvered and working fine for many years now (Fig. 13.44).

Fig. 13.44 A transducer cup holder modification for a hockey stick transducer: a piece of sticky-back plastic baseboard has been cut to size to keep the probe from falling through

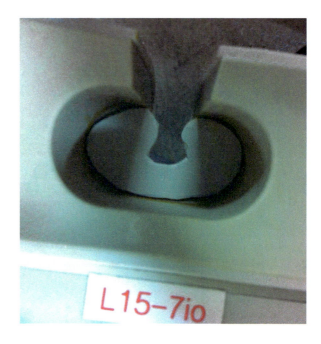

US Carts Are Not Sacrosanct!

If needed, you can customize your ultrasound cart with some conveniently located screws to attach something else to. Call the company and find out if anything important is located on the portion of the cart body that you want to drill into. Pick a structurally solid area for your point of attachment, drill and attach your cable ties or screws as needed.

Color Code Your Transducers

Like most US cart modifications, this one began as a poor design work-around. One vendor's product required that you visually follow the transducer cord back to the underside of the machine to determine which of the three available transducer switches you needed to activate to use that transducer. Color-coding the individual transducers, their respective switches and their designated cup holders made activation of the correct transducer for clinical use much easier (Fig. 13.45).

US Cart Supplies

Among the many point-of-care applications you will be using your ultrasound equipment for, you will very likely be using your machines to insert substantial numbers of US-guided peripheral lines in your difficult access patients. If this is the

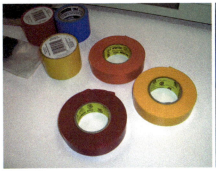
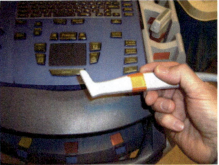

Fig. 13.45 Colored electrical tape used to make transducer activation easier and to ensure each transducer is returned to its designated up cup holder

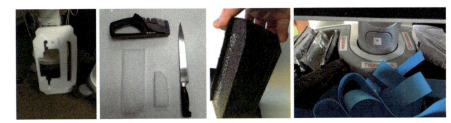

Fig. 13.46 Save the hard packing foam that arrives with a new machine. You can easily cut it into custom dividers for your storage areas. Use Velcro sticky-back tape to hold the dividers in place

case, it is most helpful to have your US carts fully stocked with all the requisite procedural supplies, roll-up and ready to go.

For efficient US PIV program operation you will want to stock your cart with tourniquets, Chloraprep skin wipes, sterile adhesive dressings (one to cover your probe and another to apply over the foam dressing at the end of the procedure), sterile surgical lubricant, a box of non-sterile gloves, a foam vein-securing device, appropriate length peripheral IV needles (48 mm and 64 mm), and benzoin swabs.

The hard packing foam that comes with a new machine and some Velcro sticky-back tape can be easily fashioned into a storage space divider to help keep your supplies neat and organized (Fig. 13.46). Get creative with what you have available. Your empty sterile adhesive dressing boxes can be trimmed and taped together with colored duct tape and be repurposed into sturdy supply organizers (Fig. 13.47). Find a suitable site on the cart to attach your new supply organizer and industrial Velcro sticky-back tape will take care of the rest (Fig. 13.48). Label the individual compartments of your storage spaces and supply box cubbies to help keep your supplies organized and facilitate restocking. Other machines might have a suitable location where you can attach a small plastic supply basket that you can purchase at any hardware store. Attach the baskets to the cart with a coiled key ring and Velcro cable ties or Velcro sticky-back tape. Location will be dictated by what free cart surfaces you have available to work with. Laminate and attach a restocking list on the side of

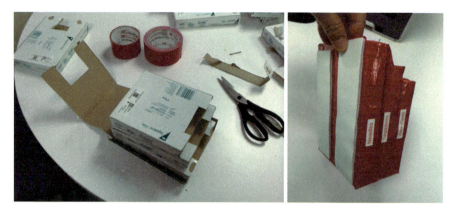

Fig. 13.47 Repurpose your empty sterile adhesive dressing boxes. Attach them together with colored duct tape, place the industrial Velcro sticky-back tape on the back, and then find a suitable place on your cart to attach it to. Label the individual cubbies to facilitate stocking and keep things neat

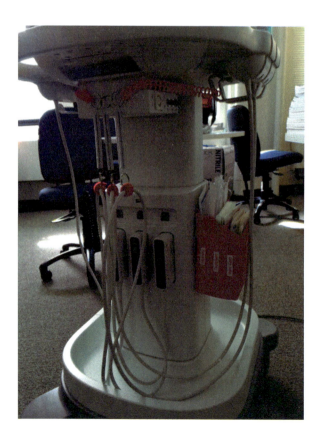

Fig. 13.48 Your new homemade supply organizer attached to the cart with industrial Velcro sticky-back tape

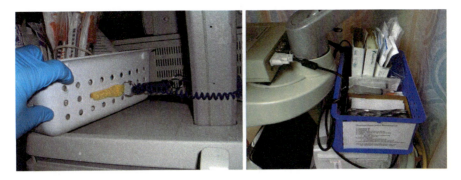

Fig. 13.49 Other supply organizer options: plastic supply baskets, attached with Velcro cable ties and coiled key rings or industrial Velcro. Add a laminated restocking list to the supply basket to remind others what needs to go on the cart

Fig. 13.50 Custom wooden bracket probe wipe holder made by a hospital carpenter, picture thanks to Dr. Hal Minnigan

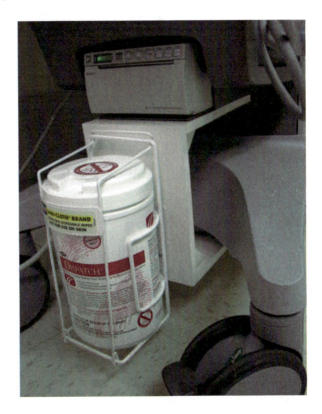

the storage basket to remind (other) people what needs to be restocked (Fig. 13.49). Your hospital carpenters may be able to help you out as well. Dr. Hal Minnigan had them build a custom bracket on his ultrasound cart to hold a container of probe wipes (Fig. 13.50).

Fig. 13.51 Industrial
Velcro: for attaching
aftermarket equipment and
supply baskets to your
carts

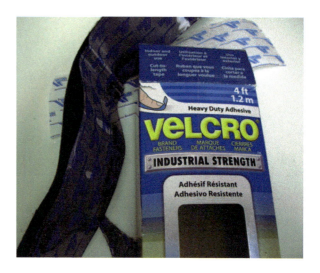

Industrial Velcro

It is amazing what Velcro can hold in place; if you have any doubts, watch the
Letterman Velcro Suit clip on You Tube sometime. You can attach all manner of
aftermarket devices to your cart with it (digital image recorders, portable wireless
access point devices, supply storage boxes, etc.) (Fig. 13.51). Now that wireless
features are built into many new US systems, however, we have less need for some
of these aftermarket add-ons.

Label Maker

Without a doubt, you should buy one. This is a relatively cheap item ($30–$100
dollars) that will give you a big bang for your buck (Fig. 13.52). It will quickly
become an essential part of your headache reduction plan. Use it to remind people
where the machine needs to be returned to, that the machine should be plugged in
when stored, and that the transducers need to be cleaned after each use (some users
still seem to think there is an automatic probe cleaning feature on board) (Fig. 13.53).
On our older machines with far too many control surface buttons, we highlighted
the seven most commonly used buttons in numerical sequence for ease of use.
Labeling your transducer cups will help remind users to return each transducer to its
designated location, thereby avoiding cord spaghetti.

Velcro and Plastic Cable Ties

Use them to keep any exposed wiring or cables neat and organized.

Fig. 13.52 A label maker: an essential part of your armamentarium. Buy one

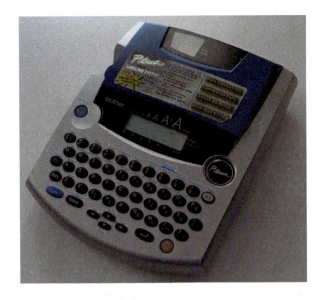

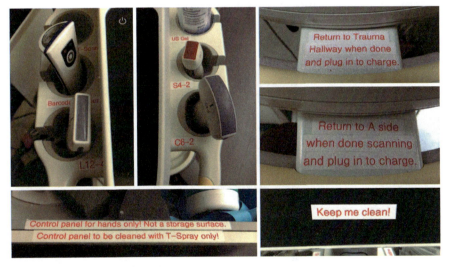

Fig. 13.53 Labels gone wild! They will help keep your fleet clean, safely stored, charged up, and help minimize avoidable damage

Midline Markers

After many years of requests to add this feature, several US vendors now have a midline mark etched onto the short axis face of their linear and curved array transducers (Fig. 13.54). This midline mark helps improve the accuracy of the many "map and mark" or free-hand ultrasound-guided procedures we perform. If you don't have them etched on your transducers already, you can add this feature

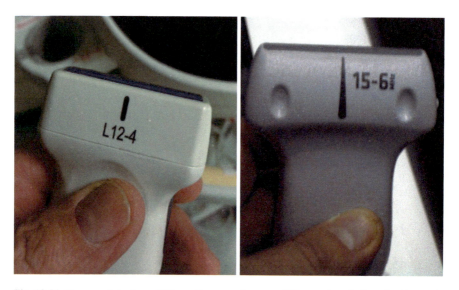

Fig. 13.54 Newer point-of-care US machines now have a midline mark etched on the short axis face of their linear array and curved array transducers. This improves your "map and mark" and free-hand procedure accuracy

Fig. 13.55 For older transducers with no midline markers, map the midline carefully, tape off with electrical tape and then mark the short axis face on both sides of the transducer with an indelible marker. Remove tape when dry

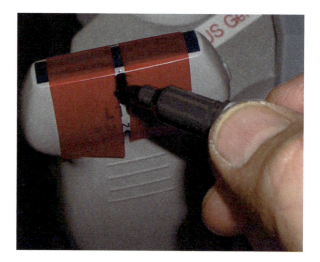

yourself. Measure carefully, mask off the short axis midline with some electrician's tape, and then mark the area yourself with an indelible marker. You will need to "repaint" the area periodically, however, since your marker ink will eventually wear off (Fig. 13.55).

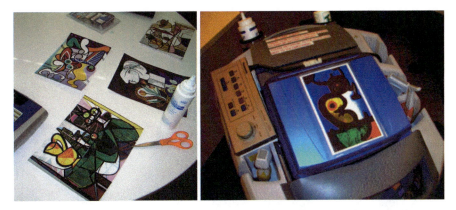

Fig. 13.56 Class up your artistically challenged work environment. Add some art to your machines with a clear self-adhesive laminating sheet or have a custom adhesive skin made as for a laptop

Artwork

Most EDs are artistically challenged places, so customize your ultrasound machines with some artwork that you and others can enjoy in your daily work life. Find some generally acceptable artwork you like and attach it with a clear self-adhesive laminating sheet (Fig. 13.56) or have a custom adhesive skin made for your machine's cart as is commonly done for laptops. Hospital CT scanners and portable X-ray machines are now often seen with artwork decals affixed to their surfaces, so why not the same for our ED ultrasound equipment?

Anthropomorphize Your Fleet

Whether you have only one machine or an entire fleet to care for, naming your machine(s) can have a number of positive downstream benefits. Surprisingly, people seem to take better care of your ultrasound machines when you anthropomorphize them. Our ED fleet's oldest machines are now affectionately known as Grandma and Grandpa; we also have Miro (with nice artwork on his laptop cover), Thing One and Thing Two (thank you, Dr. Seuss), T-Bird in our Trauma hallway, Graucho, Chico, and Harpo in our Simulation Center, and Zeppo in our Pedi ED. Our latest arrivals were bestowed with the names Yoda and Obi-Wan (May the Force be with you!). As an added benefit, when you have many machines and something goes wrong in your ultrasound family, it helps to know which one of your kids is in trouble so you can easily arrange for appropriate remediation.

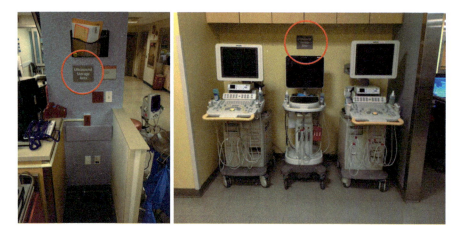

Fig. 13.57 Plant your flag. Mark your equipment storage area with appropriate signage to keep out interlopers. Have your hospital electricians place the outlets up high to save your back

Signage

Nature abhors a void, especially in a busy ED. Once you have staked out your ultrasound storage areas you should claim your turf and plant your flag with appropriate signage. Have your hospital's sign supplier make up a number of "Ultrasound Storage Area Only" signs for you to hang on the wall where your machines will be parked (Fig. 13.57). Otherwise, that storage space will quickly fill up with all manner of interlopers such as IV poles, wheelchairs, EKG machines, thermometer/BP/pulse oximetry carts, WOWs, and what have you as soon as you take your machines out to use them. As noted previously, have your hospital electricians place the outlets up high so you can easily plug the machines in and out 15–20 times a shift without wrecking your back. If you have new construction ongoing in your physical plant, make sure you are involved in the design process early on. Ensure that you will have designated storage areas constructed to protect and charge up your US machines. Proactive involvement and careful measurement of how much space will be needed to freely roll a machine in and out of a storage area cannot be overemphasized. Finding another equipment storage solution once a storage space has been lost due to poor planning can be very time consuming and most vexing.

Ultrasound Supply Storage Cabinets

If you have a large physical plant, locate several US supply cabinets on either ends of your ED/ICU/clinic for easy access to your frequently needed supplies and for easy cart restocking. Have your ED/ICU/clinic manager and medical workers help keep these storage areas stocked. With such a system in place you will be able to quickly and efficiently restock your US cart with a brief pit stop, even in the midst of a busy clinical shift (Fig. 13.58).

Fig. 13.58 Set up an US supply storage cabinet in a conveniently located area in your workplace. Have all your US cart items available in this cabinet for easy restocking

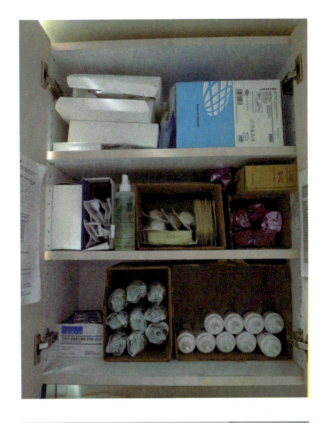

Fig. 13.59 Use a poster printer to create US educational posters for your clinical work areas and US Section posters to advertise your section's ongoing activities

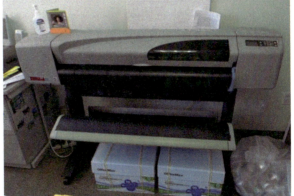

Poster Printer

If you work in an academic setting and your department either owns or has access to a poster printer (Fig. 13.59), you can use this item to advantage to create US educational posters or to advertise your US Section's ongoing activities on a

Fig. 13.60 A
representative Ultrasound
Section poster with
mission statement,
publications, ongoing
research activities,
interesting cases, etc.

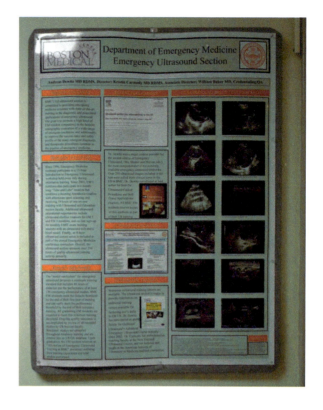

bulletin board (Fig. 13.60). Create your poster as a slide in PowerPoint using the "Page Setup" and "Custom" settings to select your poster width, height, and orientation. Once completed, the file can be easily exported to your poster printer for printing.

Service Options

What are the common service options available to you to fix the things that you cannot fix yourself? You've got five options to choose from and the relative merits of each are discussed briefly below.

Original Equipment Manufacturer

The Original Equipment Manufacturer will be more than happy to sell you a service contract. Maintenance contracts vary with the upfront equipment cost and the number of transducers covered. Read the fine print. A typical contract will run about $7000–$10,000 a year for a 3-probe machine and usually covers replacement of a damaged transducer, equipment troubleshooting, any required repairs when something breaks down, software upgrades, and 1–2 preventive maintenance visits/year. If the budget allows and money is no object, get it.

Biomed Engineering

What about your Hospital's Biomed Engineering Department? Prior to using the machine in your clinical setting, your Biomed folks are usually required to perform electrical safety testing and operational verification, after which they will place a sticker on the machine for hospital inventory and regulatory purposes. They will rarely be able to provide you with adequate coverage to deal with your inevitable equipment break-downs, however, unless they receive additional training that is specific for your machine. In some institutions, Biomed engineering personnel will be sent to the manufacturer's training site for this additional training, but this practice is not commonly the case.

Equipment Insurance

Filing an insurance claim for equipment repairs is another option, but it is cumbersome and the least user friendly of the five options mentioned. There is no on-site manager, and since the insurance provider does not handle the repairs you will have to arrange for any equipment service yourself. When the repairs are done, you will then have to submit a claim for compensation. This equipment care option leaves much to be desired.

Pay as You Go

In my experience, this is probably the cheapest service option in the long run. This can be difficult to bundle into an annual ED/ICU/hospital budget, however, since repair costs are unpredictable, it is often difficult to keep funds in an account from one year to the next, and you may end up in line behind the service contract clients in terms of your equipment repair priority. Labor rates run from $200 to $250/hr with a minimum for travel to and from the repair site. A typical minimum for any visit is $1000.

Multi-Vendor Service Providers

Large hospitals will often contract an on-site provider to bundle repair services for multiple types of machines throughout the hospital (not just ultrasound). The hospital can then consolidate the service contracts for many hundreds of pieces of hospital equipment into a single asset management solution. This option usually costs as much as the Original Equipment Manufacturer package but you will have the advantage of someone on-site who can address your equipment problems quickly. The yearly maintenance cost may vanish from your ED budget after the first year as it often gets bundled into the hospital's overall operating budget.

Breakdowns

So what do you do when one of your machines breaks down?

Have an effective communications system in place. Specific issues about a given machine can be directed to the ultrasound section director or staff by e-mail, text, a

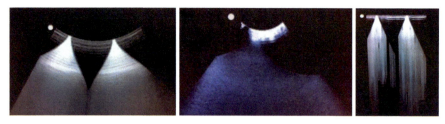

Fig. 13.61 All ultrasound probes are giving you some very unusual images: time to place a service call for help

photo, or a video clip. It can be most helpful if you have a name for each member of your ultrasound family so you know which machine is out of commission, especially if you own several of the same model: Grandpa?, Miro?, Thing One?, Yoda? Some issues can be readily resolved by phone or fixed by you in person, others will perplex you and require higher-level interventions, most likely involving a service call (Fig. 13.61). Have a list of all your ultrasound machines' names and serial numbers at the ready, and have ready access to your service provider's contact number since you will need this information to initiate any repairs. Our ED ultrasound equipment repair tech and I text message each other on a regular basis and I have found this to be a most efficient means of coordinating equipment repairs in our practice setting.

Longevity

How long should an US machine last in the ED? If you buy a well-built machine and take good care of it you should be able to get 5 years of use if appropriate daily and preventive maintenance is performed, and if you are willing to purchase the occasional transducer. The inevitable heavy wear and tear in an ED setting as well as rapid technological advances will usually propel you to purchase newer and more up to date equipment after that time.

Pitfalls

1. Failing to recognize the importance of purchasing a robust, user friendly and maintenance friendly machine.
2. Failing to recognize the importance of appropriate equipment orientation to protect your ultrasound fleet and ensure its safe and optimum use. Training should focus specifically on probe and transducer cord care as well as routine equipment cleaning expectations after each use.
3. Failing to establish protected sites for equipment storage. Clinical practice settings can be very rough on expensive multiuser equipment and you need to protect your investment. Broken equipment is very expensive to repair and keeps an essential machine out of commission or restricted in its capabilities if a

transducer or some other feature is not working. A designated storage area also improves ready access to the equipment for all users.

4. Failure to have full operational support for ultrasound equipment supply ordering, stocking and cart cleaning in place. This is a big job if you have a multi-machine practice setting. There is no such thing as shared group responsibility for this type of equipment maintenance. You will need designated personnel and dedicated time to help maintain a fleet of ultrasound machines in constant clinical use.

Key Recommendations

1. Buy the best, sturdiest machine you can afford.
2. No use without training: make sure your operators are well trained.
3. Find a safe harbor: designate a convenient and safe storage area.
4. Organize for operations: get your supply stream and distribution system organized. Advocate for dedicated personnel for this task.
5. Implement a cleaning protocol: accept the fact that you, your ultrasound staff and medical workers will likely be doing most of the daily equipment oversight and care. Outsource this task to a dedicated ED manager if possible.
6. Customize your fleet of US machines to suit your practice needs.
7. Outsource the complicated stuff to your Service Provider.
8. Get a helping hand wherever you can (Fig. 13.62).

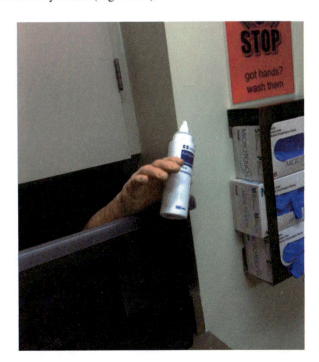

Fig. 13.62 Get a helping hand wherever you can

9. Maintain your sense of humor.
10. Be grateful you practice medicine in an era where you have access to an incredible bedside technology that allows you to peer inside your patient, helps you make more timely and correct diagnoses, and vastly expands and improves your procedural skills.

Chapter 14
Ultrasound Associated Materials and Equipment

Matthew Lipton and Robinson M. Ferre

Objectives

- Discuss the importance of various ultrasound accessories.
- Determine the optimal level of ultrasound accessories for your institution, taking into account your institution's point-of-care ultrasound budget and breadth of utilization.

Introduction

In order to run a successful point-of-care ultrasound program, there are many additional ultrasound related materials that should be in stock at all times. The most fundamental material is ultrasound gel. While it is often overlooked, this is the lifeline of ultrasound—a program cannot run without it. Besides an indispensable gel supply, there are many other ultrasound materials that can be purchased to make your point-of-care ultrasound program run more efficiently, such as barcode readers, sterile probe covers, and appropriate-length peripheral intravenous catheters. In addition, there are numerous other small pieces of equipment that may be needed as your point-of-care ultrasound program grows, such as endocavitary

M. Lipton, MD (✉) • R.M. Ferre, MD, FACEP
Department of Emergency Medicine, Vanderbilt University Medical Center,
Nashville, TN, USA
e-mail: matthew.lipton@vanderbilt.edu

probe covers, echogenic-tipped needles, needle guides, and gel warmers. We will go through each of these topics in more detail, discussing the various costs and options which will allow you to determine if they are needed for your program. Table 14.1 provides a summary of these ultrasound accoutrements, including common vendors and price ranges.

Table 14.1 Ultrasound accessories

Equipment	Brands	Approximate cost per unit	Suitable users
Ultrasound gel	Parker labs	$1–3 per 250 mL bottle	All programs
	Dynarex		
Gel warmer	Parker labs	$120–220 per warmer	Consider for added patient comfort
	Echosonics		
Endocavitary probe covers	Parker labs	$0.20–0.80 per cover	All programs performing transvaginal studies
	Various generic brands		
Sterile probe covers	Protek	$6–8 per cover	All programs performing dynamically guided sterile procedures
Echogenic needles	B. Braun	$5–20 per needle	Consider if performing nerve blocks, dynamically guided sterile procedures
	BD		
	Pajunk		
	Havel's		
Peripheral IV catheters	BD	$1.25–3.50 per catheter	All programs performing US-guided peripheral IV insertions
	B. Braun	$10–20 per catheter for those containing guidewires	
	Excel		
	Terumo		
	ARROW		
	AccuCath		
Needle guides	Civco	Varies	Consider if performing nerve blocks, dynamically guided sterile procedures
Barcode reader	Symbol LS2208	$90–120 per scanner	Consider to improve workflow
	Jadak flexpoint HS-1 M		
Cord protector	Spiral wrap	$10–20 per 100 ft	Consider for added cord durability
Cord suspension system	Various generic brands	$3 per extension spring	Consider for added durability
		$5 for 25 Velcro cable ties	
		$5 for 50 round keyrings	
		$5 for 50 zip ties	
USB hub	AmazonBasics ultra-mini-hub	$5–20	Consider if needing additional USB ports
	Various generic brands		

Machine Accessories

Most point of care ultrasound machines, while they can be portable, are attached to a cart. These carts are relatively small and can be accessorized to provide additional functionality and improved workflow efficiency. In addition, there are creative ways to improve the durability and longevity of the US machine and probes by adding additional protection to areas that are vulnerable to breakdown.

Barcode Reader

There are many barriers to inputting proper patient data into the ultrasound machine in a fast-paced Emergency Department (ED). One of these barriers is the process of manually inputting patient data into the "patient information" screen on the ultrasound machine before beginning the ultrasound exam. A barcode reader (see Figs. 14.1 and 14.2) allows a more seamless workflow process that, in our experience, improves the percentage of ultrasound scans saved, decreases data entry errors, and improves workflow efficiency. The barcode reader is a small, handheld device

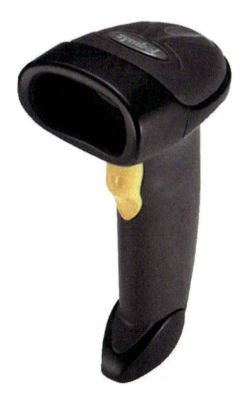

Fig. 14.1 Symbol bar code reader

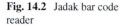
Fig. 14.2 Jadak bar code reader

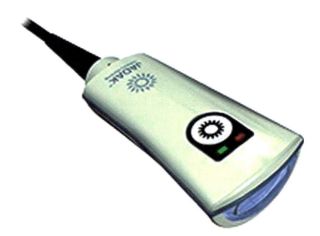

that is attached to the ultrasound machine through a USB port and allows the optical scanning of the hospital-generated barcode located on the patient's wristband.

By placing the cursor in the appropriate box on the patient information screen, the barcode reader will quickly read and input the patient's medical record number into the selected box. This bypasses the process of manually inputting the patient's full name and/or medical record number. Because different fields on the patient information screen can be uniquely "mapped" to a report or a PACS database, it is possible for a particular field on the patient information screen to be used to identify the clinician who is performing and/or supervising the exam. A barcode reader is an efficient means of inputting that data into the predetermined "mapped" location. Barcode reading software allows you to convert a clinician's name or unique alphanumeric code to a barcode that is recognized by any barcode reader. There are free and paid version online at https://barcode.tec-it.com. These barcodes can be printed on a sticker and placed on the backside of an identification badge for easy use. Most ultrasound machines will accept a variety of USB barcode scanners. However, it is important to ensure the barcode scanner is durable since it will be exposed to the same environment as the ultrasound machine. The most commonly used barcode scanners are the Symbol LS2208 and the Jadak Flexpoint HS-1 M, which typically cost $100–200 but refer to the ultrasound machine instruction manual for specific brands that are compatible with your machine.

USB Accessories

Many US machines only come with one USB port. This can be problematic if you are planning to use accessory devices that need a USB port such as a wireless dongle, a barcode reader, or simply needing to download images to a USB flash drive. A USB hub (see Fig. 14.3) is an inexpensive device that allows one USB port to be converted to a multi-port hub. An added benefit to a USB hub is that it is generally

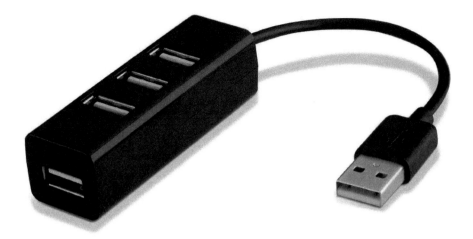

Fig. 14.3 USB hub

a more secure physical connection than a wireless dongle that protrudes from the back or side of the machine. Different hubs have different lengths of cord from the USB insertion site to the actual hub. A USB hub with a longer cord will allow you to secure the hub and any of its connecting devices (such as a wireless dongle) on the stand or under the machine, where there is less risk of inadvertent disconnection.

Probe Accessories

Endocavitary Probe Covers

A crucial component of transvaginal ultrasound is the disposable probe cover. There are essentially two types of transvaginal probe covers—inexpensive condom-type probe covers (see Fig. 14.4) and the more expensive pre-gelled, non-rolled probe covers (see Fig. 14.5). Condom-type probe covers are widely available and can be purchased from a variety of vendors. These probe covers are usually made of latex (~$0.25/cover) but latex-free versions are also available for added expense. This type of probe cover requires the sonographer to either place gel inside the cover or on the footprint of the probe prior to rolling the cover over the probe. On the other hand, pre-gelled, non-rolled probe covers have gel appropriately placed inside the cover and are generally latex-free and generally cost about $0.80/cover.

In low-resource settings, condoms or a sterile glove can also be used as a probe cover (see Figs. 14.6 and 14.7). Sterile gloves are preferred over non-sterile gloves because they are more durable, have fewer microscopic pinholes, and must meet higher levels of manufacturing standards. Because condoms are also readily available, many programs prefer to use these as endocavitary probe covers because they are less expensive and have a lower breakage rate than commercially available covers [1].

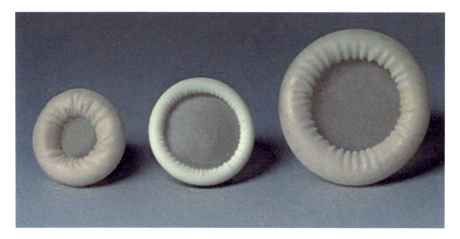

Fig. 14.4 Rolled endocavitary probe cover

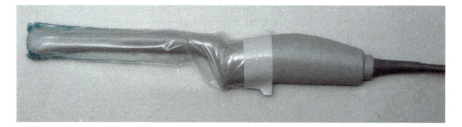

Fig. 14.5 Pre-gelled endocavitary probe cover

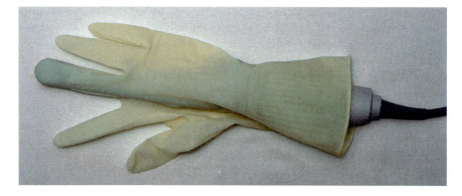

Fig. 14.6 Sterile glove used as an endocavitary probe cover: probe is placed in middle finger slot

14 Ultrasound Associated Materials and Equipment	231

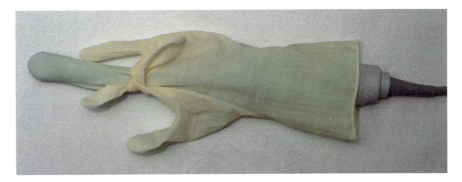

Fig. 14.7 Sterile glove used as an endocavitary probe cover: the index and ring finger slots are tied together

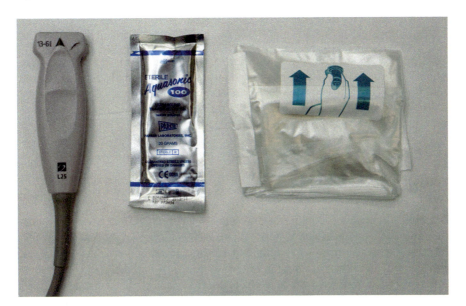

Fig. 14.8 Sterile probe cover kit contents

Sterile Probe Covers

For procedures that require sterility and use dynamic ultrasound guidance, a sterile probe cover is required. Most sterile probe cover kits include a telescopically folded probe cover, a single sterile ultrasound gel packet, along with two rubber bands (see Fig. 14.8). The are several different manufacturers of sterile probe covers and they typically cost approximately $6 per set. A sterile probe cover with PullUp™ technology uses a firm cardboard aperture with clear instructions to allow for quick probe loading and cord covering (see Fig. 14.9). One important consideration is the

Fig. 14.9 PullUp sterile
linear probe cover

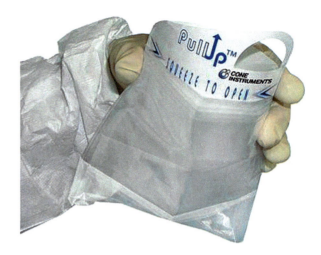

Fig. 14.9 PullUp sterile linear probe cover

type and size of the probe(s) you desire to cover, since some probe covers are uniquely tailored to the size of the probe they are covering. Finally, if a large sterile field is required, such as for central venous cannulation, it is crucial that the probe cover be at least 48 in. in length to ensure there is enough coverage of the cord to allow placement of the probe on the sterile field.

Ultrasound Gel

Ultrasonic gel acts as a coupling agent to allow sound from the probe to be transmitted into the body. Because the acoustic impedance of ultrasonic gel is nearly identical to that of the dermis, there is minimal acoustic reflection loss, thus creating an effective way to allow transmission of ultrasonic waves into the body. Ultrasound gel is composed of water, propylene glycol, a carbomer (i.e., thickening agent), and a biocide that acts as a preservative and has a pH between 6.5 and 7.0. Occasionally, gels may also contain a dye and/or scented oils.

The most common ultrasound gel used is Parker Aquasonic® 100 Ultrasound Transmission Gel (see Fig. 14.10). There are many companies that make ultrasound gel but it is important for the gel to have a few characteristics, including acoustic efficiency, high viscosity, bacteriostatic, and hypoallergenic. If a gel is acoustically efficient, then it is able to effectively transmit a broad range of sound waves with minimal or no loss of sound waves. As a practical feature, the gel should be viscous enough to allow layering of the gel on the patient. It should not be "runny" or fall off the patient once applied.

Many different ultrasound gel companies will sell their ultrasound gel in 5 L containers for a reduced price (per ounce of gel, see Fig. 14.11). However, this requires personnel to manually collect empty containers and then refill the smaller

Fig. 14.10 Ultrasound gel

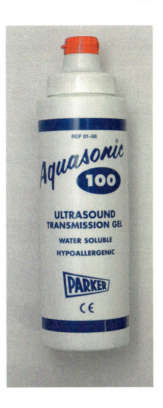

Fig. 14.11 Five-liter
ultrasound gel container

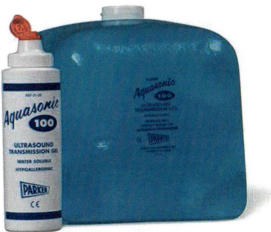

containers on the ultrasound cart on a frequent basis. The cost of an 8.5 oz (250 mL) bottle of Parker Aquasonic® 100 Ultrasound Transmission Gel is approximately $2. In comparison, the 5-L container retails for approximately $20 and is the equivalent of twenty 250 mL bottles, which effectively brings the cost per bottle down to $1, essentially reducing your ultrasound gels costs by 50%, or $1 per 250 mL bottle.

Because ultrasonic gel is bacteriostatic and hypoallergenic, there are few adverse events that are likely to occur with the use of ultrasound gel. Despite precautions used in the manufacture of these gels, contact dermatitis and bacterial contamination can still occur. There have been at least 15 cases of contact dermatitis reported in the literature as a result of the use of hypoallergenic, commercially available ultrasound gel [2]. When skin tests have been used to identify the culprit, propylene glycol and Euxyl® K 400 are the most commonly incriminated agents. There is also theoretical concern for transmission of bacteria from person to person during point-of-care ultrasound [3]. While bacteriostatic gel does not kill bacteria, its growth is reduced [4]. Wiping the exterior surface of the bottle with isopropyl alcohol or an approved cleaning wipe between examinations will theoretically reduce the possibility that the ultrasound probe becomes a vector for health care associated infections. Refilling reusable bottles is another potential method of bacterial contamination and each manufacturer has specific instructions on how to do this so as to prevent contamination. Several studies have demonstrated that the gel, gel cap, and the gel bottle can become contaminated with bacteria common to skin flora with an incidence rate between 2.5 and 6% [4].

Gel for Low-Resource Settings

In many low-resource areas, the cost and availability of commercial ultrasound gel may be prohibitive. However, locally available products are an alternative to commercially available ultrasound gel, including olive oil, mineral oil, and a mixture containing water, salt and cornstarch or cassava root [5–8]. In Africa, where cassava root is widely available, Salmon et al. found that cassava root flour (8 parts) mixed with water (32 parts) and salt (1 part) produced an acceptable gel that cost $0.09 USD per 500 mL bottle [8] (See Chap. 23 – Global Medicine Perspectives).

Ultrasound Gel Warmers

Although the process of performing an ultrasound is not painful, gel at room temperature feels cold when directly applied to the skin. It can be an uncomfortable experience for the patient each time a new batch of ultrasound gel is applied. In hospital and office based practices where an ultrasound suite is common, gel warming machines are frequently used to improve the patient's experience. These machines can be mounted on a wall or placed on a counter and can hold one to three 250 mL bottles at a time (see Fig. 14.12). The price ranges from $120 to $220 depending on the size and features of the warmer. The main drawback to using this machine in the ED or acute care setting is the lack of portability of these small machines. As a result, clinicians performing the ultrasound study would need to remove the bottle from the gel warmer from the stationary unit prior to performing

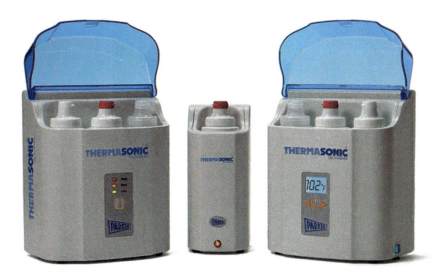

Fig. 14.12   Ultrasound gel warming machine

an ultrasound exam and then replace it when finished with the exam. This can be impractical if your department is physically large and if the ultrasound machine(s) do not have a dedicated space where a gel warming machine might be placed. If you are able to incorporate it into your practice, it will add a level of patient satisfaction that was only previously known to the radiology department.

Procedural Guidance Accessories

Procedural guidance is a significant part of a point-of-care ultrasound program. Ultrasound allows for the real-time visualization of a needle during various procedures for better accuracy, avoidance of unintended structures, and improved patient safety. The most common ultrasound-guided procedures in the ED include peripheral and central intravenous catheter placement, thoracentesis, paracentesis, and regional nerve blocks. There are a variety of accessories needed to perform ultrasound-guided procedures, including sterile probe covers, different types of needles and catheters, needle guides, and control syringes.

Echogenic Needles

Needle tip visualization can be quite difficult to the inexperienced proceduralist. A deterioration of needle visualization occurs at steeper angles of insonation due to increased reflective signal losses [9]. In an effort to improve needle tip

Fig. 14.13. Echogenic-
tipped needle

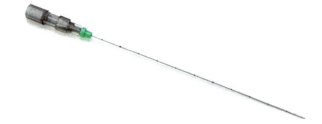

visualization, companies have created specific needles for ultrasound-guided procedures in which the needle tip has a multi-angled surface to allow for better
sound wave reflection and thus more echogenic appearance on the screen. While
not necessary to perform ultrasound-guided procedures, these needles are especially useful for dynamically guided procedures, such as regional anesthesia,
where the simultaneous visualization of the needle tip and neuroanatomy is
required for accurate placement of the local anesthetic. There are many companies that make these needles, including B. Braun, BD, Pajunk, and Havel's with a
cost ranging from $10 to $20 per needle. The only echogenic-tipped needle mar-
keted for ultrasound-guided regional anesthesia that is under $10 is Havel's
AccuTarg nerve block needle ($5–$10 per needle depending on length, gauge, and
presence of calibration markings, see Fig. 14.13). In a study of experienced
regional anesthesiologists, the Pajunk needle was preferred due to its superior
needle tip clarity [9]. For most applications of regional anesthesia performed in
the ED, it is unlikely that the clinician will need a needle with nerve stimulation
capability (which requires an insulated needle), therefore be sure to order the
appropriate needle for your program.

Control Syringes

Control of anesthetic injection is crucial to success of regional anesthesia.
Ultrasound-guided regional anesthesia has often been taught as a two-person procedure with one person controlling both the ultrasound probe and needle, while the
other person controls the injection of the local anesthetic. Regional anesthesia with
a single proceduralist has been described using various grips, including the Jedi
Grip (see Figs. 14.14, 14.15 and 14.16) [10]. However, most point-of-care ultrasound programs will not have the expensive, specialized echogenic needles with
extension tubing. Local anesthetic injections will often be performed with a needle
attached directly to a syringe (no extension tubing in between), allowing for a single
proceduralist. In this scenario, control over the needle and injection can be difficult
with a standard syringe. For improved performance, use of a control syringe may be
of benefit. A control syringe has three finger holes, two on the barrel and one on the
plunger, for maximal comfort and anesthetic control during injection and generally
cost approximately $1.50 per syringe.

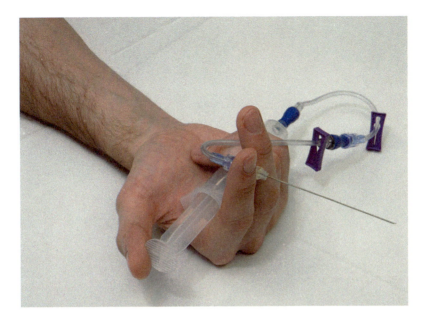

Fig. 14.14 The Jedi grip

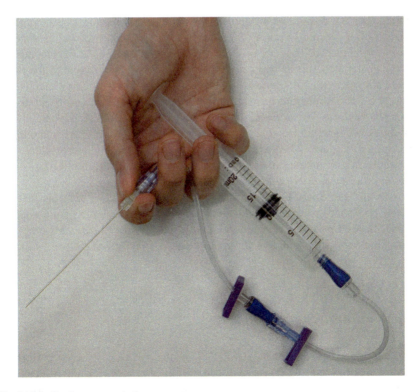

Fig. 14.15 Single person grip 1

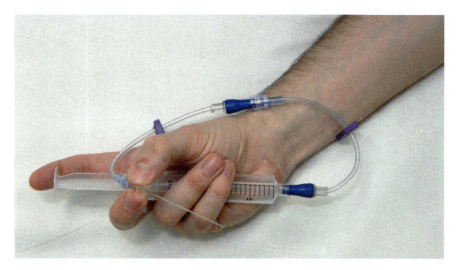

Fig. 14.16 Single person grip 2

Needle Guides

Needle guides are disposable attachments to the ultrasound probe that help guide the needle to a specific location. They attach directly to the probe after a sterile cover has been placed. They are primarily used for needle biopsies but can also be used for regional anesthesia and central line placement. These plastic probe adaptors will allow for either in-plane or out-of-plane needle localization by keeping the needle in a fixed orientation beneath the probe but allowing the proceduralist to control needle depth. While useful for deep biopsies done by interventional radiologists, they tend to be cumbersome for vascular access procedures performed in the ED. Once a proceduralist becomes familiar with the in-plane and out-of-plane needle visualization techniques, there does not appear to be much benefit of a needle guide for procedures done in the Emergency Department.

AxoTrack® and Sonix GPS® are proprietary needle guidance systems that are available on SonoSite and BK Medical systems, respectively. Both require needle kits that must be purchased for individual use. Each system allows for real-time feedback on needle depth and location, promising a more safe and effective means to ultrasound-guided procedures [11].

Peripheral Intravenous Catheters

Ultrasound-guided peripheral IV (USPIV) cannulation is a commonly performed procedure that has led to a decrease in central line placement for non-critically ill patients with difficult IV access [12]. The main difference between a standard, non-USGPIV catheter and one used under ultrasound guidance is the length of the catheter (see Fig. 14.17). The target vessels for USGPIV are the basilic, brachial, and cephalic veins of the upper arm which are deeper vessels than the palpable antecubital and superficial forearm veins. Since the target veins are deeper, the intravenous catheter must be longer than standard IV catheters to reach and remain in the vessel. To satisfy this requirement, most USGPIV catheters should be longer than IV catheters used for standard peripheral IV placement. The length of the catheter will vary based on the depth of the target vessel. For example, very small superficial veins, like those in infants and toddlers, will only require an IV catheter of at least 1.25 in. in length, whereas larger deeper veins around 1 cm deep, like those found in adolescents and adults, will need catheters of at least 2 in. in length. In adult patients, survival time of the USGPIV is dependent on the length of the catheters, with catheters at least 2.5 in. in length surviving at rates greater than those that are less than 2 in. [13, 14]. IV catheter gauge will also be dependent on patient size and vessel depth, but because of the Bernoulli effect of flow rates, catheter gauge should be at the least the same or larger than those commonly used for infants and children and at least 18–20 gauge for adolescents and adults. There are various manufactures that produce longer catheters, such as BD, B. Braun, Excel, and Terumo. More expensive catheters will have more features, such as flash chambers and needle tip protection devices and self-contained guidewires. Commonly used catheters include the B.Braun Introcan Safety® 18 gauge 2.5 in. catheter with a cost around $2.50 per catheter and the smaller 20 gauge 1.88 in. BD Insyte® Autoguard

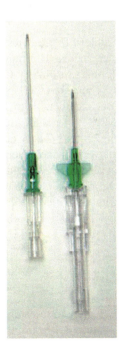

Fig. 14.17 Different peripheral IV catheter lengths (1.25 in. vs. 2.5 in.)

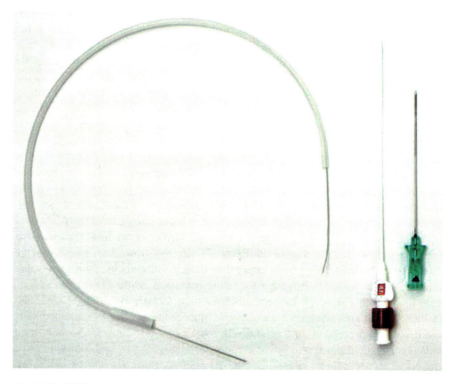

Fig. 14.18 Midline catheter set with separate guidewire

Shielded IV Catheter which costs approximately $3.50 per catheter. Other IV catheters include B. Braun Introcan Safety® IV Catheter 1.75″, Exel® IV Catheter 2″, or Terumo SurFlo® IV Catheter (which costs $1.25/catheter).

There are other options also available for US-guided peripheral IV catheters that use a guidewire to assist with cannulation. Such systems include AccuCath®, ARROW® radial artery cannulation set, and various midline catheter sets (see Fig. 14.18). AccuCath® and ARROW® brands come with an integrated wire that allows for accelerated Seldinger technique placement of the IV catheter. Both come in various sizes, including 22, 20, and 18 gauge catheters. However, the AccuCath® has a length of 2.25″ while the ARROW® radial artery cannulation set only comes with a smaller 1.75″ catheter. These integrated systems are more expensive than standard long IV catheters.

Pitfalls

• Failure to research the different options of equipment to provide the needed supplies to fit your institution's point-of-care ultrasound budget and scope.

Key Recommendations

1. Be familiar with accessories available to improve workflow, machine durability, and procedural guidance.
2. Research and obtain pricing on accessories before purchasing.
3. Do not purchase material that is unlikely to be utilized by your program.

References

1. Chalouhi GE, Salomon LJ, Marelle P, Bernard JP, Ville Y. Hygiene in endovaginal gynecologic and obstetrical ultrasound in 2008. J Gynecol Obstet Biol Reprod (Paris). 2009;38(1):43–50.
2. Chasset F, Soria A, Moguelet P, Mathian A, Auger Y, Francès C, Barete S. Contact dermatitis due to ultrasound gel: a case report and published work review. J Dermatol. 2016;43(3):318–20.
3. Lawrence MW, Blanks J, Ayala R, et al. Hospital-wide survey of bacterial contamination of point-of-care ultrasound probes and coupling gel. J Ultrasound Med. 2014;33:457–62.
4. Provenzano DA, Liebert MA, Steen B, Lovetro D, Somers DL. Investigation of current infection-control practices for ultrasound coupling gel: a survey, microbiological analysis, and examination of practice patterns. Reg Anesth Pain Med. 2013;38(5):415–24.
5. Binkowski A, Riguzzi C, Price D, Fahimi J. Evaluation of a cornstarch-based ultrasound gel alternative for low-resource settings. J Emerg Med. 2014;47(1):e5–9.
6. Luewan S, Srisupundit K, Tongsong T. A comparison of sonographic image quality between the examinations using gel and olive oil, as sound media. J Med Assoc Thail. 2007;90(4):624–7.
7. Gorny KR, Hangiandreou NJ, Hesley GK, Felmlee JP. Evaluation of mineral oil as an acoustic coupling medium in clinical MRgFUS. Phys Med Biol. 2007;52(1):N13–9.
8. Salmon M, Salmon C, Bissinger A, Muller MM, Gebreyesus A, Geremew H, Wendel SK, Azaza A, Salumu M, Benfield N. Alternative ultrasound gel for a sustainable ultrasound program: application of human centered design. PLoS One. 2015;10(8):e0134332.
9. Culp WC, McCowan TC, Goertzen TC, et al. Relative ultrasonographic echogenicity of standard, dimpled, and polymeric-coated needles. J Vasc Interv Radiol. 2000;11:351–8.
10. Pappin D, Christie I. The Jedi Grip: a novel technique for administering local anaesthetic in ultrasound-guided regional anaesthesia. Anaesthesia. 2011;66:845.
11. Ferre RM, Mercier M. Novel ultrasound guidance system for real-time central venous cannulation; safety and efficacy. West J Emerg Med. 2014;15(4):536–40.
12. Au AK, Rotte MJ, Grzybowski RJ, et al. Decrease in central venous catheter placement due to use of ultrasound guidance for peripheral intravenous catheters. Am J Emerg Med. 2012;30:1950–4.
13. Fields JM, Dean AJ, Todman RW, Au AK, Anderson KL, Ku BS, et al. The effect of vessel depth, diameter, and location on ultrasound-guided peripheral intravenous catheter longevity. Am J Emerg Med. 2012;30(7):1134–40.
14. Elia F, Ferrari G, Molino P, Converso M, De Filippi G, Milan A, Aprà F. Standard-length catheters vs long catheters in ultrasound-guided peripheral vein cannulation. Am J Emerg Med. 2012 Jun;30(5):712–6.

Chapter 15
Ultrasound Safety and Infection Control

Jason T. Nomura and Arun D. Nagdev

Objectives

- Understand the elements of the Output Display Standard for ultrasound systems
- Discuss tissue bioeffects from ultrasound and implications for clinical users
- Understand infection control principles for ultrasound systems
- Discuss the difference between the levels of cleaning and how each applies to ultrasound equipment
- Consider ultrasound gel as a safety concern with adoption of safe practices for internal and invasive procedures

Introduction

Diagnostic and procedural ultrasound utilization has rapidly expanded in different specialties and varied practice environments [1]. Ultrasound safety is not always highlighted during educational programs, but remains an important topic for all practitioners [2]. Ultrasound safety can be divided into two main areas of operator responsibility: bioeffects and infection prevention.

J.T. Nomura, MD, FACEP, FACP, FAHA (✉)
Department of Emergency Medicine, Neurosciences Service Line,
Christiana Care Health System, Christiana Hospital, Newark, DE, USA
e-mail: JNomura@Christianacare.org

A.D. Nagdev, MD
Emergency Ultrasound, Department of Emergency Medicine,
Highland General Hospital, Oakland, CA, USA

© Springer International Publishing AG 2018   243
V. S. Tayal et al. (eds.), *Ultrasound Program Management*,
https://doi.org/10.1007/978-3-319-63143-1_15

Bioeffects

Diagnostic ultrasound utilizes the transmission of sound into tissues that are then reflected back to the system for processing to produce an image. Sound waves are acoustic pressure waves that transfer energy to the patient with potential effects on biological tissue, also known as bioeffects.

Bioeffects can be divided into thermal and nonthermal effects and are dependent upon the system configuration and ultrasound physics. An in-depth review of the physics related to ultrasound and bioeffects is beyond the scope of this chapter; instead it will focus on elements related to a basic understanding of ultrasound bioeffects with a clinical user in mind.

System Power

In the 1980s, the Food and Drug Administration, FDA, began to regulate power output as part of its oversight of medical ultrasound systems [3]. At that time application specific acoustic output limitations were established based on systems in clinical use during the 1970s. In 1991, the FDA removed application specific limitations creating FDA Track 3 (used for bedside US) with an overall acoustic output limit of 720 mW/cm^2, with an exception for ocular ultrasound which was given lower limits [4]. This meant, for example, fetal exposure potentially increased from an initial limit of 46 –720 mW/cm^2 [2, 3, 5]. With the creation of the FDA Track 3, additional requirements were also instituted. The Output Display Standard, ODS, developed to promote safe practices with the increased power limitations and was required to be displayed on Track 3 ultrasound systems, see Table 15.1—Abbreviation of Key Safety Terms and Figs. 15.1 and 15.2 [4–6].

The ODS comprises the Thermal Index, an indicator of potential temperature impact, and the Mechanical Index, an indicator of potential nonthermal or mechanical effects. These parameters are affected not only by the power output of the ultrasound system but also by operator controlled parameters such as frequency, scan mode, and focus. Because of this an understanding of the Thermal Index and Mechanical Index and the potential ultrasound bioeffects are important for safe utilization of the technology.

Table 15.1 Abbreviations of key safety terms

Abbreviation	Term
ODS	Output display standard, consists of MI and TI
MI	Mechanical Index
TI	Thermal Index
TIS	Thermal Index Soft tissue
TIB	Thermal Index Bone
TIC	Thermal Index Cranial bone
ALARA	As Low As Reasonably Achievable

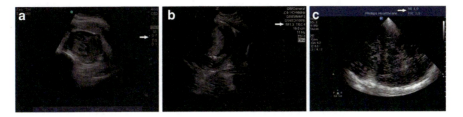

Fig. 15.1 Output Display Standard for Ultrasound Systems. The FDA requires the Output Display Standard (*ODS*) for ultrasound systems under Track 3 approval. The Mechanical Index and Thermal Index, arrows, are displayed in the ODS, location varies by manufacturer. (**a**) Abdominal aorta image with Thermal Index Soft Tissue (*TIS*). (**b**) Early Pregnancy Transabdominal with Thermal Index Bone (*TIB*). (**c**) Transcranial B Mode imaging with Thermal Index Cranial bone (*TIC*)

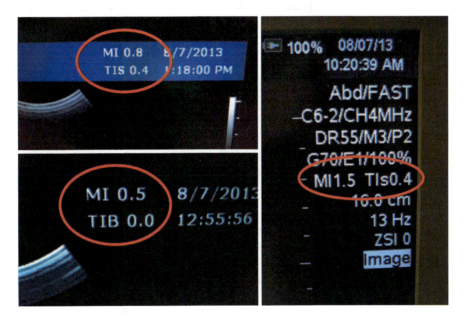

Fig. 15.2 Other examples of MI and TI displays

Thermal Index and Thermal Bioeffects

Thermal Index

The Thermal Index, TI, is a ratio of the intensity of the ultrasound beam to the relative amount of energy required to raise the tissue temperature 1 °C [5, 7].

The general formula for the TI is:

$$TI = W_O / W_{DEG}$$

where W_O is the power of the ultrasound system and W_{DEG} is power required to raise the tissue temperature 1 °C [6]. The TI is further categorized into subtypes depending on targeted tissues and the formula is then modified for the insonated tissues and attenuation. The Thermal Index Soft Tissue, TIS, assumes that there is only soft tissue insonated. Thermal Index Bone, TIB, is utilized when there is bone near the location of the focus while Thermal Index Cranial bone, TIC, is when the bone is very close to the transducer and tissue surface [2, 6, 7]. Calculations are modified due to the increased absorption of energy by bone compared to soft tissue and the differences in potential temperature changes at different sites along the ultrasound beam [6].

The TI is a relative indication of potential thermal effects during an ultrasound examination and does not represent an exact temperature rise. For example, a TI of 2 indicates a greater thermal exposure than a TI of 1, but does not necessarily mean a temperature increase of 2 °C or 1 °C [2, 5, 7].

The measurements are based on laboratory and phantom models, which do not always accurately reflect the complexity of human tissue and its interaction with ultrasound.

Based on the manufacturer system defaults, specific subtypes of the TI will be displayed for each application preset. However, some systems allow the operator to change the displayed TI appropriately for the exam being performed. For example, first trimester obstetric ultrasound would more commonly utilize the TIS while second and third the TIB. However, an obstetric preset may default to only the TIS or TIB, thus requiring the operator to change the display to the appropriate TI.

Thermal Bioeffects

Thermal bioeffects are related to the tissue scanned, scanning mode, beam focus, frequency, intensity, and exposure time [7]. The mechanical energy of the ultrasound beam is converted to heat energy as the beam is attenuated through absorption. Many point-of-care ultrasound protocols are based on grayscale or B-mode imaging which as a scanned mode has a lower potential for thermal effects of ultrasound [8]. However, increased thermal exposure occurs with utilization of Doppler during ultrasound exams [8]. The operator should be aware of the potential changes in thermal exposure as different modalities are utilized.

Thermal bioeffects are concerning in obstetrics because of the potential effect of elevated temperatures on fetal structures with particular concern during organogenesis. Maternal hyperthermia and fever have been linked to teratogenic and developmental defects [9]. There have also been studies showing ultrasound induced thermal bioeffects in experimental laboratory animals [9]. However, to date there is no evidence that medically indicated diagnostic ultrasound examinations produce thermal effects in the human fetus causing congenital anomalies [9, 10].

Diagnostic ultrasound also has the potential for heating non-fetal tissues. However, in most scanning mode applications this is usually negligible due to movement of the ultrasound beam [8]. Potential heating by diagnostic ultrasound is ameliorated in the non-fetal subject by normal physiologic dissipation of heat, such as by circulation. It has also been noted that small temperature rises of tissue can be tolerated for long periods of time without noted bioeffects [8]. For example, patients can tolerate mild fevers with no long-term tissue damage or ill effects.

Mechanical Index and Nonthermal Bioeffects

Mechanical Index

The Mechanical Index, MI, is a measure of the potential for nonthermal ultrasound bioeffects, particularly those related to cavitation, the collapse of gas bubbles in response to the ultrasonic field [5, 7]. The nonthermal effects are related to the pulse average intensity of the ultrasound acoustic wave rather than the time average intensity as is the case for thermal effects [7]. The MI is given by the formula:

$$MI = P_{r.3}\left(z_{sp}\right)/\sqrt{f_c}$$

where $P_{r.3}(z_{sp})$ is the peak rarefactional pressure derated by 0.3 dB/cm-MHz, to account for attenuation, at the point of z_{sp} where the beam has the peak pulse intensity integral and f_c is the center frequency [6]. The complex MI equation gives the operator a guide to the potential for mechanical bioeffects taking into account the frequency and pulse pressure of the beam [2]. Similarly to the TI, the MI serves as a relative guide and not an absolute measure of nonthermal bioeffects.

Nonthermal Bioeffects

Nonthermal bioeffects most commonly refers to cavitation, which is the result of the ultrasound beam interacting with gas bubbles and tissue. This was the original basis for the MI. There are two main types of cavitation, stable and inertial. Stable cavitation is when a gas bubble oscillates around an equilibrium size within the ultrasound beam [7]. This oscillation can induce microstreaming of fluid around the bubble that can also produce bioeffects such as cell membrane disruption.

Inertial cavitation is when bubbles expand and collapse or cavitation nuclei create a gas bubble that collapses [7]. The collapse or implosion of the bubble during inertial cavitation can produce large changes in pressure and temperature on a microscopic scale that has the potential to damage tissues. Inertial cavitation is believed to be a threshold effect, meaning that unless cavitation nuclei are exposed to the appropriate pressure and frequency inertial cavitation will not occur [11]. This means that dwell time does not inherently increase inertial cavitation risk, but can increase the chance that tissue will be exposed to the threshold pressure.

Cavitation bioeffects are thought to have less potential effect on fetal tissue because of the lack of in vivo gas bubbles reducing the chance for cavitation events [12]. In non-gas containing tissues, inertial cavitation effects are felt to be extremely rare with the acoustic pressure created using current diagnostic ultrasound equipment [11].

Prudent Use

While diagnostic ultrasound is widespread and generally viewed as safe, there is still the potential for bioeffects. Because of this, users should still adhere to the concept of prudent use. This means to keep ultrasound exposure to the lowest possible acoustic output for the briefest time interval possible. This is known as the ALARA principle, As Low As Reasonably Achievable, meaning to use the least power for the shortest time to gain the diagnostic information needed [5–7].

By adhering to the ALARA principle, exposure to ultrasound and potential bioeffects can be minimized.

Ultrasound Safety Education

An additional component of FDA Track 3 regulation is the distribution of educational material related to ultrasound safety [4]. Manufacturers are required to include information with their devices regarding the power output and associated TI and MI for the combinations of probes and presets that are provided. The regulation also requires inclusion of education on the ALARA principle and ultrasound safety including bioeffects [4].

Clinical users have been studied regarding their knowledge of ultrasound safety and potential bioeffects. Several studies have shown that the majority of clinical users are not knowledgeable of ultrasound safety and bioeffects beyond the ALARA statement [13–15]. Several studies have shown limited understanding of ultrasound bioeffects and the ODS with subjects being unable to answer questions about the TI and MI [13, 15, 16]. Other studies have shown that many clinical users do not know where the ODS is on their system nor monitor it during examinations [13, 14, 16]. This shows that education and retention regarding ultrasound safety can be a problem. Educational efforts need to continue with safety being incorporated into ongoing education.

Special Situations Specific to Emergency and Point-of-Care Applications

There are special situations that are of particular importance to the point-of-care ultrasound user with regard to safety and potential bioeffects. The first is ultrasound of the fetus during early pregnancy. During early pregnancy and organogenesis there is increased concern about potential bioeffects on fetal tissue. Ultrasound exposure should be limited to what is medically indicated and necessary. Fetal ultrasound in the febrile mother could lead to greater temperature elevations and dwell time should be minimized [9].

Spectral Doppler, an unscanned mode, can increase the Thermal Index and potential heating at the focal point compared to other modes. Spectral Doppler should not be the primary method used to assess the fetal heart rate. Instead M-mode, which has a lower TI, will provide the heart rate with less energy exposure. If Doppler is required for fetal assessment it should be limited to the shortest time possible [17, 18].

Ocular ultrasound has increased in utilization and provides accurate and important information that many times cannot be practically gained through a direct ophthalmologic exam of the undilated eye [19]. When the FDA created Track 3 ocular ultrasound was separated from the overall output limits. For ocular ultrasound the limits are set at a TI $\leq$ 1, MI $\leq$ 0.23 and an intensity limit of $\leq$50 mW/cm^2 [4, 5, 7].

If performing ocular ultrasound, an ocular preset should be used as it will incorporate these limitations and one should verify that the TI and MI are appropriately low.

Pulmonary and lung ultrasound in the acute and critical care setting has undergone a major paradigm shift based on the work of Lichtenstein and others [20]. This has led to an increase in pulmonary ultrasound applications and use. Aerated pulmonary tissue has a higher risk for cavitation events compared to other tissues because of the contained gas. Exposure of lung tissue to diagnostic ultrasound has produced pulmonary hemorrhage in laboratory animal models [11]. While concerning, these results are in laboratory animals only. There have been no human studies showing pulmonary hemorrhage during diagnostic sonography. A study examined preoperative TEE exams averaging 35 min and found no pulmonary hemorrhage in adjacent lung tissue [21]. Although the risk is low of pulmonary cavitation events with tissue damage during diagnostic ultrasound, care should be taken to monitor and limit exposure with particular attention to the MI.

Bioeffects and the Risk/Benefit of Using Ultrasound

The concepts of thermal and nonthermal bioeffects and the Output Display Standard with calculated Thermal Index and Mechanical Index are complex subjects, but there are take home points for the clinical users.

There is no established causal relationship between medical diagnostic ultrasound and congenital anomalies in humans [22]. Multiple groups, including the World Health Organization and the American Institute of Ultrasound in Medicine, have produced statements that medically indicated ultrasound is safe in pregnancy [10]. But they also advocate the limited use of Doppler to when medically indicated due to the increased thermal exposure [17]. Adverse thermal bioeffects have not been observed in non-fetal tissue despite prolonged ultrasound exposure if the TI is low [2].

Cavitation events are rare in non-gas containing tissues at current diagnostic ultrasound intensities [11]. The risk of cavitation is increased with insonation of gas containing tissues, but pulmonary hemorrhage has not been documented in human lungs during diagnostic ultrasound exposure.

The Output Display Standard with the Thermal Index and Mechanical Index serve as relative markers of exposure and potential risk. They do not represent absolute values of temperature rise or cavitation events. While limited they do have value to the operator to monitor and limit ultrasound exposure and risk of induced bioeffects. Ultrasound system presets will incorporate alterations in the output, as reflected by the displayed MI and TI, and should be utilized appropriately.

While the risk of bioeffects from ultrasound exposure does raise concern, this must be balanced with the clinical scenario and the risk of not obtaining the information. Cases such as the hypotensive trauma patient, the hypotensive elderly patient with a pulsatile abdominal mass, or the early pregnancy patient with pelvic pain and bleeding are frequently encountered in the emergent setting [1–3]. These are situations where the lack of the clinical information provided by ultrasound could present a greater risk to the patient than the theoretical risk of bioeffects in a standard point-of-care ultrasound exam with appropriate equipment and system settings [23].

Recently the FDA has expressed concerns about "live scanning" of human models at trade shows without a documented indication or medical benefit. After clarification between the FDA and ultrasound societies, it is clear that careful US scanning of live models with specific educational goals was not the area of concern for the FDA. Many POC specialties utilize live models in training sessions that provide education and improve the overall care of the public. In addition to obtaining consent we would advise providing models with information regarding the ALARA principle, potential bioeffects, and the overall safety of ultrasound examinations. Utilization of pregnant and pediatric models should be limited to education regarding examinations and techniques related to these special populations [24].

Infection Control

In addition to bioeffects, clinicians performing point-of-care ultrasound should understand current methods needed to maintain pathogen free transducers, as well as current recommendation for probe disinfection [23, 25, 26]. Many POC settings, especially the ED and the ICU have significant infection control challenges from bodily fluids, multiple users, and multiple scanning locations. Management solutions to increase compliance include (1) keeping the spray or wipes with towels on the machine (Fig. 15.3), (2) keeping probe barriers (both sterile and non-sterile) on

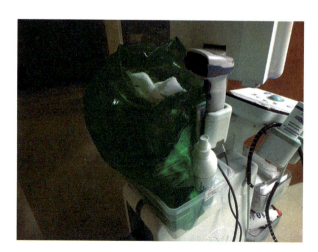

Fig. 15.3 Cleaning supplies (towels and spray cleaner) on POC US machine

Fig. 15.4 Probe barriers
on US machines

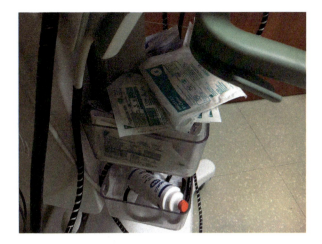

Sample US machine Daily Checklist - POC US machine #1 /Hospital Department/ Health institution

Date	US gel (full) 2 bottles	Spray Cleaner	Towels Stocked	Long IV Catheters	Tagaderm Barriers	Sterile transducer	Endocavitary barriers	Probes And probes Clean	Machine Reboot	Comments	Initials
Jan 1											
Jan 2											
Jan 3											
Jan 4											
Jan 5											
Jan 6											
Jan 7											
Jan 8											
Jan 9											
Jan 10											
Jan 11											
Jan 12											
Jan 13											
Jan 14											
Jan 15											
Jan 16											
Jan 17											
Jan 18											
Jan 19											
Jan 20											
Jan 21											
Jan 22											
Jan 23											
Jan 24											
Jan 25											
Jan 26											
Jan 27											
Jan 28											
Jan 29											
Jan 30											
Jan 31											

Fig. 15.5 US machine stocking checklist (example)

the machine (Fig. 15.4), (3) checklists for departmental personnel to check the machine on a daily or shift basis (Fig. 15.5), (4) multiple invasive probes for high volume endocavitary or invasive scanning, (5) departmental location for HLD probe cleaning (Fig. 15.6), and (6) designated responsibilities for US machine and probe care (see chapter on machine maintenance).

Fig. 15.6 Clean probe storage

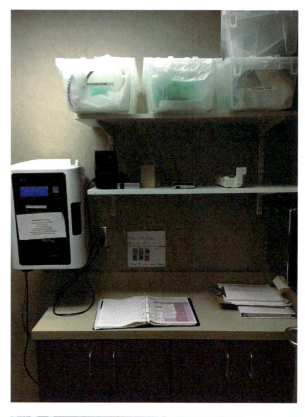

Fig. 15.7 Wiping gel off probe

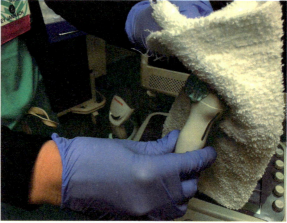

Initial Steps of Disinfection of All Probes

1. Remove barrier (if used) and dispose.
2. Wipe gel and debris off probe with towel (Fig. 15.7).
3. Wipe <u>dry</u> probe with germicidal wipes (Fig. 15.8) or spray with disinfection spray (Fig. 15.9) (or washing with soap and water prior to HLD).
4. Follow disinfection protocols based on infection control categorization below.

Fig. 15.8 Disinfecting dry external probe with germicidal wipe

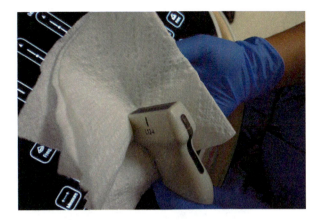

Fig. 15.9 Disinfecting dry external probe with germicidal spray

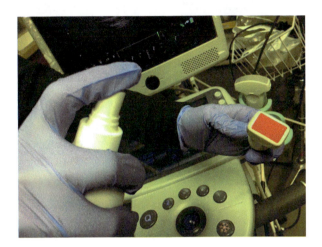

US Probe Infection Control Classification

Medical devices are classified into one of three categories: non-critical, semi-critical, and critical. This categorization informs the clinician of the type of disinfection or sterilization that must be performed to keep the device pathogen free.

Noncritical Devices (Noninvasive Probes)

Noncritical devices are those that come in contact with intact skin, which is thought to act as a barrier to most microorganisms. Ultrasound transcutaneous transducers (linear, phased array, curvilinear, etc.) are considered noncritical medical devices. Low-level disinfection (LLD) is thought to be adequate when cleaning noncritical medical devices, and should be performed between each use in a similar manner. LLD cleaning products include isopropyl alcohol (Fig. 15.10), bleach wipes

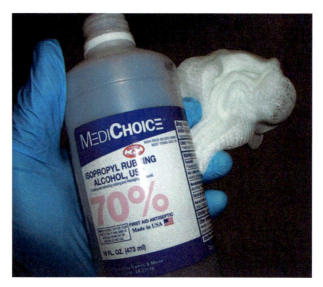

Cleaning the Distal Tip of the Transducer with Isopropyl Alcohol

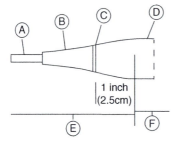

A - Cable

B - Strain Relief

C - Strain relief/housing joint

D - Housing

E - Do not use alcohol in this area

F - You may use alcohol in this area

Fig. 15.10 LLD—isopropyl alcohol

(Fig. 15.11), quaternary sprays (Fig. 15.12), ammonium chloride sprays (Fig. 15.13), and any other approved LLD cleaning solution (Table 15.2) in a standard cleaning format between transducer uses had been shown to be efficacious in removing most pathogens (bacteria, virus and fungus) [34]. Betadine is not recommended due to staining of the plastic or rubber on the probe (Fig. 15.14). Methicillin resistant Staph Aureus (MRSA) has been shown to be present on uncovered transducers, but can be easily removed with germicidal wipes cleaning (LLD) [34]. When performing ultrasound examinations on non-intact skin (cellulitis, abscess, etc.), we recommend placing a transparent dressing securely on the transducer before beginning the examination.

Fig. 15.11 LLD—bleach
wipe

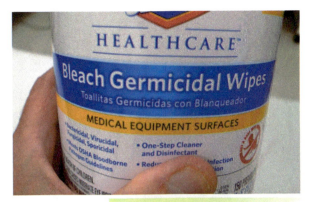

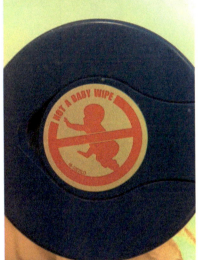

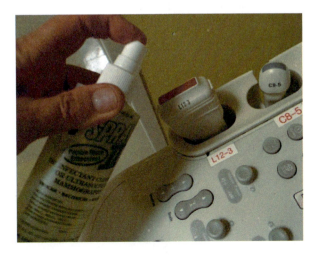

Fig. 15.12 LLD—
quaternary spray

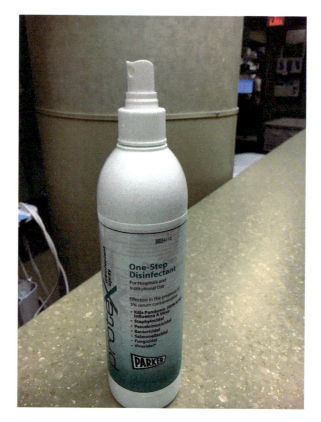

Fig. 15.13 LLD—ammonium chloride reagent

Table 15.2 Cleaning solutions for surface or noncritical devices

Ethyl or isopropyl alcohol (70–90%)
Sodium hypochlorite (5.25–6.15% household bleach diluted 1:500 provides >100 ppm available chlorine)
Phenolic germicidal detergent solution (follow product label for use-dilution)
Iodophor germicidal detergent solution (follow product label for use-dilution)
Quaternary ammonium germicidal detergent solution (follow product label for use-dilution)

Fig. 15.14 Betadine
staining of probe

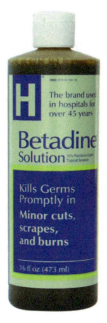 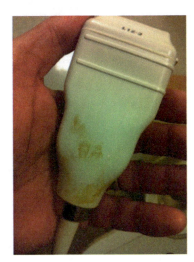

Semi-Critical Devices

Semi-critical devices are those that come into contact with non-intact skin or
mucosa. These devices include transesophageal echocardiography (TEE) transducers and endocavitary ultrasound transducers (Fig. 15.15). Even though probe covers
are always used with endocavitary transducers, preventing direct contact of the
probe surface and mucosal membranes, most governing bodies (CDC, AIUM and
ACOG, ACEP*) classify these probes as semi-critical devices [23, 25–27].

Semi-critical medical devices require high-level disinfection (HLD) in order to
eliminate all bacterial microorganisms except for a small number of bacterial
spores. Chemical disinfectants considered acceptable semi-critical medical devices
are listed (Table 15.3) and/or can be obtained from the ultrasound transducer manufacturer. Medical centers using either endocavitary or TEE transducers should
have a well-defined method for high-level disinfection or enlist the aid of hospital

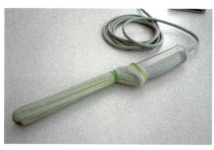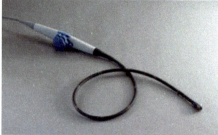

Fig. 15.15 Examples of semi-critical devices—Endocavitary and TEE probes

Table 15.3 Sterilants and high-level disinfectants listed by the FDA

Name	Composition/Action
Glutaraldehyde	Organic compound ($CH_2(CH_2CHO)_2$)
	Induces cell death by cross-linking cellular proteins; usually used alone or mixed with formaldehyde
Hydrogen peroxide	Inorganic compound (H_2O_2)
	Antiseptic and antibacterial; a very strong oxidizer with oxidation potential of 1.8 V
Peracetic acid	Organic compound (CH_3CO_3H)
	Antimicrobial agent (high oxidization potential)
Ortho-Phthalaldehyde	Organic compound ($C_6H_4(CHO)_2$)
	Strong binding to outer cell wall of contaminant organisms
Hypochlorite/ hypochlorous acid	Inorganic compound (HClO)
	Myeloperoxidase-mediated peroxidation of chloride ions
Phenol/phenolate	Organic compound (C_5H_5OH)
	Antiseptic
Hibidil	Chlorhexidine gluconate ($C_{22}H_{30}Cl_2N_{10}$)
	Chemical antiseptic

based sterile processing to ensure compliance. Obstetrics, cardiology and other services will be complying with HLD standards for their ultrasound transducers, and learning your hospital's current method for disinfection is often the first step in building a high-level disinfection method that is compliant with current recommendations.

The process of HLD involves multiple steps accomplished in either the clinical department or by hospital based sterile processing. Examples of ED department disinfection devices include glutaraldehyde-related solution hood and soaking stations (Fig. 15.16 and Fig. 15.17) and portable or mounted heated hydrogen peroxide stations (Figs. 15.18 and 15.19). There is no standard format for HLD of endocavitary probes. Rather, recommendations from transducer manufacturers in conjunction with CDC guidelines should guide the process. Documentation of a procedural log (Fig. 15.20) and replacement of disinfection solution should be standardized and in accordance with hospital and regulatory practices.

Fig. 15.16 HLD—
glutaraldehyde

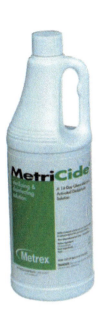
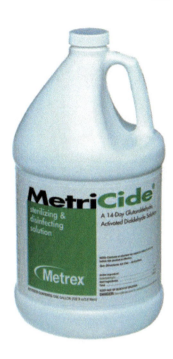

Fig. 15.17 Mounted
portable HLD soak station

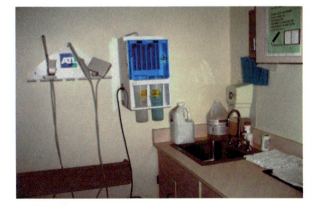

   Even though probe covers or condoms are always used with endocavitary probes
(Fig. 15.21), low-level disinfection with germicidal wipes have been shown to not
remove all bacteria and viruses [31, 32]. Probe cover perforation (Fig. 15.22) after
routine endocavitary probe use is reported to range from 1 to 9% [28]. Higher perforation rates are reported to occur with commercial probe covers as compared to
condoms, 8.3 vs. 1.7% [28]. Higher rates of condom perforation (25–815) are seen
with ultrasound-guided procedural interventions (oocyte retrieval for IVF) [29]. In
a series of 168 patients who had a TEE procedure performed, the latex condom
perforation rate post procedure was reported to be 4.4% [30]. Because of the risk of
pathogen transmission, current CDC standards mandate HDL in between patient
usage when using covered endocavitary transducers.

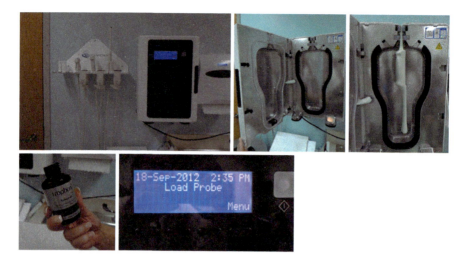

Fig. 15.18 Trophon mounted

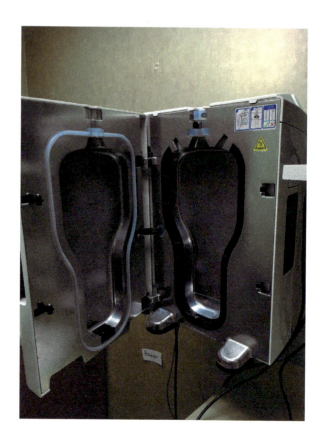

Fig. 15.19 Open Trophon

Fig. 15.20 HLD disinfection log

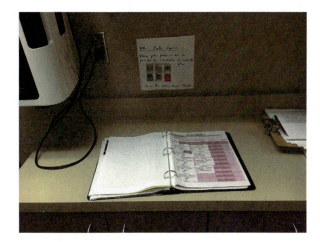

Fig. 15.21 Probe barriers

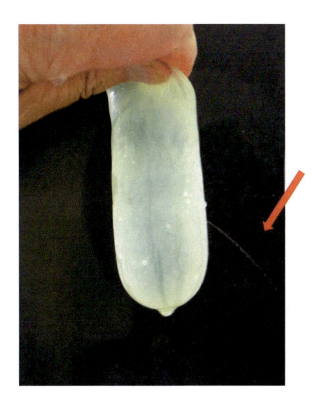

Fig. 15.22 Leakage from endocavitary barrier

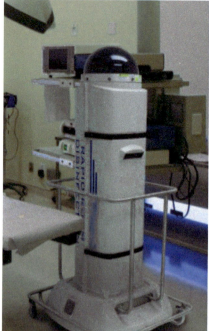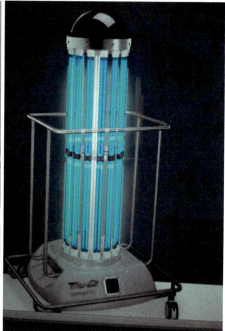

Fig. 15.23 UV disinfection equipment

Newer ultraviolet light based HLD cleaning systems (Fig. 15.23) may become more commonplace soon [33]. They employ short wave UVC light in the 100–280 nm range, have short (2–10 min) cleaning cycle, and provide HLD. These and other technological advances will allow clinicians a less cumbersome option for HLD, while maintaining patient safety. Emerging data will allow clinicians greater options for high-level disinfection, but current standards still recommend conventional practices.

Critical Devices

Critical devices are those that enter a sterile tissue or vasculature, and require sterilization. These items include surgical instruments and implantable cardiac devices. Clinicians performing POC US will most commonly not be working with medical devices that require critical sterilization.

Other Ultrasound Machine Elements

Careful attention should be paid to manufacturer instructions on cleaning of keyboards, machine, surface, probe holders, and monitors. While some germicidal sprays may be used on the plastic surfaces, other areas may be permanently damaged by strong chemicals in the spray or wipe. However, probe holders in particular should be cleaned as they accumulate dried gel and possibly bodily fluids.

Ultrasound Gel as a Safety Issue

While US gel is discussed extensively in Chap. 14 (link), a brief discussion of ultrasound gel safety practices is synergistic with the safety issues with probe cleaning. Ultrasound gel is water-based, and has been episodically associated with nosocomial infections [35, 36]. Recently the issue of when sterile US gel should be used versus non-sterile gel has been explored by regulatory bodies [37–39].

POC US directors should consider creating policies for safe use of non-sterile ultrasound gel (disposable bottles (Fig. 15.24) or filling from large US reservoirs with careful attention to lack of contact of the respective container openings), and policies for use of sterile gel. Sterile gel (Fig. 15.25) should be considered for all

Fig. 15.24 Prefilled bottles of US gel

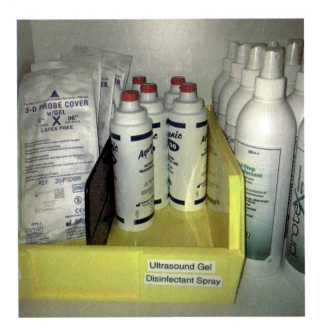

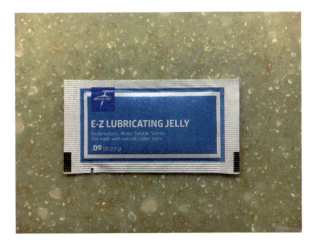

Fig. 15.25 Sterile lubricating gel packet

invasive procedures (external to the probe cover), US examinations on neonates, US examinations on non-intact skin or fresh surgical sites, endocavitary or endoscopic US procedures on internal mucous membranes, and other examinations of concern. Non-sterile gel can be used for other ultrasound examinations so long the gel is maintained per infection control guidelines. Gel warmers should only use dry heat and be serviced per infection control policies of the institution.

Summary

Bioeffects are possible with the use of diagnostic ultrasound and are related to a complex interplay of the tissues insonated, frequency, intensity, scanning mode, and dwell time. Some of these parameters are under operator control. To adhere to the ALARA principle, operators should be aware of and monitor ultrasound exposure as indicated by the Thermal and Mechanical Indices. The concept of ultrasound bioeffects is only one part of the risk-benefit analysis in the emergent setting where the lack of information presents a clear danger to the patient and impacts clinical management.

Transducer maintenance should be a priority for all clinicians to ensure patient safety. System upkeep involves fastidious cleaning for both the transducer and ultrasound system. A clear departmental infection control protocol will ensure patient safety, as well as detect early breaks in transducer surface integrity. When performing examinations on intact non-mucosal surfaces, low-level disinfection and use of non-sterile gel is adequate. When performing an ultrasound examination on non-intact skin we recommend using a transparent dressing cover over the transducer. For endocavitary examinations, transesophageal echocardiography, or internal examinations, use of sterile gel on the exterior of the probe and high-level disinfection is mandatory (via either the aide of hospital based sterile processing or an internal highly organized departmental system). Guidelines from transducer manufacturers in conjunction with the CDC can help define current standards for HLD. Clinical sonographers should be knowledgeable in regard to current disinfection and sterilization procedures to ensure infection control and patient safety.

Pitfalls

1. Nonadherence to the ALARA principle.
2. Increasing the power output of an ultrasound system from manufacturer presets without understanding the ODS and potential bioeffects.
3. Not utilizing the correct application preset with appropriate power, TI, and MI for an examination.
4. Not having a standard protocol for both noninvasive and invasive probes.

5. Not having cleaning supplies on the machine or near the machine for POC use.
6. Not having provider and POC friendly logistics for invasive probe care.
7. Not setting responsibilities and accountability for machine and probe care.
8. Not having policies for use of non-sterile and sterile gel.

Key Recommendations

1. Identify, understand, and educate users about the ODS on your ultrasound system.
2. Monitor and correct inappropriate use of MI and TI settings such as not utilizing ocular presets on ocular ultrasound or spectral Doppler for fetal heart rate measurements.
3. Create and provide cleaning protocols, logistics, and supplies for POC use.
4. When performing ultrasound examination on non-intact skin, cover the transducer with a clear adhesive dressing.
5. To ensure patient safety, a clearly defined process of HLD must be in place for endocavitary and TEE transducer cleaning.

Acknowledgment   Dr. J. Brian Fowlkes for his assistance with reviewing and editing the bioeffects data.
  Dr. Andreas Dewitz for his donation of figures for the chapter.

References

1. Moore CL, Copel JA. Point-of-care ultrasonography. N Engl J Med. 2011;364(8):749–57. doi:10.1056/NEJMra0909487.
2. Nelson TR, Fowlkes JB, Abramowicz JS, Church CC. Ultrasound biosafety considerations for the practicing sonographer and sonologist. J Ultrasound Med. 2009;28:139–50.
3. Cibull SL, Harris GR, Nell DM. Trends in diagnostic ultrasound acoustic output from data reported to the US food and drug administration for device indications that include fetal applications. J Ultrasound Med. 2013;32(11):1921–32. doi:10.7863/ultra.32.11.1921.
4. United States Food and Drugs Administration. Guidance for Industry and FDA Staff—Information for manufacturers seeking marketing clearance of diagnostic ultrasound systems and transducers. 2012.
5. Lee W, Garra B, American Institute of Ultrasound in Medicine. AIUM technical bulletin. How to interpret the ultrasound output display standard for higher acoustic output diagnostic ultrasound devices: version 2. J Ultrasound Med. 2004;23(5):723–6.
6. National Electronics Manufacturers Association, American Institute of Ultrasound in Medicine. Standard for real-time display of thermal and mechanical acoustic output indices on diagnostic ultrasound equipment, Revision 2. January 9AD:1–55.
7. American Institute of Ultrasound in Medicine. Medical ultrasound safety. 3rd ed. American Institute of Ultrasound in Medicine; 2014, pp. 1–61.
8. OBrien WD, Deng CX, Harris GR, et al. The risk of exposure to diagnostic ultrasound in postnatal subjects thermal effects. J Ultrasound Med. 2008;27:517–35.

9. Abramowicz JS, Barnett SB, Duck FA, Edmonds PD, Hynynen KH, Ziskin MC. Fetal thermal effects of diagnostic ultrasound. J Ultrasound Med. 2008;27:541–59.
10. Mr T, Vedmedovska N, Merialdi M, et al. Safety of ultrasonography in pregnancy WHO systematic review of the literature and meta analysis. Ultrasound Obstet Gynecol. 2009;33:599–608.
11. Church CC, Carstensen EL, Nyborg WL, Carson PL, Frizzell LA, Bailey MR. Nonthermal mechanisms the risk of exposure to diagnostic ultrasound in postnatal subjects. J Ultrasound Med. 2008;27:565–92.
12. Stratmeyer ME, Greenleaf JF, Dalecki D, Salvesen KA. Fetal ultrasound mechanical effects. J Ultrasound Med. 2008;27:597–605.
13. Sheiner E, Abramowicz JS. Clinical end users worldwide show poor knowledge regarding safety issues of ultrasound during pregnancy. J Ultrasound Med. 2008;27:488–501.
14. Bagley J, Thomas K, DiGiacinto D. Safety practices of sonographers and their knowledge of the biologic effects of sonography. J Diagn Med Sonography. 2011;27:252–61. doi:10.1177/8756479311424431.
15. Akhtar W, Arain MA, Ali A, et al. Ultrasound biosafety during pregnancy: what do operators know in the developing world?: national survey findings from pakistan. J Ultrasound Med. 2011;30(7):981–5.
16. Houston LE, Allsworth J, Macones GA. Ultrasound is safe… right?: resident and maternal-fetal medicine fellow knowledge regarding obstetric ultrasound safety. J Ultrasound Med. 2011;30(1):21–7.
17. World Federation of Ultrasond in Medicine and Biology. WFUMB/ISUOG statement on the safe use of doppler ultrasound during 11–14 week scans (or earlier in pregnancy). Ultrasound Med Biol. 2013;39(3):373. doi:10.1016/j.ultrasmedbio.2012.11.025.
18. American Institute of Ultrasound in Medicine. Statement on measurement of fetal heart rate. 2011:1–1. http://www.aium.org/officialStatements/43.
19. Vrablik ME, Snead GR, Minnigan HJ, Kirschner JM, Emmett TW, Seupaul RA. The diagnostic accuracy of bedside ocular ultrasonography for the diagnosis of retinal detachment: a systematic review and meta-analysis. Ann Emerg Med. 2015;65(2):199–203.e1. doi:10.1016/j.annemergmed.2014.02.020.
20. Lichtenstein D. Lung ultrasound in acute respiratory failure an introduction to the BLUE-protocol. Minerva Anestesiol. 2009;75(5):313–7.
21. Meltzer RS, Adsumelli R, Risher WH, et al. Lack of lung hemorrhage in humans after intraoperative transesophageal echocardiography with ultrasound exposure conditions similar to those causing lung hemorrhage in laboratory animals. J Am Soc Echocardiogr. 1998;11(1):57–60.
22. American Institute of Ultrasound in Medicine. Conclusions regarding epidemiology for obstetric ultrasound. 2010:1–1. http://www.aium.org/officialStatements/16.
23. American College of Emergency Physicians. Emergency ultrasound guidelines. Ann Emerg Med. 2009;53(4):550–70. doi:10.1016/j.annemergmed.2008.12.013.
24. American College of Emergency Physicians Guidance for Line Model US Scanning in Educational and conference settings http://www.acep.org/ultrasound-section-microsite/guidance for live models-us-scanning in educational-end-conference settings. Accessed 30 July 2017.
25. Guideline for disinfection and sterilization in healthcare facilities, 2008. 2015;1–4.
26. AIUM Cleaning Guidelines 2014. 2015. pp. 1–5.
27. Guideline for disinfection and sterilization in healthcare facilities, 2008. 2010;1–158.
28. Rooks VJ, Yancey MK, Elg SA, Brueske L. Comparison of probe sheaths for endovaginal sonography. Obstet Gynecol. 1996 Jan;87(1):27–9.
29. Hignett M, Claman P. High rates of perforation are found in endovaginal ultrasound probe covers before and after oocyte retrieval for in vitro fertilizationembryo transfer. J Assist Reprod Genet. 1995 Oct;12(9):606–9.
30. Fritz S, Hust MH, Ochs C, Gratwohl I, Staiger M, Braun B. Use of a latex cover sheath for transesophageal echocardiography (TEE) instead of regular disinfection of the echoscope? Clin Cardiol. 1993 Oct;16(10):737–40.

31. Casalegno J-S, Le Bail CK, Eibach D, Valdeyron M-L, Lamblin G, Jacquemoud H, et al. High risk HPV contamination of endocavity vaginal ultrasound probes: an underestimated route of nosocomial infection? PLoS One. 2012;7(10):e48137.
32. M'Zali F, Bounizra C, Leroy S, Mekki Y, Quentin-Noury C, Kann M. Persistence of microbial contamination on transvaginal ultrasound probes despite low-level disinfection procedure. PLoS One. 2014;9(4):e93368.
33. Kac G, Podglajen I, Si Mohamed A, Rodi A, Grataloup C, Meyer G. Evaluation of ultraviolet C for disinfection of endocavitary ultrasound transducers persistently contaminated despite probe covers. Infect Control Hosp Epidemiol. 2010;31(2):165–70.
34. Frazee BW, Fahimi J, Lambert L, Nagdev A. Emergency department ultrasonographic probe contaminationand experimental model of probe disinfection. YMEM. American College of Emergency Physicians; 2011;1–8.
35. Muradali D, Gold WL, Phillips A, Wilson S. Can ultrasound probes and coupling gel be a source of nosocomial infection in patients undergoing sonography? An in vivo and in vitro study. AJR. 1995;164(6):1521–4.
36. O'Rourke M, Levan P, Khan T. Current use of ultrasound transmission gel for transesophageal echocardiogram examinations: a survey of cardiothoracic anesthesiology fellowship directors. J Cardiothorac Vasc Anesth. 2014;28(5):1208–10.
37. Safety Communication: Bacteria found in other-sonic generic ultrasound transmission gel poses risk of infection. Clinician Outreach and Communication Activity (COCA). CDC Emergency communication System. April 20, 2012. Accessed 5 Jan 2017 http://emergency.cdc.gov/coca/reminders/2012/pdf/ClinicalReminder_UltraSoundGel_04_20_2012.pdf.
38. Serious risk of infection from ultrasound and medical gels—revision. Health Canada. December 14, 2004. Accessed 5 Jan 2017 http://www.healthycanadians.gc.ca/recall-alert-rappel-avis/hc-sc/2004/14289a-eng.php.
39. American Institute of Ultrasound in Medicine. Guidelines for cleaning and preparing external- and internal-use ultrasound probes between patients, safe handling, and use of ultrasound coupling gel http://www.aium.org/officialStatements/57. Accessed 31 May 2017.

Chapter 16
Ultrasound Quality Improvement

Patrick S. Hunt, Christopher David Wilbert, and Zachary T. Grambos

Objectives

- Define the purpose of Ultrasound Quality Assurance and Improvement (QI)
- Provide an overview of Ultrasound Quality Assurance and Improvement
- Define a practical and stepwise process for improvement of ultrasound quality

Introduction

Ultrasound quality assurance and improvement is the engine that drives a successful clinical US program. Every department that uses clinical ultrasound should have an integrated quality assurance and quality improvement plan (QI) [2, 27, 29]. While the details of each QI system may differ from program to program, the primary objectives of the program are to ensure a quality product, facilitate education, improve both provider and departmental performance, and to help satisfy credentialing pathways [2, 27].

P.S. Hunt, MD, MBA (✉)
Department of Emergency Medicine, Palmetto Health Richland,
Columbia, SC, USA
e-mail: huntpat@sc.rr.com

C.D. Wilbert, MD • Z.T. Grambos, MD, FAAEM
Department of Emergency Medicine, St. Thomas Rutherford/Midtown Hospital,
Murfreesboro, TN, USA
e-mail: grambos1256@gmail.com

© Springer International Publishing AG 2018   269
V. S. Tayal et al. (eds.), *Ultrasound Program Management*,
https://doi.org/10.1007/978-3-319-63143-1_16

It is the US director's responsibility to develop, monitor, and revise the QI process [2]. QI programs include the processes as well as the hardware and software that make these processes work. The process your program ultimately uses for QI will depend greatly on the hardware and software system deployed.

The US director's goals regarding QI are multifaceted. At a minimum they must evaluate images that are submitted to ensure they satisfy the minimum imaging requirements (gain/depth/focus) and confirm the images have been interpreted correctly. The director must also provide appropriate feedback to both develop good practice and change detrimental practice. This can be done at the bedside in real time or at a later time in person or electronically [27].

There are many options for QI systems currently on the market. When clinical ultrasound programs began to develop, QI generally consisted of printed images and logs. However, today there are complete digital solutions that help to integrate the QI system to the workflow of the ultrasound program. The system that works best for each institution will vary depending on how robust the program is, the amount of administrative and financial support, as well as the type of machine and support from IT. As cost for data storage and bandwidth have continued to decrease, options for dynamic video review are now more available than ever. While dynamic video is superior to static images, the increased cost, time and labor must be weighted when determining which method of image review is ideal for each program [2, 15, 27].

Process of QI

Often the QI process is developed in parallel with the credentialing process. During this process a program should determine how they will handle scans completed by both credentialed and non-credentialed sonographers with regard to QI. While most programs will review all scans by non-credentialed sonographers, programs must also decide on the percentage of cases that will be selected for review from credentialed sonographers. This can be a percentage of completed scans or a fixed number of scans per year depending on practice habits and prior training/credentialing for the group [1, 2, 28].

It is to be expected that the QI process will look slightly different for every department. Residency programs can expect a continual process given that new residents start every year and must be trained. In community programs the process may require more work at the outset and then stabilize once all the members of the group have been credentialed. However, there are five key aspects of QI that should be universal to all settings [2].

1. Images must be obtained and stored for review.
2. The sonographer must document their findings for each study completed.
3. Images must be reviewed by the QI director and feedback given on both technical and clinical grounds.
4. Feedback on images must be reviewed by the sonographer.
5. Data on the feedback given and the exams completed must be stored for later review.

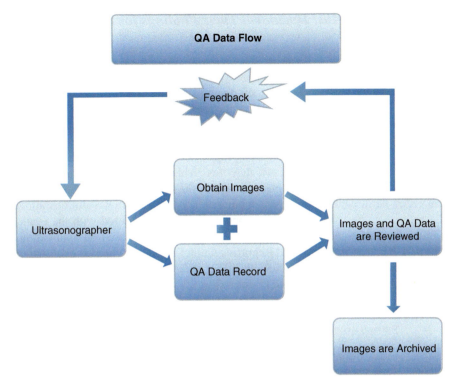

Fig. 16.1 An example QI flowsheet showing the data flow in the QI process

These five aspects of a QI program can be viewed as the flow diagram below (Fig. 16.1)

We will now look at each of these topics in more detail.

Images Must Be Obtained and Stored for Review

Given the variety of ultrasound systems and methods of capturing and storing ultrasound images it is not practical to list every option (Chaps. 17 and 18).

It is preferred that once the images are captured that they be transferred to an external archive system for review and storage. While QI can by directly completed on the ultrasound machine, ultimately the machines are not designed for long-term storage and date retrieval. Depending on the systems in place a program may prefer to use still images or video or both for review [1, 2].

The ideal image flow process allows for uploading of images and clips from the ultrasound machine directly to the EMR, to a QI system, to the ultrasound director, and back to the performing sonographer in a HIPAA compliant manner [1, 2].

The Sonologist Must Document Their Findings for Each Study Completed

After completion of an ultrasound study a sonographer should complete a US report form that corresponds with their documentation of the findings that go into the chart. This sheet should also allow the sonographer to self-reflect and comment on the adequacy of their findings. This sheet should allow the sonographer to directly answer the yes/no questions regarding findings from their examination. On the US report forms, the sonographer should identify the indication for the exam as well as which views they were able to obtain. The sonographer should also comment on their interpretation of the images [1, 2, 27]. These forms can either be in paper format or computerized. Some workflow solutions allow these forms to be filled out on the machine and then submitted with the exam, while others allow the user to complete the forms on the actual QI application. The ACEP Ultrasound Standard Reporting Guidelines [31] suggest the following data elements be included in all studies (Fig. 16.2).

Below is a simple paper-based QI form (Fig. 16.3).

Patient/ exam demographics:

Patient name: _____

Patient gender: ☐ M ☐ F

DOB: ___ / ___ / ___

MR#: _____

Bar Code/Patient Identifier: _____

Hosptial Name: _____

Date and time of exam: ___ / ___ / ___

Exam type:

    ☐ Diagnostic

    ☐ Educational

    ☐ Procedural

Clinical category:

    ☐ Resuscitative

    ☐ Symptom based

    ☐ Therapeutic

    ☐ Unknown/other

☐ Initial exam

☐ Repeat exam

Primary person obtaining/ interpreting images: _____
Secondary person obtaining/ interpreting images: _____
Additional person(s) obtaining/ interpreting images: _____

Fig. 16.2 An example of a standard patient demographic form for a limited point-of-care ultrasound examination

Physicians Code		FAST EXAM	
Hospital Code			
Patient Code			
Date			
Indication	Abdominal Pain	Trauma	Hypotension
Findings	Yes	No	Indeterminate
IPF at Morison's pouch			
IPF at spleno-renal fossa			
Pericardial fluid			
Cardiac Activity			
IPF in pelvis			

Fig. 16.3 A simple paper-based QI form for point-of-care ultrasound exams

Images Must Be Reviewed by the QI Director and Feedback Given on Both Technical and Clinical Grounds

This component of QI involves reviewing the images to ensure that they match findings that are documented. It is at this phase that the reviewer will want to comment on the technical aspects of the images obtained. Determining if features such as gain, depth, orientation, and probe position were appropriate. QI forms for each specific indication can be completed at this time and submitted back to the performing sonographer. These forms will include specific questions based on the type of study being completed. An emergency physician, who has completed an Emergency Ultrasound Fellowship or similar level of experience, preferentially performs the review of these still or video images [1, 2, 27, 28, 31]. ACEP has developed a set of Standard Reporting Guidelines including a Suggested Quality Assurance Grading Scale that can be used as a model to determine the quality of images that are submitted. This scale is included below (Fig. 16.4).

QI also includes following up on any incidental findings, incorrect interpretations, as well as any clinically relevant findings for which the patient was subsequently evaluated. In cases where there are questionable findings the reviewer may wish to contact the sonographer directly to get additional information regarding the case or the clinical outcome of the patient [1, 28, 31]. It is during this review of the patient's course that the ultrasound program really begins to improve as a diagnostic modality. By learning from "gold standards," correlation between ultrasound and other modalities helps to ensure the accuracy of findings [28]. It is important to compare the impression of the emergency ultrasound to additional data available regarding the patient. For example, a program will evaluate findings from

Suggested Quality Assurance Grading Scale

	1	2	3	4	5
Grading Scale Definitions	No recognizable structures, no objective data can be gathered	Minimally recognizable structures but insufficient for diagnosis	Minimal criteria met for diagnosis, recognizable structures but with some technical or other flaws	Minimal criteria met for diagnosis, all structures imaged well and diagnosis easily supported	Minimal criteria met for diagnosis, all structures imaged with excellent image quality and diagnosis completely supported

Image quality	1	2	3	4	5				
Accuracy of interpretation of images as presented						TP	TN	FP	FN
Accuracy of interpretation of images as compared to gold standard (ie, CT, operative report)						TP	TN	FP	FN

Fig. 16.4 ACEP's Suggested Quality Improvement Grading Scale from the Standard Reporting Guidelines

For Reviewer Use Only	Reviewer Code		
Image Acquisition	**Yes**	**No**	**Not Acquired**
RUQ			
Cardiac			
Pelivs			
LUQ			

Exam Assesment	**Agree**		**Disagree**	
Accuracy of Interpretations				
Overall Exam Adequate				

Exam Results	**True +**	**True -**	**False +**	**False -**
Exam Results				

Comments:

Fig. 16.5 An example of a simple QI review form for point-of-care ultrasound exams

surgery or other clinical studies to see if they mathch the findings of the limited emergency ultrasound exam. All of this information can be documented on the QI forms, which will be reviewed by the sonographer. Examples of a simple paper form and a more complex electronic form are included below (Figs. 16.5 and 16.6).

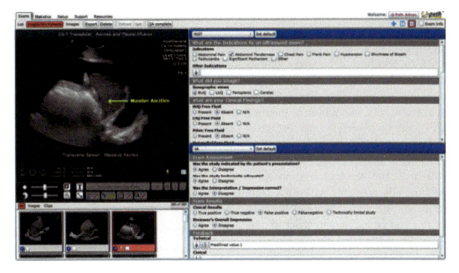

Fig. 16.6 Qpath (Telexy Healthcare, BC, Canada) sample QI worksheet and image review form

Feedback on Images Must Be Reviewed by the Sonographer

One of the most crucial components of a successful QI program is the feedback loop for the sonographer. Once the reviewer has completed their evaluation of the images and given their feedback, the sonographer should review these findings. This is the process that allows the sonographer to grow and improve their skill set. The sonographer should note that they have received and reviewed the feedback [1, 2, 27, 28].

Data on the Feedback Given and the Exams Completed Must Be Stored for Later Review

The final step in the QI process is to store all of the documentation and images in a secure location. In the past when all images were printed and QI was completed on paper forms, this type of storage required a large amount of space and was not easily searchable in the event a study needed to be located. Now with the increased availability of digital solutions, data can be stored very easily in a HIPAA compliant fashion. In addition, this data becomes very easy to search and specific cases can be located if needed [1, 2].

QI in Academic Centers

While the basic outline and functions of a QI program will be the same for both academic and community medical centers, there are some key differences that are worth noting. In a residency program the QI process may need to be more robust as you will continually have new residents with limited or no experience completing ultrasounds. Additionally, the volume of studies that require review will likely be higher than in a stable community physician group. Often as part of their training, residents will have dedicated rotations for learning emergency ultrasound. During these rotations the ultrasound director is often scanning with and/or observing the resident scanning. This allows for instant QI and rapid improvement in the resident's skill sets. In addition to the resident physicians, the ultrasound director must also continue to review a percentage of scans from credentialed faculty.

Detailed record keeping is especially important in the residency programs. Tracking resident's progress as they move through their residency helps insure they will meet the recommendation set forth in the ACEP Ultrasound Guidelines. Additionally residents will often require documentation upon completion of their residency that they have met the number of studies recommended by the ACEP Ultrasound Guidelines in order to obtain credentials in their new institutions [1, 2, 9, 27, 29].

QI in Community Hospitals

The QI process in the community setting serves many of the same roles as it does in the academic setting. The QI program should strive to keep track of the total number of exams that practicing physicians are performing. Again, a periodic sampling of all physicians' images and documentation should be reviewed. This process should also ensure that all members are performing and interpreting their ultrasound images in a quality manner. Physicians who are not yet credentialed should have all of their images reviewed. Once fully credentialed the physician group or ultrasound director should determine the percentage of the physician's images that should be reviewed yearly. It is reasonable that a performance evaluation that contains the number of scans and the adequacy of the the sampled portion be provided to credentialed physicians periodically. Similar to residents a meaningful portion of cases should contain pathology. This helps to ensure that studies are being performed on appropriate patients and therefore the performing sonographer fully understands the indications for emergency ultrasound [1, 2].

Terminology

There is some debate with regard to using the term "Quality Assurance" instead of "Quality Improvement" given that a misinterpreted scan will call the "Quality Assurance" program into question. Individually credentialed physicians are able to independently obtain and interpret their own images. Therefore, the ultrasound

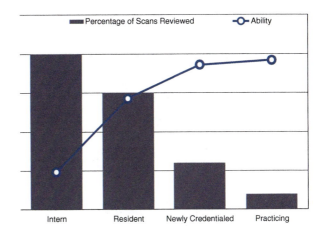

Fig. 16.7 Decreasing image review percentages based on provider skill level [21]

director is not over-reading other sonographer's images. The findings documented belong to the performing credentialed physician and should remain that way. However, a quality improvement program hopes to identify these errors and improve knowledge deficits to prevent such errors from occurring in the future. In general, the term "Quality Improvement" is preferred over "Quality Assurance" (Fig. 16.7).

Pitfalls

1. Making the QI forms too cumbersome for physicians to complete. Ideally the data should be entered when the exam in completed, and be simple enough to not impede completion of the form.
2. Failure to store data in a HIPAA compliant fashion.
3. Failure to have the trainee review the QI feedback. This final step in the QI process is critical to actually improving the trainees proficiency.

Key Recommendations

1. Invest in software that allows for review of both still and video images. Limiting yourself to one modality will limit what you are able to identify in your review process.
2. Keep the process of submitting images simple. A complex process can decrease the number of cases that are uploaded to the system.
3. Keep high standards for scans. Setting the bar too low can decrease the quality of training especially for providers that are just learning ultrasound.

References

1. American College of Emergency Physicians. ACEP emergency ultrasound guidelines-2001. Ann Emerg Med. 2001;38(4):470.
2. Tayal V, et al. Emergency ultrasound guidelines. Ann Emerg Med. 2009;53(4):550–70.
3. American Institute of Ultrasound in Medicine. Training guidelines for physicians who evaluate and interpret diagnostic ultrasound examinations (approved November 6, 2010). American Institute of Ultrasound in Medicine website. http://www.aium.org/publications/statements.aspx. Accessed 22 Mar 2011.
4. Hertzberg BS, et al. Physician training requirements in sonography: how many cases are needed for competence? Am J Roentgenol. 2000;174(5):1221–7.
5. Rose JS, et al. Physician sonography training competency. AJR Am J Roentgenol. 2001;176(3):813.
6. Kaplan D. The trouble with ultrasound's pervasive use by non-radiologists—diagnostic imaging [Internet]. Diagn Imaging. 2011 [cited 2013 Feb 18]. http://www.diagnosticimaging.com/ultrasound/content/article/113619/1814358#.
7. Shackford SR, et al. Focused abdominal sonogram for trauma: the learning curve of nonradiologist clinicians in detecting hemoperitoneum. J Trauma Acute Care Surg. 1999;46(4):553–64.
8. Lewiss RE, et al. CORD-AEUS: consensus document for the emergency ultrasound milestone project. Acad Emerg Med. 2013;20(7):740–5.
9. Jang T, Aubin C, Naunheim R. Minimum training for right upper quadrant ultrasonography. Am J Emerg Med. 2004;22(6):439–43.
10. Gaspari RJ, Dickman E, Blehar D. Learning curve of bedside ultrasound of the gallbladder. J Emerg Med. 2009;37(1):51–6.
11. Jang TB, et al. The learning curve of resident physicians using emergency ultrasonography for cholelithiasis and cholecystitis. Acad Emerg Med. 2010;17(11):1247–52.
12. Summers SM, et al. A prospective evaluation of emergency department bedside ultrasonography for the detection of acute cholecystitis. Ann Emerg Med. 2010;56(2):114–22.
13. Jang TB, et al. Learning curve of emergency physicians using emergency bedside sonography for symptomatic first-trimester pregnancy. J Ultrasound Med. 2010;29(10):1423–8.
14. Jang TB, et al. The learning curve of resident physicians using emergency ultrasonography for obstructive uropathy. Acad Emerg Med. 2010;17(9):1024–7.
15. Cook T, Hunt P, Hoppman R. Emergency medicine leads the way for training medical students in clinician-based ultrasound: a radical paradigm shift in patient imaging. Acad Emerg Med. 2007;14(6):558–61.
16. Mandavia DP, et al. Ultrasound training for emergency physicians—a prospective study. Acad Emerg Med. 2000;7(9):1008–14.
17. Ma OJ, Gaddis G. Anechoic stripe size influences accuracy of FAST examination interpretation. Acad Emerg Med. 2006;13(3):248–53.
18. Alberg AJ, et al. The use of "overall accuracy" to evaluate the validity of screening or diagnostic tests. J Gen Intern Med. 2004;19(5 pt 1):460–5.
19. Gallagher EJ. Numeric instability of predictive values. Ann Emerg Med. 2005;46(4):311–3.
20. Gallagher EJ. The problem with sensitivity and specificity…. Ann Emerg Med. 2003;42(2):298–303.
21. Pusic M, Pecaric M, Boutis K. How much practice is enough? Using learning curves to assess the deliberate practice of radiograph interpretation. Acad Med. 2011;86(6):731–6.
22. Ericsson KA. Deliberate practice and the acquisition and maintenance of expert performance in medicine and related domains. Acad Med. 2004;79(10):S70–81.
23. Robinson PJ, et al. Variation between experienced observers in the interpretation of accident and emergency radiographs. Br J Radiol. 1999;72(856):323–30.
24. Consensus. AIUM Officially Recognizes ACEP Emergency Ultrasound Guideline [Internet]. AIUM Sound Waves. 2011 [cited 2012 Nov 13]. http://www.aium.org/soundWaves/article.aspx?aId=442&iId=20111117.

25. Blaivas M, Pawl R. Analysis of lawsuits filed against emergency physicians for point-of-care emergency ultrasound examination performance and interpretation over a 20-year period. Am J Emerg Med. 2012;30(2):338–41.
26. Stolz L, et al. A review of lawsuits related to point-of-care emergency ultrasound applications. Western J Emerg Med. 2015;16(1):1.
27. Akhtar S, et al. Resident training in emergency ultrasound: consensus recommendations from the 2008 Council of Emergency Medicine Residency Directors Conference. Acad Emerg Med. 2009;16(s2):S32–6.
28. Heller MB, et al. Residency training in emergency ultrasound: fulfilling the mandate. Acad Emerg Med. 2002;9(8):835–9.
29. Moore CL, Gregg S, Lambert M. Performance, training, quality assurance, and reimbursement of emergency physician–performed ultrasonography at academic medical centers. J Ultrasound Med. 2004;23(4):459–66.
30. Stein JC, et al. A survey of bedside ultrasound use by emergency physicians in California. J Ultrasound Med. 2009;28(6):757–63.
31. American College of Emergency Physicians. "Emergency Ultrasound Standard Reporting Guidelines. 2011.

Chapter 17
Workflow and Middleware

Christopher J. Bryczkowski and Mark W. Byrne

Objectives

1. Provide contextual background illustrating the importance of a workflow solution
2. Understand workflow infrastructure and associated terminology
3. Discuss benefits to use of middleware in an ultrasound program
4. Familiarize reader with current workflow products and highlight key features

Introduction

Consider the following case: A 22-year-old male presents to the Emergency Department (ED) with a 1 day history of fever, anorexia, vomiting, and periumbilical abdominal pain. A clinical ultrasound is performed which demonstrates appendicitis. The surgeon on call is contacted, however, due to their inability to visualize the images as well as a report, a request is made to obtain a CT scan of the abdomen prior to any surgical intervention. This delays patient care by 6 h.

Clinical ultrasonography provides essential diagnostic information at the bedside. Often times this data needs to be shared with other medical providers outside the primary team. Within the current infrastructure of hospital information technology (IT),

C.J. Bryczkowski, MD, FACEP
Department of Emergency Medicine, Robert Wood Johnson Medical School,
New Brunswick, NJ, USA

M.W. Byrne, MD (✉)
Department of Emergency Medicine, Boston Medical Center, Boston University School of
Medicine, Boston, MA, USA
e-mail: mwbyrne.md@gmail.com

© Springer International Publishing AG 2018
V. S. Tayal et al. (eds.), *Ultrasound Program Management*,
https://doi.org/10.1007/978-3-319-63143-1_17

ultrasound machines and the electronic medical record (EMR) are not configured to communicate directly with one another. Similar to meaningful use initiatives in other areas of the medical record, ultrasound studies should be electronically archived and available to all providers. Instituting this in a clinical ultrasound program is frequently challenging, although establishing a workflow is paramount for a program to succeed. An effective workflow provides a coordinated approach to storing and sharing ultrasound examinations. Various workflow options exist, and the decisions which influence workflow selection may be institutionally, feature, and/or cost driven.

At present, the most common workflow setup for clinical ultrasound programs is homegrown, according to a 2013 survey by the American College of Emergency Physicians (ACEP) [1]. These setups utilize basic export standards on ultrasound machines, either digital image transfer using the universal serial bus (USB) port or by printing thermal images, which can then be attached to a paper chart. Digital image exportation onto USB flash or hard disk drives offers distinct advantages over thermal prints. Images retain their original resolution, ultrasound scans can be saved as video clips, and exams may be uploaded to digital image archive systems. Additionally, digital images will not fade over time, as occurs with thermal prints.

While these methods are readily available and inexpensive, they offer no means for organizing ultrasound exams, generating image interpretation reports, or disseminating the results. As a consequence, programs often have turned to makeshift solutions, such as archiving images on local hard disk drives and maintaining records of studies using standard spreadsheet software (e.g., Microsoft Excel®). See Chapter 18–Practical Operating Solutions.

As an ultrasound program grows, it is quite easy for such workflow solutions to outgrow their capabilities. Manual data entry and manual download and archival of studies are both tedious and time consuming, as well as introduce the potential for human error. In comparison, an effective workflow should rely upon a more automated process.

Infrastructure

Digital Imaging and Communications in Medicine (DICOM) is a standard format used for transferring imaging in healthcare, including ultrasound. This was developed in the early 1980s by the ACR (American College of Radiologists) and NEMA (National Electrical Manufacturers Association) due to inability of CT and MRI systems at that time to conform to a single image-decoding standard [2]. For ultrasound, each DICOM file incorporates the recorded images along with various other data, including patient identifiers, study date and time, hospital and department location, and the ultrasound machine used.

Ultrasound machines can communicate via DICOM to other electronic healthcare systems over a hospital network using either a wired or, when supported by the machine hardware, a wireless network. Clinical ultrasonography requires the use of portable ultrasound machines, which must be transported to the patient bedside.

This has made wireless connectivity using the Institute of Electrical and Electronics Engineers (IEEE) 802 local area network standard the preferred and most requested connection [3].

Traditional Radiology imaging workflow has been set up to send images to a hospital-based Picture Archiving and Communication System (PACS) using DICOM over a wired network. A PACS serves as a digital storage repository for hospital imaging received from multiple modalities, including CT, MRI, and ultrasound. Radiologists typically access the PACS system on stationary workstations to enter interpretation reports, which are then transferred to the hospital EMR. EMR systems contain imaging reports but at present are rarely used to store images themselves.

While ultrasound machines have the capability to send their images to a PACS server, there are factors that should be weighed when deciding whether to transfer all (or some) clinical ultrasound exams directly to the PACS. Generally speaking, studies performed by novice sonographers for either training or credentialing purposes should generally be kept off the main institutional PACS. This is primarily due to the fact that many of these scans are neither indicated for the patient's care nor are they optimally imaged. As the images acquired generally should not be used for medical decision-making, they shouldn't be archived on an institutional PACS. Alternatively, credentialed, clinical exams should be shared with the medical staff and utilizing the PACS can be cost effective and powerful. As staff members are likely familiar in its use, reviewing clinical ultrasound exams would be no different than visualizing radiology-based studies.

Novice scans should still be retained for many reasons including quality assurance, teaching, and credentialing which must and can be solved independently of traditional PACS image retention.

Middleware

Enter middleware. Middleware, also known as US Management systems or workflow solutions, is software with the goal of organizing and streamlining workflow in a clinical ultrasound program. Middleware products are capable of intercommunicating with various hospital data systems to seamlessly transfer scan data. They provide functionality for image archival and generation of interpretation reports, as well as track provider credentialing and aid in quality assurance and feedback. Middleware products can work either in tandem with or in place of a PACS server. A middleware solution is usually hosted on a server within the hospital network, although also may reside in the cloud and be remotely accessed. A local server is generally utilized for departments within a single hospital site, whereas a cloud-based setup may aid organizations with multiple sites, each within different hospital networks, to centralize storage. Middleware solutions have been tailored for clinical ultrasounds performed at the point of care, and accordingly serve to simplify workflow in several key areas (Fig. 17.1).

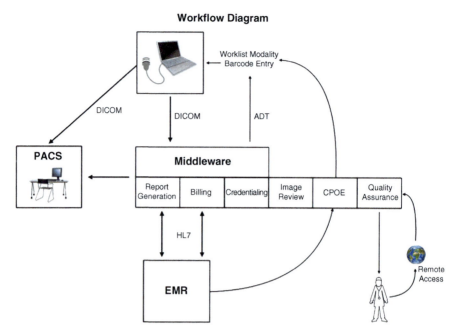

Fig. 17.1 Workflow overview diagram

Data Entry

Upon initiating an ultrasound exam, various demographic information needs to be entered into the ultrasound machine in order to link the study to the patient's hospital record. This usually consists of the patient's name and medical record number and may also include additional information such as the date of birth. Likewise, the provider performing the scan has to input his or her name. Manual entry of this data is both tedious and more importantly prone to human error. Automated solutions exist to streamline this workflow process.

The admissions, discharge, and transfer (ADT) system serves as the framework for most hospital IT systems. It holds essential patient information including full name, date of birth, and medical record and account numbers. When patients enter a healthcare facility, their registration information is linked to and stored within the ADT. The ADT system is then utilized for patient tracking and throughput as well as billing purposes. The ADT shares relevant patient data (such as demographics or isolation precautions) with other hospital IT systems such as the EMR [4].

One function of DICOM protocols is a modality worklist, whereby ultrasound orders submitted into computerized physician order entry (CPOE) are transferred to the ultrasound machine in a worklist format. When beginning a scan on a patient, the corresponding order within the modality worklist on the ultrasound machine may be selected, which then autopopulates multiple demographic fields using information from the ADT system. While this process is native to any ultrasound machine with DICOM functionality, middleware products can be utilized to facilitate modality worklist generation. Using information from the ADT system, middleware can create a worklist of all patients currently residing within the ER, bypassing the need to place an initial CPOE order.

Another means of autopopulating patient information onto the ultrasound machine is via barcode scanners. Healthcare institutions encode patient information onto barcodes residing on patient identification bracelets. Most ultrasound vendors support barcode scanners that can then be used to transmit information from the patient barcode into fields on the ultrasound machine. Often these barcode scanners are proprietary and specific to the individual ultrasound machine vendor, although on certain machines a standard barcode scanner (e.g., Motorola Symbol series) can be attached to the machine's USB port. It is important to recognize that the information that the patient barcode encodes for varies across different institutions. While often the barcode contains the medical record number, it may also encode for different patient data, such as the visit number.

Report Generation

Middleware user interfaces are designed to allow for a high degree of customization. Categorizing studies by patient, the performing provider, date of scan, or the machine used should all be easily configurable options (Fig. 17.2).

After an ultrasound study is complete, images and scan data can be sent via DICOM to middleware. Interpretation of the ultrasound exam can then be entered into an electronic worksheet on a computer workstation. Interpretation worksheets should be fully customizable by the administrator in order to tailor to the needs of the individual hospital site (Fig. 17.3). In certain circumstances, depending on the specific middleware product and ultrasound machine vendor, worksheets can be completed directly on the ultrasound machine. This streamlined approach of performing and interpreting ultrasound studies at the point of care has been a frequently requested feature for many users of clinical ultrasound.

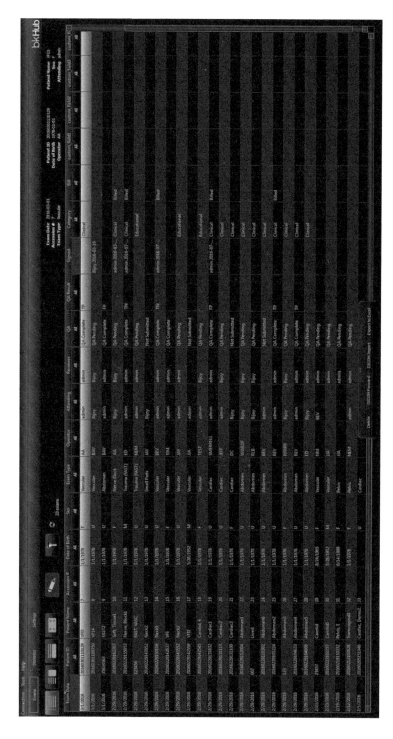

Fig. 17.2 Sample middleware worklist. © 2016 BK Ultrasound

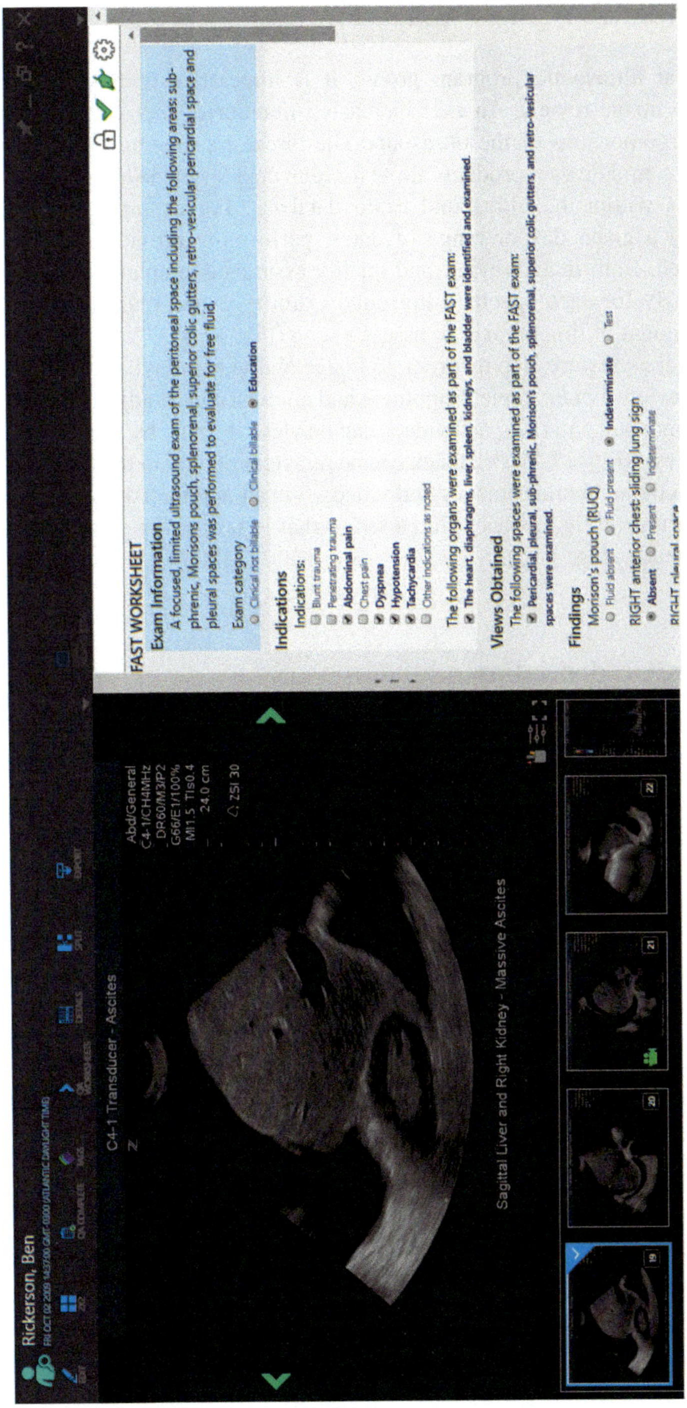

Fig. 17.3 Sample exam report. © 2016 Telexy Healthcare Inc

Image Review/Quality Improvement

As a clinical ultrasound program grows, it is imperative to have a structured approach to image review. An ever-increasing number of images to review may consume large portions of the ultrasound site director's time and efforts. As discussed above, middleware products allow for high degrees of customization in organizing scans within the ultrasound exam database. For example, scans can be reviewed by a given day or range of dates, performing provider, or ultrasound machine used. Both image review and quality assurance templates can be viewed simultaneously for each specific ultrasound exam type and thus significantly cut down the amount of time it takes to assess a scan (Fig. 17.4).

Middleware software also incorporate image and video playback tools to facilitate image review. For example, brightness and contrast can be adjusted, images can be zoomed into and enlarged, and videos can be viewed frame by frame to allow for precise analysis (Fig. 17.5). Feedback can be relayed not only in the form of written text but also by annotating images and videos. Via an automated process, the software can then compile feedback into a report that is sent to the clinician who performed the study (Fig. 17.6).

Education/Credentialing

Timely feedback is particularly important when trainees are involved. Some ultrasound clips may contain common findings, while others subtleties. In both instances, valid teaching points regarding scan technique, image interpretation, or medical management may be important to make. Accordingly, middleware software provides a means for image and video exportation into commonly used file formats. Automated removal of patient identifiers from ultrasound scan images avoids potential violation of the Health Insurance Portability and Accountability Act (HIPAA). Exported images and video clips can subsequently be used in publications or presentations to share with the broader medical community.

As providers submit increasing numbers of scans, it is important to track individual provider scan numbers. Resident scan numbers must be followed in order to ensure they meet ultrasound milestones, and attending physician scan numbers must be tracked for hospital credentialing purposes. All ultrasound scans already reside within the middleware exam database, and middleware software provides functionality to easily generate reports of number of scans performed by each individual provider (Fig. 17.7).

Furthermore, data obtained from worksheets can be used as a part of a robust research database. Interpretation worksheets may be refined to identify specific data points (for example, ultrasound-guided peripheral intravenous access placed in transverse approach), which can be an invaluable aid when planning and performing research projects. Data can then be easily exported and compiled to standard spreadsheet software (Microsoft Excel®) for further analysis.

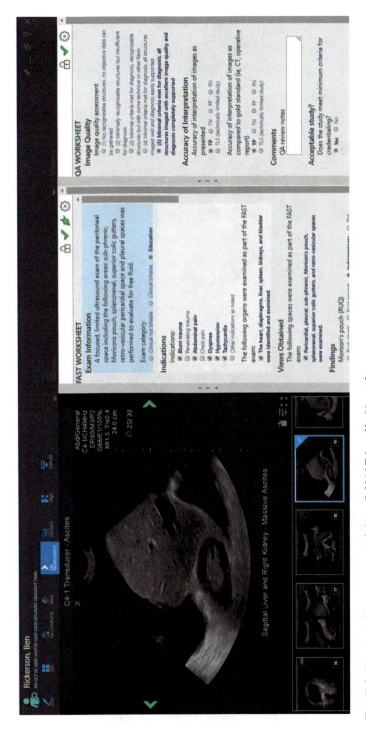

Fig. 17.4 Sample quality assurance worksheet. © 2016 Telexy Healthcare Inc

C.J. Bryczkowski and M.W. Byrne

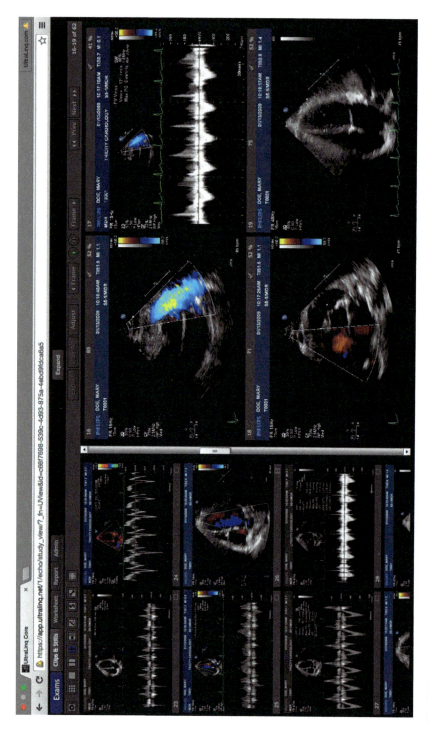

Fig. 17.5 Sample image viewer. © 2016 UltraLinq Healthcare Solutions Inc

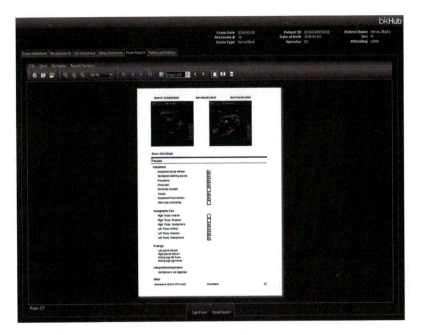

Fig. 17.6 Sample exam report. © 2016 BK Ultrasound

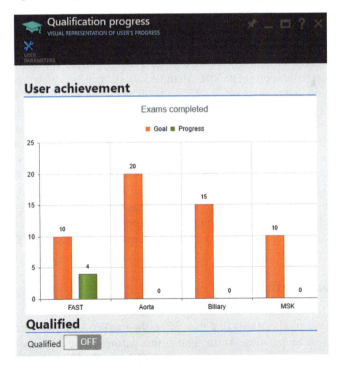

Fig. 17.7 Sample statistics report. © 2016 Telexy Healthcare Inc

Order Entry/Billing

The method of billing for clinical ultrasound exams varies greatly across different institutions. In some instances, the billing interface may be built directly into the EMR, while in others it may be independent. In either case, the use of middleware to facilitate ultrasound billing can capture substantial revenue, which may rapidly pay for the cost required for initial software implementation.

Analogous to ultrasound machines communicating with middleware via DICOM, middleware has the capability to interact with EMRs using what is known as Health Level 7 (HL7). HL7 refers to a set of standards used in the transfer of administrative and clinical data among various healthcare software applications. It serves to enhance interoperability, giving electronic systems the ability to exchange information [5].

Any bill generated from an ultrasound exam has to first start with a request, or an order to perform the study in the first place. Via the use of HL7 connectivity, the request for the completion of the ultrasound exam can be accomplished in various ways.

The order to perform a clinical ultrasound exam can be placed using the CPOE functionality of an EMR. Middleware software can be configured to receive this request and send the ordered study to a modality worklist on the ultrasound machine. The provider can then select the corresponding study from the modality worklist on the ultrasound machine as previously discussed. After images have been obtained and a study interpretation has been entered, the middleware software will then automatically generate a billing report.

Through the use of middleware, this task can also be accomplished retrospectively. For instance, if a patient presents in extremis, an ultrasound is often performed at the point of care without any known demographics. Once the ultrasound examination is complete, the appropriate MR (Medical Record) number can be placed within the middleware and then all other relevant fields including name, age, and account number will autopopulate. A report worksheet can then be filled out and subsequently submitted for billing. In this scenario, middleware can automatically communicate with the EMR and place an order for the completed ultrasound exam on the back-end. As a result, when a bill is generated it is directly tied to a request for it.

In either scenario, the middleware can also facilitate billing inquiries. It can check whether appropriate sections of a report were filled out in order to generate a bill. Likewise, it can be set to flag studies that, for instance, don't have indications or appropriate charge codes selected. This can aid an administrator in understanding why certain examinations were not successfully billed and in some cases perform a simple fix in order to resubmit.

Middleware Vendors

Given the distinct advantages that they offer, the market for middleware management systems is blossoming. At the time of this writing, there are three major vendors that offer workflow systems: Q-path™ (Telexy Healthcare), BkHub™ (BK ultrasound), and UltraLinq®. Additionally, there are many upcoming software companies such as Tricefy™ (Trice Imaging, Inc.), which will further add diversity to a growing market segment. Until recently, SonoSite™ (Fujifilm Inc.) ultrasound systems had made their own workflow solutions software "SonoSite SWS" but have since advertised support to the use of Q-path. At the time of this writing, Q-path seems to have the largest point of care market share [6].

All middleware workflow solutions have the overall goal of facilitating the user in the archive, review, and dissemination of clinical ultrasound examinations. Nevertheless, there are distinct differences among them, which must be assessed in detail prior to a purchasing decision. While comparing and contrasting each individual feature is beyond the scope of this chapter, some key differences, current at the time of this writing, will be reviewed.

Q-path and BkHub are installed on local servers within a medical institution (Figs. 17.8 and 17.9) They can both send images to PACS, but may also work independent of one for clinical ultrasound exams. Both are HL7 compatible and are interlinked to other hospital data systems via the hospital network. They have a robust interface for reviewing examinations and allow the administrator to customize worksheets for both report generation as well as quality assurance/feedback. They both support integrated worksheets, but this depends on the ultrasound machine vendor. For instance, BkHub supports worksheets only on Bk ultrasound systems. Remote access is achievable with both Q-path and BkHub through the use of a point-to-point connection. Depending on the healthcare institution this may be via the use of a hospital-based virtual private network (VPN) or a commercially available solution such as Citrix™ (Citrix Systems, Inc.). In essence, a user connects to the middleware for remote viewing by having to first connect to the hospital network and accessing the software through it.

UltraLinq as well as Tricefy are cloud-based storage systems in which examinations are hosted on a server external to the medical institution. Much like any other website, they offer the advantage of easy access from any Internet enabled device—there is no need for connecting to the hospital network. However, as the workflows are web-based, UltraLinq and Tricefy both do not offer support for integrated worksheets on ultrasound systems. Furthermore, there is no ability to send images from the worklist directly to a PACS, if needed. They do offer feedback reporting, but do not offer the customizable worksheets to the degree that the locally stored middleware allow (Figs. 17.10 and 17.11).

Of note, Q-path also has a cloud-based storage option "Q-path Cloud" which offers the dual benefit of having a locally installed server, along with off-site storage hosted by Q-path. This hybrid model may be beneficial to share image data for those within a healthcare system that has more than one site.

Generally, middleware that is locally hosted, such as BkHub and Q-path, have a much higher upfront cost versus web-based workflow platforms. This cost can range in the ballpark of $10,000 to $20,000+. Web-based solutions, such as UltraLinq or Tricefy, are typically based on a flat fee per scan cost model. Deciding on a middleware platform is much like expanding an emergency department—one has to anticipate growth. If clinical ultrasound studies are only going to be performed by credentialed providers and billed, then paying a small cost is cheaper and

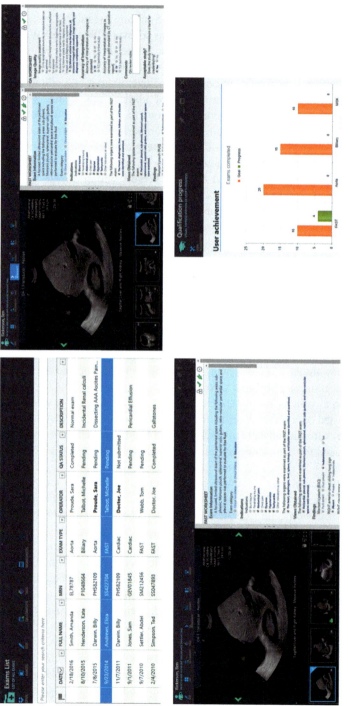

Fig. 17.8 Telexy Qpath solution sample images. © 2016 Telexy Healthcare Inc

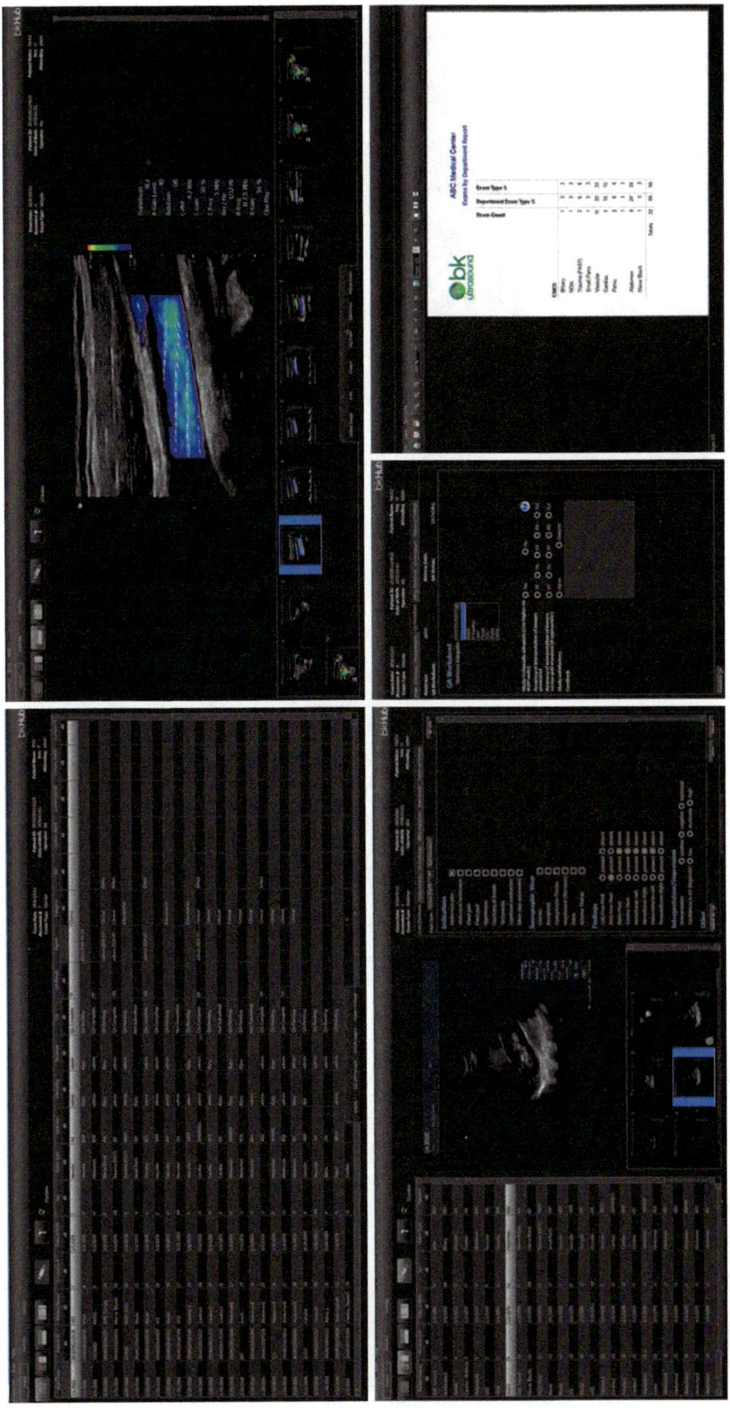

Fig. 17.9 BkHub solution sample images. © 2016 BK Ultrasound

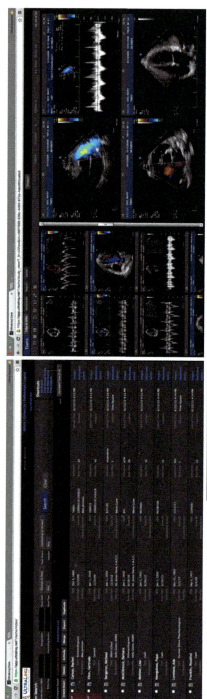

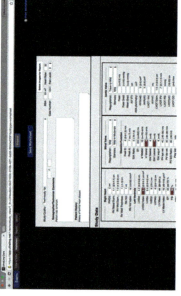

Fig. 17.10 Ultralinq solution sample images. © 2016 UltraLinq Healthcare Solutions Inc

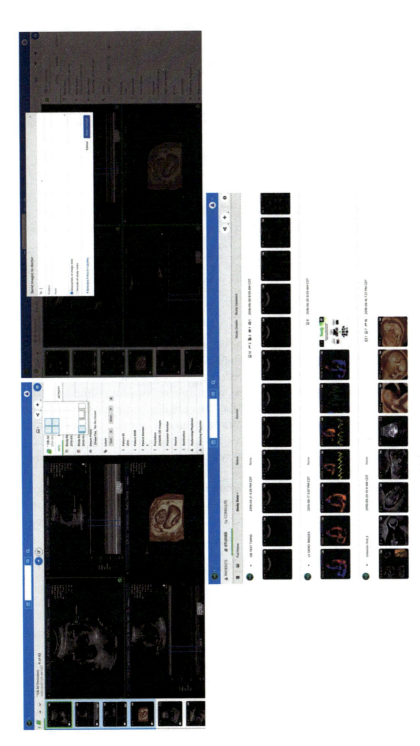

Fig. 17.11 Tricefy solution sample images. © 2016 Trice Imaging Inc

Key Definitions	
ADT	Admissions, Discharge, Transfer system. Computer system holding patient data points including: registration, medical record and account numbers. Intercommunicates amongst medical records systems.
CPOE	Computerized Physician Order Entry.
DICOM	Digital Imaging and Communications in Medicine. standard for handling, storing & sharing imaging in medicine.
EMR	Electronic Medical Record.
HL7	Health Level 7. Set of standards used in transfer of administrative/clinical data among software applications
Middleware	Software that acts as a bridge between a database and applications
PACS	Picture Archiving and Communications System. medical images storage system that stores multiple imaging modalities in a healthcare setting.
Front End	Where information about the patient is gathered and put into the ultrasound machine
Back End	Getting reports and images into the EMR

Fig. 17.12 Key definitions

can be recuperated in their billing. On the other hand, if clinical scans are to be done at an academic center (or one anticipating a residency program), for instance, then the cost associated with the storage of educational or teaching scans may quickly negate a cheaper upfront cost. The caveat to this rule is that while UltraLinq as well as Q-path cloud are web-hosted, UltraLinq does not charge for the storage of educational scans and Q-path bases their costs on estimated monthly usage, rather than a fee per scan model. Further differences in workflow solutions can be located on the ACEP ultrasound section's workflow systems comparison guide and are subject to change at any time [7].

Ultimately, a clinical ultrasound program is only as strong as the infrastructure supporting it. A good workflow system based on middleware is currently the most optimal solution in facilitating image archival, report generation, quality assurance, and billing (Fig. 17.12).

Pitfalls

1. Lack of appreciation that ED-specific workflow solution programs provide many functionalities beyond the image archival of a traditional Radiology PACS.
2. Not purchasing an ultrasound machine that is compatible with your hospital Wi-Fi network. Wireless connectivity is essential to a seamlessly functioning ED workflow.
3. Not seeking the support and backing of your department chair before approaching hospital IT about the implementation of a workflow solution in the ED.

4. Not acknowledging the potential improved billing capture and resultant increased ultrasound revenue when considering the cost of purchasing a workflow solution.

Key Recommendations

1. Ultrasound utilization at the point of care presents unique challenges for clinicians performing ultrasound as well as ultrasound program directors. Establishing a well-structured ED workflow is a key component in the overall success of an emergency ultrasound program.
2. An ED-specific workflow solution automates numerous tasks within an emergency ultrasound program, resulting in improved clinician compliance, reduced potential for human error, and invaluable time savings for the program director.
3. A workflow solution seamlessly tracks clinician scan numbers for credentialing purposes and facilitates an effective quality assurance program, providing clinicians with timely feedback about their scan technique and image interpretations.
4. ED workflow must provide that ultrasound images and reports be available within the medical record in real-time for review by other treating clinicians and consultant services in order to ensure safe, efficient, and timely patient care.

References

1. Byrne M, Geria R. ACEP emergency ultrasound workflow survey. Survey. American College of Emergency Physicians Ultrasound Section. Web. 2013.
2. Doctor line art vector illustration. Doctor line art vector illustration | Public domain vectors. N.p., 22 Mar. 2015. Web. 15 Jan. 2017.
3. Strategic document. DICOM. 14 Apr. 2014. Web. 26 Apr. 2015. http://medical.nema.org/dicom/geninfo/Strategy.pdf.
4. Byrne M, Geria R, Kummer T, et al. ACEP emergency ultrasound: workflow white paper. Web. 27 Apr. 2015. http://www.acep.org/uploadedFiles/ACEP/memberCenter/SectionsofMembership/ultra/Workflow%20White%20Paper.pdf.
5. McGonigle D, Mastrain K. Nursing informatics and the foundation of knowledge. 2nd ed. Sudbury: Jones & Bartlett; 2009.
6. Introduction to HL7 standards. Web. 4 May, 2015. http://www.hl7.org/implement/standards/index.cfm?ref=nav.
7. Byrne M. Workflow Systems Comparison. Web. 28 Apr. 2015. http://www.acep.org/uploadedFiles/ACEP/memberCenter/SectionsofMembership/ultra/Workflow%20Systems%20Comparison%202013.pdf.

Chapter 18
Practical Operating and Educational Solutions

Petra E. Duran-Gehring and Alfredo Tirado-Gonzalez

Objectives

- Discuss noncommercial methods for image acquisition and storage
- Describe options for low cost quality assessment and archival
- Review tools for creation of digital education content

Introduction

Although the implementation of a point-of-care ultrasound program first begins with the equipment needed to perform the ultrasound examinations, the supporting structure of any successful program should include an operating solution to store images for quality, education, and credentialing. Commercial solutions include software for image capture, image storage, and the ability to edit images for download or education. See Chapter 17–Workflow and Middleware. Although newer US machines typically include electronic transfer of images as part of the standard package, they will still require a system for storage. However, when older machines are used the capacity to wirelessly transfer images for electronic storage may not be included and alternate methods will need to be employed for storage. Although many commercial products can simplify this process with a single system approach,

P.E. Duran-Gehring, MD (✉)
Department of Emergency Medicine,
University of Florida College of Medicine-Jacksonville, Jacksonville, FL, USA
e-mail: Petra.Duran@jax.ufl.edu

A. Tirado-Gonzalez, MD, FACEP
Department of Emergency Medicine,
Florida Hospital-East Orlando, Orlando, FL, USA

© Springer International Publishing AG 2018
V. S. Tayal et al. (eds.), *Ultrasound Program Management*,
https://doi.org/10.1007/978-3-319-63143-1_18

this may not be a feasible option for a new or unfunded program that is just starting. Therefore, a low cost system can be created to ensure that images are appropriately captured, stored, and available for review, modification, and education in the future. In this chapter we will discuss the options for the creation of a system to include the above elements with low cost or free hardware and software to achieve image storage and review, as well as the elements needed to create cost-effective e-learning. See Chapter 17–Workflow and Middleware.

Media Acquisition Options

Although ACEP recommendations state that a hard copy of all ultrasound images should be saved for all point-of-care ultrasound studies, the manner in which those images are saved is left to each department. The options for image storage include thermal paper prints, videotape, and digital storage. Depending on the method of storage, additional hardware equipment will be needed to save these images besides the ultrasound machine itself. Images and video may be saved temporarily on the machine's hard drive or externally via another piece of hardware [1].

Internal Image Acquisition

Internal methods for image acquisition actually store the images on the US machine's hard drive. Once stored on the hard drive, the images can be removed and sent to storage. The images may be offloaded from the machine in either a PC or DICOM format, which will be discussed in more detail later in this chapter. Depending on the ultrasound machine make and model, the images may be offloaded from the machine wirelessly or through an Ethernet or USB connection. An Ethernet cable is a wired option that requires the machine to be plugged into an Ethernet port to make the connection and requires time to download the images. Images can also be downloaded from an ultrasound machine with a USB port to an external thumb drive. This is an easy method, but one must ensure that great care is taken with the thumb drive unless images are deidentified prior to removal from the machine. Both of these options may place the machine out of service for the time it takes to download images, so it is best to schedule these downloads in low volume times of day.

Lastly, wireless download is a quick and efficient way to transfer data from ultrasound machine to server. Ultrasound machines that do not have inherent wireless downloads may be made to transmit images wirelessly with software upgrades and the addition of a wireless dongle that acts as a router to wirelessly transmit images. This software can often be added to older machines at a minimal cost and can improve workflow since the machine can wirelessly upload images while the machine is still in use. Check with your ultrasound manufacturer to see if this is an option for your model machine, since older machines may lack the capability for this upgrade.

External Image Acquisition

In older ultrasound machines lacking the ability to perform any of the internal image acquisition methods, an external recorder can be used to save the images as a screen capture (Table 18.1). An external recorder does not save the images or video on the machine's hard drive, but copies the images off of the ultrasound machine screen while scanning. Images can only be saved as video files and are not available in a DICOM format. Although these may not be ideal in the modern digital world, these options are a low cost method to record the images as they are being performed.

Thermal printers are the original method for cataloging images. Thermal printers are small black and white printers that are attached to the US machine and require a roll of special thermal paper. The printer uses heat to create the images, so the paper will discolor and the images will fade when the paper is exposed to heat. Therefore, care must be taken to store the images in a climate controlled location to prevent exposure to excessive heat. Even in the best temperature controlled locations, the images will still degrade over time. This method is only good for still images and images cannot be edited after they are printed. The benefits to this method is that images can be printed and placed on the patient's chart and can be scanned into the medical record at a later time. The downside of this method is that the images only are available as a hard copy and can be easily lost.

Video screen recorders are a step up from the thermal printer. The images are still saved as a screen capture, but both stills and videos may be saved. The original screen recorders were small video tape recorders that were placed on the ultrasound machine. The VHS recorder would record the entire scan session, which could be quite cumbersome. The benefits of this modality were that it could be used for multiple ultrasound examinations, tapes could easily be removed and stored and the tapes could be watched on any video player. Due to the extinction of video cassette

Table 18.1 Comparison of external image acquisition modalities

Imagining modality	Pros	Cons
Thermal prints	Small images that can be attached to chart	Degrade over time and increased temperature
		Only still images
		Images easily misplaced
VHS/DVD	May store still and video images	VHS modality obsolete
	May record entire ultrasound evaluation	VHS studies require additional hardware to convert to digital
	May be used for multiple exams	
	DVDs may be viewed on computer	
External hard drive	May be rewritten after image transfer	More expensive that DVD recorder
	Connect easily to computer	

recorders, these machines are no longer made. However, if your machine already has one in place, know that it can be a useful image storage option and a low cost VHS to CD/DVD converter machine will convert VHS tape to CD/DVD modalities until an upgrade to digital modalities can be made.

DVD recorders have now taken the place of the VHS recorders. DVD recorders have the same benefits of the VHS recorder, but have the added benefit of using removable media (DVDs) that can be stored and reviewed in a much less cumbersome manner. The DVDs can be viewed on a computer, allowing the media to be viewed without the need for another piece of hardware (VHS viewer). Small DVD recorders initially cost in the $2000–3000 range, but now one can find a small recorder on the internet for as little as $150! These machines work best as a small format machine that can be placed on the ultrasound machine cart and plug into the back of the machine. Some options may include a remote for easy start and stop or may require a button to be pushed on the machine to begin recording. The DVD can be removed and the images can be downloaded to a computer and the DVD reused, making this a cost-effective option for repeat use.

A step above the DVD recorder is the external hard drive. Images are still saved via the screen capture method, but instead of using a tape or disc to store the media, images and video are saved directly onto a hard drive. The external hard drive would ideally be a small machine placed on the ultrasound machine cart that would have a removable component that would connect to a computer via a USB or firewire cable. The hard drive could be emptied once the images and video were removed and then used again. This option may be slightly more expensive than the DVD recorder, but the ability to rewrite the drive and connect easily to any computer make this an excellent option when internal image storage is not an option. Regardless of which option you use, ensure that image and video storage are accessible for future use.

QA and Archival

Once the images have been saved, whether it be on DVD, picture or video files, they must be stored for future use. Images should be stored to allow for quality review, credentialing, and billing purposes. Therefore, they will need to be kept in a safe location with redundant backup in case of initial storage failure. The storage of images should allow for: (1) easy viewing of the images, (2) image formatting, (3) archival of images and video, and (4) editing of images and video.

Image Viewing and Archiving

The simplest method for image storage is simply to download them to a computer. A single computer can be dedicated to image archival and is a secure way to keep the images HIPPA compliant. The set up can be extremely simple. Image storage can be performed by simply using the preloaded picture storage software included in the preloaded standard computer software. The drawbacks of this system are that a single station will require you to be physically present to view images and manage storage. It will also require system backup to prevent data loss. This may be a viable inexpensive option to begin image archival.

A single computer station can be expanded to include a computer network to improve the ability to view images from more than one location. This option would allow for more than one workstation and may be included in a VPN network access. This system will be more complex to set up and may require IT assistance. A hybrid system would allow of a single computer workstation to be the hub and to use one of the internet-based "cloud" networks to backup images and allow for viewing in other locations. More discussion of internet cloud use will be made later in this chapter.

Image Format

Ultrasound images and video can be saved in one of two formats depending on your image acquisition hardware: DICOM and PC modalities.

DICOM is the Digital Imaging and Communications in Medicine format which is a standard way to handle, store, print, and transmit medical images across manufactures. The imaging file contains the patient identifying information within the image itself so that the two pieces of data cannot be separated. This can be useful so that there is never a concern of mixing up patient information. These files therefore tend to be larger than the PC format, so will need more time to download and more space for image storage. Furthermore, DICOM files cannot be stored or viewed without a specific program to view the images. The Picture Archiving and Communication System (PACS) needed for DICOM images need not be a large and expensive system. Any system that performs these duties is considered a PACS; therefore, a small PACS can be created on any computer with the correct software and storage capacity. Since DICOM images require a specific viewer, a mini-PACS can be created by using one of the free downloadable DICOM viewers. There are several choices available depending on the computer's operating system.

OsiriX is a DICOM viewer that is available for Mac users and can easily be downloaded from the web (http://www.osirix-viewer.com). It is used worldwide and is available for all apple devices including a mobile version. This software can store all DICOM images, becoming its own self-contained PACS. Images can be viewed, sorted, edited, emailed, and manipulated for future use. It has a free version to download, OsiriX Lite, that may be a good starting point for new ultrasound systems as it has many features. The Osirix MD upgrade does cost $699, but it is a one-time cost and would be a worthwhile investment as it expands functionality with improved speed, unlimited user limits, email support and is FDA-cleared for medical usage. The mobile version, OsiriX HD ($49.99 in App store) is a basic

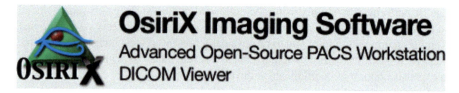

Fig. 18.1 Osirix Imaging Software. Advanced Open-Source PACS Workstation DICOM viewer

DICOM viewer that allows users to perform basic image manipulation (zoom, pan, etc.) on any iOS devices (iPhone, iPod Touch, and iPad) [2] (Figs. 18.1 and 18.2).

There are also DICOM views for the windows PC users. The most well known of these windows-based DICOM viewers is Showcase, which is available in two versions depending on the functionality needed [3]. Other PC-based DICOM viewers include Micodicom and I Do Imaging, to name a few [4, 5].

Despite the benefits of DICOM, using a more user-friendly image format might be an easier and more economical solution for programs with limited funding. Ultrasound studies can be saved in a PC image format such as a .jpg or .png format for ease of viewing and editing on any basic computer. Video formats may be saved as .mov, .m4v, .mp4, or .flv files depending on the computer software available. The ease of use of these file types when compared to DICOM is significant. Normal computer software can be used to view and edit the images and images can be saved with far less file size requirements. The drawbacks of using PC formats for images and video is that the file type varies from machine to machine and may require a conversion program to put them all in the same format. The image quality will also be slightly less when compared to DICOM. Lastly, the patient identifying information is not imbedded into the images/video; therefore, if care is not taken, the associating patient information could be lost.

While discussing PC versions of image storage, it is important to ensure that all ultrasound studies are saved in a HIPPA compliant manner. If studies are stored on a single server, then the server must be HIPPA compliant, with the proper safeguards taken to prevent unauthorized users from accessing the images on the machine. If a cloud-based system is used, then deidentification of images may be required prior to upload or the use of an encryption program may be required to keep data safe. Always refer to your compliance office to ensure that image storage is meeting HIPPA and your hospital standards.

Internet Cloud Storage

When considering a web-based solution or cloud storage of non-DICOM images or video, one could use any of the free or low cost services for home photo storage. Services such as Picasa, Flickr, and Shutterfly are just a few of the online image storage solutions available for photo storage [6, 7]. However, none of these services

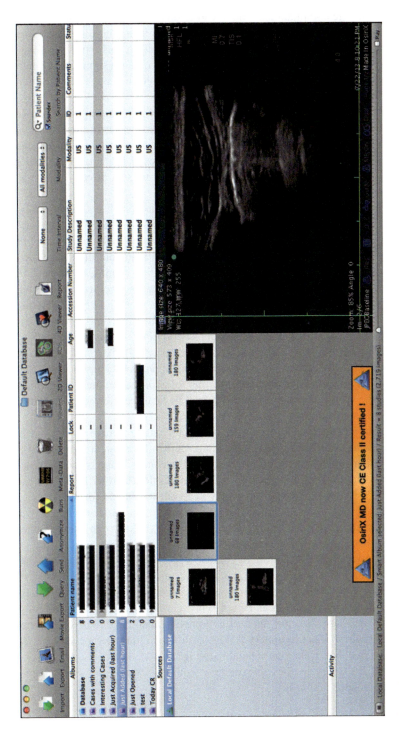

Fig. 18.2 Screenshot of Osirix imaging software

are HIPPA storage compliant and could lead to unauthorized users viewing private health information. Therefore, care must be taken in using these services. Images may be deidentified and a "dummy" number assigned to each study to allow for upload to one of these commercial services. This does create a significant amount of work on the front end, but these services provide storage and image editing software that may outweigh the initial limitations.

Image storage cloud programs such as Picasa (www.Picasa.google.com), for example, allow images to be sorted into folders to ease organization. Images and video can be starred to identify important images for another time. Images can be cropped and edited for brightness and contrast. Images and videos can be exported for lecture or case presentations. Lastly, images can be sent directly via email to allow reviewers to send feedback to users.

There are also purely web-based cloud storage options such as Dropbox, Google Drive, Amazon Cloud Drive, iCloud, and Symform [8–12]. These programs do not offer editing of images or video, but are purely a file storage solution. Most of these cloud storage solutions are low cost and offer a certain amount of storage for free even. However, only a few of these options are HIPPA compliant. To be HIPPA compliant a program must have a Business Associate Agreement (BAA) which ensures that files are encrypted on the way in and out. Google Drive and Symform are both HIPPA complaint right out of the box. Dropbox in its basic form does not have a BAA, but when used with Sookasa, an encryption program made specifically for Dropbox, then it does meet the requirements to be HIPPA compliant. Sookasa (www.sookasa.com) creates a folder within Dropbox or Google Drive that is encrypted. Any patient files are placed in this folder are encrypted, although they remain in the cloud of the storage platform. Files can be viewed on any mobile device that contains the Sookasa application [13].

Cloud services such as Dropbox are purely for image storage and do not have editing software within the program, so image deidentification, cropping, and editing must be performed outside of this program. The cloud storage is good for backup storage and to allow for files to be viewed from multiple locations. It can be a useful mini-PACS for your program or to simply keep all files handy for use outside the department. It may also be a good way to communicate and share images within your department as files can be sent directly via email. Folders can also be shared to allow other users to view those images or videos.

Google Drive is another option for cloud storage. It also uses the Sookasa format to encrypt files within the cloud storage. Folders can be made and permissions can be given to users for viewing, editing, and commenting. When allowing others to access your files, permissions can be set to prevent download, printing, or copying of the files you share. This may be useful to prevent unauthorized image sharing.

Lastly Symform is a proprietary HIPPA compliant cloud storage service. Basic services are free, but when a certain data limit is reached, then costs apply. As it has a BAA, this cloud service does not require any other software programs to maintain HIPPA compliance (Table 18.2).

Table 18.2 Cloud storage HIPPA compliance

Storage program	HIPPA compliance	Requires additional program for HIPPA compliance
Dropbox	No	Yes, Sookasa
Google drive	No	Yes, Sookasa
iCloud	No	No
Symform	Yes	No

Video Editing Software

There are many low cost video editing software that can be used to edit ultra-sound video clips. Using a program that is already on your computer is an inexpensive way to repurpose a program that you already have. iMovie and Windows Movie Maker are free programs what come standard with new computers. Software such as Quicktime Pro, Final Cut Express, and CyberLink Power Director II Deluxe are other video editing software that may also be used with limited cost.

All of these video editing software can be used to crop video clips, splice several clips together for a lecture or adjust the contrast on the video. Each of these programs will allow creation of folders to better organize video clips into categories. Some will allow for text to be placed within the video, arrows and music to be added for extra effects.

There are also several sites that provide free software for video editing. Ultrasound specific video editing programs are few, but the Ultrasound of the Week website has a free clip deidentifier available (http://www.ultrasoundoftheweek.com/clipdeidentifier/) for download [14]. This tool will batch deidentify video clips with drag and drop ease. Files are dragged into the program and a grid is used to exactly denote how much the videos will be cropped to ensure that all patient identifying information has been removed. The program will remember the amount cropped from the last video and use that as the default for future videos.

The Ultrasound of the Week site also supplies an innovative tool to create an m-mode image from any video to allow measurement of time and distance which may be useful, especially in cardiac imaging (http://www.ultrasoundoftheweek.com/m-mode-ify) [15]. This useful tool can be used when an m-mode image was not obtained to get further information from a video clip.

Sonocloud (www.sonocloud.org) is an online ultrasound specific video sharing site. Not only can you share your cool ultrasound videos with others, but you can download videos to use in your multimedia presentations. Photos and videos are sorted by type and you can even select favorites to keep your favorite videos easily accessible. Also videos are deidentified to maintain HIPPA compliance [16].

Ultrasound Education Creation

Education is an integral part of Point-of-Care Ultrasound (POC US). Depending on your group, you will likely spend a lot of time teaching attendings and advanced practitioner providers the basics of ultrasound. As the needs of the program continue to grow you will probably be asked to expand your role to teach others like residents, medical students, nurses, and other physicians from other specialties. While doing regular class room education might seem as a cost-effective alternative, it requires one of the most limited resources, the instructors time. Not only that, coordinating to have all the learners in the same room at the same time might be a real challenge to any emergency department, requiring multiple sessions. An excellent alternative can be e-learning. E-learning basically stands for all learning using electronic technologies to access a curriculum outside of a traditional classroom. Research results appear to be promising as a potentially time saving alternative to live classroom lectures and offer similar educational benefits for the postgraduate learner with adequate e-learning resources and a web-based curriculum in POC US [17–19].

E-learning has the potential to transform how we deliver content to our learners helping us integrate education and making accessible to our learners. It offers the ability to share knowledge in a wide variety of formats such as videos, documents, PDFs, and slideshows. The ACEP 2016 guidelines describe the role of emergency ultrasound instructors as curators of information and online courses should effectively teach the objectives established in the guidelines before being introduced into an Emergency Ultrasound (EUS) Curriculum [20]. While there are multiple online resources for ultrasound education, both free open source and commercial resources, we will be discussing the process to start your own e-learning platform as well as the tools you will need to establish e-learning as part of a practical operating solution.

To institute e-learning you will need some basic tools to create an online course. These tools include: content development tools, screencasting software, repurposing video sharing programs, content authoring tools and learning management systems (LMS). The best foundation to an effective online course will always be its content, for this you need to know your subject material well and it needs to appeal to all learning styles. Once you have determined your goals, you can start creating professional presentations without extraneous software.

Presentation software such as Powerpoint, Keynote (for Mac users), and Google Slides each have the ability to create pictures, animations, and videos to be used in your educational content. These software modalities can be used for more than just lecture presentations. You can create your own drawings (Fig. 18.3) and animations that can help your learners understand different concepts. Animations can easily be created using your drawings and a series of transitions, with effects added as well.

Once you have created your content, you can start creating educational videos using simple software, to digitally record your computer screen's output. This is referred to as screencasting or video capture. Depending on the software you use you can add narration to it as well using your computer's internal microphone or

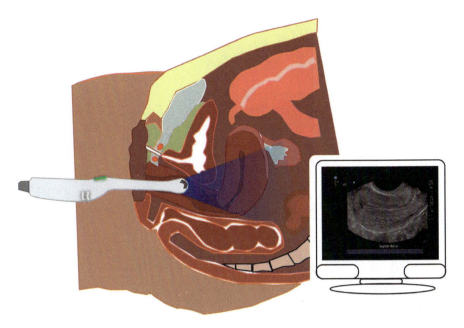

Fig. 18.3 Pelvic Ultrasound drawings for POC US learning

adding an external mic. Depending on your engagement you could start with free open screen capture software such as QuickTime player (if you own a mac, Fig. 18.4) and screencast-o-matic. Other commercial options give you more features like video and audio editing, animations, engaging videos and sharing (youtube). Some that need mention are Camtasia (both Mac and PC users Fig. 18.5) and Screenflow (Mac Users) [21, 22].

Repurposing video sharing programs such as Vimeo and Youtube can be a great way to spread your educational message to a group. Each of these programs can provide you with a free platform to share your deidentified ultrasound videos and educational materials. Your content can be categorized to create folders for ease of use and even made private to share just among your users. You can also create links and add them to your favorite blog, website, and even into your own LMS. Although these video sharing sites do not offer editing, they are a great option to share content once it has been created.

Depending on how comprehensive you want your course, you might consider starting with a content authoring tool. A content authoring tool is software used to create multimedia content available on the internet or as format files such as CDs (compact discs). While Flash and Power Point, could be consider authoring tools, only a few support Shareable Content Object Reference Model (SCORM) to package your entire content in a format that's easy to work and upload to your LMS. A couple examples of known programs that are available with such capabilities are: Articulate, Adobe Authorware, and Camtasia [22–24]. As you work more on projects, you will find a solution that will be easy to use and can adjust to your budget.

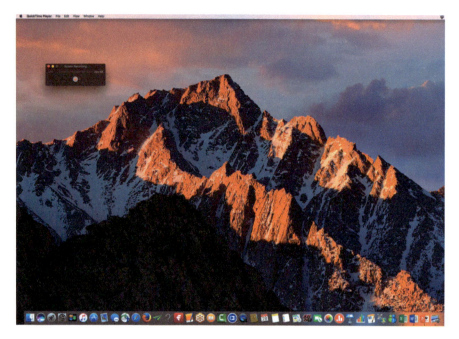

Fig. 18.4 QuickTime Player Screen recording option

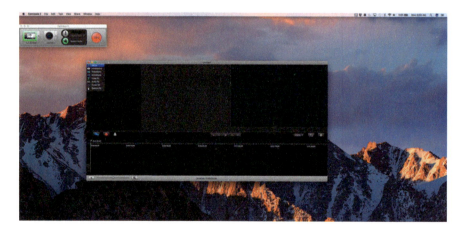

Fig. 18.5 Camtasia video capture solution

Once you have created your content, you will need a way to manage the online course, distribute material, monitor progress, keep records of training, and allow collaboration between learner and instructor. The Learning management system is a computer system developed for those specific needs. The LMS will allow you to manage every aspect of a course from the registration to keep in touch with your students to deliver assignments and test students to assess their grasp of the material and knowledge, Fig. 18.6.

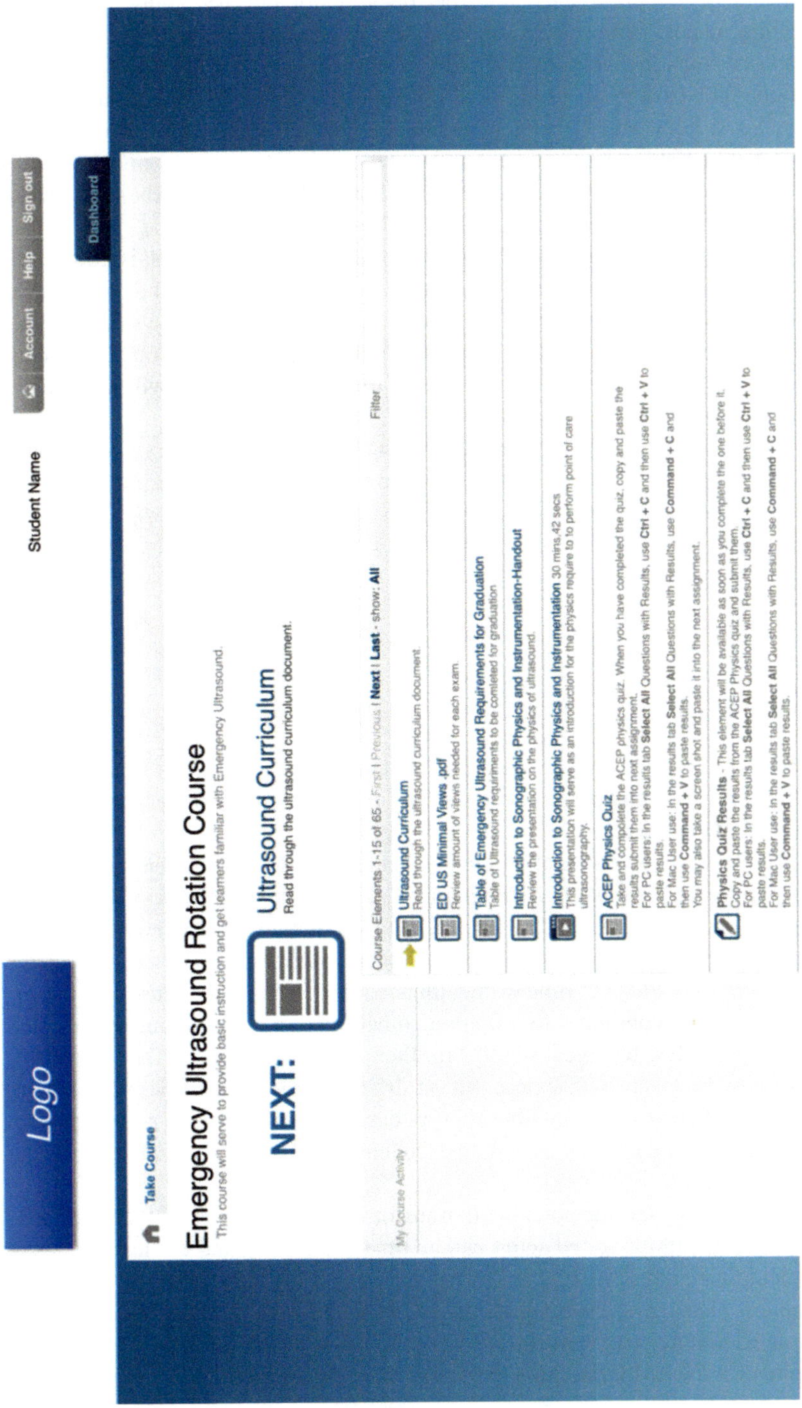

Fig. 18.6 Example of Online Curriculum using LMS and different course elements

There are lots of options available when deciding for an LMS. Things to consider are teaching needs, format they support, ease of use, and budget. There are free opens source software solutions and commercial products. It's very likely that your institution will be using some type of LMS to monitor CME and continuous medical training. So, a good way to start your process is to evaluate what solutions they already have available, support and evaluate if it covers your needs. Common examples of both free open and commercial LMS are: Moodle, Blackboard, Absorb LMS, Docebo, Litmos, Mindflash, and DigitalChalk [25–31].

If no structured LMS is available or if it doesn't cover your needs, is good practice to review different LMS before your committing to a product and assess functions (like social media integration), ease of use, will it be a hosted system (leaving in the cloud) or will it need to be a deployed solution, set up in a computer or internal server within the hospitals firewall. All of these considerations will help you to decide which product works best for you.

As a conclusion, e-learning is here and most of our current learners expect this to be the norm not the exception. While on the front end, creating all the infrastructure seems to be complicated, on the back end it provides the instructor with more time to do hands on training, reach more people in a cost-effective manner, and improve efficiency of day to day operations.

Pitfalls

1. Internal methods for image acquisition are temporary measures of image storage within the ultrasound system's hard drive; this makes it inefficient as a permanent storage solution.
2. Manual system download of studies and safekeeping of documentation can be time consuming, and likely need ancillary staff to help with process.
3. Thermal printed images and VHS recording suffer as long-term archiving solutions (unless digitized), they require a physical space for safe storage, and image quality can degrade over time even with adequate room temperature control.
4. As technology continues to improve, other modalities continue to become extinct, hence less technical support for them (e.g., VHS and DVD).
5. Care must be taken with external hard drive and cloud solutions to maintain HIPA compliance and if possible encrypt data to meet institution requirements.
6. Cloud storage and PACS viewers are excellent ways to safe keep information but need IT support.
7. While e-learning has the potential to transform how we deliver and monitor educational content, the initial setup can be time consuming and carries a progressive learning curve.
8. E-leaning also carries costs to maintain content and will depend of the software's use and learning management systems (LMS) annual licenses. The more the features for the LMS, the more expensive will likely it be.

Key Recommendations

1. The supporting structure of any successful program should include an operating solution to store images for quality, education, and credentialing.
2. Practical operating solutions can help create a workflow process in programs that are starting with limited or no resources by keeping the cost low.
3. Once a workflow has been established, consistency will help promote the process.
4. Automatization of process should be a goal to help with compliance of the end users.
5. Creating a team consistent of IT, PACS administrators, documentation (EMR if applicable), and revenue can help streamline process, with goals of review and improve process.
6. Education is an integral part of POC US, so content development and delivery should be a priority to impart knowledge and use as a tool to improve process.
7. Exploring all resources of your institution, such as current software being used or LMS systems in place, can help minimize cost and gain support.

References

1. American College of Emergency Physicians, Policy Statement. Ultrasound Guidelines: Emergency, Point of Care and Clinical Ultrasound Guidelines in Medicine. June 2016.
2. OsiriX Dicom Viewer. www.osirix-viewer.com.
3. Showcase DICOM Image Viewing Software. www.triltech.com.
4. MicroDicom Image viewing Software. www.microdicom.com.
5. I Do Imaging DICOM viewing software. www.idoimaging.com.
6. Picasa. www.picasa.google.com.
7. Flickr. www.flickr.com.
8. Dropbox. www.dropbox.com.
9. Google Drive. www.drive.google.com.
10. Amazon Cloud Drive. www.amazon.com/clouddrive.
11. iCloud. www.icloud.com.
12. Symform. www.symform.com.
13. Sookasa. www.sookasa.com.
14. Ultrasound of the Week Clip Deidentifier. www.ultrasoundoftheweek.com/clipdeidentier.
15. Ultrasound of the Week M-mode Creator. www.ultrasoundoftheweek.com/m-mode-ify.
16. Sonocloud. www.sonocloud.org.
17. Kang TL, Berona K, Elkhunovich MA, Medero-Colon R, Seif D, Chilstrom ML, Mailhot T. Web-based teaching in point-of-care ultrasound: an alternative to the classroom? Adv Med Educ Pract. 2015;6:171–5.
18. Turner EE, Fox JC, Rosen M, Allen A, Rosen S, Anderson C. Implementation and assessment of a curriculum for bedside ultrasound training. J Ultrasound Med. 2015 May;34(5):823–8.
19. Lewiss RE, Hoffmann B, Beaulieu Y, Phelan MB. Point-of-care ultrasound education: the increasing role of simulation and multimedia resources. J Ultrasound Med. 2014;33(1):27–32.
20. American College of Emergency Physicians, Policy Statement. Ultrasound Guidelines: Emergency, Point of Care and Clinical Ultrasound Guidelines in Medicine. June 2016; 6–7.

21. Screenflow: http://www.telestream.net/screenflow/.
22. Camtasia Screencast: https://www.techsmith.com/camtasia.html.
23. Adobe Authorware: http://www.adobe.com/products/authorware.
24. Articulate: https://articulate.com.
25. Moodle: https://moodle.org.
26. Blackboard: http://www.blackboard.com.
27. Absorb LMS: https://www.absorblms.com.
28. Docebo: https://www.docebo.com.
29. Litmos: http://www.litmos.com.
30. Mindflash: https://www.mindflash.com.
31. DigitalChalk: https://www.digitalchalk.com.

Chapter 19
Politics of Point of Care Ultrasound

Paul R. Sierzenski

Objectives

- Discuss the political landscape at the departmental, hospital, regional, state and federal levels.
- Understand and dispel common misconceptions of point-of-care (POC) ultrasound politics.
- Highlight major ultrasound milestones, events, policies, and documents affecting point-of-care ultrasound.
- Understand looming hurdles such as accreditation and value based medicine.

Introduction

What makes politics both exciting and frustrating is that the issue to be negotiated or resolved represents a topic for which two or more parties are intensely passionate. Politics can be defined as: "activities that relate to influencing the actions and policies of a government/or governing body" [1]. In this chapter, we will discuss the concept of clinician-performed point-of-care ultrasound instead of specialty specific ultrasound, since thinking in this broadest sense helps understand political challenges and opportunities.

Interestingly, emergency physicians have used, researched, and developed emergency ultrasound for decades, yet many emergency providers still lack access to the technology. One would think agreement would be fairly simple, especially when supporting a patient centered approach. Yet we repeatedly see that progress takes

P.R. Sierzenski, MD, MS HQS, FACEP
Acute Care Services, Renown Health, Reno, NV, USA
e-mail: peski71@icloud.com

© Springer International Publishing AG 2018   317
V. S. Tayal et al. (eds.), *Ultrasound Program Management*,
https://doi.org/10.1007/978-3-319-63143-1_19

time since much of the opposition and support for clinician-performed ultrasound are rooted in deep biases and have the propensity to acutely reoccur as might a chronic relapsing medical condition.

Departmental Aspects

There still exist and may always exist individuals in your departments, offices, or clinics who are opposed to the use of clinical ultrasound. In fact some of their concerns are likely based on valid points. They will cite issues with work flow, risk management, competency, cost, and patient experience. We certainly can't dismiss these concerns, rather we have to understand them, their motivation, and feel comfortable that we're able to address them in order to optimize patient care in our high-risk environment. If we cannot adequately respond to such concerns it is likely that we do not fully comprehend why ultrasound is of benefit at the patient bedside. This chapter and textbook will strategically address each of these issues, any of which may be the leverage point for or against the initiation or expansion of a Point-of-care Ultrasound program.

There is a departmental component that will evaporate over time, and that is the general resistance to technology. It is a generational problem. The status quo is often comfortable. In a world that is moving to pay for value, from payment for performance (RVU based), we must be able to address the real concerns of point-of-care ultrasound critics. The traditional position is that a team is only as strong as its weakest link. As you develop concepts for a program or its expansion, challenge yourself with the feedback and views of the individuals most opposed to point-of-care ultrasound.

Interdepartmental Aspects

There are a number of departments, which the Point-of-care Ultrasound Director will need to successfully engage including cardiology, medicine, critical care, emergency medicine, and obviously radiology. Some of these specialties will align with your needs and others might be obstructive. The opportunity exists since early point-of-care ultrasound adopters are well positioned in this space to leverage your background, passion, knowledge, and time to gain support such as assisting anesthesiology in training staff for ultrasound guided access, or assisting OBGYN in the development of a documentation pathway, or aiding trauma in their ACS trauma site visit through E/FAST exam QA documentation. The assets you bring are extensive.

An important trend to recognize among our colleagues in Radiology is they are beginning to understanding the use of this technology from our standpoint.

Both Emergency and Radiology Residencies have a mandated ACGME Milestones for residents to perform "ultrasound." However the Radiology Residency Milestone document sites the term "ultrasound" only once [2], and others are likely to follow in time the Emergency Medicine Residency Milestone document lists "ultrasound" 11 times with details in "Other Diagnostic and Therapeutic Procedures: Goal-directed Focused Ultrasound (Diagnostic/Procedural) (PC12)" and has done so since 2012 [2], a powerful fact that deserves publicity and duplication in other areas of practice.

National Organizational Aspects

When is it obvious that an issue in healthcare has reached a significant level importance? When everyone has a statement, position, or policy about the issue. The following is a prominent list of well-known organizations that have publically discussed, supported, or raised concern or outright objection to Point-of-care ultrasound:

AAEM—American Academy of Emergency Medicine
AAFP—American Academy of Family Physicians
ABEM—American Board of Emergency Medicine
ACC—American College of Cardiology
ACOG—American College of Obstetrics and Gynecology
ACOEP—American College of Osteopathic Emergency Physicians
ACEP—American College of Emergency Physicians
ACGME—American College of Graduate Medical Education
ACR—American College of Radiology
ACS—American College of Surgeons
AHRQ—Agency for Healthcare Research and Quality
AIUM—American Institute of Ultrasound in Medicine
AMA—American Medical Association
ARDMS—American Registry of Diagnostic Medical Sonographers
ASE—American Society of Echocardiography
The Blues: Blue Cross and Blue Shield
CMS—Centers for Medicare and Medicaid Services
CQU—Coalition for Quality in Ultrasound
JC—The Joint Commission
MedPac—Medicare Payment Advisory Commission
RRC-EM—Residency review Committee for Emergency Medicine
SAEM—Society for Academic Emergency Medicine
SHM—Society of Hospitalists Medicine
SRU—Society of Radiologists in Ultrasound Congress
NQF—National Quality Forum

Misconceptions Regarding Point of Care Ultrasound

There are many misconceptions with Point-of-care ultrasound and here we will focus on 10 most commonly seen ones. Realistically, these are mainly "straw man arguments."

1. **Clinicians are not competent at using ultrasound**. This remains a pervasive misconception at all organizational levels and within hospitals and health systems. Hospital medical executive boards may not hold a current world view or realize the rapid integration of clinical ultrasound since 2010, and it is our challenge and duty to educate them. Substantial evidence exists about training rates, competency curves for emergency physicians, PAs, nurses and other clinical specialties' safe use of ultrasound.

2. **Point-of-care ultrasound will increase costs**. Arguably this misconception could be the number one challenge, as this is rapidly becoming the default position after research disproved concerns regarding competency. There are two points to consider, first that clinical ultrasound examinations are typically billed as "limited codes" and thus are only a fractional cost compared to "complete codes" billed by traditionally imagers. Second, as medicine continues to move away from pay for volume to pay for value, the lower expense of the limited ultrasound and its real-time performance can reduce variable costs across the health system. These variable costs include reducing transportation, staffing (traditional sonographers) and improved efficiency leading to reduction of time to clinical decision-making. Additionally as a move away from traditional imaging processes can result in repurposing of care spaces such dedicated ultrasound rooms.

3. **Point-of-care Ultrasound is not best clinical practice.** From procedural guidance to diagnosis in pregnancy, shock, soft-tissue, renal colic, biliary colic, trauma, ocular, thoracic, venous thrombosis point-of-care US is considered a de facto standard of care [3].

4. **Point-of-care Ultrasound is not a residency standard.** This is an ACGME/ABEM Milestone in EM, and mentioned in multiple other specialties in procedures or knowledge competencies (see residency chapter).

5. **Point-of-care Ultrasound will increase misdiagnosis/risk.** Point-of-care Ultrasound has been shown to reduce and focus the differential diagnosis of emergency physicians, especially in the critically ill hypotensive patients.

6. **Self-referral issues represent a Stark violation.** Studies and documentation should meet CMS documentation and clinical indication requirements. A procedure by the examining physician is not self-referral during the visit.

7. **Point-of-care Ultrasound is unnecessary as other services are available.** Though other consultative services may be available, they are not contemporaneous to real-time clinical care. Hypotensive, septic and ultrasound guided procedures alone debunk this myth.

8. **Point-of-care Ultrasound decreases physician performance**. Point-of-care ultrasound actually improves physician decision-making, reduces differential diagnosis, reduces time to diagnosis, improves patient satisfaction, and improves safety.

9. **Point-of-care Ultrasound is a fad**. This has been said repeatedly since 1994! At some point, perhaps after a few decades, things can no longer be just fads.

10. **Point-of-care Ultrasound is an extension of the physical exam**. Now this is a politically difficult myth as many have used it to justify gaining Point-of-care Ultrasound clinically or for medical student training. Yet the fact remains that ACEP has recognized that ultrasound is a focused imaging service as detailed in the 2013 ACEP Council passed resolution 33 which states:

Resolution 33 Clinical Ultrasound is a Specific Imaging Modality (as amended).

RESOLVED, That ACEP define Clinical Ultrasonography as a diagnostic modality; and be it further.

RESOLVED, That ACEP recognizes that Clinical Ultrasonography goes beyond clinically important data not obtainable by inspection, palpation, auscultation, or other components of the physical exam; and be it further.

RESOLVED, That ACEP recognize Clinical Ultrasonography as a unique clinical modality, distinct from the physical examination, and not an adjunct to or extension of the physical examination [4].

The Contrarian's Viewpoint

There remains a significant disconnect between what providers or clinicians in various specialties do every day when taking care of patients; on nights, on weekends, on holidays, and the challenges and variability of resources that are available to care for patients. Point-of-care Ultrasound is an attempt by clinicians to advocate for patients to have a consistent standard of care that meets our commitment to serve the healthcare need of society 24/7/365. It's a disconnect from the work we do, we need to do and the current realities of the system, or future system of care to develop.

Point of Care Ultrasound Political Backstory

In 1991, the emergency ultrasound shot was heard around the organized medical world. The next several graphs depict the key public position statements by organizations for and against Clinician-Performed Ultrasound from the 1990s through 2012. These documents and their impact are too vast to discuss in detail for this chapter. However, they should be known or accessible to any proponent of point-of-care ultrasound.

Paramount for individuals seeking to initiate a new point-of-care ultrasound program are the following five documents:

1. The 1999 AMA HR 802-Privileging in Ultrasound Imaging, the resolution from the house of medicine that unequivocally states that clinicians have the right to use ultrasound, be trained in ultrasound and develop specialty specific guidelines and criteria for hospital privileging and credentialing (Fig. 19.1).
2. The 2001 (and updated) ACEP Emergency Ultrasound Guidelines.

3. 2001 AHRQ Evidence Report No. 43. Making Healthcare Safer; Ultrasound Guidance for Central Venous Cannulation.
4. 2010 ACEP/ASE; Focused Cardiac Ultrasound in the Emergency Setting.
5. 2011 AIUM Officially Recognizes ACEP Ultrasound Guidelines.
6. SCCM Hospital Credentialing pathway published in 2014 (Figs. 19.2, and 19.3).

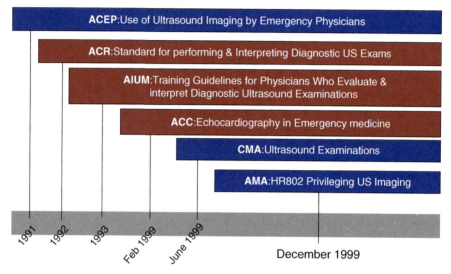

Fig. 19.1 EUS Events 1990s

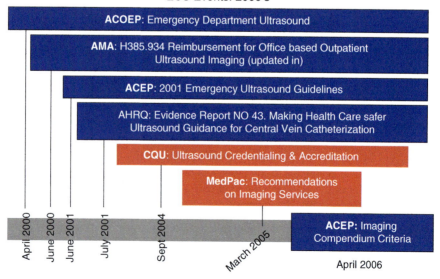

Fig. 19.2 EUS Events 2000s

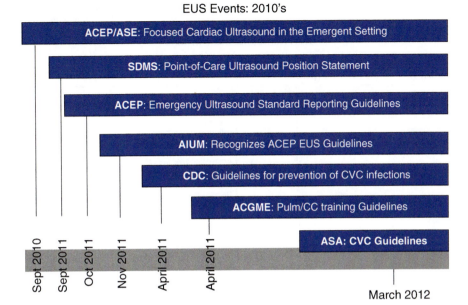

Fig. 19.3 EUS Events 2010s

Recent Developments to Know

Late in 2012, the American College of Radiology in its ACR Appropriateness Criteria ® rated highly the Focused Assessment in Sonography for Trauma (E/FAST) exam. The FAST received an eight out of ten rating, five points higher than a CT abdomen and pelvis with or without contrast, which scored a 3 as noted below (Fig. 19.4):

In 2013, AMA House Resolution 507–2013 titled; Diagnostic Ultrasound Utilization and Education supports the integration and use of ultrasound throughout the continuum of medical education. At the time of publication it is estimated that over 40 medicals schools include clinician-performed ultrasound within their 4-year medical school curriculum, with a constant increase in this number.

Reimbursement for POC Ultrasound

Fair payment for fair work is reasonable. During the early phases of negotiation, raising issues of payment for point-of-care ultrasound can be a "third rail" risking turmoil and frustration. This is not to say it should be taken off the table, as that is potentially problematic. As noted by the AMA, it is unethical for other specialties and stakeholders to suggest such a concept. Other chapters will discuss the detail,

Date of origin: 1996
Last review date: 2012

American College of Radiology
ACR Appropriateness Criteria®

<u>Clinical Condition:</u>   **Blunt Ab-dominal Trauma**

<u>Varlant 1:</u>   **Unstable patient.**

Radiologle Procedure	Raing	Comments	RRL*
X-ray chest:	8	To evaluate for fracture, pneumomediastinum, and abnormal air collection or gas collections, patient condition permitting. Chest radiograph, KUB, and Fast scan are complementary examinations. All are commonl performed in this setting, patient condition permitting.	☢
US chest abdomen and pelvis (FAST scan)	8	Rapid assessment of free fluid, patient condition permitting. Chest radiograph, KUB, and FAST scan are complementary examinations. All are commonly performed in this setting. patient condition permitting.	O
X-ray abdomen and pelvis (KUB)	8	To evaluate for fracture, free intraperitoneal air or abnormal fluid or gas collections. Chest radiograph, KUB, and FAST scan are complementary examinations. All are commonly performed in this setting.patient condition permitting.	☢☢
Arteriography with possible embolization abdomen and pelvis	5	Not appropriate as initial imaging modality but may become more appropriate if additional clinical information or imaging suggests possibility of active hemorrhage.	Varies
CT abdomen and pelvis without contrast	3	Not appropriate for critically unstable patients. Appropriateness rating may increase if clinical condition of patient improves and becomes hemodynamically stable. Would only consider in setting of prior serve contrast reaction or renal failure.	☢☢☢☢
CT abdomen and pelvis with contrast	3	Not appropriate for critically unstable patients. Appropriateness rating may increase if clinical condition of patient improves and becomes hemodynamically stable.	☢☢☢☢

Fig. 19.4 ACR appropriate criteria—Blunt Abdominal Trauma

regulations and options related to billing and payment for point-of-care ultrasound. However one aspect is clear, a quality program developed with the patient as the focus is critical. Once reimbursement is raised as a topic, the altruistic high-ground can be lost, it is best to focus on the patient and move to discuss the support of the program and the development of a self sustaining point-of-care ultrasound program.

Of course clinicians are right to obtain fair pay for their work effort, however that can take many forms (fee-for service, fair-market-value flat rate payments for services, etc.) and with a healthcare system in transition, over-fixation on reimbursement can backfire.

That POC Ultrasound can represent the ideal venue to demonstrate a payment for value metric. Probably every facility has credentialed and non-credentialed providers who, in real-time, use ultrasound for risk stratification to determine further actions. For example, identification of a pericardial effusion and specifically pericardial tamponade aids in rapid treatment, consultation, and disposition for this high-risk patient population derived from those with trauma, cancer, dialysis, sepsis, and iatrogenic therapies such as anticoagulation.

Regulatory Issues and Accreditation for Clinical Ultrasound

Regulation is ingrained in healthcare to assure that care provided to patients is safe and of high quality. Regulation is fundamentally a function of government. The establishment of Medicare, within the Social Security Act of 1965, resulted in the development of an industry respective to the appropriate payment for services, under Medicare. The primary organization that grew out of this is The Joint Commission (TJC), the organization for accreditation for hospitals, hospital services and quality for Medicare payment. The TJC states, "In order to make the decision of privileging more objective and continuous, in 2007 The Joint Commission introduced its Ongoing Professional Practice Evaluation (OPPE) and Focused Professional Practice Evaluation (FPPE) processes." OPPE and FPPE [5] are combined to assure that providers granted privileges, especially as relates to new skills or procedures, are performed safety and to assure quality through evaluation at regular intervals such as every 2 years. From the POC US standpoint this means that departments and organizations must have established means to assess providers use of POC US. Though this may seem overly burdensome, the same quality processes that occur for any department can be adapted for POC US (see credentialing and training chapters).

Of critical importance is that the United States Congress, which provides oversight to the Department of Health and Human Services (HHS) which administrates CMS, requires certification and/or accreditation for many imaging modalities for payment. The Medicare Improvements for Patients and Providers Act of 2008 (MIPPA) [6] required all nonhospital suppliers of "advanced imaging services" be accredited by organizations designated by the Secretary of HHS by January 1, 2012, to be qualified to provide such services to Medicare beneficiaries. Though ultrasound is not on the list of advanced imaging services, HHS reports that it can be "added" in the future. Accreditation in ultrasound and POC US is inevitable. MIPPA currently recognizes three organizations for accreditation, the American College of Radiology (ACR), the Inter-Societal Accreditation Commission (IAC), and The Joint Commission (TJC). Some private payers also require accreditation for imaging services and have added ultrasound, expanding the accreditation bodies to include the American Institute for Ultrasound in Medication (AIUM), Anthem Blue Cross, and Blue Shield. Several states are aggressively moving forward with this initiative and obtaining background information.

Accreditation

If accreditation is inevitable then POC US must identify a pathway that understands the challenges of our environment, resources, and the breadth practice as clinical ultrasound specialists in emergency, critical care, anesthesia, primary care, and surgical specialties. As a result and following the spirit of AMA HR 802, ACEP established the Clinical Ultrasound Accreditation Program (CUAP), as a pathway for emergency departments to gain accreditation for their emergency/POC US program. The process assures that the program meets ACEP Ultrasound Guidelines and the ACEP Emergency Ultrasound Imaging Compendium to assure quality performance and practice of POC US. It remains to be seen if payers will accept this. However, as a principle architect and catalyst for the POC US ultrasound revolution, ACEP is in excellent position to advocate for patients and providers of acute care services and imaging.

Future Considerations

The world is ever changing, and this is the same for point-of-care ultrasound, imaging and the politics that surround these changes. The move toward a "value based, not volume based" healthcare system is more than a political sound bite. Leveraging its significant buying power through the Medicare and Medicaid programs, the federal government has developed multiple programs to demonstrate and facilitate this pivot to reduce costs and improve value for patients and payers of healthcare services through the landmark 2010 Patient Protection and Affordable Care Act (PPACA) [7], commonly called the Affordable Care Act (ACA). Bundled payments seek to collapse the line item payments for hospital services. With this new approach a single payment should cover the care of a patient during a given event such as surgical repair of a hip fracture, which may extend to 30 days post operative for that patients care. In such or similar cases the value of POC US grows immensely to reduce overall costs as a focused and limited study, improve efficiency, and reduce fixed costs. As we consider how we can adapt to this shifting landscape, focus on advocating for patients, demand for clinical excellence and competency, supported by fair pay should continue to guide us. POC US is a powerful means to demonstrate value in clinical care.

Conclusion

In conclusion, the politics of Point-of-care Ultrasound is critical to understand and dynamic in nature. Clinicians are well positioned to leverage our role as patient advocates in gaining support of the use of this powerful real-time diagnostic and procedural guidance tool. As you move forward with your launch, expansion, or evaluation of your POC US program consider the following potential pitfalls and recommendations.

Pitfalls

1. Lack of understanding of the core knowledge, and goals of point-of-care US
2. Lack of understanding of the historical developments that contributed to point-of-care US
3. Failure to acknowledge the political landscape locally, regionally, and nationally
4. Lack of knowledge of economic issues associated with Point-of-care US
5. Go it Alone strategy (unless absolutely last resort)
6. Failure to use specialty specific guidelines for your program
7. Failure to lobby and educate decision-makers in regard to point-of-care ultrasound
8. Failure to incorporate ultrasound into value processes such as quality indicators, accreditation, and payment

Key Recommendations

1. Negotiations related to clinical ultrasound can become intense and unfortunately at time personal, so stay composed and patient focused, but stay passionate. No one else can provide the breadth of ultrasound services truly needed in their clinical setting but a clinician trained to use point-of-care ultrasound.
2. Be certain to bring like minds to your side: emergency medicine, surgery, critical care, medicine, family medicine, cardiology, risk management, and nursing.
3. Meet with your radiology and other consultative imaging colleagues, put a face and a name to your interaction, and display the respect and understanding of their views, even though we may disagree. Keep records, emails, and notes of meetings to be certain you have clear evidence of communication and your intent to collaborate. You would be amazed what some will write or say and always keep composure.
4. Executive support is essential, so learn the executive (CEO/CMO) lexicons and priorities for your organization and demonstrate how clinical ultrasound can help attain those goals. As with your clinical practice, know the landmark literature, both within and outside our specialty as we are challenged to be responsible to this reality every day.
5. Though difficult, try not to recoil from errors, but embrace them. Be transparent, since mistakes will be made and each set back can serve as an opportunity to leap forward. Open accountability will gain you and your program respect over time.

6. Finally be your own advocate. Use public relations with your use of technology for the care of your patients, clinical cases bring the challenge of emergency care and impact of point-of-care ultrasound to patients, colleagues and healthcare leaders alike.

References

1. Politics. Merriam Webster at http://www.merriam-webster.com/dictionary/politics. Accessed 3 Sept 2012.
2. The Emergency Medicine Milestone Project: A Joint Initiative of the Accreditation Council for Graduate Medical Education and The American Board of Emergency Medicine. July 2015. http://www.acgme.org/Portals/0/PDFs/Milestones/EmergencyMedicineMilestones.pdf. Accessed 4 Apr 2016.
3. American College of Emergency Physicians. Ultrasound Guidelines: Emergency, Point-of-Care, and Clinical Ultrasound Guidelines in Medicine [policy statement]. Approved June 2016. https://www.acep.org/Clinical---Practice-Management/Ultrasound/. Accessed 8 Sept 2016.
4. Summary of 2013 Council resolutions. ACEP. https://www.acep.org/uploadedFiles/2013%20Resolutions%20Adopted%20by%20the%20Council%20and%20Board.pdf. Accessed May 2014.
5. OPPE and FPPE: Tools to help make privileging decisions. Wise R. 2013. http://www.joint-commission.org/jc_physician_blog/oppe_fppe_tools_privileging_decisions/. Accessed 20 Apr 2016.
6. Public Law 110–275—July 15, 2008. Medicare Improvements for Patients and Providers Act of 2008. https://www.gpo.gov/fdsys/pkg/PLAW-110publ275/pdf/PLAW-110publ275.pdf. Accessed 20 Sept 2009.
7. Public Law 111–148—Patient Protection and Affordable Care Act. https://www.gpo.gov/fdsys/granule/PLAW-111publ148/PLAW-111publ148/content-detail.html. Accessed 30 Mar 2010.

Chapter 20
Credentialing and Privileging

Robert Jones

Objectives

1. Define credentialing, privileging, and competence.
2. Describe the credentialing and privileging processes.
3. Discuss the effect of scope of practice controversies (turf battles) on credentialing and privileging.
4. Discuss methods of obtaining privileging in point-of-care ultrasound.
5. Discuss the complicated privileging process.

Introduction

Credentialing and privileging of health care practitioners within a health care organization or hospital is essential to ensure accountability and competence. Prior to 1965, the hospital and its medical staff were considered separate entities with distinct missions. A malpractice case in 1965 resulted in significant changes in hospital's credentialing and privileging processes and established the hospital's corporate liability for the quality of the medical staff. Hospitals now have an inherent liability to ensure that health care practitioners are competent to practice and to perform the procedures granted in the credentialing and privileging process, and they have accepted The Joint Commission's (TJC) quality monitoring requirements as the legal standard. The credentialing and privileging process, while complex and challenging, must be fair and impartial. Unfortunately, scope of practice

R. Jones, DO, FACEP
Department of Emergency Medicine, MetroHealth Medical Center,
Case Western Reserve University, Cleveland, OH, USA
e-mail: jones2174@me.com

© Springer International Publishing AG 2018
V. S. Tayal et al. (eds.), *Ultrasound Program Management*,
https://doi.org/10.1007/978-3-319-63143-1_20

issues frequently arise during the process that pits one specialty against the other. No specialty owns any privilege or procedure but this fact is frequently forgotten during the process and a turf battle ensues. These issues are economically and politically motivated due to a perception that another specialty is encroaching into their area of practice and the process is no longer about whether or not the applicant is appropriately trained and can provide high-quality patient care. This chapter will define terms, discuss the history, describe both the complicated and uncomplicated processes for providers, and suggest strategies for a successful program.

Key Terms

The terms credentialing and privileging are often used interchangeably even though they have different meanings. The American College of Emergency Physicians (ACEP) defines physician credentialing as the process of gathering information regarding a physician's qualifications for appointment to the medical staff [1]. In the credentialing process, the physician's qualifications, such as residency training and board certification, are verified.

The delineation of clinical privileges is the process by which the hospital determines the specific procedures that may be performed by each medical staff applicant and appointee in the hospital. TJC mandates that every individual who is permitted by law and by the hospital to provide medical care in the hospital have delineated clinical privileges. ACEP believes that the exercise of clinical privileges in the emergency department is governed by the rules and regulations of the department (Table 20.1).

At the heart of the credentialing and privileging processes is the issue of competence. Competence refers to having the technical, cognitive, and integrative skills to perform a procedure or group of procedures and it is very context-dependent [2]. Competence is easy to define but can be difficult to accurately measure in clinical practice.

Table 20.1 ACEP policy statement on credentialing and privileging [1]

The American College of Emergency Physicians believes that
• The exercise of clinical privileges in the emergency department is governed by the rules and regulations of the department
• The ED medical director is responsible for periodic assessment of clinical privileges of emergency physicians
• When a physician applies for reappointment to the medical staff and for clinical privileges, the reappraisal process must include assessment of current competence by the ED medical director
• The ED medical director will, with the input of department members, determine the means by which each emergency physician will maintain competence and skills and the mechanism by which to monitor the proficiency of each physician

Historical Background

Prior to 1965, the hospital and its medical staff were considered to be separate entities with distinct missions. Hospitals were solely responsible for the day-to-day operations within the institution while the medical staff was responsible for patient care issues. In 1965, the case of *Darling v. Charleston Community Memorial Hospital* changed hospital liability jurisprudence forever [3].

The patient in this case had presented to the emergency department with a leg injury and was diagnosed with a fracture. He was subsequently placed in a cast and discharged home. The following day he returned to the emergency department and it was determined that the cast was too tight. The patient had already suffered significant vascular compromise and ultimately underwent amputation of the leg.

The facts of this case are not extraordinary or unique from a medicolegal standpoint. However, the legal decision in this case effected two key changes in hospital liability jurisprudence. First, liability theory has been extended to hospitals for their role in patient care. Second, violation of competent duties of care to a patient can result in direct liability to a hospital.

Today, emergency physicians are considered agents of the hospital, irrespective of whether they are hospital employees, employed by a separate group, or independent contractors. The relationship between a physician and the hospital is legally referred to as an agency relationship.

Scope of Practice Controversies

There is currently a view of scope of practice within the medical community that is conceptually flawed and potentially damaging. Medical specialties first to perform a specific procedure often feel that they own the procedure and therefore block other specialties from performing the procedure. Rarely is this done based on sound medical facts but is most commonly guided by political and economic motives.

Privileging disputes are common in specialties such as emergency medicine and family medicine since our practices overlap with numerous specialties [4]. In addition to point-of-care (POC US) ultrasound, procedural sedation is a common cause of privileging disputes for emergency medicine physicians. The literature on procedural sedation in the emergency department has been favorable and there is no evidence to support claims that morbidity or mortality for the procedure is higher if done in the ED as opposed to the operating room [5–7]. Yet despite appropriate clinical training by emergency physicians and overwhelmingly supportive literature, these turf battles have gone for years for a lot of emergency medicine groups. The same applies to POC US ultrasound, so it is imperative that these concerns not be taken lightly when approaching the privileging process.

Obtaining Point-of-Care Ultrasound Privileges (Step-by-Step)

1. *Assess internal commitment*: Not uncommonly, physicians get excited about procedures after attending conferences or short courses and want to incorporate the procedure(s) into their clinical practice. They, however, fail to recognize the time commitment required to become privileged and then quit before completing the process.
2. *Appoint an ultrasound director*: Running an ultrasound program within a busy emergency department is challenging and it is essential that a lead person be appointed to deal with clinical, political, and machine issues.
3. *Determine allies and enemies*: The best way to guarantee you or your group never loses a privileging conflict is to never have one in the first place. Identifying and addressing controversial issues that may arise during the application process should ideally be handled prior to submitting the application for privileging. Gathering support from other departments at this point can be helpful in preventing a privileging dispute. An uncomplicated privileging process may take up to 6 months to complete, while a complicated privileging process can take years to complete so pre-empting the battle is important.
4. *Follow current ACEP guidelines*: The policy on privileging for ultrasound imaging from the AMA identifies that ultrasound has wide-ranging applications and can be beneficial to multiple clinical specialties (Table 20.2) [8]. The policy affirms that ultrasound imaging is within the scope of practice of appropriately trained physicians. Additionally, the policy states that each hospital medical staff should review and approve criteria for granting ultrasound privileges based upon background and training for the use of ultrasound technology and strongly recommends that these criteria are in accordance with recommended training and education standards developed by each physician's respective specialty. Within the specialty of emergency medicine, we are fortunate to have comprehensive specialty-specific ultrasound guideline to follow [9]. In the event of a privileging dispute, the AMA policy statement as well as the ACEP ultrasound guidelines should be referenced and compliance with the specialty-specific guidelines noted. Currently there are no national certification criteria pertaining to the use of point of care ultrasound by emergency physicians. Additionally, there are very few studies that have been published looking at requirements to achieve competency so the current ACEP guidelines play an important role.

Table 20.2 AMA policy H-230.960 on privileging for ultrasound imaging [8]

(1) AMA affirms that ultrasound imaging is within the scope of appropriately trained physicians.
(2) AMA policy on ultrasound acknowledges that broad and diverse use and application of ultrasound imaging technologies exist in medical practice.
(3) AMA policy on ultrasound imaging affirms that privileging of the physician to perform ultrasound imaging procedures in a hospital setting should be a function of hospital medical staff and should be specifically delineated on the Department's Delineation of Privileges form.
(4) AMA policy on ultrasound imaging state that each hospital medical staff should review and approve criteria for granting ultrasound privileges based upon background and training for the use of ultrasound technology and ensure that these criteria are in accordance with recommended training and education standards developed by each physician's respective specialty society

5. *Review medical staff bylaws*: Be familiar with the medical staff bylaws. It is not uncommon to find older statements in medical staff bylaws that were appropriate for the time period written, but are no longer applicable and could be used by other specialties in a turf battle. Statements such as "the department of radiology controls all hospital-based imaging" could easily be used to support a privileging dispute, so it is best to have these types of statements removed in advance.

6. *Submit application*: In an uncomplicated process, the application along with the supportive documents is submitted to the credentialing committee. Verification that physicians have or will successfully complete either the residency/fellowship-based pathway or the practice-based pathway prior to consideration for privileging should be documented. Both competency-based pathways can be found in the current ACEP ultrasound guidelines [9]. The specific ultrasound examinations being requested for clinical privileging will need to be documented. Whether to apply for all ultrasound examinations listed in the ACEP ultrasound guidelines or to request specific ultrasound examinations should be based on the group's training and clinical needs as well as the political environment [9]. Provided there are no quality of care issues identified or objections raised, the credentialing committee will forward their recommendation on to the medical executive committee and the trustees for final approval. Privileges are usually granted for time periods of 1–2 years at which time a reappointment process is initiated.

You Were Denied Privileging, Now What?

If the above steps are followed and you or your department are denied clinical privileging in POC ultrasound, don't give up. Ask the credentialing committee for a written explanation for the denial. The hospital has an obligation to the community as well as to the medical staff to provide a fair credentialing and privileging process. Hospitals are not looking to deny privileges to qualified medical staff members, but when other departments bring political and economic motives into the process and create a turf battle hospitals frequently take a passive role in hopes that the two departments can work the issues out. The reason for denial may be minor due to a paperwork error and these would be easy to remedy, as opposed to those due to a turf battle.

All hospital privileging processes must be fair and awarded or denied solely on documented training, experience, and current clinical competence. Privileging based on any other factors is contrary to the written standards of TJC. Requesting a written explanation of the denial may help the hospital realize that they deviated from TJC's standards. When privileging battles go to court, they are won principally because the privileging process deviated from this standard.

With that being said, it is unlikely that many emergency physicians or groups would want to enter into a lawsuit with the hospital for fear that this would jeopardize their group's contract with the hospital. It is important to first exhaust all local avenues of appeal. Gather support from other departments since they may be going through the same denial process. Working together may help to improve the chances for success. Additionally, hospitals are very interested in keeping up with the local competition. If other emergency departments within the local area utilize POC US ultrasound, emphasize this to the hospital administration and provide them with cases where POC ultrasound could have improved patient outcome or minimized chance of a procedural adverse outcome.

Maintenance of Competency

TJC required re-credentialing once every 2 years by medical staff and hospitals utilized the no news is good news approach to evaluate competency and to identify performance issues. In 2008, TJC implemented a new standard that mandates detailed evaluation of the practitioner's professional performance as part of the process of granting and maintaining practice privileges in a hospital or health care organization.

Ongoing Professional Practice Evaluation (OPPE) and Focused Professional Practice Evaluation (FPPE) are the two evaluation processes that TJC is now supporting as the new standard. OPPE is intended as a means of evaluating professional performance on an ongoing basis to monitor professional competency, identify areas for possible performance improvement by individual practitioners, and obtain objective data in decisions regarding continuance of practice privileges. Evaluations must be done more frequently than annually. Entry of practitioner's OPPE performance data can be done monthly, every 3 months, or every 6 months.

FPPE involves more specific and time-limited monitoring of a practitioner's practice performance and is utilized when a provider is initially granted practice privileges, new privileges are requested for an already privileged provider or performance non-conformance involving an already privileged provider is identified. TJC does not specify the time period length of a FPPE. For commonly performed procedures, a 3–6 month period would be reasonable. For infrequently performed procedures, a longer period of monitoring such as 6–12 months would be required.

Obtaining OPPE and FPPE data for an emergency medicine group is a time-consuming process and emphasizes the need for an emergency ultrasound director within the group. Further information on the ultrasound director can be found in that chapter.

Pitfalls

1. Granted privileges should be in line with what you do clinically.
2. Competency goes beyond the number of examinations performed.
3. Avoid turf battles.
4. The OPPE process should be in place to identify clinicians who are delivering an unacceptable quality of care.

Key Points

- No one department/specialty owns any privilege.
- AMA policy on ultrasound affirms that ultrasound imaging is within the scope of practice of appropriately trained physicians. Training criteria should be based on specialty-specific guidelines
- Follow the current ACEP ultrasound guidelines during the credentialing and privileging process
- ACEP supports that emergency physicians obtain privileges consistent with their documented training, experience, and current clinical competence. The recommendations for clinical privileging should come from the director of the emergency department.
- The credentialing and privileging process must be fair and unbiased.
- The best way to guarantee never losing a privileging conflict is to never have one in the first place.

References

1. American College of Emergency Physicians. Physician credentialing and delineation of clinical privileges in emergency medicine. Ann Emerg Med. 2006;48:511.
2. Epstein RM, Hundert EM. Defining and assessing professional competence. JAMA. 2002;287(2):226–35.
3. Ill. Sup. Ct., 33 Ill.2d 326, 211 N.E.2d 253 (1965).
4. Hirsch EA. Establishing a fair privileging process in your hospital. Fam Pract Manag. 1996;3(4):22–40.
5. Burton JH, Miner JR, Shipley ER, et al. Propofol for emergency department procedural sedation and analgesia: a tale of three centers. Acad Emerg Med. 2006;13:24–30.
6. Green SM, Roback MG, Krauss B, et al. Predictors of airway and respiratory adverse events with ketamine sedation in the emergency department: an individual-patient data meta-analysis of 8,282 children. Ann Emerg Med. 2009;54:158–68.
7. Pena BMG, Krauss B. Adverse events of procedural sedation and analgesia in a pediatric emergency department. Ann Emerg Med. 1999;34:483–90.
8. American Medical Association. House of Delegates. Privileging for ultrasound imaging. 2001:H-230.960.
9. American College of Emergency Physicians. Emergency ultrasound guidelines. Ann Emerg Med. 2009;53:550–70.

Chapter 21
Accreditation in Point of Care Ultrasound

Michael P. Mallin

Objectives

– Describe and Define Accreditation in Medicine
– Why Accreditation for Clinical Ultrasound
– The Accreditation process

Introduction

The concept and process of accreditation has seen significant growth in medicine in recent years. Each year it seems additional sites, procedures, and applications of healthcare are seeking accreditation from governing bodies, private companies, and nonprofit organizations.

The concept of accreditation in healthcare began in 1951 with the formation of the Joint Commission on Accreditation of Hospitals (JACH, later known as JACHO) [1]. In 1965 Medicare tied conditions of participation (reimbursement) to JCAH accreditation and changed healthcare forever.

Since 1951 accreditation by external entities has become the accepted norm for validation and scrutiny of the credibility of a healthcare system, process, or group. Hospitals now often seek accreditation to become a Stroke Center, a STEMI receiving center, or a Trauma Center. Many hospital radiology based ultrasound departments, Vascular ultrasound Labs, Echocardiography labs, and Maternal and fetal medicine

M.P. Mallin, MD, FACEP
Division of Emergency Medicine, Department of Surgery, University of Utah School of
Medicine, Salt Lake City, UT, USA
e-mail: michaelmallin@gmail.com

© Springer International Publishing AG 2018   337
V. S. Tayal et al. (eds.), *Ultrasound Program Management*,
https://doi.org/10.1007/978-3-319-63143-1_21

ultrasound departments are already receiving accreditation from groups such as the American College of Radiology [2], The American Institute of Ultrasound in Medicine [3], and the Intersocietal Accreditation Commission [4]. Yet no external entity had created an appropriate accreditation process for clinical based, point-of-care ultrasound.

In 2007 the American College of Emergency Physicians passed Council Resolution 32:

RESOLVED, That ACEP, in cooperation with all established College liaisons and relationships with other medical specialty societies, the American Medical Association, the Alliance for Specialty Medicine, the Coalition for Patient-Centric Imaging, and other interested parties actively and fully opposes the imposition upon the specialty of Emergency Medicine of any accreditation programs developed, offered, and/or governed solely by other specialties; and be it further.

RESOLVED, That the Board of Directors of ACEP submit a comprehensive report to the Council at the 2008 Council Meeting regarding the adoption and execution of a strategic plan to address the long and short-term accreditation issues relating to the performance and interpretation of imaging studies by emergency physicians and, specifically, emergency ultrasound [5].

From 2007 to 2015 the ACEP Accreditation Subcommittee of the Ultrasound Section was tasked in developing what eventually became The Clinical Ultrasound Accreditation Program or CUAP (http://cuap.acep.org). In 2015 CUAP first started accepting application and accrediting hospitals in the performance of clinical ultrasound. This program includes standards such as administration of ultrasound program, education and training of healthcare providers, performing and interpreting ultrasound examinations, equipment management, transducer disinfection, image acquisition and retention, and confidentially and privacy.

What Is Accreditation?

Definition: Accreditation is a process of review that healthcare organizations participate in to demonstrate the ability to meet predetermined criteria and standards of accreditation established by a professional accrediting agency. Accreditation represents agencies as credible and reputable organizations dedicated to ongoing and continuous compliance with the highest standard of quality.

Accreditation, credentialing, and privileging are often confused and used interchangeably within the healthcare setting. Yet each of these is quite different. As it pertains to medicine and specifically physician oversight:

"What CUAP Does……" Accreditation is a self-assessment and external peer assessment process used by a healthcare entity to accurately assess the facility's level of performance in relation to established standards and to implement ways to continuously improve.

"What the Ultrasound Director Does……" Credentialing is the process of gathering information regarding a physicians qualifications and capacity for appointment to the medical staff and those procedures implied by that appointment.

What the Hospital Medical Board Does……. Privileging is the authority granted to a physician by a hospital governing board to provide patient care in the hospital. Clinical privileges are limited by the individual's professional license, experience, and competence.

Thus, when we are discussing the process of providing credibility to the process by which an ultrasound division within a hospital entity is directed, we are talking about accreditation. CUAP or any other form of accreditation does not credential or privilege healthcare providers to perform ultrasound, but may approve the process by which the ultrasound director may credential them.

Why Do We Need Accreditation?

There are many reasons why accreditation can benefit your group, hospital, and ultrasound program. These include standardization, quality assurance, and recognition. At its essence, though, accreditation is meant to give you direction and organization in establishing and maintaining an exceptional ultrasound program.

One of the greatest advantages of accreditation is organization. Most accreditation programs such as CUAP outline necessary requirements for a successful, well-run, and standardized ultrasound program. Guidelines such as machine maintenance, credentialing standards, and probe cleaning are often created by the accrediting body and prevent "from-scratch" protocol creation for the ultrasound director. A secondary advantage to this is that in meeting these requirements, directors can often ask for hospital, departmental, or division support.

Take, for example, endocavitary probe cleaning. It can be difficult convincing your chair or hospital administrators to enact a complicated and expensive probe cleaning policy or purchasing the necessary equipment to run such a policy. If, however, that policy is necessary to gain accreditation, the ultrasound director can use those requirements and accreditation itself as leverage to meet the minimum standards created by that accreditation.

Other reasons commonly mentioned to justify accreditation are [6]:

- Exhibit your commitment to clinical excellence.
- Display your commitment to the highest quality patient care.
- Provide credibility to peers and patients.
- Demonstrate that your practice meets the quality assurance requirements of a growing number of insurance companies.

These are all reasonable reasons to seek accreditation. In the case of ACEP and the Clinical Ultrasound Accreditation Program, it was also advantageous to create a non-specialty specific accreditation process for point-of-care ultrasound or clinical ultrasound so that emergency physicians and emergency departments did not have to try to fit into the mold of non-point of care, consultative ultrasound accreditation programs.

What Is the Clinical Ultrasound Accreditation Program?

The Clinical Ultrasound Accreditation Program (CUAP) is an ACEP-governed national accreditation organization with an understanding of clinical bedside ultrasound and a purpose of establishing a system of review for emergency departments performing clinical, point-of-care ultrasound. This accreditation system promotes the goals of quality, patient safety, communication, responsibility, and clarity regarding the use of clinical ultrasound. As the use of ultrasound has become mainstream in clinical medicine, a need has emerged to promulgate and support national standards for clinical ultrasound programs as detailed in the American College of Emergency Physicians' Ultrasound Guidelines [7].

CUAP has been developed with the express purpose of providing assistance to those looking to implement a point-of-care ultrasound program, so that new programs can take advantage of expert experience to ensure they are meeting best practice standards.

This program includes standards in the areas of administration of ultrasound programs, education and training of healthcare providers, performing and interpreting ultrasound examinations, equipment management, transducer disinfection, image acquisition and retention, and confidentiality and privacy.

What Are the Requirements of CUAP Accreditation?

CUAP, being governed by ACEP, has set the minimum standard for accreditation in an effort to match the ACEP Ultrasound Guidelines [7]. The ACEP 2016 Ultrasound Guidelines are used in multiple specialties as the standard for point-of-care ultrasound. Further validity to these guidelines was gained in 2011 when American institute of Ultrasound In Medicine officially recognized them [8].

CUAP includes standards for administration of an ultrasound program, education and training of healthcare providers, performing and interpreting ultrasound examinations, equipment management, transducer disinfection, image acquisition and retention, and confidentiality and privacy.

Each Institution Will Be Expected to Meet the Following Criteria [9]:

- Every licensed healthcare provider using point-of-care ultrasound either meets ACEP credentialing guidelines or is in the process of meeting these guidelines.
- An emergency ultrasound coordinator/director must oversee the maintenance, education, and monitoring of the ultrasound program.
- The program must also meet minimum standards of continuous quality management (CQM).
- Each healthcare provider must complete a minimum amount of continuing medical education (CME) in each ultrasound credentialing cycle.
- All ultrasound equipment must meet state and federal guidelines and undergo regular maintenance and cleaning.
- A policy must be in place for infection control following the local institution's standards.
- Periodic review of each healthcare provider must be performed.
- Reports must be generated for ultrasound exams and be included in the medical record, and the images must be archived.
- Each institution should follow storage guidelines, respect patient confidentiality and HIPAA guidelines, and follow the ALARA Principle.

In summary, CUAP is designed to be clinician-relevant, bedside-focused, efficient, and complementary of current hospital processes and accreditation.

Other Ultrasound Imaging Accreditation Organizations

AIUM American Institute of Ultrasound in Medicine covering consultative and specific areas including Abdominal/General, Breast, Musculoskeletal (Diagnostic), Musculoskeletal (Ultrasound-Guided Interventional Procedures), Dedicated Thyroid/Parathyroid, Fetal Echocardiography, Gynecologic (with or without 3D), Head and Neck, Obstetric or Trimester-Specific Obstetric, OB with Adjunct Detailed Fetal Anatomic US, Urologic, Ultrasound-Guided Regional Anesthesia

ACR American College of Radiology - for radiology based consultative ultrasound

IAC Intersocietal Accreditation Commission - for consultative vascular and cardiology imaging

Decision to Seek Accreditation

Accreditation may not be for everyone. Some groups are so small that they may not benefit from the standardization and quality assurances gained through the economies of scale associated with larger ultrasound divisions and accreditation. While we encourage these groups to still strive for excellence in point-of-care ultrasound, accreditation should by no means be set as an absolute requirement for emergency departments practicing well within the standard of care, especially if those groups are adhering to the ACEP Ultrasound Guidelines.

Established ultrasound divisions that are already meeting the accreditation minimum standards, are not receiving reimbursement denials for lack of accreditation, and don't need the guidance or leverage of applying for accreditation may also choose to continue along their current path without seeking accreditation. However, there is still recognition to be gained through accreditation.

Pitfalls

1. New US programs with basic elements of machine or director but without basic elements of accreditation (e.g., scope of practice, clinical or infection control protocols, credentialing, machine maintenance or QA) may not be ready for accreditation processes.
2. Not reading or understanding the standards of the accrediting organization.
3. Choosing accreditation from an organization that is unfamiliar with the type of your US practice.
4. Expecting accreditation to be a one time process. Accreditation is time limited recognition that requires programs to maintain standards.
5. Expecting accreditation to resolve all program issues. Accreditation set a bar of quality but other issues may occur.

Key Recommendation

1. Ultrasound accreditation should be a desired quality recognition for clinical ultrasound programs.
2. Ultrasound accreditation can offer you guidance in developing a top-notch ultrasound program, all without having to start from scratch.
3. Develop your US program with awareness of the standards and expectation of accreditation bodies.
4. Use accreditation to your program's advantage including obtaining resources, recognition, and personnel.

References

1. Roberts JS, Coale JG, Redman RR. A history of the Joint Commission on Accreditation of Hospitals. JAMA. 1987;258(7):936–40.
2. ACR Accreditation Modalities: Ultrasound. ACR Web 12 July 2015.
3. AIUM Ultrasound Practice Accreditation: What is AIUM accreditation. Accreditation. AIUM. Web 12 July 2015.
4. Intersocietal Accreditation Commision: Echocardiography. IAC Web 12 July 2015.
5. Action on 2007 Resolutions. Actions on Council Resolutions. ACEP. 23 August 2010. Web 12 July 2015.
6. "AIUM Ultrasound Practice Accreditation: Why should my practice seek AIUM accreditation" Accreditation. AIUM. Web 12 July 2015.
7. ACEP policy statement: ACEP Ultrasound Guidelines. ACEP Policy Statements. ACEP October 2008. Web 12 July 2015.
8. Sound Waves Weekly. Sound Waves Weekly. AIUM, 17 Nov. 2001. Web. 12 July 2015.
9. About the Accreditation Process. Clinical Ultrasound Accreditation. ACEP, n.d. Web. 04 Jan. 2016.

Chapter 22
Point of Care Ultrasound Reimbursement and Coding

Jessica R. Goldstein and Stanley Wu

Objectives

1. Become familiar with coding lexicon
2. Understand how both clinicians and the facility get reimbursed for commonly performed point of care ultrasounds
3. Understand requirements for compliant billing

Introduction

Clinicians use point of care ultrasound as a lean, patient-centered approach to guide therapies, distill differential diagnoses, and confirm clinical impressions. Providers perform focused ultrasounds based on their clinical examination of the patient and communicate real-time results to the patient and family. Point of care ultrasound delivers value to patients by expediting throughput, decreasing patient exposure to radiation, improving safety of invasive procedures, and lowering costs [1–9]. Patients have more favorable opinions of physicians when point of care ultrasound is performed [10].

Reimbursement for diagnostic and procedural ultrasound in the United States as a separately identifiable and billable procedure follows from the American Medical

J.R. Goldstein, MD, FACEP (✉)
Department of Emergency Medicine, University Hospitals Ahuja Medical Center, Case Western Reserve University, Cleveland, OH, USA
e-mail: jessica.goldstein4@uhhospitals.org

S. Wu, MD, MBA, FACEP
Department of Emergency Medicine, Baylor College of Medicine, Houston, TX, USA

© Springer International Publishing AG 2018   345
V. S. Tayal et al. (eds.), *Ultrasound Program Management*,
https://doi.org/10.1007/978-3-319-63143-1_22

Association's *Current Procedural Terminology* (CPT) annual publication [11]. Billing is essential to support the work required to deliver this service to emergency patients and maintain a quality ultrasound program.

CPT Coding

Regardless of specialty and setting, all physicians use CPT codes to compliantly bill for procedures. Appropriately trained clinicians credentialed and privileged by their medical staff to perform a procedure described by CPT may bill for ultrasound.

The American Medical Association's Specialty Society Relative Value Scale Update Committee (RUC) assigns relative value units (RVUs) annually to each CPT code. These updates are published through the CMS website as the Medicare Physician Fee Schedule (MPFS) [12]. The RUC reviews both old and new CPT codes and makes adjustments in RVUs according to the assumed resources required to perform the work. Many private carriers reimburse services based on a multiple of what CMS reimburses on the MPFS.

Global vs. Professional vs. Technical

Clinicians use five-digit CPT codes to bill for a variety of diagnostic and procedural ultrasounds. The MPFS lists three distinct ways to code for these CPT codes: (1) global codes, (2) professional component (PC), and (3) technical component (TC). The legal determination of the practice setting determines how the medical practice bills for professional and facility (technical) services.

Office Setting

A traditional private practice office that is independent from the hospital is a "non-facility" setting. Non-facility offices typically bill global radiology codes. The office pays for equipment, sonographer, physician interpretation, malpractice, and any other overhead required. In return, the office receives a global payment to cover these expenses (Table 22.1).

Table 22.1 Professional and technical fees, site of service, and bundling

	Office setting (non-hospital)	ED (hospital outpatient)	Inpatient
Professional fee	Included in global fee	Billed separately by physician	Billed separately by physician
Technical fee	Included in global fee	Billed by hospital, may be subject to bundling under OPPS or DRG if admitted	Billed by hospital, bundled into DRG

Facility Setting

Hospital-run Emergency Departments, including free-standing hospital-owned Emergency Departments, inpatient and outpatient hospital departments including operating rooms and intensive care units, ambulatory surgery centers, and radiology departments within hospitals are considered "provider based" or "facility" settings. Facility settings split the global code into a professional and technical code. In a facility setting, physicians may not bill global codes, even if they own the ultrasound equipment. In all of the departments listed above, physicians must bill professional CPT codes for diagnostic and procedural ultrasound (Table 22.1).

Professional Component

The professional component (PC) covers the work of the physician's interpretation of an ultrasound image. Only licensed physicians or privileged licensed independent practitioners can bill the PC for interpreting ultrasounds. Though the concept of point of care ultrasound centers on the clinician performing and interpreting the images at the bedside, CPT does not require the interpreting physician to be present during the image acquisition process for diagnostic ultrasound. Local privileging guidelines determine who may obtain images in the Emergency Department that are archived and used to generate the PC interpretation for billing.

Billing for procedural ultrasound follows slightly different requirements from diagnostic ultrasound. The professional component of procedural ultrasound involves interpreting the diagnostic image associated with the procedure that the same physician is performing [13]; therefore the physician must be personally performing the procedure in order to bill compliantly. The five digit CPT code is listed with a PC modifier (-26) on the CMS 1500 professional charge sheet to indicate the charge is for the interpretive work and not the global charge.

Technical Component

The technical component (TC) covers the practice expense of machine and equipment purchase, ultrasound technician salary, archiving expenses, and overhead involved in maintaining space for the service. The hospital bills for the technical component on a UB04 billing sheet. The UB04 lists the revenue center code to identify where the service took place. When a 24/7 ED bills for the TC of the ultrasound, the ED lists the ED revenue code 450 to identify the location of the procedure and the five-digit ultrasound CPT code with a TC modifier (-TC). In the ED setting, the hospital typically bills the TC component because they typically pay for the machine and ultrasound procedure supplies.

Centers for Medicare and Medicaid Services and POC US Coding and Billing

Medicare Patients: Hospital Outpatient Prospective Payment System

Medicare patients treated in outpatient hospital departments such as the Emergency Departments and observation units, as well as ambulatory surgery centers, are considered outpatients. Billing for these outpatient Medicare patients follows the Outpatient Prospective Payment System (OPPS). While the professional fees are unaffected by inpatient and outpatient status, the facility fees are affected. Facilities list the same CPT code the physician is billing for professional services, and the CPT code is matched to the appropriate ambulatory payment classification (APC) code. While most diagnostic radiology codes are reimbursed separately under their associated APCs, the TC of image-guidance procedures are bundled into packaged services for the actual procedure performed. For example, a clinician performs an ultrasound-guided peripheral IV on a challenging patient in the ED. The physician bills the professional fee for the venous access and add-on ultrasound-guided vascular access code. The technical payment gets bundled into the payment for the line placement service—no additional technical payment is generated. An anesthesiologist performs an ultrasound-guided axillary nerve block prior to an orthopedic case. The physician bills the professional service for the ultrasound-guided procedure and the nerve block procedure. The hospital bundles the facility fee for the ultrasound-guidance procedure into the overall fees for the nerve block procedure.

Medicare Patients: Inpatient Versus Outpatient

With Medicare patients, payment of the TC fee differs depending if the patient is an outpatient or inpatient. When a patient is seen and discharged from the Emergency Department or observation status from the hospital, the patient is an outpatient. The technical charges for the ultrasound remain with the department that performed the service. For example, a patient presents to the ED with abdominal pain. The ED physician performs a limited abdominal ultrasound to evaluate for gallstones. The patient is discharged home. The ED physician bills for the professional services and the ED facility bills for the TC of the ultrasound.

If the same Medicare patient has evidence of cholecystitis and requires admission to the hospital, the ED physician bills the professional component but the ED facility does not get reimbursed for the TC as a separately identifiable procedure. When this patient is admitted to the hospital, the hospital is paid a prospective payment based on the diagnosis-related group (DRG) for cholecystitis (Table 22.1). The technical fee for the ultrasound and other ED facility charges are bundled into the DRG payment to the hospital. Many private insurers also use DRGs to determine a bundled payment to the hospital.

RVUs

Within both the professional and TC, the RUC assigns RVUs for work (wRVU), practice expense (PE RVU), and malpractice expense (MP RVU). The RUC assumes the same overall work-flow for diagnostic and procedural ultrasound regardless of the practice setting (i.e., Radiology Department versus Emergency Department versus private practice Obstetric office) (Table 22.2).

Sample table excerpted from 2017 National Physician Fee Schedule Relative Value File January Release for CPT 76705 [12]. Technical Component Medicare Allowable = (work RVU + practice expense RVU + malpractice RVU) * Conversion Factor. Professional Component Medicare Allowable = (work RVU + practice expense RVU+ malpractice RVU) * Conversion Factor. The Status code "A" indicates a code that is paid separately under the physician fee schedule. PC/TC Indicator 1 identifies diagnostic tests for radiology services that have both a professional and TC.

The work flow for point of care ultrasound is distinct from the work flow of consultant radiology ultrasound. The point of care ultrasound clinician determines the medical necessity for the ultrasound, obtains appropriate images, interprets the images, archives the images, and documents a report. Reimbursement for the professional component of ultrasound covers only the physician interpretation of the ultrasound images. Currently, CPT does not have a list of point of care clinician performed CPT codes for diagnostic ultrasound that accurately describe and reimburse for the work of point of care ultrasound in a facility setting (Fig. 22.1).

Table 22.2 Example of work components of CPT US codes and global RVUs

Modifier	Description	w RVU	PE RVU	MP RVU	Total	CONV factor	Status code	PC/TC indicator
TC	Echo exam of abdomen, limited	0.00	1.75	0.01	1.76	35.7751	A	1
PC	Echo exam of abdomen, limited	0.59	0.22	0.03	0.84	35.7751	A	1
Global	Echo exam of abdomen, limited	0.59	1.97	0.04	2.60	35.7751	A	1

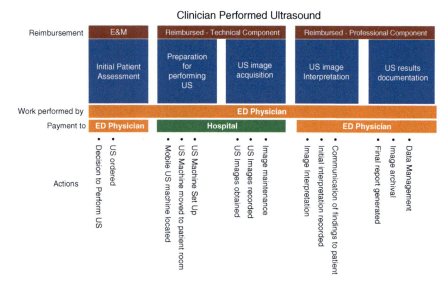

Fig. 22.1 Work-flow for clinician performed ultrasound highlights the work performed versus the payments made to clinicians and facilities (hospital) [14]

Machine Purchase

There are specific circumstances that may permit a physician or physician group in a facility setting to purchase ultrasound equipment and receive compensation for both the professional and TC [15]. Any consideration of this relationship between a physician group and a hospital to allow the physician group to bill technical services requires experienced legal counsel to review physician-self referral (Stark Law) implications as well as the complicated process for bundling facility radiology fees when an emergency patient becomes admitted to an inpatient status.

Hand-Held Ultrasound Devices

Hand-held ultrasound devices are becoming affordable for individual provider purchase. These machines fall under the same billing guidelines for other portable ultrasound machines. CMS/CPT billing requirements remain the same: an order for the ultrasound, an archived representative image of the study must be maintained, a statement of medical necessity, a written report and interpretation and the physician's signature. Site of service payment rules in a facility setting still require a split in professional and technical charges, even if the physician owns the equipment.

Several particular areas raise questions and concerns which merit further discussion: (1) archiving, (2) HIPAA, and (3) Stark Law/Anti-Kickback Statute. Access to image archival is required for both billing and quality purposes. Images must be present in the patient's medical record, whether scanned into the actual record, or available on an archiving system that is available at all hours. If the machine travels with the physician, image archiving on the actual machine is unacceptable.

With regard to HIPAA hand-held ultrasound devices that record patient information are also subject to HIPAA regulations. Patients have a right to privacy and security regarding any data collected with patient identifiers and hand-held ultrasound devices are no exception.

The Stark Law governs physician self-referral for Medicare and Medicaid patients and generally prohibits a physician from referring patients for certain designated health service ("DHS"), to a medical facility in which the referring physician maintains some ownership interest. "Ultrasound services" is one such defined DHS. Under the Stark Law's definition of "referral" a physician should be permitted to both order, perform and bill for scans using a hand-held ultrasound device. However, because the law often lags behind the advent of technology, and because CMS has not yet issued a specific advisory opinion which limits or restricts billing Medicare for hand-held ultrasound devices, it remains to be seen whether this situation could create any Stark law implications.

Similarly, the Anti-Kickback Statue ("AKS") prohibits any individual from receiving anything of value for purposes of inducing referrals. Although CMS has not issued any specific opinion regarding the impact of AKS on hand-held ultrasounds, providers should avoid any incentive, bonus, or compensation structure which is derived from or directly linked to the performance of these ultrasound services.

Limited vs. Complete Ultrasound

Since 2005, CPT has defined the work required for complete and limited diagnostic ultrasounds. Complete ultrasounds include all of the structures present in an anatomical region and are specifically listed in the CPT manual. Clinicians may bill for complete ultrasounds if medical necessity supports a complete ultrasound should take place and all of the elements required for a complete ultrasound are included in the report. For example, many clinicians are comfortable documenting all of the elements required for a complete first trimester obstetric transabdominal ultrasound (76801). Requirements for 76801 include the following: determination of the number of gestational sacs and fetuses, gestational sac/fetal measurements appropriate for gestation (younger than 14 weeks 0 days), survey of visible fetal and placental anatomic structure, qualitative assessment of amniotic fluid volume/gestational sac shape and examination of the maternal uterus and adnexa [11]. If an element that is required by CPT for a complete ultrasound is not visualized, a reason is required. In the diagnostic ultrasound section, CPT instructs: "For those anatomic regions that have 'complete' and 'limited' ultrasound codes, note the elements that comprise a 'complete' exam. The report should contain a description of these elements or the reason that an element could not be visualized (e.g., obscured by bowel gas, surgically absent)." [11].

Most point of care ultrasound exams are limited in scope because clinicians perform ultrasounds to answer focused questions or guide procedures. For example, a provider evaluating a multiparous woman with epigastric pain performs an ultrasound with a focused question: "Does this person have gallstones to explain their discomfort?" Rather than performing a complete abdominal ultrasound, a clinician would evaluate the gallbladder for gallstones and if gallstones are present, he/she would look for signs of cholecystitis. A complete ultrasound (76700) requires evaluation of the following: real-time scans of the liver, gallbladder, common bile duct, pancreas, spleen, kidneys, and the upper abdominal aorta and inferior vena cava including any demonstrated abdominal abnormality. A focused ultrasound for gallstones falls under 76705, a limited abdominal ultrasound. For limited studies, CPT has no specific requirements on elements included in the study.

CPT Modifiers

CPT modifiers are used to provide additional coding information on the type of study performed. The table below lists the most common CPT modifiers used in the Emergency Department. A complete list of modifiers can be found in CPT 2017 [11] (Table 22.3).

Table 22.3 CPT Modifier commonly used in POC US

CPT modifier number	CPT modifier	Definition
-26	Professional component	Professional interpretation of the ultrasound study with a signed written report and accompanying archived images in a facility/hospital-owned setting. With procedural ultrasound the professional component is the clinician performing the procedure personally with either real-time ultrasound-guidance or ultrasound assistance [13].
-TC	Technical component	Technical portion of the global ultrasound fee that covers the cost of the machine, the technician salary, other overhead. The facility typically bills for the TC because they own the hospital equipment and maintain it.
-52	Reduced services	Used when a procedure is performed but the work that was done was less than what is detailed in the CPT description. The availability of limited CPT codes obviates the need for this modifier in most circumstances. An example when the -52 modifier should be used is when a physician's skill is required to place a midline angiocatheter into a deep vein due to inadequate peripheral venous access. It would be appropriate to code 36556, the code of inserting a PICC in someone 5 years or older, with the 59 modifier, because the tip of the catheter lies close to the axillary vein instead of a central vein [16].
		Typically reimbursement is reduced 50% for this modifier and in some cases reimbursement is denied.

Table 22.3 (continued)

CPT modifier number	CPT modifier	Definition
-59	Distinct procedural service	This modifier is used to report procedures that are distinct from a non-evaluation and management code on the same date of service. For example, if a patient had multiple foreign bodies in both the right upper and lower extremities, the 76882 code for ultrasound extremity, nonvascular, real time with image documentation, would be used twice, with a -59 modifier.
-76	Repeat procedure by the same physician	Same ultrasound procedure performed on the patient on the same date of service or patient encounter. Practitioners in the same specialty, same group and during the same encounter are viewed from a billing perspective as the "same physician." Payment is based on the group's Medicare provider number, not the unique physician identifier number. For example, if a patient with blunt abdominal trauma and a negative initial FAST exam becomes hemodynamically unstable, a repeat examination may be medically necessary by the same physician or a partner (76705-26 initial, 76705-26,-76 for repeat).
77	Repeat procedure by different physician	Repeat procedure done by a physician in a different billing group, for example, a trauma surgeon repeating the FAST examination for ongoing hypotension. If two bills are submitted for the same procedure and neither has a repeat modifier, the first bill received will likely be reimbursed and the second will be rejected. To avoid this conflict, providers should communicate with each other who is billing for the initial and repeat procedures. Limited ultrasound studies which are subsequently sent to radiology for complete studies or repeat limited ultrasound studies also require a modifier in order for both departments to get reimbursed. A limited ultrasound is subsumed in a complete ultrasound so medical necessity is imperative for the repeat study. An example would be performing a limited abdominal ultrasound for suspected gallstones and finding a liver mass unexpectedly. Billing for the complete ultrasound and the limited ultrasound in the same encounter may be rejected initially. Unless arrangements are made with radiology to bill for a repeat study, the first department to submit the bill will receive payment and the second department will likely get rejected. Inter-departmental agreements on how to handle these situations should be agreed upon ahead of time.

Diagnostic vs. Procedural Codes

Diagnostic and procedural ultrasounds may be billed on the same day during the same encounter as long as each one is not subsumed in the other. For example, ultrasound-guidance for vascular access (76937) specifically states that diagnosing potential sites is subsumed in the procedure [11]. For other procedures, such as ultrasound-guided pericardiocentesis, if a focused cardiac ultrasound was performed to diagnose the tamponade, then a diagnostic code (limited echocardiogram, 93308) and a procedural code (ultrasound-guided pericardiocentesis, 76930) would be appropriate.

In addition to the ultrasound-guided procedural codes, the surgical code for the actual procedure being performed is applied when it is not subsumed in the ultrasound-guided code. In the pericardiocentesis example, the surgical procedure itself (33010, pericardiocentesis; initial) and the ultrasound-guidance procedure (76930, ultrasound-guidance for pericardiocentesis) are both coded. A more common example would be ultrasound-guided central venous access in which the surgical procedure (36556, Insertion of a non-tunneled central venous catheter, age > 5 yo) would be coded in addition to the ultrasound-guided vascular access procedure (76937).

Over the past 5 years, CPT has added new codes to describe specific image-guided procedures such as ultrasound-guided paracentesis (e.g., 49083 paracentesis with imaging, new to CPT in January 1, 2012). When a specific ultrasound-guided procedure is not available, then the generic ultrasound-guidance code 76942 can be added to the primary surgical code. For example, ultrasound-guided lumbar puncture to evaluate for meningitis would include both the primary surgical code (62270) and the ultrasound-guidance code (76942) because currently no ultrasound-guided lumbar puncture code exists.

Add-on Codes

Most CPT codes can be billed as unique stand-alone codes. Others are considered add-on codes to a primary procedural code. Add-on codes are procedures that the same physician performs during one patient encounter in addition to a primary procedure. A commonly used add-on code is 76937, ultrasound-guidance for vascular access. This code must accompany a primary code such as 36410 (venipuncture, age 3 or older, necessitating skill of physician or other qualified health care professional) or 36556 inserting a non-tunneled central line into a patient older than 5 years. Add-on codes have a specific icon in the CPT manual (+).

Nonphysicians Performing Ultrasounds

RN/Medics Performing Ultrasound-Guided Procedures

With appropriate competencies, nurses and medics can place ultrasound-guided IVs. Since a licensed independent practitioner is not involved in these procedures, no professional component can be billed.

Licensed Independent Practitioners

With appropriate state license, scope of practice, and hospital privileging, licensed independent practitioners with their own National Provider Identifiers can perform, interpret, and bill professional fees for ultrasounds. Credentialing requirements for licensed independent practitioners would be expected to be equal to physician requirements. Billing for licensed independent practitioners follows billing for any other procedure they perform in the ED.

Insurance Payment Policies

Private insurance and Medicare may require documentation of specialized training in certain ultrasound areas prior to reimbursement for diagnostic and procedural ultrasound charges. Billing departments must review local insurance carrier policy requirements.

Technical Billing

Understanding basic aspects of technical billing help clinicians develop the business case for creating departmental and institutional ultrasound programs. When professional and TC are split such as in the ED facility setting, revenue from the technical TC of ultrasound exceeds the professional component by a ratio of approximately 2:1 [14]. Billing for the TC is critical to cover the cost of machine investment and deliberate growth of departmental or institutional point of care ultrasound. Technical billing follows the same billing requirements as professional billing and uses the same CPT codes. A professional interpretation or procedure note must accompany a TC bill.

Point of Care Ultrasound CPT Codes

Core Emergency Ultrasound CPT Codes

Emergency physicians have been pioneers in the field of point of care ultrasound, so it is not surprising that ACEPs published guide of core and advanced applications may be helpful to clinicians outside of emergency medicine. ACEP Emergency Ultrasound Guidelines (2006 and 2015) describe core and advanced emergency ultrasound applications [17]. Each application and the accompanying CPT code are described below. CMS carriers in specific geographic coverage areas publish Local coverage determinations (LCDs) which describe clinical utility for a specific CPT code. LCDs are listed when available following the ACEP recommended application. Exhibit 1 from the ACEP Coding and Reimbursement Document provides a table of commonly used POC US codes and their descriptions.

Diagnostic POC US

Trauma Ultrasound 93308, 76705, 76604

ACEP describes the clinical guidelines for performing the Focused Assessment by Sonography in Trauma (FAST) exam in the 2006 ACEP Ultrasound Imaging Criteria Compendium [17]. These guidelines are also supported by the joint AIUM/ACEP Guidelines for the Performance of the FAST Exam published in 2008 [18]. The above documents outline the traditional four-window abdominal and cardiac examination plus anterior pleural windows and additional cardiac views to evaluate for hemoperitoneum, pneumothorax, hemopericardium, and hemodynamic status.

There is no CPT code that specifically describes the extended FAST as this is not a single ultrasound procedure, but rather a clinical approach to the trauma patient that utilizes a group of distinct limited ultrasound examinations described by several CPT codes. Currently, there are three CPT codes that reflect separately identifiable elements of the FAST exam as described by the AIUM/ACEP documents: (1) cardiac 93308, (2) abdomen 76705, and (3) chest 76604. Despite the availability of three codes which describe a full trauma torso ultrasound evaluation, physicians and coders should list only those appropriate for the individual patient with supporting medical necessity. More detailed descriptions for CPT codes 93308, 76705, and 76604 follows below.

LCD: see LCDs for 93308, 76705, and 76604 below

Female Pelvic Ultrasound: Pregnant 76815, 76817; Nonpregnant 76857, 76830

Evaluation of the pregnant female with abdominal pain or vaginal bleeding is a common scenario in the Emergency Department. The primary objective in this setting is to identify a clear intrauterine pregnancy and therefore decrease the likelihood of an ectopic pregnancy. Physicians with advanced skills may evaluate the adnexa and identify pelvic masses. The scope of practice for pelvic ultrasound will vary depending on clinician skill-level and departmental policies [17].

The coding of pelvic ultrasound depends upon knowing if the patient is pregnant prior to ultrasound examination. When the patient is known by any means to be pregnant, including a positive pregnancy test, and the physician is utilizing ultrasound to evaluate the pregnancy or a suspected complication of pregnancy, then the obstetric pelvic codes would be utilized (e.g., complete (76801) or limited (76815) pelvic ultrasound in a woman known to be pregnant; and/or transvaginal pelvic ultrasound in a woman known to be pregnant (76817)). The obstetric pelvic codes would apply to the "known to be pregnant patient" even in the absence of an intrauterine pregnancy identified by the subsequent ultrasound and even if the patient was found to have an ectopic pregnancy, spontaneous abortion, molar pregnancy, or a non-pregnancy-related condition.

If pregnancy is documented to be absent prior to the ultrasound examination, properly trained clinicians may utilize advanced pelvic ultrasound to evaluate pelvic pain, amenorrhea, vaginal bleeding, or non-gynecologic pelvic pathology. In these cases, the non-obstetric pelvic codes would be utilized (e.g., complete (76856) or limited (76857) pelvic ultrasound not pregnant and/or transvaginal ultrasound not pregnant (76830)). This code selection would hold true even if the result of the subsequent ultrasound examination was an intrauterine or ectopic pregnancy.

If both transabdominal and transvaginal examinations are medically necessary and performed, both can be coded. If both are complete examinations, the complete codes can be used (76801, 76817 if pregnant; 76856, 76830 if not pregnant). If both are limited examinations, the limited obstetric or non-obstetric code may be used in conjunction with the transvaginal approach (76815, 76817 if pregnant, 76857, 76830 if not pregnant). The planned sequencing for every transabdominal ultrasound to be followed by a transvaginal ultrasound would be inappropriate. Based on clinical requirements, the transvaginal examination may be the only ultrasound performed and coded. If the transvaginal examination is limited, the limited pelvic ultrasound can be used (76815 or 76857) or the transvaginal exam (76817 or 76830).

LCD Pregnant Uterus: NA

LCD Nonpregnant Uterus: L34280, L30054

Abdominal Aortic Aneurysm (AAA), Urinary Tract 76775, Screening AAA 76706, Bladder 76857

An emergency ultrasound of the abdominal aorta in a patient presenting with symptoms concerning for AAA or an emergency ultrasound of a patient with suspected hydronephrosis would be coded for by 76775, a limited retroperitoneal ultrasound. This study consists of fewer elements than a complete retroperitoneal ultrasound (76770). According to CPT 2017 [11], a complete retroperitoneal ultrasound would require evaluation of "kidneys, abdominal aorta, common iliac artery origins, and inferior vena cava, including any demonstrated retroperitoneal abnormality. If clinical history suggests urinary tract pathology, complete evaluation of the kidneys and urinary bladder also comprises a complete retroperitoneal ultrasound." If sectional views of the kidney were imaged in this same patient, the limited retroperitoneal code (76775) would still apply and would not be separately billable from the ultrasound of the aorta.

One of the additions to the 2017 CPT is the new code, 76706, for ultrasounds performed to screen for the presence of AAA. This code cannot be used with 76770 (complete retroperitoneal ultrasound), 76775 (limited retroperitoneal ultrasound), 93978, or 93979 (complete and limited duplex scan of the aorta or IVC). CMS will reimburse for a one-time screening ultrasound for AAA on men between 65 and 75 years old who have smoked at least 100 cigarettes in their lifetime or have a family history of AAA [11].

Bladder volume measurement can be performed using nonimaging or imaging ultrasounds. Many hospitals and Emergency Departments now utilize a three-dimensional volumetric probe (e.g., The Bladderscan) to measure bladder volumes. The mechanical probe auto-steers to obtain consecutive sectional images of the bladder and automatically calculates a volume. These devices produce no image to detect abnormalities such as bladder diverticula, enlarged prostate, bladder mass, or hematoma. For these types of instruments which do not produce ultrasound images and are used solely to obtain a bladder volume, the 51798 code is appropriate. CPT describes code 51798: "Measurement of post voiding residual urine and/or bladder capacity by ultrasound, non imaging" [11]. Transadbominal pelvic ultrasound (76857) should be utilized when an actual image of the bladder is obtained and interpreted.

LCDs on Retroperitoneal Ultrasound: L31601, L34577

Cardiac 93308

Primary emergency indications for performing transthoracic ultrasound include shock, dyspnea, penetrating thoracic trauma with the goals of: "detection of a pericardial effusion and/or tamponade, estimation of gross cardiac activity in the setting of cardiopulmonary resuscitation or estimation of global left ventricular function." [17]. More extended techniques include: "gross estimation of intravascular volume and cardiac preload: identification of acute right ventricular dysfunctions and/or acute pulmonary hypertension in the setting of acute and unexplained chest pain, dyspnea, or hemodynamic instability; identification of proximal aortic dissection or thoracic aortic aneurysm; and procedural guidance of pericardiocentesis, or pacemenaker wire placement and capture." [17]. Each of these scenarios codes as a limited transthoracic echocardiogram (93308). A complete transthoracic echocardiogram would require 2-D and M-mode examination of all atria and ventricles, all valves, the pericardium, adjacent portions of the aorta, and a functional assessment of the heart. Additional structures that may be visualized including the inferior vena cava are included in the complete study.

LCDs for echocardiography: L27630, L27536, L28565, L28997, L29296, L29402, L31794, L31848, L32675, L33472, L33577, L33768, 34338, L34637, L34852, L35017

Biliary, Bowel, Hemoperitoneum, Appendix 76705

A complete ultrasound of the abdomen would include evaluation of the liver, gallbladder, common bile duct, pancreas, spleen, kidneys, and the upper abdominal aorta and inferior vena cava. Limited abdominal ultrasound (76705) evaluates fewer elements than a complete examination. Evaluation of the gallbladder for gallstones codes to 76705. Bowel ultrasound (76705) consists of a B-mode scan with image documentation. Bowel ultrasound can be limited to either a single organ, such as appendix, or a single quadrant for ileus or intussusception. Evaluation for focused intra-abdominal pathology such as hemoperitoneum, portal venous gas or free air also codes to 76705.

The abdominal portion of the FAST exam codes to 76705. Visualization of the diaphragm and sectional views above the diaphragm on the hepatorenal or splenorenal windows is included in 76705 and does not warrant a separate bill for chest ultrasound. Similarly, visualization of the bladder when looking for hemoperitoneum in the cul-de-sac view does not warrant a separate bill for a pelvic ultrasound.

Abdominal Ultrasound LCDs: L31572, L34572

Deep Venous Thrombosis (DVT) 93971

A clinician's primary application of venous ultrasound is in the "evaluation of deep venous thrombosis of the proximal lower extremities." [17] Providers perform compression ultrasound of the lower extremity veins (93971). This study consists of fewer elements than a complete duplex study of the extremity veins which requires integrating B-mode 2-D vascular structure with spectral and/or color flow Doppler mapping or imaging. While looking primarily for venous thrombosis, POC US of lower extremity veins may also reveal other etiologies for lower extremity swelling such as edema, lymphadenopathy, baker's cyst, or superficial venous thrombosis. These findings may warrant additional imaging but can be listed in the limited examination results section without requiring billing for two separate POC US exams.

Noninvasive duplex ultrasound studies LCDs: L27355, L28586, L28936, L28999, L29234, L30040, L30046, L33693, L33479, L33627, L34229, L34267, L34714, L34721, L35451, L34714, L35451, L35751.

Soft Tissue/Musculoskeletal

Soft tissue/musculoskeletal ultrasound is one of the rapidly growing areas of emergency ultrasound. The most common use for soft tissue ultrasound is to distinguish between cellulitis and abscess. Though no specific code exists for soft tissue ultrasound, the May 2009 CPT Assistant provides guidance on appropriate coding for these studies [19]. These codes would also be used for evaluation of foreign body or other superficial mass. Correct coding for evaluation of a palpable soft-tissue mass is based on the location of the mass. According to May 2009 CPT Assistant, reduced service modifier (-52) is not required for any of these codes [19].

Neck	76536-26
Upper extremity, limited	76882-26
Axilla, limited	76882-26
Chest wall	76604-26
Breast limited[a]	76642-26
Upper back	76604-26
Lower back	76705-26
Abdominal wall	76705-26
Pelvic wall, limited	76857-26
Lower extremity, limited	76882-26
Other soft tissue	76999-26

[a]CPT 2017 distinguishes complete and limited breast ultrasound codes [11]

Coding for musculoskeletal ultrasound is not well developed. The only codes that exist are extremity ultrasound, nonvascular, B-scan and/or real time with image documentation (76882), complete infant ultrasound hip, and limited infant ultrasound hip (76886). Ultrasounds for miscellaneous musculoskeletal indications including fracture evaluation, tendon rupture, or muscle tear are coded with 76882.

LCDs for nonvascular extremity ultrasound: L28178, L33619, L34673, L34716, L35222, L35409, L35469.

Thoracic Ultrasound 76604

CPT 2017 describes Ultrasound Chest succinctly: "Ultrasound, chest (includes mediastinum), real time with image documentation." CPT assistant May 2009 provides additional guidance for billing requirements: An ultrasound of the chest for pleural fluid or pneumothorax does not require examination of the mediastinum in order to bill for a complete study. (22) Evaluation of the chest for lung sliding in a patient with shortness of breath and a history of pneumothorax would be appropriately coded by 76604 without a -52 modifier. In the setting of a critical traumatically injured patient, medical necessity supports scanning the anterior chest pleura separately from the hepatorenal and splenorenal fossa to evaluate for pneumothorax.

LCD: NA

Ocular Ultrasound 76512

Ocular ultrasound is primarily used in the "detection of retinal detachment with or without vitreous detachment." [17]. Advanced studies include "measurement of intracranial pressure indirectly via measuring the optic nerve sheath diameter, visualizing a vitreous hemorrhage, lens dislocation, intraocular foreign body, globe rupture, retrobulbar hemorrhage, central retinal artery/vein occlusion, subretinal hemorrhage, posterior vitreous detachment and/or visualizing the presence or absence of a direct and consensual light reflex." [17]. All of these studied are coded with 76512, ophthalmic ultrasound, diagnostic, B-scan (with or without superimposed non-quantitative A-scan). Ocular foreign body has a separate code (76529).

LCD: L33904, L29082

Ultrasound-Guided Procedures

There are three main categories of ultrasound-guided procedures:

1. Ultrasound-guidance for vascular access (76937).
2. Specifically named ultrasound-guidance for needle placement with or without leaving a catheter in place for drainage for specific organs.
3. Miscellaneous Ultrasound-guided procedures without leaving a catheter (76942).

Ultrasound-guidance for vascular access (76937-26) requires written documentation of real-time ultrasound-guidance for vascular access and a representative image. This image need not capture the needle entering the vessel due to obvious safety concerns due to obvious safety concerns of a single operator in the ED insertnig a needle and not having a free hand to freeze an image. Nonetheless, documentation must account for real-time ultrasound guidance. This code is an add-on code (see section on add-on description).

With the rise in ultrasound-guided procedures, CPT has added several organ specific ultrasound-guided procedures with associated RVUs.

The following are organ specific, ultrasound-guided procedures in which a catheter is not left in place after the procedure:

Ultrasound-guided Paracentesis (49083)
Ultrasound-guided Thoracentesis (32555)

Ultrasound-guided Pericardiocentesis (76930)—This code is an image-only code. The surgical code for pericardiocentesis (33010) should be added.

Ultrasound-guided Joint aspiration of small (20604), medium (20606), and large (20611) joints.

The following are organ specific, ultrasound-guided procedures in which a catheter is left in place after the procedure:

Ultrasound-guided Thoracentesis while leaving a catheter for drainage (32557)

Ultrasound-guided Soft tissue drainage leaving a catheter in place for drainage (10030)

Ultrasound-guided Suprapubic aspiration and catheterization, leaving a catheter in place for drainage (49405)

Ultrasound-guided Peritoneal or retroperitoneal fluid collection drainage, and leaving a catheter in place for drainage (49406)

CPT code 76942 describes all the other needle placement procedures not specifically named in CPT in which a physician uses ultrasound to guide needle placement without leaving a drainage catheter. Guidance need not be real time. Examples of using 76942 as a separately identifiable code in addition to the primary surgical code include: Ultrasound-guided abscess drainage, peritonsillar abscess drainage, lumbar puncture, suprapubic aspiration, and foreign body removal.

Advanced Emergency Ultrasound Codes

Advanced emergency ultrasound studies described by ACEP Ultrasound Section documents 2006 and 2015 include the following: transesophageal, adnexal, and scrotal pathology including torsion, transcranial doppler, and contrast ultrasound studies [13]. Point of care clinicians should receive additional training in these advanced modalities.

1. Transesophageal echocardiogram (93312) includes transesophageal B-mode echo, with image documentation (with or without M-mode recording). The code description includes probe placement, image acquisition, interpretation and a report.
2. Female Adnexa: 76857, 76830, 93975, 93976

See female pelvic ultrasound section above for detailed discussion on nonpregnant female pelvic ultrasound coding. A separately billable complete duplex scan of the ovaries to evaluate for torsion includes both venous and arterial waveform measurements (93975). The limited duplex code is 93976.

LCD Non-obstetric Pelvic US: L30054, L34280

3. Scrotal and male pelvis ultrasound

Men with scrotal pain or swelling are evaluated using scrotal ultrasound (76870) to diagnose scrotal cellulitis, abscess, or mass. The scrotal ultrasound code is a complete code, so a limited study requires a reduced service modifier (-52). A separately billable complete duplex scan of the testicular vasculature, such as to evaluate for testicular torsion, includes both venous and arterial waveforms measurements (93975). The code for a limited duplex testicular ultrasound is 93976.

LCD Scrotal US: NA

Outpatient vs. Inpatient

Bundling of facility services takes place when a Medicare patient is hospitalized on an inpatient unit. While professional charges for ultrasound are not bundled, the technical charges for radiology services are bundled into the diagnostic-related category for the admission diagnosis. The hospital is incentivized to streamline care and avoid unnecessary testing for inpatients because there is one standard facility payment made to the hospital regardless of how many tests are ordered. When discussing hospital investments in ultrasound development such as wireless archiving systems and aligning other department leaders to support point of care ultrasound, it is critical to understand participants' motivation for archiving or setting up compliant billing templates. Inpatient departments and OB departments which already face major bundling challenges for reimbursement may be more motivated to set up archiving and billing structures to optimize quality assurance programs rather than solely to meet requirements for billing.

Government ABCs

Medicare

Medicare Part B covers Emergency Department professional services, including professional component for Radiology services. Medicare Part A covers the TC of Emergency Department and Radiology services.

MACs

Medicare delegates regional administrative duties to Medicare Administrative Contractors (MAC). MACs develop local coverage determinations (LCDs) to describe groups of similar CPT codes and requirements for reimbursement. For example, there are several LCDs on transthoracic echocardiography. Information on LCDs relevant to clinician billing includes the following: State jurisdiction, effective coverage dates, coverage indications/medical necessity, and training requirements.

It is important to be familiar with your regional MAC's LCDs because the content may vary between MACs. An important example of MAC LCD variability is transthoracic echocardiogram training requirements. CGS Administrators LLC, which has jurisdiction in Kentucky and Ohio, refers to LCD L31848. CGS lists training criteria for professional services to be billed for 93308 as "(1) Board certified in Cardiovascular Diseases or (2) The physician has Level II training in TTE as defined by the ACC/AHA/American College of Physicians Task Force on Clinical Competence in Echocardiography or the equivalent of Level 2 training as set forth in that document." Level 2 training requires performing 150 transthoracic echocardiograms and interpreting 300 transthoracic echocardiograms [20, 21].

In contrast, Wisconsin Physicians Service Insurance Company, which has jurisdiction in Kansas, Missouri, Iowa, Nebraska, Indiana, Michigan, publishes LCD L28565. Regarding training criteria, L28565 states, "Medicare does expect a satisfactory level of competence from providers who submit claims for services rendered…It is expected that based on their experience and/or training, that such images will be submitted for interpretation. Providers of the professional component must provide proper interpretation, based on their experience and/or training."

With advocacy from Emergency and Critical Care Physicians to expand credentialing bodies beyond ACA, this particular LCD may continue to evolve.

Medical Necessity/ICD

Title XVIII of the Social Security Act refers to medical necessity when ordering tests: Section 1862 a(1) (A) The Social Security Act "excludes expenses incurred for items or services which are not reasonable and necessary for the diagnosis or treatment of illness or injury or to improve the functioning of a malformed body member." [22]. International Classification of Diseases (ICD) is the nomenclature used to describe medical signs, symptoms, and diagnoses. For example, an provider evaluates a hypotensive elderly man with periumbilical abdominal pain for an abdominal aortic aneurysm with ultrasound. The CPT code 76775 would be used for the ultrasound and the ICD-10 code would be R10.33 (periumbilical abdominal pain). Medicare publishes local coverage determinations (LCDs) for many frequently used CPT codes. The LCDs contain a list of approved ICD-10 codes. Clinicians must remember that the LCDs apply to patients seen in all clinical settings. The broad list of ICD codes contains only several that are relevant to emergency patients. Screening ultrasound examinations, i.e., in the absence of abnormal signs, symptoms, laboratory tests, or pathologic diagnosis, are not reimbursable by most insurance carriers (a future exception may be for abdominal aortic aneurysms).

Payment Edits

Physician billing is typically an electronic process that associates a CPT code with an ICD code. When an insurance carrier such as Medicare receives the CMS 1500, the standard professional billing form, an automated process takes place that checks for appropriateness of billing as a front end edit. One of the front-end edits is matching an ICD code with an ultrasound CPT code. If an ICD code is used that is not on the published LCD for a CPT code, the bill will likely be rejected on a front-end edit. Many ultrasound CPT codes do not have a published LCD, and private insurance carriers are not required to follow Medicare rules for reimbursement. Communication with your local insurance carrier or MAC is helpful to determine requirements for reimbursement when an LCD or National Coverage Determination (NCD) is not available or being followed.

Multiple Procedure Payment Reduction (MPPR)

Starting January 1, 2012, CMS reduced professional reimbursement for multiple radiology studies performed by the same physician on the same date of service and in the same "family" by 25% [23]. MPPR had already been applied to the TC since

2006. The imaging family relevant to physicians performing point of care ultrasound is Family 1 (Ultrasound) and includes the following CPT codes:

76604 US chest
76700 US Abdomen, complete
76705 US Abdomen, limited
76770 US Retroperitoneal, complete
76775 US Retroperitoneal, limited
76856 US Pelvis transabdominal, nonpregnant, complete
76870 US Scrotum
76857 US Transabdominal nonpregnant male or female pelvis, limited

Ultrasound Procedure Requirements for Billing

1. **Permanently recorded images** are required for all diagnostic and procedural ultrasound bills. CPT does not specify the method of archival or the minimum number of images. The method of archival can be as basic as a thermal print to as advanced as hospital supported picture archiving and communication system (PACS). The number of images required should follow local departmental guidelines.
2. **A final written report** is required by CMS for all radiology studies. Documentation for a procedural ultrasound should be included in the procedure note.
3. **Order** for the procedure from a clinician caring for the patient [24]. Best practice is for EDs to develop an order set for point of care ultrasound. In the absence of an order set, a clear description of the procedure and the reason for performing it within a procedure note should suffice in the event of an audit.
4. **Medical necessity** (see above section on medical necessity)

Billing Optimization

Cooperation between physicians and coders is essential for billing optimization. Physician documentation should be structured to meet the requirements for billing in addition to conveying a meaningful report. Coders benefit from basic education on point of care ultrasound. In turn, coders provide invaluable feedback to ultrasound directors on opportunities for improvement in chart documentation.

Responding to insurance payment denials is integral to any coding department. The decision to appeal should be based on a pattern of rejections from a particular insurance company. If a particular insurance company is consistently denying payment for ultrasounds, it is worth taking the time to write an appeal and request an explanation for the pattern of rejection. Common reasons for nonpayment include the following:

1. **Incidental to primary procedure.** This denial is the insurance company bundling the ultrasound into the evaluation and management code or bundling the ultrasound-guidance code into the primary surgical procedure. If ultrasound is a significant part of a department's business plan, negotiating with an insurance company to reimburse specific limited ultrasound CPT codes in addition to evaluation and management may be helpful. Evidence for the value that point of care ultrasound brings to the patient (expedite care, reduce radiation, improve safety with procedures, improve patient satisfaction, etc.) is detailed elsewhere and critical to this negotiation.

2. **Not covered diagnosis.** This denial may be a first pass edit set up by an insurance company to reject ultrasounds that do not meet their list of diagnosis codes. An example may occur when coding a FAST exam and using a diagnosis code that is not included on the insurance company's list of common diagnosis codes that support medical necessity for a limited abdominal ultrasound. In reviewing Medicare's LCD for 76705 (LCD 31572), traumatic shock (ICD-9968.4) is not listed as an ICD-9 code that supports medical necessity, but fecal impaction (ICD-9560.32) is listed. Clinicians performing a point of care ultrasound have to remember that CPT codes are used for all physicians, so the most common reasons for performing these studies will be slanted towards outpatient radiology testing. Clinicians should continue to use the correct CPT codes with diagnoses that support medical necessity for performing these tests regardless of their practice setting. ACEP's ultrasound section provides substantial. documents to assist in writing appeals when needed.

Quick Guide to Professional Coding for Point of Care Ultrasound

1. Know your site of service to determine global versus professional billing.
2. List the appropriate CPT code for the diagnostic or procedural ultrasound with associated modifiers. Refer to the current CPT publication for current guidelines.
3. List the ICD-10 code that supports medical necessity for the ultrasound performed.
4. Know your updated local insurance carrier rules for reimbursement on commonly billed ultrasounds.

Conclusion

Billing for point of care ultrasound is critical to continued growth of emergency ultrasound. When physician leaders better understand the legal definitions and federal requirements for coding in different settings, they can strategize how to deliver the most effective business case for a departmental or institutional point of care ultrasound program. Strong relationships between physician leadership, the coding departments of the emergency group and the hospital, and the hospital's compliance department optimizes compliant coding and reimbursement.

Pitfalls and Key Recommendations

1. Local guidelines determine which independently licensed practitioners can obtain images to generate the PC bill for interpretation or procedural guidance.
2. Due to the mismatch between physician work and physician reimbursement, the hospital and physician group should collaborate to support physician resources required to meet governing credentialing bodies for clinician performed ultrasound.
3. Obtain legal counsel when considering billing both professional and technical charges for ultrasound in a facility setting.
4. Medical Necessity must accompany each separate ultrasound CPT code. Screening ultrasounds are not billable except for Abdominal Aortic Aneurysm which received a new CPT code 76706 in 2017.
5. All procedural ultrasounds require permanently archived images.
6. The TC cannot be billed without a professional component.
7. Requirements for professional ultrasound billing:

   (a) Permanently recorded images
   (b) Signed written diagnostic report or procedure note
   (c) Documentation of missing elements for complete examinations
   (d) Order
   (e) Medical Necessity

Glossary/Abbreviations Centers for Medicare and Medicaid Services (CMS)—US federal agency which oversees Medicare, Medicaid, and Children's Health Insurance Program

CMS 1500—standard physician billing form

Current Procedural Terminology (CPT)—AMA publication on procedural codes that physicians use to identify services rendered

Diagnosis-related group (DRG)—system used to categorize hospital inpatients based on diagnosis code for reimbursement purposes.

Global codes—Codes that either 1. Cannot by definition be broken down into professional and TC or 2. Due to the practice setting in which the procedure is occurring, include both the professional and the TC.

International Classification of Diseases (ICD)—categorization system listing signs, symptoms, and diseases for billing purposes

Local coverage determinations (LCDs)—CMS description of clinical utility for a common CPT code which applies locally to providers in a particular geographic coverage area

Medicare Administrative Contractors (MAC)—Private companies hired by CMS to administer the responsibilities of Medicare Part A or B.

Medicare Physician Fee Schedule (MPFS)—annual publication by CMS on RVUs and for varying CPT codes

Multiple Procedure Payment Reduction (MPPR)—bundling for radiology procedures in the same family

National coverage determination (NCD)—CMS description of clinical utility for a common CPT code which applies nationally

Professional component—professional work involved in a procedure. With diagnostic ultrasound, the professional work is the interpretation of the images and creation of a report.

Prospective Payment System (PPS)—a method of reimbursement in which Medicare payment is made based on a predetermined, fixed amount. The payment amount for a particular service is based on the DRG.

Relative Value Scale Update Committee (RUC)—multiply-specialty group reviews RVUs for approved CPT codes.

Relative value units (RVUs)—measure of value used to weight physician services

Technical component—technical work involved in performing a procedure. With diagnostic ultrasound, the technical component covers the cost of equipment, technician salaries, image archiving, overhead, etc.

UBO4 Form—medical insurance claim forms used by "facilities" to bill insurance companies for services rendered.

NOTE: Medicare administrative carriers frequently update their local coverage determinations. The AMA publishes the reference book, Current Procedural Terminology, and the Medicare Physician Fee Schedule annually. Please refer to these references for the most up to date rules and reimbursement information.

Exhibit 1
Emergency Ultrasound Coding Guide 2017

Core emergency ultrasound codes

US study	CPT code	CPT description	wRVU 2017
Fast: Scan for hemopericardium and hemoperitoneum; may include lung us for pneumothorax	93308	Echocardiography, transthoracic, real-time with image documentation (2D), with or without M-Mode recording; follow-up or limited	0.53
	76705	Echography, abdominal, B-scan and/or real time with image documentation, limited (eg, single organ, quadrant, follow-up)	0.59
	76604	Ultrasound, chest, B-scan (includes mediastinum) and/or real time with image documentation	0.55
Intrauterine pregnancy			
Pregnant uterus limited (TA)	76815	Ultrasound, pregnant uterus, real time with image documentation, limted (eg fetal heart beat, placental location, fetal position and/or qualitative amniotic fluid volume), one or more fetuses	0.65
Pregnant uterus complete (TA) <14 weeks	76801	Ultrasound, pregnant uterus, real time with image documentation, fetal and maternal evaluation, <14 weeks, single or first gestation; complete	0.99

US study	CPT code	CPT description	wRVU 2017
Pregnant uterus complete (TA) ≥ 14 weeks	76805	Ultrasound, pregnant uterus, real time with image documentation, fetal and maternal evaluation, ≥14 weeks, single, or first gestation; complete	0.99
Pregnant uterus transvaginal (TV)	76817	Ultrasound, pregnant uterus, real time with image documentation, transvaginal	0.75
AAA	76775	Echography, retroperitoneal (eg renal, aorta, nodes); B-scan and/or real time with image documentation; limited	0.58
Screening AAA	76705	Ultrasound, abdominal aorta, real time with image documentation, screening study for abdominal aortic aneurysm	0.59
Cardiac	93308	Echocardiography, transthoracic, real-time with image documentation (2D), with or without M-Mode recording; follow-up or limited;	0.53
Biliary, Bowel	76705	Echography, abdominal, B-scan and/or real time with image documentation, limited (eg, single organ, quadrant, follow-up)	0.59
Thoracic, lung, or upper back	76604	Ultrasound, chest, B-scan (includes mediastinum) and/or real time with image documentation	0.55
Pelvic wall	76857	Ultrasound, pelvic (nonobstetric), B-scan and/or real time with image documentation, limited or follow-up	0.5
Urinary tract/Renal	76775	Echography, retroperitoneal (eg renal, aorta, nodes); B-scan and/or real time with image documentation; limited	0.58
Post-void residual	51798	Measurement of post-voiding residual urine and/or bladder capacity by bladder volume measurement machine	0
Bladder imaging	76857	Imaging of bladder anatomy, including bladder volume measurement using an ultrasound machine	0.5
Focused DVT study	93971	Duplex scan of extremity veins including responses to compression and other maneuvers; unilateral or limited study.	0.45
Soft tissue ultrasound			
Neck	76536	Ultrasound, soft tissues of head and neck (eg, thyroid, parathyroid, parotid), B-scan and/or real time with image documentation	0.56
Musculoskeletal (extremities, non-vascular), including axilla	76882	Ultrasound, extremity, non-vascular, B-scan and/or real time with image documentation, limited	0.49
Chest wall	76604	Ultrasound, chest, B-scan (includes mediastinum) and/or real time with image documentation	0.55
Breast	76642	Ultrasound, breast, B-scan and/or real time with image documentation, limited	0.68

US study	CPT code	CPT description	wRVU 2017
Abdominal wall or lower back	76705	Echography, abdominal, B-scan and/or real time with image documentation, limited (eg, single organ, quadrant, follow-up)	0.59
Pelvic wall	76857	Ultrasound, pelvic (nonobstetric), B-scan and/or real time with image documentation, limited or follow-up	0.5
Infant hip, static	76886	Ultrasound, infant hips, real time with imaging documentation; limited, static (not requiring physician manipulation)	0.62
Ocular	76512	Ophthalmic ultrasound, diagnostic; B-scan (with or without superimposed non-quantitative A-scan)	0.94
Ocular FB	76529	Ophthalmic ultrasonic foreign body localization	0.57
Miscellaneous ultrasound	76999	Unlisted ultrasound procedure (ex, diagnositc, interventional)	0

Advanced emergency ultrasound codes 2017 (recommend advanced training)

US study	CPT code	CPT description	wRVU 2017
Advanced echo	93308	Echocardiography, transthoracic, real-time with image documentation (2D), with or without M-Mode recording; follow-up or limited	0.53
Transesophageal echo	93312	Echocardiography, transesophageal, real time with image documentation (2D) (with or without M-mode recording); including probe placement, image acquisition, interpretation and report	2.55
Adnexal pathology			
Nonpregnant uterus TA complete	76856	Ultrasound, pelvic (nonobstetirc), complete B-scan and/or real time image	1
Nonpregnant uterus TA, limited	76857	Ultrasound, pelvic (nonobstetric), B-scan and/or real time with image documentation, limited or follow-up	0.5
Nonpregnant nonuterus TV	76830	Ultrasound, transvaginal (nonobstetric) and/or real time with image documentation can be used for complete or limited study	0.69
Focused duplex scan of ovaries or testes for torsion	93976	Duplex scan of arterial inflo and venous outflow of abdominal, pelvic, scrotal contents or retroperitoneal organs; limited or unilateral	0.8
US scrotum and contents	76870	Ultrasound internal anatomy of scroum and scrotal contents; to evaluate for hydrocele, azoospermia, oligospermia, orchitis and epididymitis	0.64

Ultrasound guided procedure codes 2017

US-guided procedure	CPT code	Notes	wRVU 2017	Additional CPT code
US-guided pericardiocentesis[1]	76930	Requires image of site to be localized but does not require image of needle in site	0.67	33010

US-guided procedure	CPT code	Notes	wRVU 2017	Additional CPT code
US guided vascular access placement	+76937[3]	Requires written documentation of real-time ultrasound guidance and a representative image but does not require image of needle in site. This is an add- on code and must be used in conjuction with a primary code[*]	0.3	36000, 36555, 36556, 36557, 36558
US-guided thoracentesis[2]	32555	Requires image of site to be localized but does not require image of needle in site	2.27	
US-guided paracentesis[2]	49083	Requires image of site to be localized but does not require image of needle in site	2	
Miscellaneous ultrasound-guided procedure without catheter—non organ specific[1]	76942	Requires image of site to be localized but does not require image of needle in site	0.67	
US-guided abscess drainage[1]	76942	Requires image of site to be localized but does not require image of needle in site	0.67	10160 OR 10061
US-guided peritonsillar abscess drainage[1]	76942	Requires image of site to be localized but does not require image of needle in site	0.67	42700
US-guided lumbar puncture[1]	76942	Requires image of site to be localized but does not require image of needle in site	0.67	62270
US-guided suprapubic aspiration[1]	76942	Requires image of site to be localized but does not require image of needle in site	0.67	51100
US-guided FB removal[1]	76942	Requires image of site to be localized but does not require image of needle in site	0.67	10120 OR 10121
US-guided joint aspriation[2]	20604	Arthrocentesis of small joint	0.89	
	20606	Arthrocentesis of medium joint	1.00	
	20611	Arthrocentesis of large joint	1.10	
Ultrasound guided regional nerve blocks				
Femoral[1]	76942	Requires image of site to be localized but does not require image of needle in site	0.67	64447
Brachial plexus (includes interscalene, supraclavicular, infraclavicular, axillary, and intercostal nerve blocks)[1]	76942	Requires image of site to be localized but does not require image of needle in site	0.67	64415 (brachial plexus); 64417 (axillary), 64418 (suprascapular), 64420/64421 (intercostal)

US-guided procedure	CPT code	Notes	wRVU 2017	Additional CPT code
Ulnar[1]	76942	Requires image of site to be localized but does not require image of needle in site	0.67	64450
Radial[1]	76942	Requires image of site to be localized but does not require image of needle in site	0.67	64450
Sciatic[1]	76942	Requires image of site to be localized but does not require image of needle in site	0.67	64445
Saphenous[1]	76942	Requires image of site to be localized but does not require image of needle in site	0.67	64450

[1]These codes are imaging codes only. They do not include the charge for the surgical procedure

[2]These codes include both the imaging code, as well as the surgical code

[3]CMS designated add-on codes are procedures that are performed in conjunction with another primary procedure/service. These are designated by the "+" symbol in front

Ultrasound guided procedure (leaving a catheter in place) codes 2017

US-guided procedure	CPT code	Notes	wRVU 2017
US-guided thoracentesis	32557	Thoracentesis and catheter placement. Requires image of site to be localized but does not require image of the needle in site	3.12
Image guided fluid collection drainage by catheter, soft tissue	10030	(eg, abscess, hematoma, seroma, lymphocele, cyst), soft tissue (eg, extremity, abdominal wall, neck), percutaneous, includes moderate sedation when used. Must leave catheter in place for drainage. Requires image of site to be localized but does not require image of needle in site	2.75
Image guided fluid collection drainage by catheter, visceral percutaneous	49405	(eg, abscess, hematoma, seroma, lymphocele, cyst), visceral (eg, bladder), percutaneous, includes moderate sedation when used. Must leave catheter in place for drainage. Requires image of site to be localized but does not require image of needle in site	4.00
Image guided fluid collection drainage by catheter, peritoneal/ retroperitoneal percutaneous approach	49406	(eg, abscess, hematoma, seroma, lymphocele, cyst), peritoneal/retroperitoneal percutaneous, includes moderate sedation when used. Must leave catheter in place for drainage. Requires image of site to be localized but does not require image of needle in site	4.00
Image guided fluid collection drainage by catheter, peritoneal/ retroperitoneal transvaginal/ transrectal approach	49407	(eg, abscess, hematoma, seroma, lymphocele, cyst), peritoneal/retroperitoneal transvaginal/ transrectal includes moderate sedation when used. Must leave catheter in place for drainage	4.25

Separately billable CPT codes for ultrasound guided procedures (in numerical order)

CPT code	Description	wRVU 2017
10120	Incision and removal foreign body simple	1.22
10121	Incision and removal foreign body complicated	2.74
10160	Incision and drainage of abscess simple	1.25
10061	Incision and drainage of abscess complicated	2.45
33010	Pericardiocentesis, initial	1.99
36000	Place needle in vein	0.18
36555	Insertion of non-tunneled central venous catheter age <5 YO	2.43
36556	Insertion of a non-tunneled central venous catheter agE >5 YO	2.50
36568	Insertion of a non-tunneled picc age <5 YO	1.67
36569	Insertion of a non-tunneled picc age >5 YO	1.82
42700	Drainage of tonsil or peritonsillar abscess	1.67
51100	Aspiration of bladder by needle	0.78
62270	Diagnostic lumbar puncture	1.37

Disclaimer: wRVU are for 2017 only and may change in future years

References

1. Blaivas M, Adhikari S, Lander L. A prospective comparison of procedural sedation and ultrasound-guided interscalene nerve block for shoulder reduction in the emergency department. Acad Emerg Med. 2011;18(9):922–7. https://doi.org/10.1111/j.1553-2712.2011.01140.x.
2. Blaivas M, Harwood RA, Lambert MJ. Decreasing length of stay with emergency ultrasound examination of the gallbladder. Acad Emerg Med. 1999;6(10):1020–3.
3. Blaivas M, Sierzenski P, Plecque D, Lambert M. Do emergency physicians save time when locating a live intrauterine pregnancy with bedside ultrasonography? Acad Emerg Med. 2000;7(9):988–93.
4. Brass P, Hellmich M, Kolodziej L, Schick G, Smith AF. Ultrasound guidance versus anatomical landmarks for internal jugular vein catheterization. Cochrane Database Syst Rev. 2015;1:CD006962. https://doi.org/10.1002/14651858.CD006962.pub2.
5. Chiem AT, Chan CH, Ibrahim DY, et al. Pelvic ultrasonography and length of stay in the ED: an observational study. Am J Emerg Med. 2014;32(12):1464–9. https://doi.org/10.1016/j.ajem.2014.09.006.
6. Elikashvili I, Tay ET, Tsung JW. The effect of point-of-care ultrasonography on emergency department length of stay and computed tomography utilization in children with suspected appendicitis. Acad Emerg Med. 2014;21(2):163–70. https://doi.org/10.1111/acem.12319.
7. Melniker LA, Leibner E, McKenney MG, Lopez P, Briggs WM, Mancuso CA. Randomized controlled clinical trial of point-of-care, limited ultrasonography for trauma in the emergency department: the first sonography outcomes assessment program trial. Ann Emerg Med. 2006;48(3):227–35. https://doi.org/10.1016/j.annemergmed.2006.01.008.
8. Panebianco NL, Shofer F, Fields JM, et al. The utility of transvaginal ultrasound in the ED evaluation of complications of first trimester pregnancy. Am J Emerg Med. 2015;33(6):743–8. https://doi.org/10.1016/j.ajem.2015.02.023.
9. Smith-Bindman R. Ultrasonography vs. CT for suspected nephrolithiasis. N Engl J Med. 2014;371(26):2531. https://doi.org/10.1056/NEJMc1412853.
10. Howard ZD, Noble VE, Marill KA, et al. Bedside ultrasound maximizes patient satisfaction. J Emerg Med. 2014;46(1):46–53. https://doi.org/10.1016/j.jemermed.2013.05.044.

11. American Medical Association. Current procedural terminology 2017 Professional. American Medical Association; 2016.
12. Physician Fee Schedule January 2017. Accessed online May 17, 2017. http://www.cms.gov/apps/physician-fee-schedule.
13. FAQ: Surgery: Cardiovascular System. CPT Assistant. 2014;24(9).
14. Ultrasound Guidelines: Emergency, Point-of-Care and Clinical Ultrasound Guidelines in Medicine. Ann Emerg Med. 2017;69(5):e27–e54. https://doi.org/10.1016/j.annemergmed.2016.08.457.
15. Department of Health and Human Services Chapter IV: Centers for Medicare and Medicaid Services, Department of Health and Human Services. Subchapter B – Medicare Program Part 415 – Services Furnished by Physicians in Providers, Supervising Physicians in Teaching Settings, and Residents in Certain Settings Subpart C – Part B Carrier Payments for Physician Services to Beneficiaries in Providers Section 410.42 Limitations on coverage of certain services furnished to hospital outpatients. Section 415.102 – Conditions for fee schedule payment for physician services to beneficiaries in providers. Section 415.120 – Conditions for payment: Radiology Services. Accessed online May 31, 2015. http://www.ecfr.gov.
16. FAQ: Surgery: Cardiovascular System. CPT Assistant September. 2014;24(9).
17. American College of Emergency Physicians. Emergency ultrasound imaging criteria compendium. American College of Emergency Physicians. Ann Emerg Med. 2006;48(4):487–510. https://doi.org/10.1016/j.annemergmed.2006.07.946.
18. Bahner D, Blaivas M, Cohen HL, et al. AIUM practice guideline for the performance of the focused assessment with sonography for trauma (FAST) examination. J Ultrasound Med. 2008;27(2):313–8.
19. CPT Assistant. Reporting ultrasounds. CPT Assistant 2009;19(5).
20. Ryan T, Armstrong WF, Khandheria BK, American Society of Echocardiography. Task force 4: training in echocardiography endorsed by the American Society of Echocardiography. J Am Coll Cardiol. 2008;51(3):361–7. https://doi.org/10.1016/j.jacc.2007.11.012.
21. Ryan T, Berlacher K, Lindner JR, Mankad SV, Rose GA, Wang A. COCATS 4 Task Force 5: Training in Echocardiography: Endorsed by the American Society of Echocardiography. J Am Soc Echocardiogr. 2015;28(6):615–27. https://doi.org/10.1016/j.echo.2015.04.014.
22. Administration SS. Compilation of the social security laws. Secondary compilation of the social security laws. http://www.ssa.gov/OP_Home/ssact/title18/1862.htm.
23. Department of Health and Human Services. CMS Manual System Pub 100-20. One-time notification transmittal 1040, February 3, 2012.
24. Medicare payments for diagnostic radiolgoy services in emergency departments. Office of the Inspector General. Department of Health and Human Services, April 2011.

Chapter 23
Global Medicine Perspectives

Sachita P. Shah

Objectives

- Describe ultrasound program management issues encountered in limited resource settings including low and middle-income countries (LMICs), and rural, austere settings
- Desired features of ideal equipment and maintenance plans
- Step by Step strategies for program implementation including needs assessment, education program options, interdisciplinary approach, and sustainability
- Funding, billing and infrastructure in LMICs
- Unique safety and supply chain considerations including gel, sanitation, and storage

Introduction

As the field of clinical ultrasonography continues to grow, there has been a rapid expansion in new applications of point of care ultrasound (POC US) in global and rural health. Diseases cited as the leading causes of death in low and middle-income countries (LMICs) each have ultrasound-diagnosable features (Fig. 23.1) and the growth of POC US use globally has garnered interest of major stakeholders in global health such as the World Health Organization (WHO) [1], high impact nonprofit organizations (e.g., Partners In Health [2], Medecins Sans Frontieres [3], International Medical Corps [4]), and ministries of health (e.g., Rwanda Medical Council Continuing Professional Development course [5]). While some

S.P. Shah, MD, FACEP
Department of Emergency Medicine, University of Washington,
Harborview Medical Center, Seattle, WA, USA
e-mail: sachita.shah@gmail.com

© Springer International Publishing AG 2018
V. S. Tayal et al. (eds.), *Ultrasound Program Management*,
https://doi.org/10.1007/978-3-319-63143-1_23

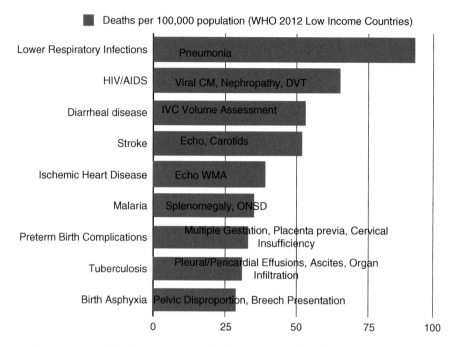

■ Deaths per 100,000 population (WHO 2012 Low Income Countries)

Lower Respiratory Infections — Pneumonia

HIV/AIDS — Viral CM, Nephropathy, DVT

Diarrheal disease — IVC Volume Assessment

Stroke — Echo, Carotids

Ischemic Heart Disease — Echo WMA

Malaria — Splenomegaly, ONSD

Preterm Birth Complications — Multiple Gestation, Placenta previa, Cervical Insufficiency

Tuberculosis — Pleural/Pericardial Effusions, Ascites, Organ Infiltration

Birth Asphyxia — Pelvic Disproportion, Breech Presentation

0   25   50   75   100

Fig. 23.1 Ultrasound for Identification of Top Causes of Mortality. Source http://www.who.int/mediacentre/factsheets/fs310/en/index1.html

ultrasound program management principles are applicable globally, a thoughtful and unique approach to expansion of POC US to LMIC's and even within rural, underserved areas of the United States should be used. New programs for ultrasound training are increasing in frequency, and a recent website www.globalsono. org, sponsored by an ACEP (American College of Emergency Physicians) section grant, is attempting to connect and register all POC US programs in LMICs (Fig. 23.2. GlobalSono.org Map of registered programs for POC US education in LMICs).

POC US, or use of sonography by the treating clinician, appears to be the main method of rapid expansion for ultrasound use worldwide. This is multifactorial, including the worldwide shortage of radiologists and sonographers [6, 7], general barriers to patient transport for imaging studies from rural areas to higher level of care in LMICs with poor infrastructure, and lack of access to advanced imaging such as computed tomography (CT). For example, in the West African country of Liberia, population 4.3 million with only 50–150 practicing physicians in the country only a handful of whom are specialists of any kind, there is frequently not a single functioning computed tomography (CT) or Magnetic Resonance Imaging (MRI), making ultrasound the most detailed level of diagnostic imaging available for millions. The WHO has suggested that ultrasound is the ideal imaging modality for limited resource settings due to its versatility for diagnostic use, and increasing portability, affordability, and durability. In 1998 the WHO published consensus-based, ultrasound

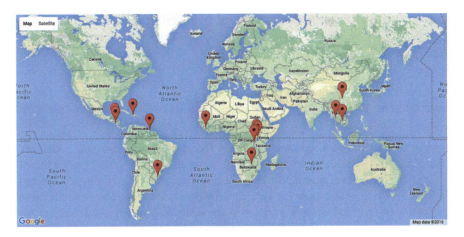

Fig. 23.2 Marker = Collaborating site for POC US education and training in resource-limited setting. From http://www.globalsono.org/AllSites.aspx

training guidelines to assist LMICs in ultrasound program development [8], however the literature suggests that the major barrier to adoption of ultrasound worldwide is lack of training in its use [9].

Despite the challenges of ultrasound program development in LMICs, successful implementation of sustainable ultrasound services has been undertaken by several organizations. Their models have helped to guide many other programs to begin needs assessments and fledgling training programs worldwide and the leadership of each of these listed organizations are receptive to collaboration.

- PURE: Point-of-care Ultrasound in Resource Limited Environments (www. pureultrasound.org). This nonprofit organization is dedicated to enhancing ultrasound education and use in the developing world, with current focus in Africa. PURE has created sustainable ultrasound programs at the district hospital level in Rwanda and has developed a Training of Trainers Course to promote long-term partnership.
- Partners In Health: (www.pih.org) This nonprofit has ultrasound programs in nearly all of its locations including Mexico, Haiti, Rwanda, Lesotho, Malawi, Liberia, and Sierra Leone including over 40 machines in use and hundreds of clinicians trained in ultrasound [10].
- Global Emergency Care Collaborative: (www.globalemergencycare.org) This unique nonprofit focuses on development of Emergency care training programs for nurses practicing in East Africa. It has a novel published ultrasound curriculum for nonphysician clinicians [11].
- WINFOCUS: This multinational organization leads training and educational programs in many middle-income countries worldwide including Brazil, India, and within Eastern Europe, with the mission of enhancing education in POC US for treatment of "critical" patients, from the out-of-hospital realm to emergency departments to intensive care units [12].

Ultrasound Management in Global Medicine: Key Concepts

Equipment

Procurement of ultrasound equipment that will function well and last for years in limited resource settings can be a challenge. When seeking ultrasound machines for use in a district hospital or health center, consider these features:

- *Portability*: Hand-carried machines have the advantage of extreme portability making them invaluable for use on home visits and also between hospital buildings. Perhaps more importantly, hand-carried machines can be easily transported back to the manufacturer for service. However, extremely portable machines have a risk of theft or loss if not properly secured, therefore a mechanism for signing out the machine from a secure location within the hospital is recommended.
- *Durability*: How much heat can the machine withstand? How much moisture? How much dust? What if the machine or probes get dropped or jostled? What is the battery life? We suggest purchase of a service contract for ongoing machine maintenance as well as loaner machine options. Consider asking the manufacturer to provide in-service training to the regional site biomedical engineer in commonly encountered equipment problems and their solutions.
- *Electrical concerns:* Long battery life and short boot-up time are ideal. Consider adding extra batteries and power cords at the time of original purchase, as some power cords are sensitive to the frequent power surges and non-grounded electrical outlets found in many developing countries.
- *Options for remote QA*: Even with adequate training, clinician sonographers in any program sometimes require image interpretation assistance, and should be encouraged to maintain quality assurance image review procedures. Ease of image upload via PACS or flash disc should be considered with ultrasound machine procurement.
- *Probes*: Studies demonstrate that obstetric and abdominal ultrasound exams are the most frequent application in many LMICs, and thus a low frequency curved abdominal probe is a must [13, 14]. In addition, the WHO and United Nations have recently recognized noncommunicable diseases (NCDs) such as hypertension and diabetes mellitus as a major challenge for sustainable development, therefore a phased array probe is suggested for diagnosis of NCD complications including heart and renal failure [15]. If there is ability to secure multiple probes, a linear, high frequency probe can be quite useful for procedural guidance and deep venous thrombosis assessment in areas with high prevalence of tuberculosis (e.g., Tuberculous pericardial and pleural effusions and ascites requiring drainage) and HIV (which increases the risk of deep venous thrombosis).

Many of the major ultrasound manufacturers produce ultra-mobile equipment for use in LMIC settings (See Chap. 12 – Ultrasound Equipment and Purchase).

Table 23.1 Example options for sonography equipment geared for LMIC use

Company	Product
Sonosite Inc. (Fujifilm)	Soundcaring program (refurbished): Nanomaxx and M turbo
	New release 2016: iViz (handheld tablet)
Phillips	VISIQ, Lumify (tablet-based with lease option)
Terason	t3200, t3300 (PC laptop based machines)
Mindray	M5, M7, M9
Siemans	Acuson P300, freestyle (wireless probes)
GE	Vscan (portable, handheld)

While not exhaustive, the table below provides an example of the different types of options currently in use internationally or newly available (Table 23.1).

Financial constraints often preclude purchase of new ultrasound equipment for use in LMICs. However, refurbished or slightly older equipment is often of high enough quality to be useful and is more affordable. If procuring a machine to leave or donate in an LMIC, many of the major manufacturers have charitable arms (e.g., Soundcaring program, Sonosite Inc.) [16] which may accept applications for low cost or free machines. Another option is to ask for donation of refurbished machines from your local hospitals. Most major companies will loan extra equipment for training purposes for periods of up to a few months with enough lead time, and this can often be arranged by your local representative. Careful reading of loan agreements is recommended, and consideration of additional insurance for loaned equipment by your hospital's underwriter is sometimes necessary. When traveling with loaned equipment, a letter stating the value of the equipment and that it is for use on loan should be hand-carried from the international host hospital in case of customs interrogation.

Maintenance

Implementation of ultrasound programs should include plans for maintenance before equipment fails. In LMICs, if local biomedical engineering is available, consider requesting the equipment manufacturer to host a training for the engineer to learn more about their machine, or providing a service contract for repair with the equipment. Consider paper and electronic copies of the user manuals on site, as well as extra cords/batteries on hand.

Despite thoughtful consideration in the procurement of ultrasound equipment, there are known points of weakness even in the most durable machines. Hand-carried machines stored in bags with probe cords curled will suffer fraying of cords at the junction of cord and probe as well as cord and connector plate over time. Consider establishing a safe area to hang probes while they are not in use to avoid this problem. Another common issue arises from the sensitivity of the equipment to voltage surges which can burn the power boxes and cords, which is completely avoidable by use of voltage stabilizers and grounding of outlets used to charge equipment.

Program Implementation

Ultrasound services will only flourish if they address the immediate patient care needs of the clinicians and impact patient care substantially to offset time and human resources needed for training/implementation. To create this scenario, the program must include attention to the question of what happens when a surgical or medical emergency is diagnosed with ultrasound. Ultrasound programs are often most impactful when plans for rapid transfer to higher level of care, or to operative or transfusion services are arranged simultaneously or otherwise established. Therefore, we recommend beginning with a needs-assessment to discern which ultrasound applications will be most useful for each specific setting (Table 23.2: Needs Assessment sample questions) [17]. Once a needs-assessment has been performed, development and delivery of a tailored curriculum can begin.

Education Strategies

Even the best ultrasound equipment will collect dust in storage or be quickly rendered medical waste by misuse without proper training. Ultrasound technology implementation without training is, to borrow a Haitian proverb, like washing your hands and drying them in the dirt. To manage a successful ultrasound program in an under-resourced setting, we suggest the following key considerations:

Table 23.2 Needs Assessment sample questions

Ultrasound Machine Available? Type? Probes?	Establish plan for Maintenance, Service, Bring loaner/update probes
Current use of ultrasound? Indications? Background training of users? Logging scans?	Create log system, expand indications of current use, use established experts to help train (if any)
Hospital characteristics: OR? L&D?Xray? Electricity? Internet?	Establish communication for sending images for review if needed, establish protocols for how to transfer patients based on ultrasound findings to OR if needed
Top 10 causes of death in this region, top causes of in-hospital mortality	Use this to build your curriculum for life-saving POC US exams first
Hospital politics? Will trainers need a medical license?	Consider training administrators/MD's first, obtain local licenses, permission from ministries of health
Yes or no questionnaire for diseases present: Heart failure, renal failure, sepsis, pneumonia, ascites/effusions, TB, HIV, trauma, unexplained Dyspnea	Use this to create your curriculum tailored to what clinicians will encounter on their wards
Contact list: Obtain names/emails for medical director, clinical director, head of nursing, radiographers, prior US trained clinicians	Begin contact well before introducing ultrasound and training to establish rapport and enthusiasm

Henwood P, Mackenzie D, Rempell J, Murray A, Leo M, Dean AJ, Liteplo A, Noble V. A Practical Guide to Self-Sustaining Point-of-Care Ultrasound Education Programs in Resource-Limited Settings. Annals of Emerg Med 2014 Sept;64 (3):277–85 [17]

- *Train an ultrasound champion*: Choose an enthusiastic clinician with leadership skills to be your local ultrasound coordinator in charge of arranging trainings, keeping equipment safe and functioning, and establishing a quality assurance program.
- *Sustainability*: Training programs should include both initial trainings, refresher courses within 6 months, ongoing email contact for case discussion and quality assurance, and eventual training of local trainers through mentorship and separate coursework. Establish ability for image upload and distance learning options, such as webinars or image based case reviews at timely intervals, as early as possible after initial training.
- Consider an *interdisciplinary approach* to use the clinical skills of physicians from varied specialties and other health professionals who will be able to offer different training perspectives and assist with integration of the newfound ultrasound knowledge into clinical care.
- *Train administrators and publicize*: Train not only the clinicians who interface directly with patients whether they are physicians, nurses, or clinical officers, but also physician/nurse administrators so they understand the scope and importance of POC US and will advocate for continuation of the services once they are established. Consider widely publicizing the training and presence of ultrasound services once established, to draw patients to services and alert referral hospitals of the new diagnostic option.
- *Sample Curricula*: Sample curricula exist and learning resources for training courses do not need to be reinvented. While published data suggest training length varies substantially, consider building a curriculum to address the main causes of mortality (Table 23.3: PIH Ultrasound Curriculum).

Table 23.3 PIH ultrasound curriculum

Ultrasound exam topic	Focus
Safety, physics	ALARA principle, cleaning/sanitation, common artifacts, machine knobs and modes of scanning, quality assurance process
Cardiac/volume assessment	Pericardial effusion, chamber size, heart failure, endocarditis, rheumatic valvular disease, inferior vena cava collapsibility and IVC: Aorta ratio
Trauma	Hemothorax, hemopericardium, Hemoperitoneum (eFAST exam), pneumothorax (PTX)
Thoracic	Pleural effusion, PTX, pneumonia
Abdominal	Liver cirrhosis/cysts/abscess, ascites, hydronephrosis, chronic renal failure, gallstones, cholecystitis
Obstetrics	Ectopic and intrauterine pregnancy, molar pregnancy, estimation of gestational age, multiple gestation, placenta previa, amniotic fluid index, abnormal fetal presentation, fetal heart rate
Procedural guidance	Thoracentesis, paracentesis, pericardiocentesis
Soft tissue/bone	Cellulitis, abscess, pyomyositis, fracture
Deep venous thrombosis	2 point exam for DVT in femoral or popliteal vein

Advanced topics: Testicular torsion/masses, thyroid, biopsy guidance, regional Anesthesia
Adapted from Partners In Health Ultrasound Curriculum (copyright 2011), http://www.pih.org/library/manual-of-ultrasound-for-resource-limited-settings

Politics: Funding, Billing, Infrastructure

Despite good will and intentions, it can be a struggle to find funding for development of ultrasound services in LMIC countries. Potential donated equipment should be thoroughly inspected before acceptance to ensure it is within the required specifications with respect to durability and functionality, and should always be deployed with a training plan in place which will likely require its own funding. Research in POC US use for specific indications in LMICs is an area rich for exploration [18]. Funded research studies can help to build local capacity both by engaging local providers in academic pursuits and by financing general ultrasound training and equipment. The knowledge gained by local practitioners along with the ultrasound equipment remains long after the study period.

While still uncommon, some developing countries (e.g., Rwanda, Uganda) have established POC US billing which when paired with national insurance, can establish a steady revenue stream for the hospital to ensure continuation of services.

Sanitation, Storage, and Safety

Providing sanitary medical care and ultrasound services can be a challenge in areas of the world where medical waste is burned or dumped near water supplies, and chemical agents such as Cidex and sterilization options are limited. For sanitation of probes, alcohol should be avoided, however diluted bleach solutions can be used for sanitation of most probes. Intracavitary probes consistently used with probe covers and bleach water and sterilized between uses should ideally not transmit disease. Nevertheless, local customs for sanitation of sensitive equipment should be followed [19, 20]. To encourage safe and responsible use of ultrasound, training should begin with the ALARA (as low as reasonably achievable) principle. Trainers should also be familiar with local ultrasound laws and regulations, including cultural and social issues, before embarking on ultrasound training missions. For example, teaching gender identification is illegal and punishable in areas of the world known for sex-selective abortion and female infanticide (e.g., China and India) [21, 22]. Archiving options are uncommon in LMICs, limited currently to PACS wireless upload and cumbersome mechanical downloading, however secure, cloud-based options are on the horizon. For example, Sonosite Inc. has partnered with Trice Imaging for Sonosite's newly released iViz, which has embedded software to allow rapid, secure, cloud-based image transfer from remote locations using WiFi or cellular service.

Discussion

The field of POC US in resource-limited settings is ever-changing, and clinicians from many disciplines of medicine are finding leadership in this field to be both rewarding and challenging. While the equipment is rapidly evolving to meeting the technological needs of worldwide users, best practices with regard to training and program management are quickly being established. Leaders in POC US with interest in developing ultrasound services in LMICs can successfully overcome commonly encountered challenges with advanced planning discussed in this chapter and further details from other sections in this book. While unanticipated obstacles often crop up when working in LMIC's, creative solutions are generated in discussion with the small but growing community of clinicians with expertise in this field.

Pitfalls

Unfortunately, many potential pitfalls exist when implementing any program in a LMIC in addition to the ultrasound-specific challenges. Potential pitfalls and techniques for avoiding them include:

- Administrators do not understand scope or importance of POC US and can feel ashamed that less experienced clinicians have skills they do not: Train the administrators first, publicize the training, and suggest billing for services once established.
- Ultrasound training is completed, but then adoption is slow: Train high impact exam types first (e.g., saving lives through rapid diagnosis of life-threatening diseases such as ruptured ectopic and traumatic hemoperitoneum), integrate time scanning on the clinical wards to discuss ways that ultrasound could be used to explore almost every chief complaint and emphasize how the findings change patient management.
- Ultrasound services begin, but then referrals don't increase and practice continues in a silo: Consider public outreach to make referral centers and tertiary care centers aware of the training and new ultrasound programs.
- Staff turnover leaves no one trained after implementation of the ultrasound program: Timely refresher courses can ensure knowledge transfer even with staff turnover. Establishing a cadre of local trainers who can easily return to the site for future training sessions will reduce need for foreign trainers.

Key Recommendations

- Ultrasound should be introduced as part of an overall health systems strengthening package, including training and human resources for improvement of clinical care.
- Highest impact of ultrasound is attained when POC US is paired with improvement of surgical services and ability for emergency transport of critical patients.
- Introducing ultrasound services means more than just choosing an ideal machine; it involves ongoing partnership for training and education and a curriculum tailored to meet the needs of the resource-limited setting.

References

1. http://www.who.int/diagnostic_imaging/imaging_modalities/dim_ultrasound/en/.
2. http://www.pih.org/blog/a-new-resource-for-using-ultrasound-in-developing-countries.
3. http://www.doctorswithoutborders.org/news-stories/field-blog-doctor-what-about-my-brother.
4. http://internationalmedicalcorps.org/page.aspx?pid=1906.
5. http://www.rmdc.rw/spip.php?article159.
6. Kawooya M. Training for rural radiology and imaging in sub-Saharan Africa: a mismatch between services and population. J Clin Imaging Sci. 2012;2:37.
7. http://www.diagnosticimaging.com/articles/radiologist-sightings-drop-around-world.
8. Training in diagnostic ultrasound: essentials, principles and standards. Report of a WHO Study Group. World Health Organ Tech Rep Ser. 1998;875:i-46.
9. LaGrone LN, Sadasivam V, Kushner AL, Groen RS. A review of training opportunities for ultrasonography in low and middle income countries. Tropical Med Int Health. 2012;17(7):808–19.
10. Shah S, Epino H, Bukhman G, Dushimiyimana JMV, Umulisa I, Reichman A, Noble V. Impact of the introduction of ultrasound services in a limited resource setting: rural Rwanda 2008. BMC Int Health Hum Rights. 2009;9:4.
11. Stolz L, Muruganandan KM, Bisanzo M, Dreifuss B, Hammerstedt H, Nelson S, Nayabale I, Shah S. Point-of-care ultrasound education for non-physician clinicians in a resource-limited emergency department. Trop Med Int Health. 2015;20(8):1067–72.
12. www.winfocus.org.
13. Steinmetz JP, Berger JP. Ultrasonography as an aid to diagnosis and treatment in a rural African hospital: a prospective study of 1,119 cases. Am J Trop Med Hyg. 1999;60(1):119–23.
14. Sippel S, Muruganandan K, Levine A, Shah S. Review article: use of ultrasound in the developing world. Int J Emerg Med. 2011;4:72.
15. http://www.who.int/global-coordination-mechanism/ncd-themes/sustainable-development-goals/en/.
16. http://www.sonosite.com/about/global-health/soundcaring.
17. Henwood P, Mackenzie D, Rempell J, Murray A, Leo M, Dean AJ, Liteplo A, Noble V. A practical guide to self-sustaining point-of-care ultrasound education programs in resource-limited settings. Ann Emerg Med. 2014;64(3):277–85.
18. Moresky R, Bisanzo M, Rubenstein B, Hubbard S, Cohen H, Ouyang H, Marsh RH. A research agenda for acute care services delivery in low- and middle-income countries. Acad Emerg Med. 2013;20(12):1264–71.
19. Talan D, Partida CN. Emergency department ultrasound infection control: do unto (and into) others. Ann Emerg Med. 2011;58(1):64–6.
20. Frazee BW, Fahimi J, Lambert L, Nagdev A. Emergency department ultrasonographic probe contamination and experimental model of probe disinfection. Ann Emerg Med. 2011;58(1):56–63.
21. Oomman N, Ganatra BR. Sex selection: the systematic elimination of girls. Reprod Health Matters. 2002;10(19):184–8.
22. Complilation and Analysis of Case-Laws on Pre-conception and Pre-natal Diagnostics Techniques (Prohibition of Sex Selection) Act, 1994. www.countryoffice.unfpa.org/india/drive/Compilation_and_Analysis_of_Case_Laws_on_Pre_Conception.pdf.

Chapter 24
Pediatric-Specific Point of Care US Management

Jennifer R. Marin

Objectives

- Discuss reasons why ultrasound is favorable in pediatric patients
- Highlight specific point-of-care ultrasound exams in pediatric patients and the limitations of each
- Describe strategies to reduce anxiety and pain associated with particular point-of-care ultrasound examinations
- Describe how to demonstrate need and obtain funding for ultrasound equipment in the pediatric setting

Introduction

Point-of-care ultrasound in pediatric patients has several unique and important considerations, beyond the typical advantages of ultrasound (rapid, bedside, non-invasive, less costly), making it a favorable imaging modality. First, children have higher water content and smaller body habitus relative to adult patients resulting in high quality images. Second, ultrasound can be performed without the child being completely still, and thus requires less cooperation than with other imaging modalities. Third, when considering diagnostic imaging in pediatric patients, ultrasound, compared with computed tomography (CT), is often the preferred modality, given the lack of radiation and in keeping with the As Low As Reasonably Achievable (ALARA) principle. Radiation exposure from medical imaging is particularly

J.R. Marin, MD, MSc
Departments of Pediatrics and Emergency Medicine,
Children's Hospital of Pittsburgh of UPMC, Pittsburgh, PA, USA
e-mail: jennifer.marin@chp.edu

© Springer International Publishing AG 2018
V. S. Tayal et al. (eds.), *Ultrasound Program Management*,
https://doi.org/10.1007/978-3-319-63143-1_24

relevant in pediatric patients, as they are more sensitive to radiation compared to adults [1]. Recent epidemiological studies support the increased relative risk of future malignancies from childhood exposures to CT [2].

Pediatric-Specific US Examinations and Considerations

Many of the point-of-care ultrasound examinations performed in adult patients can be translated to use in pediatric patients. For example, torso trauma, pregnancy, cardiac instability, and appendicitis are also seen in pediatric patients. Therefore, many core emergency ultrasound applications should be learned for use for the pediatric population [3]. However, there are several exams that are particularly relevant and in some cases, unique, to children and worthy of discussion (Table 24.1).

Most pediatric emergency visits are to general EDs [4] that may not have around-the-clock radiology ultrasound. Further, if ultrasound examinations are available, ultrasound technicians may not be skilled in pediatric-specific exams. For some examinations, point-of-care ultrasound may obviate the need for other imaging modalities, such as computed tomography and radiography. These point-of-care ultrasound examinations may also be important to guide further evaluation and management strategies as well as decrease emergency department lengths of stay. Therefore, it behooves the emergency physician to become adept at performing these exams. It should be noted that the overall incidence of disease and pathology in children presenting to the emergency department is much less than that of adults, therefore, physicians should be conscientious about getting enough experience with "positive" studies in order to be competent in a particular application.

Table 24.1 Key point-of-care ultrasound exams in pediatric patients

Exam[a]	Indications
Bladder volume	Pre-urethral catheterization
Soft tissue	Distinguishing abscess from cellulitis; evaluating for foreign body
Hip effusion	Limp, leg pain, refusal to bear weight
Elbow fracture	Fall on outstretched arm
Skull fracture	Closed head trauma
Ultrasound-guided venous access	Need for vascular access
Pneumonia/parapneumonic effusion	Symptoms concerning for pneumonia; lower lobe consolidation
Intussusception	Colicky abdominal pain; bilious emesis, hematochezia
Pyloric stenosis	Non-bilious emesis in a 1-month old
Appendicitis	Right-sided abdominal pain, fever, vomiting

Exams ordered by increasing difficulty
[a]A linear array transducer is appropriate for all exams listed

Pediatric Abdominal Complaints

Abdominal pain is one of the most common complaints of children presenting to the emergency department, with appendicitis being the most common surgical diagnosis. Although appendicitis is not exclusive to pediatric patients, the clinical diagnosis in children can be particularly challenging, given the difficulty of examining pre-verbal children, as well as the overlap of symptoms with other, more benign etiologies. Studies of point-of-care ultrasound for the evaluation of pediatric appendicitis have demonstrated high specificity, thereby making the point-of-care ultrasound a "rule-in" exam [5, 6]. Point-of-care ultrasound diagnoses of pyloric stenosis and intussusception have also been studied with findings suggesting the exams can be learned easily and diagnoses made accurately [7, 8].

Pre-urethral (Bladder Size) Catheterization

The standard of care for obtaining sterile urine from children unable to provide a clean catch specimen is urethral catheterization. Initial catheterization attempts may result in a 28% failure rate due to lack of urine in the bladder at the time of catheterization [9]. Chen, et al. demonstrated an increase in the rate of successful catheterizations with the use of point-of-care ultrasound prior to catheterization [9].

Given the frequency of urethral catheterization in pediatric patients, bedside nurse-use of point-of-care bladder ultrasound may also be an opportunity to improve care and patient flow and deserves further study.

Head Trauma

In children with head trauma, the presence of a skull fracture is associated with significantly increased odds of intracranial injury [10]. Two studies have demonstrated high specificity of point-of-care ultrasound for the evaluation of skull fractures in head-injured children [11, 12].

Musculoskeletal Complaints

Musculoskeletal complaints are common reasons for pediatric emergency care. Atraumatic leg pain or limp in the pediatric patient can be a manifestation of several disease processes. Although not specific to the type of effusion, point-of-care ultrasound of the hip can be used to determine if a hip effusion is present and potentially narrow the differential diagnosis [13]. A common mechanism of injury for children is a "fall on an outstretched hand" (FOOSH), with the pediatric elbow being particularly vulnerable to this mechanism. In the setting of most elbow fractures, hemarthrosis will lead to displacement of the posterior fat pad. Point-of-care ultrasound has been shown to be a sensitive screening tool for the evaluation of an elevated fat pad in pediatric patients with upper extremity trauma [14]. In addition, point-of-care ultrasound may be particularly useful to evaluate for forearm fractures in children with arm pain, but no obvious deformity [15, 16], as well as for assessment of fracture realignment during fracture reduction [17].

FAST

The Focused Assessment with Sonography in Trauma (FAST) is widely accepted as standard of care in the evaluation of the adult trauma patient. Numerous studies highlight the accuracy as well as utility of the FAST exam in rapidly identifying hemoperitoneum. The evidence in pediatric patients is not as robust. While the specificity is quite high (98%), the sensitivity (20%) and negative predictive value (78%) are not sufficient for the FAST to be used as a screening tool in children [18]. The inconsistency in the performance of and utility of the FAST exam in children is due to several factors. First, up to 37% of pediatric abdominal injuries lack hemoperitoneum as evaluated by CT [19]. Therefore, a lack of free fluid does not exclude intraabdominal injury. In addition, the presence of free fluid during the FAST exam may not obviate the need for CT imaging, even in the hemodynamically unstable patient. This is because the FAST does not distinguish between solid organ and hollow viscous injuries, which often require different management strategies. Specifically, the vast majority of solid organ injuries are managed conservatively without surgical intervention, while many hollow viscous injuries require operative intervention [20, 21]. Improvements in the accuracy of the FAST have been noted with combining the FAST with physical examination findings, [22] transaminase levels, [23] and performing serial FAST exams [24]. At this time, more research is needed into the utility of the FAST for pediatric trauma as measured by patient-relevant outcomes.

Soft Tissue Infections

Soft tissue infections represent a spectrum of disease from a cellulitis treated with systemic antibiotics to an abscess requiring incision and drainage. Given the potential need for sedation particularly in very young patients, an accurate diagnosis is important. Several studies have demonstrated the utility and improved diagnostic accuracy of point-of-care ultrasound compared with clinical examination in children [25–27].

Pneumonia

An adequate lung exam can be difficult in young children presenting with respiratory distress, fever, and/or hypoxemia. Point-of-care ultrasound has been shown to be highly specific for pneumonias in pediatric patients and may reduce the number of chest radiographs in some cases [28, 29]. In addition to identifying pneumonias, point-of-care ultrasound may also be valuable in assessing for parapneumonic effusions.

Venous Access

Infants, children with complex medical conditions, and those with hypovolemia can present challenges when trying to obtain venous access. Ultrasound-guidance for peripheral venous access may be particularly useful in pediatric patients with difficult access [30]. In addition, although not yet studied in pediatric patients, point-of-care ultrasound may be an additional adjunct for bedside nurses placing intravenous catheters.

Equipment

Physicians who perform pediatric point-of-care examinations should have access to appropriate equipment to perform these exams. Despite the reduction in the cost of portable ultrasound machines in the last decade, the cost remains significant enough that physicians should plan to delineate the value of point-of-care ultrasound for departments and/or hospitals. In addition to the return costs from billing revenue, there are improvements in quality benchmarks worth highlighting, such as reduced lengths of stay, [6] complication rates, [31] and improved patient satisfaction [32]. Further, use of some point-of-care ultrasound examinations may translate into fewer computed tomography scans [6, 33] and, therefore, radiation exposure. In pediatrics, specifically, there are often hospital foundations, or donor programs, which may be valuable sources of funding for such equipment. One strategy is for departments to begin use of point-of-care ultrasound as a quality improvement initiative with initial focus on a single exam that is widely applicable to the patient population and easy to learn, such as bladder volume assessment.

For most examinations (e.g., appendicitis, intussusception, pyloric stenosis, hip effusions, fractures, vascular access, soft tissue) in pediatric patients, a high frequency, linear array transducer will provide ideal resolution and sufficient penetration. In addition, for point-of-care ultrasound examinations in infants and toddlers, it is useful to have different sized linear transducers available (Fig. 24.1) with different lengths. This is such that for smaller surface areas, the operator can ensure the entire surface of the probe makes contact with the skin (e.g., infant arm for peripheral vascular access).

The FAST and cardiac examinations require use of a low frequency phased array or curvilinear transducer, as well as for select examinations in obese or older adolescents. For infants and toddlers, the optimal frequency range may be higher, so frequencies of 3–7 MHz, for example, may be considered.

Regardless of the probe, review of the near-field and far-field resolution in a variety of patient size is even more important in pediatrics. With ages from newborn to 21 years, the acoustical transmission will vary tremendously, especially in the near field.

In addition to equipment needed in order to perform point-of-care ultrasound examinations, departments should invest in training equipment, such as ultrasound-compatible phantoms and simulators. This equipment represents an opportunity for collaboration and cost-savings through resource sharing with other specialties in the hospital (See Chap. 12 – Ultrasound Equipment and Purchase).

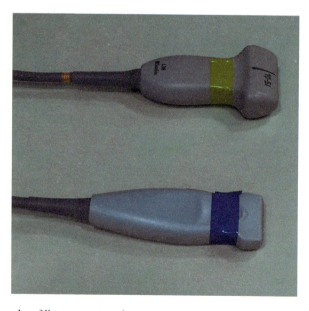

Fig. 24.1 Examples of linear array transducers

Managing Anxiety/Pain

Depending on the child and examination being performed, a point-of-care ultrasound examination may provoke anxiety and/or cause discomfort or pain. Depending on the age of the child, it is often helpful to explain the examination and compare it to things the child can relate to such as a computer game or comparing the image screen with a television. Having the child hold the transducer and apply it to himself or herself or a family member can also ameliorate fears. Other tools to reduce anxiety include child life specialists who are trained to distract and redirect patients for procedures. Toys, smartphones, or tablets which a parent or guardian can help hold can also serve as distraction tools. Use of warm ultrasound gel is imperative when performing point-of-care ultrasound in children, as it reduces the shock of the cool gel applied. In cases of particularly painful exams (e.g., soft tissue infections), stand-off pads, or alternatively, copious gel (Fig. 24.2) can be used as a barrier between the transducer and the patient's skin and may make for a pain-free

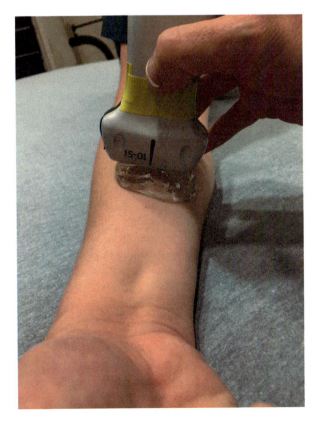

Fig. 24.2 Copious gel can be used over tender areas to reduce pain from the ultrasound exam

experience. For exams where direct pressure is unavoidable, and necessary, such as with the evaluation for appendicitis, it is important to provide systemic analgesia to the patient prior the exam in order to obtain adequate images. There are occasions where, despite efforts to reduce anxiety and pain, the child will not remain still for the examination. In these cases, the child should be appropriately restrained, as with other procedures, such as intravenous line placement or lumbar puncture, in order to obtain quality images worthy of interpretation.

Point-of-Care Ultrasound by Pediatric Emergency Medicine Physicians

In the last decade, there has been tremendous growth in pediatric emergency medicine (PEM) physician-performed point-of-care ultrasound. Nonetheless, the field is relatively new and still growing. In contrast to emergency physicians who receive training in point-of-care ultrasound during residency, point-of-care ultrasound training has only recently been incorporated into PEM fellowship training programs [34]. Comparable to the American College of Emergency Physicians Ultrasound Guidelines [3], and Council of Emergency Medicine Residency Directors recommendations for residency training [35], guidelines are now available for PEM physicians and fellow trainees. Vieira et al. [36] described educational guidelines and a sample curriculum for PEM fellowship training programs. In 2014, the American Academy of Pediatrics, in collaboration with the Society for Academic Emergency Medicine, American College of Emergency Physicians, and the World Interactive Network Focused on Critical Ultrasound, published the first national statements on PEM-performed point-of-care ultrasound [37, 38]. These documents outline considerations for those seeking to begin a PEM point-of-care ultrasound program. For those seeking additional ultrasound training, many programs offer one-year PEM-specific ultrasound fellowships. Finally, physicians who perform pediatric point-of-care ultrasound are encouraged to join the P2 Network, an international organization dedicated to pediatric point-of-care ultrasound (p2network.com).

Interdepartmental Considerations and Credentialing

It is useful to collaborate with other pediatric subspecialties, particularly when initiating a pediatric point-of-care ultrasound program. Depending on the practice environment, physicians outside of emergency medicine may not be familiar with the concept of emergency medicine-performed ultrasound. As its use remains relatively new in PEM, it is important to educate others regarding the precedent already set forth in emergency medicine as well as the aforementioned PEM guidelines. Additionally, other pediatric specialties, such as cardiology and radiology, may be valuable resources for those seeking to learn pediatric exams.

Credentialing considerations for the PEM physician include applications unique to the pediatric patient, inclusion of ultrasound applications that affect the range of pediatric patients (neonate to adolescent), and the point-of-care paradigm versus comprehensive ultrasound examinations, such as those done in radiology departments (See Chap. 20 – Credentialing and Privileging).

Pitfalls

1. Failure to understand the test characteristics of pediatric point-of-care ultrasound examinations and the utility of the exam. Specifically, most exams are used to rule-in pathology, and therefore should not be used as screening exams.
2. Failure to appreciate size-specific considerations in children. An appropriate transducer should be selected for very small children in order to adequately and optimally visualize anatomy and successfully perform procedures.
3. Failure to distract a patient sufficiently or keep a patient still during the exam in order to obtain adequate images.
4. Failing to gain sufficient experience with positive exams given the relatively low incidence of certain pediatric pathology.

Key Recommendations

1. Ultrasound should often be considered as the first imaging modality in pediatric patients and is in keeping with the ALARA principle of reducing radiation exposure.
2. Emergency physicians should consider point-of-care ultrasound in children with abdominal complaints, prior to urethral catheterizations, in the evaluation for a skull fracture, for children with a limp or fall on an outstretched arm, for soft tissue infections, and for children with respiratory distress.
3. Different from adult POC US, a linear array transducer is the optimal transducer for the majority of pediatric-specific examinations and departments should have multiple sizes available to accommodate different patient ages. One curvilinear or phased array probe should be available for torso applications such as cardiac and FAST examinations.
4. Utilize tools such as distraction techniques, child life specialists to assuage fears and anxiety, and take steps, such as the application of copious warm gel, to minimize pain and discomfort of certain ultrasound exams.

References

1. Brenner DJ. Estimating cancer risks from pediatric CT: going from the qualitative to the quantitative. Pediatr Radiol. 2002;32(4):228–31.
2. Pearce MS, Salotti JA, Little MP, McHugh K, Lee C, Kim K-P, et al. Radiation exposure from CT scans in childhood and subsequent risk of leukaemia and brain tumours: a retrospective cohort study. Lancet. 2012;380:499–505.
3. Ultrasound guidelines: emergency, point-of-care, and clinical ultrasound guidelines in medicine. Ann Emerg Med. 2017; 69(5):e27–e54.
4. Gausche-Hill M, Schmitz C, Lewis RJ. Pediatric preparedness of US emergency departments: a 2003 survey. Pediatrics. 2007;120(6):1229–37.
5. Sivitz AB, Cohen SG, Tejani C. Evaluation of acute appendicitis by pediatric emergency physician sonography. Ann Emerg Med. 2014;64(4):358–364.e4.
6. Elikashvili I, Tay ET, Tsung JW. The effect of point-of-care ultrasonography on emergency department length of stay and computed tomography utilization in children with suspected appendicitis. Acad Emerg Med. 2014;21(2):163–70.
7. Sivitz AB, Tejani C, Cohen SG. Evaluation of hypertrophic pyloric stenosis by pediatric emergency physician sonography. Acad Emerg Med. 2013;20(7):646–51.
8. Riera A, Hsiao AL, Langhan ML, Goodman TR, Chen L. Diagnosis of intussusception by physician novice sonographers in the emergency department. Ann Emerg Med. 2012;60(3):264–8.
9. Chen L, Hsiao AL, Moore CL, Dziura JD, Santucci KA. Utility of bedside bladder ultrasound before urethral catheterization in young children. Pediatrics. 2005;115(1):108–11.
10. Quayle KS, Jaffe DM, Kuppermann N, Kaufman BA, Lee BCP, Park TS, et al. Diagnostic testing for acute head injury in children: when are head computed tomography and skull radiographs indicated? Pediatrics. 1997;99(5):e11–1.
11. Rabiner JE, Friedman LM, Khine H, Avner JR, Tsung JW. Accuracy of point-of-care ultrasound for diagnosis of skull fractures in children. Pediatrics. 2013;131(6):1757–64.
12. Riera A, Chen L. Ultrasound evaluation of skull fractures in children: a feasibility study. Pediatr Emerg Care. 2012;28(5):420–5.
13. Vieira RL, Levy JA. Bedside ultrasonography to identify hip effusions in pediatric patients. Ann Emerg Med. 2010;55(3):284–9.
14. Rabiner JE, Khine H, Avner JR, Friedman LM, Tsung JW. Accuracy of point-of-care ultrasonography for diagnosis of elbow fractures in children. Ann Emerg Med. 2013;61(1):9–17.
15. Barata I, Spencer R, Suppiah A, Raio C, Ward MF, Sama A. Emergency ultrasound in the detection of pediatric long-bone fractures. Pediatr Emerg Care. 2012;28(11):1154–7.
16. Chaar-Alvarez FM, Warkentine F, Cross K, Herr S, Paul RI. Bedside ultrasound diagnosis of nonangulated distal forearm fractures in the pediatric emergency department. Pediatr Emerg Care. 2011;27(11):1027–32.
17. Dubrovsky AS, Kempinska A, Bank I, Mok E. Accuracy of ultrasonography for determining successful realignment of pediatric forearm fractures. Ann Emerg Med. 2015;65(3):260–5.
18. Fox JC, Boysen M, Gharahbaghian L, Cusick S, Ahmed SS, Anderson CL, et al. Test characteristics of focused assessment of sonography for trauma for clinically significant abdominal free fluid in pediatric blunt abdominal trauma. Acad Emerg Med. 2011;18(5):477–82.
19. Taylor GA, Sivit CJ. Posttraumatic peritoneal fluid: is it a reliable indicator of intraabdominal injury in children? J Pediatr Surg. 1995;30(12):1644–8.
20. Davies DA, Pearl RH, Ein SH, Langer JC, Wales PW. Management of blunt splenic injury in children: evolution of the nonoperative approach. J Pediatr Surg. 2009;44(5):1005–8.
21. Streck CJ, Lobe TE, Pietsch JB, Lovvorn HN III. Laparoscopic repair of traumatic bowel injury in children. J Pediatr Surg. 2006;41(11):1864–9.
22. Suthers SE, Albrecht R, Foley D, Mantor PC, Puffinbarger NK, Jones SK, et al. Surgeon-directed ultrasound for trauma is a predictor of intra-abdominal injury in children. Am Surg. 2004;70(2):164–7; discussion 167–8.

23. Sola JE, Cheung MC, Yang R, Koslow S, Lanuti E, Seaver C, et al. Pediatric FAST and elevated liver transaminases: an effective screening tool in blunt abdominal trauma. J Surg Res. 2009;157(1):103–7.
24. Blackbourne LH, Soffer D, McKenney M, Amortegui J, Schulman CI, Crookes B, et al. Secondary ultrasound examination increases the sensitivity of the FAST exam in blunt trauma. J Trauma. 2004;57(5):934–8.
25. Marin JR, Dean AJ, Bilker WB, Panebianco NL, Brown NJ, Alpern ER. Emergency ultrasound-assisted examination of skin and soft tissue infections in the pediatric emergency department. Acad Emerg Med. 2013;20(6):545–53.
26. Sivitz AB, Lam SHF, Ramirez-Schrempp D, Valente JH, Nagdev AD. Effect of bedside ultrasound on management of pediatric soft-tissue infection. J Emerg Med. 2010;39(5):637–43.
27. Iverson K, Haritos D, Thomas R, Kannikeswaran N. The effect of bedside ultrasound on diagnosis and management of soft tissue infections in a pediatric ED. Am J Emerg Med. 2012;30(8):1347–51.
28. Shah VP, Tunik MG, Tsung JW. Prospective evaluation of point-of-care ultrasonography for the diagnosis of pneumonia in children and young adults. JAMA Pediatr. 2013;167(2):119–25.
29. Samson F, Gorostiza I, González A, Landa M, Ruiz L, Grau M. Prospective evaluation of clinical lung ultrasonography in the diagnosis of community-acquired pneumonia in a pediatric emergency department. Eur J Emerg Med. 2016 Aug 17.
30. Doniger SJ, Ishimine P, Fox JC, Kanegaye JT. Randomized controlled trial of ultrasound-guided peripheral intravenous catheter placement versus traditional techniques in difficult-access pediatric patients. Pediatr Emerg Care. 2009;25(3):154–9.
31. Brass P, Hellmich M, Kolodziej L, Schick G, Smith AF. In: Brass P, editor. Ultrasound guidance versus anatomical landmarks for internal jugular vein catheterization. Cochrane Database of Systematic Reviews: Chichester; 2015.
32. Claret P-G, Bobbia X, Le Roux S, Bodin Y, Roger C, Perrin-Bayard R, et al. Point-of-care ultrasonography at the ED maximizes patient confidence in emergency physicians. Am J Emerg Med. 2016;34(3):657–9.
33. Doniger SJ, Kornblith A. Point-of-care ultrasound integrated into a staged diagnostic algorithm for pediatric appendicitis. Pediatr Emerg Care. 2016 Jun 14.
34. Marin JR, Zuckerbraun NS, Kahn JM. Use of emergency ultrasound in United States pediatric emergency medicine fellowship programs in 2011. J Ultrasound Med. 2012;31(9):1357–63.
35. Lewiss RE, Pearl M, Nomura JT, Baty G, Bengiamin R, Duprey K, et al. CORD-AEUS: consensus document for the emergency ultrasound milestone project. Acad Emerg Med. 2013;20(7):740–5.
36. Vieira RL, Hsu D, Nagler J, Chen L, Gallagher R, Levy JA. Pediatric emergency medicine fellow training in ultrasound: consensus educational guidelines. Acad Emerg Med. 2013;20(3):300–6.
37. Marin JR, Lewiss RE, American Academy of Pediatrics, Society for Academic Emergency Medicine, American College of Emergency Physicians, World Interactive Network Focused on Critical Ultrasound. Technical report: point-of-care ultrasonography by pediatric emergency medicine physicians. Pediatrics. 2015;135(4):e1113–22.
38. Marin JR, Abo AM, Doniger SJ, Fischer JW, Kessler DO, Levy JA, et al. Policy statement: point-of-care ultrasonography by pediatric emergency physicians. Ann Emerg Med. 2015;65(4):472–8.

Chapter 25
Ultrasound in Disaster and Pre-hospital Use

Haley Cochrane and Heidi H. Kimberly

Emergency POC Ultrasound During Disaster and Mass Casualty Incidents

Objectives

- Review the utility and limitations of emergency ultrasound during disaster and mass casualty incidents
- Understand the importance of including emergency ultrasound during disaster preparation and protocol development

Introduction

Disaster and mass casualty incidents (MCI) are unfortunately becoming more common worldwide. These events, while unpredictable, can be prepared for with emergency management plans and disaster drills. Point of care US (POC US) can be a valuable tool in patient triage, evaluation and management during disaster scenarios both in the prehospital and hospital environment. Its use has been driven by the established role of ultrasound in emergency and trauma evaluation and the widened availability and portability of ultrasound technology. Emergency ultrasound should be included as part of comprehensive disaster preparedness planning.

H. Cochrane, MBBS (✉)
Department of Emergency Medicine, Massachusetts General Hospital, Boston, MA, USA
e-mail: HCOCHRANE@PARTNERS.ORG

H.H. Kimberly, MD, FACEP
Department of Emergency Medicine, Brigham and Women's Hospital, Boston, MA, USA

© Springer International Publishing AG 2018
V. S. Tayal et al. (eds.), *Ultrasound Program Management*,
https://doi.org/10.1007/978-3-319-63143-1_25

Ultrasound During Triage

Mass casualty triage often occurs in two stages. The first is onsite triage by emergency providers to identify patients on scene that require immediate transport or evacuation, and the second is hospital-based triage of arriving patients to direct the timing of access to care. There are various triage scoring systems. The most commonly recognized and utilized triage scoring system in the United States is START, but all variations follow very similar principles with regard to categorization based on severity (see Table 25.1).

The core principle behind triage scoring systems is the rapid evaluation and appropriate triage of sick patients to definitive care and appropriate utilization of resources. These categorization systems are typically based on the physical exam and assessment of vital signs. However, this evaluation with limited available data can increase the risk of over- or under-triage of patients to higher levels of care.

The most heterogeneous patient group within the triage categories is the urgent but not immediately life-threatening (yellow) category of patients. Because of its diversity, this group could benefit from a secondary evaluation using ultrasound to identify subgroups with potentially life-threatening injuries that would benefit from re-triage. There is an opportunity to design new triage-based protocols involving ultrasound, both for identifying occult life-threatening injuries within this category and further subclassifying stable ambulatory patients with extremity injuries in order to streamline further diagnostic evaluation (see Table 25.2). Focused assessment with sonography in trauma (FAST) incorporated into the START triage algorithm has been used to identify yellow category patients with hemoperitoneum [1, 2]. Stawicki et al. have also proposed a triage-specific ultrasound protocol for evaluation of mass casualty patients focused on a modified E-FAST (Extended FAST incorporating thoracic ultrasound for pneumothorax), IVC, and limited musculoskeletal evaluation [3]. Many of these triage protocols have been made with adults in mind, but could likely be extrapolated to children and other unique populations. Given the unpredictable nature of disaster events, it may be difficult to empirically demonstrate a potential mortality benefit with the use of ultrasound.

Table 25.1 Triage categories	Modified triage categories
	Expectant, unsalvagable or deceased—Black
	Immediate life threatening—Red
	Urgent, not immediately life threatening—Yellow
	Ambulatory or delayed care—Green

Modified from START triage algorithum—START TRIAGE. Available at http://www.start-triage.com. Accessed 20 July 2016.

Table 25.2 Ultrasound incorporated into triage algorithm

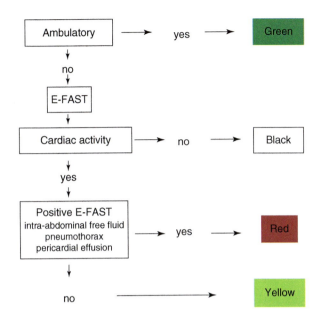

Trauma and Diagnostic Ultrasound

Ultrasound is an ideal modality for initial diagnostic workup during domestic and international natural and manmade disasters [4–7]. Typically, the E-FAST exam is the most valuable diagnostic tool to rapidly evaluate for life-threatening intrathoracic and intra-abdominal pathology when performed by experienced providers. Some disaster response teams currently utilize portable ultrasound and this use will likely expand with increased training opportunities. We recommend EMS services have a portable ultrasound available for MCI assessment performed in the field by reliable trained personnel. In addition, hospital radiology resources are often quickly overwhelmed leaving portable clinician performed ultrasound an ideal diagnostic modality in the emergency department for patients awaiting advanced radiology imaging.

There exists a significant patient injury burden that does not fall into the initially life-threatening category and a bedside E-FAST exam can help to rule out significant intrathoracic or intra-abdominal trauma and potentially avoid further imaging. The majority of patients presenting for evaluation and care after MCIs will fall into the yellow and green categories, with a significant proportion of injury burden from extremity, soft tissue, and orthopedic injuries. From the experience after the Boston Marathon Bombings, approximately 74% of patients presenting to two level one hospitals had shrapnel injuries [8]. Unique to organized terrorist attacks with shrapnel containing explosive devices and mass shootings, radiographic images are vital for potentially radiolucent foreign body identification. However, radiation-based modalities can often miss radiopaque substances such as glass and wood. Non-radiopaque foreign body identification is enhanced with ultrasound and a recent meta-analysis reports that ultrasound is approximately 72% sensitive and 92% specific in detecting foreign bodies [9].

The development of US-based protocols for triage assessment could also be extended to modified bedside reassessment protocols during the longitudinal emergency department evaluation. Repeat targeted FAST exams or modified shock ultrasound protocols, such as the RUSH exam [10], are potential tools for monitoring evolving cases within the initially less critically injured appearing patient population, that subsequently develop physical exam or vital sign abnormalities.

Ultrasound for Procedural Guidance

In addition to triage and diagnostic evaluation, ultrasound can be used therapeutically to guide procedures such as vascular access and peripheral nerve blocks. Lippert et al. suggest that the use of US-guided interscalene, forearm, femoral, and popliteal nerve blocks are potentially valuable procedures that could improve pain control in a disaster setting [11]. Ultrasound-guided peripheral nerve blocks are well described in the emergency medicine literature as being within scope of practice of emergency physicians competent in ultrasound. These procedures can provide pain relief during wound washout and repair as well as orthopedic reduction and splinting when procedural sedation would have been otherwise indicated, but nearly impossible due to significant resource and time constraints. A systematic review of multiple earthquakes victims found that on average 68% of patients presented with extremity injuries [12]. Providers caring for patients after the earthquake in Haiti utilized ultrasound-guided nerve blocks for pain relief and to assist with orthopedic procedures and wound care [13]. Basic information regarding the types of blocks as well as limitations and challenges of each proposed procedure are listed in Table 25.3.

Incorporating Ultrasound into Disaster Planning

Protocols and procedures for emergency ultrasound performed both in the field and in emergency department settings should be included in comprehensive disaster planning. A well-documented bottleneck in the ED evaluation of MCI injuries is the high demand on diagnostic radiology. From military data we know that combined X-ray, CT, and US evaluations may be required for complete injury evaluation [14]. The number of radiology studies and the report response times after the Boston Marathon Bombing were both noted to be significantly increased compared to baseline [8]. Brunner et al. suggest "radiology departments should maintain a

Table 25.3 Ultrasound-guided nerve blocks in mass casualty incidents

US-guided nerve block	Injuries	Difficulty	Challenges	Estimated procedural time, minutes[a]
Femoral	Knee	Basic	Risk of inadvertent arterial puncture; partial pain control	10
	Femoral neck Proximal femur			
Popliteal (distal sciatic nerve just proximal to the popliteal fossa)	Distal tibial fracture	Advanced	Excludes saphenous innervation of the medial foreleg, ankle, and foot; increased level of difficulty if patient unable to move to prone position; inadequate block without targeted anesthetic deposition	10
	Fibular fracture			
	Majority of foot and ankle injuries Soft tissue injuries lower leg			
Forearm (median, ulnar, radial nerves)	Isolated hand injuries	Basic	Radial nerve can be difficult to visualize in forearm	5
Interscalene (brachial plexus)	Shoulder dislocation Humerus fracture Elbow dislocation	Intermediate	Complex anatomy in the neck. Higher risk of complications: Pneumothorax, phrenic nerve paralysis	10

Reproduced from Lippert et al. [10]
[a]Estimated procedural time includes ultrasound setup, nerve identification, preparation of the injection site, and deposition of local anesthetic around the peripheral nerve identified.

comprehensive mass casualty plan to address the surge in imaging needs that arise from blast injuries. This may require mobilization of additional portable imaging equipment or cancellation of non-emergent imaging on CT scanners or nearby fixed X-ray units to create additional capacity" [8].

POC US can be used to expand diagnostic evaluation of patient injuries while awaiting operative care or advanced diagnostic radiology, and the same principles apply in regard to a preparing a comprehensive mass casualty plan. Mobilization of resources including personnel trained in ultrasound and additional ultrasound systems from other locations, such as radiology departments or ICUs, should be prepared and planned for in advance. There should also be a yearly comprehensive review of the available equipment within emergency department to ensure that there is easy identification and regionalization of necessary equipment, such as spare battery packs or functional probes, and that each machine has a linear and curvilinear probe available for the most common imaging modalities. There is also a role for review and education of providers in obtaining necessary imaging with suboptimal probe availability, such as obtaining eFAST with a phased array probe, in the event of equipment damage or unavailability of ideal probes (see equipment chapter).

IMAGING STUDIES

☐ EFAST: _____

_____

XRAY	CT
☐ C-spine: _____	☐ Head: _____
☐ Chest: _____	☐ C-spine: _____
☐ Pelvis: _____	☐ Chest: _____
☐ T/L/S spine: _____	☐ Abd/Pelvis: _____
☐ Extremities: _____	☐ T/L/S-spine: _____
☐ Other: _____	☐ Other/Incidental: ____

Fig. 25.1 Example of paper MCI and downtime documentation

Communication between emergency department providers and specialists during MCIs can be challenging, potentially putting patient care at risk. Emergency departments must weigh heavily on the strength of their information systems for patient flow, resource allocation, ordering, proper documentation of point of care imaging, and procedures. Disaster planning must include documentation systems such as the use of paper versus electronic medical records, or a hybrid system for the timely collection and sharing of valuable findings between team members [15]. If paper charting is utilized during down time or disaster scenarios, it should include an area for ultrasound documentation (see Fig. 25.1), a lesson learned during the Boston Marathon Bombing experience [16, 17]. Pertinent ultrasound findings are only valuable if the results are easily communicated between the medical and surgical teams. This is particularly important if ultrasound is being used in the prehospital environment or on scene where diagnostic information or specific diagnoses may have already been obtained prior to ED arrival. Pertinent positive findings could be documented either directly on the patient or via an adhesive such as masking tape, to ensure that this information does not get lost in transit, during triage, or patient decontamination.

Equipment

Ultrasound systems for use during disaster and MCI should be portable, durable, and function on battery power. Use of both linear and curvilinear transducers allows for a range of applications from procedural guidance to E-FAST. In addition to the appropriate ultrasound machines, comprehensive disaster planning must include easy availability of backup battery packs or alternative energy sources as well as equipment such as gel, cleaning solution, and probe covers. In case of hazmat scenarios, machines and equipment may become compromised and we recommend including protocols for identification of potentially contaminated equipment, training personnel on appropriate procedures, and having backup equipment readily available (See Chap. 12 – Ultrasound Equipment and Purchase).

Conclusion

Ultrasound is increasingly being utilized during disaster and MCI incidents throughout the world. Evaluation of life-threatening traumatic injuries and reevaluation of undifferentiated patients is important for the triage and management of large numbers of patients in a short period of time. Even the most robust emergency departments quickly mirror any resource limited setting with a large and rapid influx of sick undifferentiated patients. Emergency departments as well as disaster management teams must be prepared with the appropriate ultrasound equipment including plans for portable, battery-powered, machines, trained personnel, and understanding of disaster scenario documentation and communication.

Key Recommendations

- Ultrasound can be incorporated into triage algorithms and utilized for both diagnostic and therapeutic indications during disasters.
- E-FAST is the most common application utilized during disaster and MCI situations.
- US-guided regional anesthesia can be used for extremity injuries and to facilitate wound care and orthopedic procedures.
- Expect and plan for a surge in imaging utilization during disasters.
- US machines used in disaster scenarios must be portable and rechargeable.
- Develop reliable disaster protocol documentation for ultrasound results to facilitate team communication.
- Emergency ultrasound should be included in comprehensive disaster response planning.

Ultrasound in the Prehospital Setting

Objectives

- Understand the utility and limitations of ultrasound in the prehospital setting
- Describe the role of telemedicine for prehospital ultrasound

Table 25.4 Principles of prehospital ultrasound

Principles of ultrasound application in the United States prehospital environment
1. Ultrasound training and skill maintenance EMS personnel
2. Development of prehospital ultrasound protocols and guidelines based on available evidence
3. Regular imaging QA by ultrasound credentialed director or establish prehospital US director
4. Research and innovation for adaptive prehospital ultrasound practice

Introduction

The incorporation of ultrasound into the prehospital environment varies worldwide with different prehospital models of care delivery. It is more common in places like Europe, Scandinavia, and Australia where physicians typically staff prehospital transport and remains in the early stages of utilization in North America. Ultrasound has been utilized in the field by emergency medical services to assist in appropriate prehospital triage, diagnosis, management, and resuscitation of critically ill and injured patients. Increasing adoption of this technology will likely occur as ultrasound machines become even smaller and more durable, training opportunities expand, and the potential benefits to patient care are realized.

Currently the use of ultrasound in the American prehospital setting has focused mainly on air transport and some advanced paramedic units. General use by local EMS is limited but growing. A 2014 survey of EMS directors in North America found that only 4% of EMS systems were using ultrasound, primarily for trauma and cardiac arrest evaluations, but an additional 20% were considering implementation [18]. The expanding role for ultrasound within the American system will be centered on applications that are simple to teach, are reliable and answer clinical questions that have the potential change patient management (see Table 25.4).

Trauma Evaluation

The E-FAST examination is a valuable tool in the evaluation of trauma patients in both in the emergency department and in the prehospital setting. E-FAST can provide early identification of life-threatening injuries such as pneumothorax, hemoperitoneum, or cardiac tamponade. Prehospital providers can perform E-FAST exams reliably and quickly after brief training programs [19–22]. There is emerging literature to suggest that prehospital ultrasound has the potential to change patient management including prehospital therapies and altering hospital transport decisions [23–26].

In addition to an initial E-FAST exam, ultrasound can be used to guide vascular access and provide augmented reassessment of trauma patients during prolonged transfer. For example, monitoring for pneumothorax in ventilated patients, repeated FAST exam for the development of intra-abdominal free fluid, and management of fluid resuscitation management could be valuable data for receiving hospitals or for critical care transport teams to monitor between hospitals settings.

Limitations to wide spread adoption of EUS includes the costs of equipment and training as well as lack of specific guidelines and protocols. Likely this technology will be adopted first by advanced paramedics, aeromedical transport, and local units with prolonged transport times. With improvements in technology and recognition of improvements in clinical management of patients, we will likely see an expansion of ultrasound use locally with prehospital crews that have access to physician trainers who can create specific polices and guidelines that take into account experience of providers and local transport times.

Cardiac Arrest

Ultrasound is increasingly being incorporated into cardiac arrest resuscitation. EUS can diagnose potential etiologies of cardiac arrest such as pericardial effusion with tamponade, massive pulmonary embolism resulting in RV strain, or pneumothorax. The 2015 European resuscitation counsel guidelines now include ultrasound stating, "Peri-arrest ultrasound may have a role in identifying reversible causes of cardiac arrest" [27]. In addition, ultrasound can provide prognostic information. In a large multi-center trial of 793 cardiac arrest patients, in those with asystole, lack of cardiac activity on ultrasound had a sensitivity of 90% and positive predictive value of 99% for non-survival to hospital discharge [28].

Telemedicine

Another expanding field within the prehospital setting is the opportunity to combine telemedicine and ultrasound. Incorporation of tele-ultrasound for onsite personnel could provide valuable diagnostic resources to EMS providers with limited US experience, and in turn supply receiving hospitals with vital patient data prior to hospital arrival. This could provide time to prepare to arrange or resources such as massive transfusion protocol activation or operating room setup. Military, space, and civilian studies have demonstrated that the transmission of US images is both feasible and reliable with respect to specific imaging modalities [29, 30]. If the equipment is available, but the providers on scene have limited training, appropriate images could be obtained through coaching using remote guidance from experienced emergency providers. While concerns regarding patient confidentiality and image quality are limitations to its widespread implementation, it is an area of potential growth and innovation.

Limitations

Obstacles to the widespread adoption of ultrasound in the prehospital setting include the cost and resources necessary for equipment and training and lack of large-scale data demonstrating clinical outcome benefits. However, with advances in technology ultrasound machines will continue to become cheaper and more portable. A proliferation of online resources provides ample opportunities for education. The adoption of EUS within American prehospital systems will need to be symbiotic with the primary focus on short scene time and rapid transport to definitive care. Systems with short transportation intervals between scene and hospital may find limited uses for US such as trauma, cardiac arrest, and vascular access. Rural locations with longer transport times or critical care transport teams will likely have expanded indications for ultrasound. The acquisition of this new skill set for emergency medical providers will require a time and financial commitment, training and competency assessment, outcomes assessments, and a significant frequency of use to maintain proficiency. This process has been well delineated for emergency physicians in the 2016 ACEP Emergency Ultrasound guidelines and could be adapted for prehospital providers. Emergency physicians with advanced ultrasound training will be crucial in facilitating the development of prehospital POC US.

Conclusion

Ultrasound use in the prehospital setting is an emerging frontier with increased interest and adoption of this technology. Emergency physicians trained in ultrasound have a unique opportunity to pair with local EMS providers to develop training protocols and procedures unique to regional EMS systems. Protocols will need to take into account the unique practice environment of medical transportation including time, space, and training constraints. New solutions and applications will be possible with advancing technology including a potential role for telemedicine. Lastly, ongoing research is needed into the role of prehospital POC US regarding the potential to change patient management and outcomes.

Key Recommendations

- Ultrasound is increasingly utilized in the prehospital setting, especially for trauma and cardiac arrest patients as well as patients with prolonged transport times.
- Challenges to widespread incorporation include costs and logistics of training and equipment as well as need for protocol development.
- Use of telemedicine has the potential to advance the use of ultrasound in the prehospital environment.

References

1. Sztajnkrycer MD, Baez AA, Luke A. FAST ultrasound as an adjunct to triage using the START mass casualty triage system. Prehosp Emerg Care. 2006;10(1):96–102.
2. Hu H, et al. Streamlined focused assessment with sonography for mass casualty prehospital triage of blunt torso trauma patients. Am J Emerg Med. 2014;32(7):803–6.
3. Stawicki SP, et al. Portable ultrasonography in mass casualty incidents: the CAVEAT examination. World J Orthop. 2010;1(1):10–9.
4. SARKISIAN AE, et al. Sonographic screening of mass casualties for abdominal and renal injuries following the 1988 Armenian earthquake. J Trauma Acute Care Surg. 1991;31(2):247–50.
5. Dan D, et al. Ultrasonographic applications after mass casualty Incident caused by Wenchuan Earthquake. J Trauma Acute Care Surg. 2010;68(6):1417–20.
6. Shorter M, Macias DJ. Portable handheld ultrasound in austere environments: use in the Haiti disaster. Prehosp Disaster Med. 2012;27(02):172–7.
7. Wydo SM, Seamon MJ, Melanson SW, et al. Portable ultrasound in disaster triage: a focused review. Eur J Trauma Emerg Surg. 2016;42(4):151–9.
8. Brunner J, et al. The Boston marathon bombing: after-action review of the Brigham and women's hospital emergency radiology response. Radiology. 2014;273(1):78–87.
9. Davis J, et al. Diagnostic accuracy of ultrasonography in retained soft tissue foreign bodies: a systematic review and meta-analysis. Acad Emerg Med. 2015;22(7):777–87.
10. Perera P, et al. The RUSH exam: rapid ultrasound in SHock in the evaluation of the critically ill. Emerg Med Clin North Am. 2010;28(1):29–56.
11. Lippert SC, et al. Pain control in disaster settings: a role for ultrasound-guided nerve blocks. Ann Emerg Med. 2013;61(6):690–6.
12. Missair A, et al. A matter of life or limb? A review of traumatic injury patterns and anesthesia techniques for disaster relief after major earthquakes. Anesth Analg. 2013;117(4):934–41.
13. Shah S, Dalal A, Smith RM, et al. Impact of portable ultrasound in trauma care after the Haitian earthquake of 2010. Am J Emerg Med. 2010;28:970–1.
14. Raja AS, Propper BW, Vandenberg SL, et al. Imaging utilization during explosive multiple casualty incidents. J Trauma. 2010;68:1421–4.
15. Landman A, et al. The Boston marathon bombings mass casualty incident: one emergency department's information systems challenges and opportunities. Ann Emerg Med. 2015;66(1):51–9.
16. Eyre A, Stone M, Kimberly HH. Point-of-care ultrasonography in a domestic mass casualty incident: the Boston marathon experience. Emerg Med Open J. 2016;2(2):32–5.
17. Kimberly HH, Stone MB. Clinician-performed ultrasonography during the Boston marathon bombing mass casualty incident. Ann Emerg Med. 2013;62(2):199–200.
18. Taylor J, et al. Use of prehospital ultrasound in North America: a survey of emergency medical services medical directors. BMC Emerg Med. 2014;14(1):1–5.
19. Kim CH, Shin SD, Song KJ, Park CB. Diagnostic accuracy of focused assessement with sonography for trauma (FAST) examinations performed by emergency medical technicians. Prehosp Emerg Care. 2012;16(3):400–6.
20. Heegaard W, et al. Prehospital ultrasound by paramedics: results of field trial. Acad Emerg Med. 2010;17(6):624–30.
21. Chin EJ, Chan CH, Mortazavi R, Anderson CL, Kahn CA, Summers S, Fox JC. A pilot study examining the viability of a Prehospital Assessment with UltraSound for Emergencies (PAUSE) protocol. J Emerg Med. 2013;44(1):142–9.
22. Rooney KP, Lahham S, Anderson CL, Bledsoe B, Sloane B, Joseph L, Osborn MB, Fox JC. Pre-hospital assessment with ultrasound in emergencies: implementation in the field. World J Emerg Med. 2016;7(2):117–23.
23. Walcher F, et al. Prehospital ultrasound imaging improves management of abdominal trauma. Br J Surg. 2006;93(2):238–42.

24. Rudolph SS, et al. Effect of prehospital ultrasound on clinical outcomes of non-trauma patients—a systematic review. Resuscitation. 2014;85(1):21–30.
25. Jorgensen H, Jensen CH, Dirks J. Does prehospital ultrasound improve treatment of the trauma patient? A systematic review. Eur J Emerg Med. 2010;17(5):249–53.
26. O'Dochartaigh D, Douma M. Prehospital ultrasound of the abdomen and thorax changes trauma patient management: a systematic review. Injury. 2015;46(11):2093–102.
27. European Resuscitation Council Guidelines for Resuscitation. 2015. https://cprguidelines.eu/. Accessed 14 Oct 2016.
28. Gaspari R, et al. Emergency department point-of-care ultrasound in out-of-hospital and in-ED cardiac arrest. Resuscitation. 2016;109:33–9.
29. Adhikari S, et al. Transfer of real-time ultrasound video of FAST examinations from a simulated disaster scene via a mobile phone. Prehosp Disaster Med. 2014;29(03):290–3.
30. Boniface KS, et al. Tele-ultrasound and paramedics: real-time remote physician guidance of the Focused Assessment With Sonography for Trauma examination. Am J Emerg Med. 2011;29(5):477–81.

Chapter 26
Community Ultrasound

Rajesh N. Geria and Robert J. Tillotson

Objectives

- Explain the history and current state of POC US in the community hospital
- Discuss what challenges are unique to the community hospital
- Discuss strategies to solicit department leadership support for ultrasound in the group and community setting
- Discuss tips for training and credentialing the community physician
- Discuss the importance of image archival and overall workflow to program success
- Discuss the role of certification and accreditation in community practice
- Discuss solutions/resources for implementation and management of ultrasound in the community hospital

R.N. Geria, MD, FACEP (✉)
Department of Emergency Medicine, Robert Wood Johnson Medical School, New Brunswick, NJ, USA
e-mail: rgeria@mac.com

R.J. Tillotson, DO, FACEP
Northwest Wisconsin Emergency Medicine, Mayo Clinic Health System, Eau Claire, WI, USA
e-mail: tillotson.robert@mayo.edu

© Springer International Publishing AG 2018
V. S. Tayal et al. (eds.), *Ultrasound Program Management*,
https://doi.org/10.1007/978-3-319-63143-1_26

Introduction

Nationwide there is a total of 5627 hospitals. Of these hospitals, there are 1007 designated teaching hospitals and only 400 academic medical centers. Consequently, the vast majority of medicine is practiced in community hospitals. It is in these community hospitals that point of care ultrasound can have its greatest impact on patient care. The greatest potential for growth of point of care ultrasound is also found in community hospitals.

The focus of academic centers is typically threefold: education, research, and patient care. But the real impact of these centers' research and new innovations is dependent upon the implementation of these advancements into the medical community at large. Successful implementation and management of a point of care ultrasound program in community hospitals ensures that patients receive the benefits that ultrasound provides at the bedside.

Physicians practicing in the community setting face unique challenges in developing and maintaining point of care ultrasound programs. Community physicians have clinical demands without the advantages of physicians in training, mandated training requirements, and protected nonclinical time. Training in ultrasound is challenging as shown in a community ultrasound survey by Moore et al. in 2006, which found lack of training as the biggest reason for not integrating point of care ultrasound into community practice [1].

Community physicians face evolving standard of care issues as ultrasound is adopted for diagnosis and procedural guidance and feeling behind can add to the pressure of adopting ultrasound. Community physicians may not be getting the full benefit of postgraduate ultrasound fellowships according to Society of Clinical Ultrasound Fellowships (SCUF) database. Most fellows graduating from ultrasound fellowships are joining academic groups further contributing to the expertise void in the community setting. Community physicians may have more justification for ultrasound adoption due to lack of availability of consultative ultrasound from traditional providers and increased pressures for efficiency and risk management. Community physicians also have a more collegial relationship with their colleagues and face less political battles. Physicians practicing in this setting can build successful ultrasound programs by following national guidelines and strategies outlined in this chapter.

History of POC US in Community Setting

Emergency Medicine was early in implementing point of care ultrasound (POC US), but the challenges Emergency Medicine encountered in the community setting mirror the challenges other specialties face. In Emergency Medicine residencies, the initial training of residents in the use of point of care ultrasound varied by institution. For these reasons, many physicians practicing in community hospitals have limited experience in point of care ultrasound, nor do they have anyone to train, mentor, or administrate the implementation of ultrasound into these community hospitals.

In the 2000s, it became evident from the academic centers that ultrasound was going to be a new standard of care for many clinicians. Following this trend, there was a resulting spike in sales of ultrasound machines to community hospitals. Soon, most community emergency departments were equipped with an ultrasound machine for point of care evaluation. Many community-based emergency physicians took introductory ultrasound courses under the assumption that the course would adequately prepare them to effectively implement point of care ultrasound into their practice. Now possessing an ultrasound machine, emergency physicians assumed that learning to utilize the machine and incorporating it into their practice would be simple, similar to incorporating the Gluidescope or Ez-IO.

Unfortunately, many physicians failed to understand that, in addition to the foundational training obtained in introductory courses, full implementation of point of care ultrasound also required having a number of proctored or over-read studies until the clinician mastered acquisition and recognition of both normal and abnormal images. Most community emergency departments did not provide, or have access to, the additional oversight and mentorship necessary to ensure physician competency in point of care ultrasound. Incomplete image acquisition and inconsistent image quality resulted in ineffective integration of bedside ultrasound. This effect was magnified in low volume community Emergency Departments because of the lack of available patients and pathology. Consequently, the benefit of clinical ultrasound as a diagnostic modality was not realized in most community hospitals, and ultrasound machines were banished to the corner to collect dust. In fact, the challenges faced by emergency medicine in this respect offer great lessons for other specialties.

Although some community hospitals were able to successfully implement emergency ultrasound into the emergency department, most of these hospitals had no consistent workflow to follow. Archived images for education, credentialing, and patient records were printed pictures and videos; few had electronic storage solutions. There was no established workflow or QA process, so most borrowed from academic centers or created their own. Inconsistency in interpretation and documentation of results was common, undermining credibility of EUS with the medical staff. This resulted in ineffective integration into patient care workflow. Therefore, use of ultrasound was sporadic and inconsistent. Unfortunately, many community hospitals attempting to implement EUS into the practice of emergency medicine did not reach their full potential.

There have been additional obstacles to the implementation of EUS in community hospitals from both within and outside the emergency department. Medical staff challenges arose both as turf battles and a lack of confidence in the results obtained by emergency physicians. Many community hospital emergency departments are not uniformly staffed, which creates challenges in EUS implementation and consistency within emergency department groups. Navigating the political structure of the group to obtain participation and support was difficult, especially since most of these physicians had practiced successfully for years using radiology consultants for ultrasound and did not appreciate the benefit of doing ultrasounds themselves. After all, it was easier to check a box than to try and do an ultrasound oneself.

Finally, community hospitals do not have the benefit of an academic program to support and perpetuate complex advances in medicine, such as point of care ultrasound. There is a paucity of dedicated funds for training, ultrasound directors, and equipment expenditures. Early on many champions encountered uphill battles with administration to justify allocating funds for developing an ultrasound program. Administrators, often viewed EUS as a duplication of services and did not understand the need to dedicate physician resources to manage an ultrasound program in their emergency departments. However, much of this has or is now changing.

Creating a Successful Ultrasound Program in the Community Setting

The core of a successful ultrasound program in the community hospital is making ultrasound an effective tool in the hands of the practicing physicians in those hospitals. This quintessential statement is the key to having ultrasound integrated successfully. This book gives detailed instructions on how to implement a successful ultrasound program. The principles detailed apply to both academic and community hospitals. This chapter will focus on the obstacles that are unique to the community setting and their possible solutions (Table 26.1).

Commitment

In order for point of care ultrasound to become an effective tool in the community hospital setting, an ultrasound program committed to following established guidelines must be implemented. There is no academic drive, competition, or curriculum to fuel implementation of an ultrasound program in a community hospital. Therefore, someone has to be the impetus to make this happen. To make matters worse, there will be many obstacles to building this program. Commitment is the key to

Table 26.1 Community management obstacles and solutions

Community management obstacles	Solutions
Department chair commitment	Demonstrate safety, quality, value, standard of care additional benefits: Recruiting, innovation
Ultrasound director training	Take management course, recruit fellowship trained physician, attend preceptorship (mini-fellowship)
Funding	Demonstrate reimbursement potential, decrease cost of procedural complications, approach donors
Physician training	Imported courses, curated online medical education, scanning shifts, functional quality assurance program
Credentialing	Follow ACEP guidelines [5]
Quality improvement	Workflow middleware

overcoming these obstacles. This commitment starts with an ultrasound champion. That champion could be the medical director, department chair, nurse director, an emergency physician who took an ultrasound course, a new physician out of residency that was trained in ultrasound, or an Ultrasound Director. The champion's first objective is to foster support from their physician group. If the group does not show commitment to implementing ultrasound, it will be an uphill battle. Typically, the group will support the idea if it is framed in a way that shows physicians how ultrasound will improve their clinical practice.

This champion will also need to obtain commitment from hospital administration. Keep in mind that many hospital administrators invested money in an ultrasound machine in the early 2000s that ultimately sat in the corner; they will need to be convinced that commitment is sincere. After all, an ultrasound machine with a workflow solution, ongoing expenses for supplies and maintenance, and compensation for an ultrasound director, will be one of the biggest single item expenditures brought to the hospital as a capital request.

Soliciting Department Chair/Director Support

Support from the chair or director is critical to the success of any ultrasound program. Most chairs recognize the positive impact bedside ultrasound has had on patient care. This section is designed to assist the practitioners who may find themselves up against stiff chairmen resistance to developing an ultrasound program. Academic chairs often implement what is right for the residency program and as mentioned in the introduction, involves an aggressive ultrasound curriculum in order fulfill RRC mandates. Chairmen of community ED's and contract groups do not have this incentive so it falls on the ultrasound director to develop a creative approach to attain support to move forward. Community chairs may not need to adhere to residency guidelines but they do need to ensure patients are getting high quality care. In the current healthcare climate, all chairs face pressures from the hospital to comply with the Affordable Care Act to deliver high quality, cost-effective, and safe care. It is important for ultrasound directors to leverage these goals and build the following equation into any conversation with a Chair when trying to attain program support:

Quality = Safety/Cost
Value = Quality

Safety

This is the lowest hanging fruit with the biggest impact. Multiple studies have demonstrated that ultrasound guidance improves the success rates and safety of invasive procedures including central lines, paracentesis, and thoracentesis. Using ultrasound guidance to insert central venous catheters is not a novel concept anymore. In fact, it is essentially standard of care and any community ED not using this is practicing suboptimal care that could result in grave consequences for the patient. Complications resulting from blind attempts at central venous access have been well documented inclusive of pneumothorax, arterial hemorrhage, CVA, pericardial tamponade, hemothorax, and central line associated blood stream infections (CLABSI). In 2011, the CDC released guidelines to reduce CLABSI and number 7 is the use of ultrasound guidance to place central venous catheters to reduce the number of cannulation attempts and mechanical complications. In 2013, CMS released its finalized payment reduction program for Hospital Acquired Conditions (HAC), which essentially states that 1% of Medicare payments to hospitals performing in the bottom 25th percentile will be at risk. The Agency for Healthcare Research and Quality (AHRQ) lists ultrasound guidance for central venous catheters as a top 10 recommendations for clinicians to make healthcare safer for patients. The Joint Commission (JC) lists using ultrasound for central line insertion in Chap. 3 of the Central Line Associated Blood Stream Infections CLABSI toolkit. Any reluctant chair could be reminded that from a pure safety perspective in 2016 ultrasound use will be mandated for central line guidance by the National Quality Forum (NQF). Another useful strategy illustrating the importance of safety that may be even more effective than external evidence and supporting literature is leveraging complications that occurred at the home institution such as the dreaded sentinel event. Keep track of cases where ultrasound guidance was not used that resulted in poor outcomes and show administrators. Medical directors interested in improving safety for patients can easily accomplish this by supporting the purchase of smaller scale machines with one transducer. The linear transducer is capable of doing a large percentage of basic procedural ultrasound applications and is the recommended entry point into the world of point of care ultrasound for any community ED practice because it is clearly the path of least resistance.

Cost

Cost-effective care is the new focus for today's administrators and healthcare leaders. The fee for service model is being phased out and replaced with fee for quality. Point of care ultrasound is helping reduce hospital and patient expenses by reducing the cost to the health system and the time required for diagnosis and treatment. The increasing utilization of CT is an area of concern in this country as it continues to burden the healthcare system with high cost while also leading to radiation induced cancer. There is a national movement led by AIUM to promote an "Ultrasound Approach" for common conditions like trauma, renal colic and undifferentiated abdominal pain in order to cut down the number of CT scans being ordered. Another way to look at cost in the eyes of the community or large group director is LOS and impact on practitioner RVU. Some critics of bedside ultrasound in this setting argue that it will slow them down and directly impact their compensation. If ultrasound slows them down fewer patients will be seen resulting in increased LOS. One study evaluated this theory by looking at a community group where compensation was entirely RVU based. The investigators found that the practitioners categorized as the highest performers of bedside ultrasound actually had the highest RVU's in the group [2]. Plain and simple, ultrasound allows rapid narrowing of the differential diagnosis and often cuts down the workup required to safely treat and disposition the patient. Community directors will have to be convinced that bedside ultrasound can actually increase physician productivity while leading to safer higher quality care.

There is a general perception that ordering more CT scans may prevent frivolous malpractice lawsuits. In addition, using bedside ultrasound may expose clinicians to medicolegal risk. It is important for ultrasound directors to discuss the rise in cases in the malpractice legal literature where guilty verdicts are being given for failure to use ultrasound in the ED when it was available specifically with relation to vascular access.

Training and Credentialing the Community Physician

The lack of these resources and inherent motivation of community physicians to come in on "days off" to scan in order to meet credentialing guidelines set forth by ACEP create a challenging problem for the chair unique to this setting. The first consideration must be what training does the "ultrasound director" have? Is this individual a recent graduate of a residency program or a seasoned community physician that may have grandfathered into this role with minimal ultrasound experience? The chair should consider investing resources to develop the "ultrasound director" if he/she falls into the latter category. Ultrasound preceptorships or mini-fellowship programs are available and excellent ways to gain experience of running an ultrasound program while fulfilling the ACEP requirements to become credentialed in the process. A listing of these programs can be found on the ACEP Ultrasound Section website and range from anywhere between 4 and 7 K/month (Table 26.2).

Table 26.2 Ultrasound preceptorship sites

(CA) University of California	(NC) Carolinas Medical Center
(DE) Christiana Care Health System	(NJ) Morristown Memorial Hospital
(GA) Medical College of Georgia	(NY) Albany Medical Center
(IL) John H. Stoger Hospital of Cook County	(NY) Mount Sinai School of Medicine
(MA) Massachusetts General Hospital	(NY) NY Hospital-Queens/Weill Cornell Med Coll
(MA) Tufts Medical Center	(NY) New York Methodist Hospital
(MA) University of Massachusetts	(NY) North Shore University Hospital
(MD) Johns Hopkins Hospital	(NY) St. Luke's—Roosevelt Hospital Center
(OH) Mid-Ohio Emergency Services	

Adapted from ACEP.org

The initial didactic component of training can easily be accomplished by an internal or external course but ongoing hands on scanning and pattern recognition are crucial to developing real skill (See Chap. 5 – Introductory Education and Chap. 6 – Continuing Education). There are several strategies that community chairs can try to encourage physicians to partake in the experiential phase of credentialing. A dedicated number of scan shifts with and without the ultrasound director is a good start. This will fail unless physicians are held accountable for this process. It is critical for the chair to emphasize the importance of this to the overall mission of the department and build language into re-appointment contracts that reflect ultrasound-credentialing expectations. An example may be Dr. X will not be re-appointed after year 2 if not credentialed in at least 2 of the 5 core applications of bedside ultrasound. The other approach could be strictly monetary. Each ultrasound performed as part of the credentialing process holds some monetary value in terms of annual bonus. Physicians in the group that perform more ultrasound will effectively make more bonus money. How much is each ultrasound worth? Do physicians really want to come in on a "day off" to make a few extra bonus dollars? Maybe a better strategy is to link the entire bonus to ultrasound performance? A study by Budhram et al. showed the successful implementation of ultrasound training using monetary incentives [3]. It is often only after physicians perform high volumes of scans that they begin to see the true value of the technology. It may take 15 FAST exams to see a positive but that single case may be enough evidence to convince the physician to use it in the future for a similar patient. After a time, there may not be a need to link ultrasound performance to financial incentives because credentialing requirements will have been met and ultrasound will be perceived as part of good care rather than a hindrance. In this era of Free Online Access to Medical Education (FOAM), there are countless resources available online for community physicians to learn the didactics of ultrasound. The motivated community chair should be aggressive to stimulate physician training and credentialing so that the group can begin billing for point of care ultrasound and get direct return on investment for the hospital.

Ultrasound Director Support

The role of ultrasound director is almost always undervalued regardless of academic or community practice settings. Sometimes it is hard to find justification to take the ultrasound director position in the community setting. Attractive titles, book chapters, and research grants are scarce in nonacademic settings. So how then can the community ultrasound director make the case that he/she should be supported in terms of monetary compensation, protected time, or both. It starts with educating and training faculty (See Chap. 2 – Ultrasound Directors).

How much time will the ultrasound director be spending up front training the group and what is this worth? The chair should consider providing annual stipends to cover educational time until x % of faculty are credentialed in the majority of core complications. This maybe kept as simple as a 1 year guaranteed stipend for procedural guidance alone since vascular access is the low hanging fruit and then renegotiating after that goal is met. If procedural guidance is the focus of year 1, it may be smart to bundle nurse training into the deal as additional support may come from the hospital as this is clearly high priority for the delivery of safe care. Placement of more peripheral lines may reduce number of central lines leading to an overall decrease in cost while ensuring safe patient care. The biggest challenge most community ultrasound directors eventually have to deal with is what happens when all the education and training of the group are completed. Can a stipend still be justified? The answer is yes. The common denominator between academic and community ultrasound director time requirements is quality assurance. As the credentialed physicians in the group start billing for studies there needs to be an even higher level of quality assurance in place. The one common denominator that ultrasound directors must accomplish in both academic and community settings is quality assurance. As physicians become credentialed they will begin documenting and billing for studies. A percentage of these exams will still need to be reviewed for ongoing quality and of course re-credentialing. Recommendations on numbers are given in the ACEP Ultrasound Guidelines.

Time spent performing quality assurance must be tracked and used as justification to community chairs to provide ongoing protected time even though the training period is over. In academic settings, there are new people to train every year as a new resident class starts and therefore ongoing protected time is granted regardless of QA volume. A common question in the community setting is how much protected time is fair to ask for. This varies depending on number of faculty in the group, baseline experience with ultrasound, and depth of ultrasound division. Is the ultrasound director a fresh residency grad or fellowship trained? One may be able to negotiate a higher salary, stipend and/or protected time with fellowship experience. If the ultrasound director is starting a new program from scratch, there is a lot more room for negotiation. It is important the community chair understands that before any billing can be done for ultrasound a critical mass of physicians must be trained. Furthermore, a solid infrastructure must be built from the ground up with heavy emphasis on front and back end workflow. Purchasing a machine is just the first step. How will findings be documented? How will consultants review images and reports? Who is responsible for ongoing machine maintenance? Who will perform daily checks that images are being transferred? Will there be a database for easy query for teaching and tracking purposes? All of this fall on the ultrasound director and will require significant time commitment. A solid infrastructure and critical mass of trained clinicians may take several years to build, so the chair must be ready to provide multiple years of support for the ultrasound director.

Importance of Workflow

The true power of ultrasound becomes evident when there is complete institutional transparency. It is important to diagnose a ruptured ectopic pregnancy within minutes of arrival to ED. But if the OB can't see the images in PACS or report in the EMR, will there still be delay in care? It would be great if consultants just took the clinicians at their word when it comes to ultrasound findings but the reality is they usually ask for "formal" Radiology studies. This is especially true in the community setting where many specialties do not have residents in house to see consults and need good objective reasoning to come in to see the patient in the middle of the night. It is important to recognize that Centers for Medicare and Medicaid Services (CMS) mandates minimal documentation requirements when performing diagnostic ultrasound in order to be considered for reimbursement.

An *ultrasound workflow system* generally involves software that allows bedside ultrasound studies to be retained, reviewed, feedback can be provided, and then be used for privileging, study documentation and billing. These new software programs perform these tasks in an electronic format that are consistent with the trend and direction of electronic medical records and "Meaningful Use" goals. Meaningful use is using certified electronic health record (EHR) technology to: Improve quality, safety, efficiency, and reduce health disparities. A workflow system differs from a Picture Archiving and Communication System (PACS) in many ways. In most hospitals, the PACS is currently being used to store studies done by credentialed providers for radiologist review. A new paradigm with POC US studies is that many new users must perform studies to obtain ultrasound privileges (credentialing). Therefore, it is commonplace to have a non-credentialed provider performing POC US studies for training purposes only, thereby putting those studies into a separate category. POC US studies also require a real-time interpretation of the study, followed by a peer review by a credentialed provider. The peer review component of POC US is essential given the new Joint Commission (JC) guidelines for Focused Provider Performance Evaluations and Ongoing Provider Performance Evaluations (FPPE and OPPE) respective to medical staff privileging and credentialing [4]. This same process of review can benefit all levels of users from those credentialed, seeking credentials, residents and other practitioners.

Regulatory bodies such as the Office of the National Coordinator of Health Information Technology (ONC-HIT) have begun recognizing the need for workflow systems through its focus on transferability and storage of radiologic imaging. This focus will only expand as healthcare information technology comes under additional scrutiny. The Center for Medicare and Medicaid Services (CMS) mandates that all ultrasound images must be stored for a minimum of 5 years—strengthening the need for a computer ultrasound study archiving system. Thermal paper prints are not storable for long periods of time, and do not provide information to adequately review and critique the study. US workflow systems are gradually being adopted in hospitals throughout the United States. The solution to the documentation, compliance, and regulatory aspects for the transparent integration of POC US is the adoption of **ultrasound workflow systems** (See Chap. 17 – Workflow and Middleware). Hospital IT is usually the rate-limiting step to workflow implementation as they are usually overwhelmed with other hospital IT jobs. This may change as hospitals are forced to demonstrate meaningful use of technology and may be a smart play for the ultrasound director to remind them of this to speed up the process. The author recommends setting up a meeting with the department chair, hospital IT leadership and the middleware vendor via webinar format during which the product features can be viewed and questions can be answered. Most hospital IT departments are concerned about slowing down the native EMR applications and HIPPA compliance. If there is still resistance or delay in implementation it may be necessary to meet with the hospital CEO to discuss the importance of a middleware or PACS system to facilitate image archival, documentation, reporting, and quality assurance of billed ultrasound studies being done by clinicians on a daily basis. You may be surprised how little hospital leadership knows about any imaging being done outside the confines of Radiology.

Role of Certification and Accreditation in Community Practice

Certification is an official document attesting to achievement of a level of training. In the past, physicians obtained certification from organizations outside their specialty in an effort to lend credibility to their training and skill. This seemed useful in the fledgling era of emergency ultrasound where many administrators were unfamiliar with physicians performing bedside ultrasound. Having a certificate that sonographer technicians achieved would add, many maintained, legitimacy. This was especially true in the community hospitals where few emergency physicians were trained in this modality during residency or were self-taught.

However, today's physicians are trained in point of care ultrasound, some receiving training as early as medical school. Specialties are establishing training guidelines for both residency and practice-based pathways for their physicians. For example, the ACEP Ultrasound Guidelines (first approved in June 2001 and currently in its 3rd update in June 2016) delineates the specific recommendations for an emergency physician to learn clinical ultrasound specific to its specialty. Since physicians practice within their own specialty, the respective national specialty organizations should be responsible for regulating their skill set and not rely on outside organizations to do so.

Physician specialties are developing methods for demonstrating excellence in ultrasound. Although not designed for physician individuals, ACEP supported the development of Clinical Ultrasound Accreditation Program (CUAP) to demonstrate that a program satisfies the quality requirements of the national specialty organization of emergency physicians. A program applies for CUAP accreditation through an online process attesting to key elements of their program such as machine maintenance, image retention, documentation, training, credentialing, and other components. This thorough method of substantiating a program's excellence is one of the best ways to further legitimize an already established skill clinicians use every day (See Chap. 21 – Accreditation in POC US).

Making Ultrasound an Effective Tool

A community hospital will have physicians with a broad span of ultrasound experience, ranging from no experience to those with considerable expertise. Each of these physicians has different needs. An ultrasound program should be able to address the various levels of ultrasound skills, as well as strive to achieve the ultimate goal of ensuring that every physician is at least competent in the core uses of ultrasound in their department. A computerized workflow solution is needed to assure that the volume, quality, and type of studies being done by each physician can be tracked and reviewed. This will give the ultrasound director the essential information required to help each individual physician develop and integrate ultrasound into his or her practice.

History tells us that most physicians in the community hospital, when left to their own accord, frequently fail to successfully integrate point of care ultrasound into their practices. Most fail in the experiential phase of learning ultrasound because of the lack of mentoring and teaching. Unlike academic institutions, community hospitals usually do not provide time set aside for training and education. Therefore, a conscious effort needs to be made to develop proctored scanning time, tailored to each physician's needs addressing: physician requests, deficiencies noted in quality review, and core competencies not yet developed or implemented. Implementing an educational program for the group by reviewing interesting cases, focused teaching on core ultrasound skills, and practice guidelines will help the physician group to integrate ultrasound successfully into their workflow. They also need to understand how taking the time to do an ultrasound will actually create more time for them by expediting patient flow. For example, the physician won't have patients waiting for hours for DVT studies or fetal viability verification.

Engaging the nursing staff is also important. They can be your greatest assets to promote US in the group and hospital. Nurses are often the first to recognize the disparity in patient care between physicians who can use ultrasound effectively and those who cannot. Recognizing the disparity, the nursing staff encourages the entire physician group to develop their ultrasound skills. Nurses can also be engaged in the ultrasound program by teaching them ultrasound guided vascular access. Optimally, to facilitate patient care and flow, the staff will recognize the opportunity to use ultrasound and have the machine in, or near, the room when the physician sees the patient.

Following Guidelines

There are established guidelines for point of care ultrasound programs, especially in Emergency Medicine. Unlike academic medicine, there is no mechanism in place to ensure that these guidelines are followed. If ultrasound is to be used in the care of patients, the medical community expects you to be competent in the acquisition and interpretation of ultrasound images and to be able to demonstrate that competency.

If US studies are done without patient and physician identifiers, they provide little, if any, value to the consulting physician. This will undermine the credibility of point of care ultrasound with the medical staff and administration. An ultrasound program needs to define and ensure quality and consistency among the physician group. Following established guidelines and protocols when setting up your ultrasound program is essential for this to happen. In Emergency Medicine, the ACEP Ultrasound Guidelines, Standard Reporting Guidelines, Ultrasound Compendium, and the Coding and Billing papers were developed to facilitate the appropriate use of point of care ultrasound. Following the guidelines is the short cut to building a quality program. If you follow these guidelines, you can face any credibility challenge with a solid foundation.

Conclusion

While clinical ultrasound remains pervasive among academic medical centers in this country, there continues to be a large void in community practice. Many ultrasound applications are considered standard of care and should be performed at every institution. But there are unique challenges to developing an ultrasound program in the community setting. These obstacles can be overcome by following a systematic approach built around commitment from a director and administration, adherence to established guidelines, and a smooth workflow process (Table 26.3).

Pitfalls

1. Failure to recognize that recommendations and guidelines used in academic centers translate well into community centers.
2. Failure to leverage procedural guidance as catalyst to start program.
3. Failure of chair to hold faculty accountable for lack of ultrasound performance and credentialing.
4. Failure to build solid workflow infrastructure prior to billing for ultrasound.
5. Lack of commitment from Hospital Administration and the Emergency Department group.

	Community ultrasound management action items
Table 26.3 Community ultrasound management action items	Department chair commitment
	Ultrasound director/lead financial support and shift buy down
	Machine purchase funding
	Feasible physician training plan/program
	Workflow solution integrated into plan from the onset, with plan for funds and implementation

Key Recommendations

1. The ultrasound director should attend a management course and/or a preceptorship if there is a training or experience gap.
2. Understand the unique challenges and efficiencies of community practice settings.
3. Integrate education, workflow, and reimbursement into the ultrasound program management plan.

References

1. Moore CL, Molina AA, Lin H. Ultrasonography in community emergency Departments in the United States: access to ultrasonography performed by consultants and status of emergency physician-performed ultrasonography. Ann Emerg Med. 2006;47(2):147–53. Epub 2005 Nov 21.
2. Sierzenski PJ, Geria R, O'Connor RE. Emergency physicians who use emergency ultrasound demonstrate higher patient charges, patients seen, and relative value units per hour when compared with colleagues who are rare or non-users of emergency ultrasound [abstract]. Acad Emerg Med. 2006;13(s5):193.
3. Budhram G, Elia T, Rathley N. Implementation of a successful incentive-based ultrasound credentialing program for emergency physicians. West J Emerg Med. 2013;14(6):602–8.
4. Ziaya et al. Joint Commission Blog: using OPPE as a performance improvement tool National Quality Forum (#0666) Ultrasound guidance for Internal Jugular central venous catheter placement, 2011.
5. Tayal et al. ACEP emergency ultrasound guidelines. 2008.

Chapter 27
Critical Care Medicine

Aliaksei Pustavoitau and Erik Su

Objectives

1. Discuss ultrasound management in an ICU setting, both adult and pediatric.
2. Understand the training and skill acquisition process typically encountered when building an ICU ultrasound program.
3. Discuss program infrastructure for an ICU ultrasound program.
4. Discuss available pathways to hospital credentialing and competency for ICU ultrasound program.

In this chapter, we describe ultrasound program building and management in Critical Care Medicine (CCM) based on up-to-date principles outlined in published statements, recommendations, and guidelines.

Ultrasound in CCM has been used extensively during the last several decades, with expansion largely attributable to the increasing portability of ultrasound machines, overall decrease in cost of equipment, development of guiding documents, and easy access to educational courses. American Medical Association (AMA) resolution 802 passed in 1999 [1], stating that ultrasound was within the scope of practice for appropriately trained physicians of varied disciplines, opened a door in the United States into widespread ultrasound use by specialties other than classically associated with ultrasound technology. As a body of knowledge, ultrasound in CCM was first summarized in two supplements to Critical Care Medicine in 2007 [2, 3]. Ongoing development of recommendation statements

A. Pustavoitau, MD, MHS (✉) • E. Su, MD
Department of Anesthesiology and Critical Care Medicine,
Johns Hopkins Hospital, Baltimore, MD, USA
e-mail: apustav1@jhmi.edu

© Springer International Publishing AG 2018   423
V. S. Tayal et al. (eds.), *Ultrasound Program Management*,
https://doi.org/10.1007/978-3-319-63143-1_27

included the American College of Chest Physicians (ACCP) and the Société de Réanimation de Langue Française (SRLF) publishing a Statement on Competence in Critical Care Ultrasonography [4] in 2009. Additionally, the World Interactive Network Focused on Critical Ultrasound (WINFOCUS) has provided guiding documents on the practice of Critical Care Echocardiography [5] and a group of experts representing 12 critical care societies worldwide have described training standards for Critical Care Ultrasonography [6], and specifically Advanced Critical Care Echocardiography [7]. In response to evolving body of literature, the Society of Critical Care Anesthesiologists (SOCCA) published recommendations for education in critical care ultrasound during formal training in critical care medicine [8]. Finally, the Ultrasound Certification Task Force on behalf of Society of Critical Care Medicine (SCCM) has developed comprehensive recommendations on competence and credentialing in Critical Care Ultrasound and Advanced Critical Care Echocardiography [9].

Progress in ultrasound in CCM has been relatively slow compared to some other medical specialties; this is largely due to a multitude of the United States and international critical care societies having variable approaches to ultrasound program development. There are additional discrepancies in terminology as one may notice in titles of documents; therefore in this chapter terminology consistent with SCCM recommendations [9] is used:

– Critical Care Ultrasound (CCUS) includes noncardiac ultrasound applications as well as focused cardiac ultrasound.
– Advanced Critical Care Echocardiography (ACCE) includes both focused cardiac ultrasound and advanced applications of echocardiography.

Applications

Ultrasound applications in CCM can be divided into diagnostic and procedural. In turn diagnostic applications can be subdivided into cardiac and noncardiac applications, and procedural applications can be divided into guidance for vascular access and other procedures requiring needle guidance. Commonly accepted core applications and potential applications for further development are summarized in Table 27.1. Classification is somewhat arbitrary; it is based partially on Statement by ACCP and SRLF [4] and on recommendations by SCCM [9].

While efforts have been made in the chapter to accurately summarize applications, ultrasound in CCM is very dynamic. As other applications are tested in the clinical arena, additional core applications will develop and become part of the armamentarium of the critical care provider.

In cardiac ultrasound, commonly used modalities include transthoracic (TTE) and transesophageal echocardiography (TEE). In some environments (e.g., cardiac surgical intensive care units) TEE is commonly used and both TTE and TEE are utilized in focused cardiac ultrasound and ACCE [4, 6–9]. The only caveat being that TEE as part of focused cardiac ultrasound should be performed on anesthetized, tracheally intubated patients only [9].

Table 27.1 Core and additional promising applications of ultrasound in CCM

Categories	Major areas	Applications
Diagnostic ultrasound	Cardiac ultrasound	Focused cardiac ultrasound[a]
		Advanced critical care echocardiography[b]
	Noncardiac ultrasound	Pleural ultrasound
		Pulmonary ultrasound
		Focused abdominal ultrasound
		Vascular ultrasound
Procedural ultrasound	Vascular access guidance	Central venous access guidance
		Arterial access guidance
		Peripheral venous access guidance
	Other procedures requiring needle guidance	Thoracentesis
		Pericardiocentesis
		Paracentesis
		Arthrocentesis
		Other procedures
Additional potential applications	Diagnostic ultrasound	Ophthalmic ultrasound
		Hepatic and biliary tree ultrasound
		Renal and urinary system ultrasound
	Procedural ultrasound	Airway management
		Regional anesthesia

[a, b]Both focused cardiac ultrasound and advanced critical care echocardiography may include use of transesophageal echocardiography in addition to transthoracic echocardiography

Education

Medical Knowledge

CCM Ultrasound is an imaging modality applied in conjunction with acquiring fundamental clinical knowledge of a patient, in particular, hemodynamic and respiratory data. We emphasize the use of CCUS and ACCE only in the context of a clinical situation after collecting patient history, performing a physical examination integrating information from other diagnostic tests and studies. Clinical competence in caring for critically ill patient is paramount, therefore critical care providers should have completed their primary specialty education and received adequate training in care of critically ill and/or injured patients in order to employ ultrasound in the ICU [9].

Pathways

When specifically discussing education and training in ultrasound, we acknowledge the existence of two pathways: fellowship-based and practice-based. A fellowship-based pathway is best suited for postgraduate trainees. In this paradigm the trainee achieves competence in ultrasound either as part of CCM training, or completes an ultrasound fellowship [9]. CCM providers already in practice can train in ultrasound while continuing their normal clinical activities under supervision of an ultrasound educator. Providers should obtain 20 h (for CCUS) or 40 h (for ACCE) of AMA PRA Category 1 continuing medical education credits or their equivalent [6, 7, 9]. Credits should also be obtained while acquiring practical experience in ultrasound. Additionally, it is expected that providers in either pathway perform an adequate number of examinations to achieve competence (detailed under section "Skills Acquisition").

Ultrasound Knowledge and Skills

Practice of both CCUS and ACCE involves skills of ultrasound technician for adequate image acquisition and knowledge of a specialist to interpret the image. Both CCUS and ACCE share similar knowledge base and skills in general aspects of ultrasound as described in Table 27.2.

Table 27.2 Knowledge and skills common to both CCUS and ACCE

Domain	Descriptions
Knowledge	Physical principles of ultrasound image formation and pulse-wave, continuous, and color Doppler
	Artifacts and pitfalls
	Operation of ultrasound machines, including controls and transducers
	Equipment handling, infection control, and electrical safety
	Data management, including image storage, integration with hospital image management systems, reporting, quality assurance process
	Ergonomics of performing an ultrasound exam in the intensive care unit environment
	Indications, contraindications, limitations, and potential complications of CCUS and ACCE
	Normal ultrasound anatomy of evaluated organ system and surrounding structures
	Standard windows and views for each ultrasound application
Skills	Recognize common ultrasound artifacts (e.g., reverberation, side lobe, mirror image)
	Operate ultrasound machines and utilize their controls to optimize image quality
	Ability to differentiate normal from markedly abnormal anatomic structures and their function
	Ability to perform systematic ultrasound evaluation at the anatomic location of interest and organ system of interest and surrounding structures
	Ability to select an appropriate transducer for a given ultrasound examination
	Ability to communicate ultrasound findings to other healthcare providers, the medical record, and patients
	Recognize when consultation with other specialists is necessary
	Ability to recognize complications of various critical care ultrasound applications

CCUS critical care ultrasound (includes focused cardiac ultrasound), *ACCE* advanced critical care echocardiography

Because CCUS and ACCE differ in complexity of both knowledge and skills, they are reviewed separately in this chapter. Table 27.3 describes core applications of CCUS and is based on the Statement by the ACCP and SRLF [4], SOCCA recommendations [8], and on recommendations by SCCM [9]. Unlike the ACCP and SRLF statement [4], abdominal ultrasound applications (hepatic and biliary ultrasound, renal and urinary system ultrasound, assessment of large vessels) are not included, and they are classified as potential

Table 27.3 Core applications of CCUS and knowledge and skills required for successful execution of corresponding application

CCUS applications	Knowledge	Skills
Focused cardiac ultrasound	Normal ultrasound anatomy and sizes of the heart structures, major blood vessels and surrounding anatomic structures	Ability to differentiate normal from markedly abnormal heart structures and function
		Ability to identify signs of chronic cardiac disease
	Standard windows and views[a]	Ability to perform TTE, insert a TEE probe and perform TEE in an anesthetized, tracheally intubated patient[b]
	Integration with other modalities of cardiopulmonary monitoring	Ability to incorporate ultrasound examinations in the bedside management of critically ill or injured patients in shock
	Identify abnormal atrial size, and manifestations of severe valvular abnormalities	Ability to recognize grossly obvious valvular lesions and dysfunction
	Identify abnormal right and left ventricular size and systolic function	Ability to recognize marked changes in global left systolic function
	Identify large pericardial effusion/ tamponade and understand limitations of ultrasound in diagnosis of tamponade	Ability to detect significant pericardial effusions
	Understand ultrasound manifestations of septic shock	Ability to assess the entire spectrum of cardiovascular abnormalities in patient with shock
	Understand ultrasound manifestations of severe hypovolemia and limitations of assessment of "volume status" with ultrasound	Ability to recognize severe hypovolemia
	Estimation of central venous pressure and understand limitations of ultrasound estimation	Ability to evaluate size and variation in size of IVC to approximate central venous pressure
	Incorporation into ACLS protocols	Ability to meaningfully incorporate TTE/ TEE in patient resuscitation without interfering with ACLS protocols or interrupting chest compressions

(continued)

Table 27.3 (continued)

CCUS applications	Knowledge	Skills
Pleural ultrasound	Understand ultrasound manifestations of pneumothorax and understanding of the limitation in diagnosis of pneumothorax	Ability to rule out and to rule in pneumothorax
	Understand ultrasound characterization of pleural effusion and limitations of ultrasound evaluation	Ability to assess pleural effusion characteristics: Size, location, degree of loculation
Pulmonary ultrasound	Understand ultrasound manifestations of lung consolidation	Ability to assess consolidated lung
	Understand ultrasound manifestations of extravascular lung water	Ability to assess alveolar/ interstitial syndrome
Focused abdominal ultrasound	Understand ultrasound characterization of intraabdominal fluid and limitations of ultrasound evaluation	Ability to assess intraabdominal fluid characteristics: Size, location, volume, presence of debris septae
Vascular ultrasound	Understand ultrasound manifestations of large DVT in femoral veins	Ability to recognize large DVT in femoral veins
Procedural ultrasound	Principles of needle/wire guidance with ultrasound for bedside procedures, including vascular access, thoracentesis, paracentesis, etc.	Ability to guide bedside procedures with ultrasound (e.g., vascular access, thoracentesis, paracentesis)

CCUS critical care ultrasound (includes focused cardiac ultrasound), *ACLS* advanced cardiac life support, *TTE* transthoracic echocardiography, *TEE* transesophageal echocardiography, *IVC* inferior vena cava, *DVT* deep venous thrombosis
[a]Both TTE and TEE windows and views as required by specific needs of a provider
[b]TEE is required only for providers with specific needs in their patients

future applications, because as mentioned in recommendations by the SCCM [9] the critical care community does not universally use them.

Table 27.4 describes knowledge and skills required for successful execution of ACCE.

There are naturally other additional potential future applications, as some are performed at select centers depending on their practitioners' skillsets and needs.

Skills Acquisition

While there is no number of ultrasound examinations that definitively ensure competence, currently available guidance documents in critical care provide some numeric targets. The targets are based either on expert consensus opinion [6, 7] or on standards in emergency medicine [10] and anesthesiology [11]. In fact, documents from these specialties require the same number of performed echocardiographic examinations: 30 examinations for basic cardiac ultrasound and 200 for ACCE. A difference between the statements is that the SCCM recommendations require examinations to be interpreted in addition to ones personally performed:

Table 27.4 Knowledge and skills required for successful execution ACCE

Knowledge	Skills
Comprehensive TTE and/ or TEE views	Ability to perform comprehensive TTE/ TEE exam
Qualitative and quantitative echocardiography	Ability to quantify flows and pressures across various cardiac chambers
Heart-lung interactions in spontaneously breathing and mechanically ventilated patients	Ability to acquire comprehensive hemodynamic data
Diseases of the heart relevant to care of critically ill or injured patients (e.g., dynamic left ventricular outflow tract obstruction, systolic anterior motion of the mitral valve)	
Normal and abnormal left ventricular systolic function, including segmental wall motion abnormalities	Ability to quantify systolic left ventricular function
Normal and abnormal left ventricular diastolic function	Ability to quantify diastolic left ventricular function
Normal and abnormal right ventricular function	Ability to quantify right ventricular systolic function
Commonly encountered complications of acute coronary syndrome	Ability to recognize subtle left ventricular wall motion abnormalities, and evaluate complications of acute coronary syndrome
Valve dysfunction and its hemodynamic consequences	Ability to quantify normal and abnormal native and prosthetic valvular function
Tamponade physiology	Ability to evaluate hemodynamic consequences of pericardial effusion and tamponade
Comprehensive evaluation of fluid responsiveness	Ability to assess fluid responsiveness in spontaneously breathing and mechanically ventilated patients using validated dynamic indices of preload
Anatomy, physiology, and implications of intracardiac and intrapulmonary shunts	Ability to assess for the presence of intracardiac and intrapulmonary shunts
Echocardiographic manifestations of intracardiac masses and thrombi	Ability to assess for intracardiac masses and thrombi
Detailed knowledge of other diagnostic modalities relevant in hemodynamic management of critically ill or injured patients	Ability to recognize limitations of ACCE and identify additional diagnostic modalities necessary for the management of a critically ill patient

ACCE advanced critical care echocardiography

total of 50 for basic cardiac ultrasound and total of 400 for ACCE (these numbers including examinations personally performed). The SCCM recommendations also specify targets for diagnostic noncardiac CCUS:

- Twenty examinations performed for pleural and pulmonary ultrasound, with total of 30 examinations interpreted.
- Twenty examinations performed for limited abdominal ultrasound, with total of 30 examinations interpreted.
- Twenty examinations performed for vascular ultrasound, with total of 30 examinations interpreted.

In regard to procedural ultrasound, vascular access guidance (central venous access in particular) is the most fundamental needle guidance skill; achieving competence requires at least 10 personally performed ultrasound-guided procedures. Once vascular access guidance skills are acquired, any additional needle guidance procedure (thoracentesis, paracentesis, pericardiocentesis, and others) requires five additional ultrasound-guided performances.

Certification

The general consensus in critical care medicine community is that CCUS does not require certification to establish competence in its applications. ACCE, on the other hand, is a more complex application and requires certification [6, 7, 9]. Certification involves an external agency validating competence through a set of requirements. This commonly involves an examination. Currently, there is no established certification process in ACCE, and the SCCM recommends achieving certification status in the National Board of Echocardiography's examination of special competence in adult echocardiography (ASCeXAM) or perioperative transesophageal echocardiography (advanced or basic PTEeXAM), until an ACCE-specific process is developed.

Credentialing and Maintenance

Credentialing is the process of qualifying providers as competent for performance of certain skills within the scope of practice of medical staff in a given health system. The process of credentialing requires an institutional commitment to document the ultrasound activities of practitioners and structure their clinical conduct with regard to the technology. Credentialing standards will naturally differ by institution, and can range from informal agreements between institutional departments to requirements for practical and didactic education, certification, as well as requirements for ongoing education. See Chapter 20–Credentialing and Privileging.

A baseline of mandatory didactic and practical education, followed by proctored scanning has been pioneered by specialties such as emergency medicine and is mentioned above. Such a regimen is easily translated to the ICU arena in institutions where emergency medicine providers already have an established program in point-of-care ultrasound. However in other hospital systems where clinical imaging is predominated by other specialties which may use and teach ultrasound primarily practically in clinical settings, such as urology, the landscape may differ. In settings where credentialing requirements are less structured, a greater level of specialty collaboration is necessary for prompt study verification. Ultimately a mutually accepted agreement on credentialing standards (with or without concrete requirements) is useful and necessary for determining when clinicians are ready to perform ultrasound in CCM practice environments.

Maintenance of skills is also relevant for ongoing practice in terms of skill upkeep and reception of new developments in the field. Little is published on what degree of ongoing training is necessary among ICU providers, though some have proposed recommendations such as World Interactive Network Focused on Critical Ultrasound. The WINFOCUS echocardiography recommendation statement [5] advises that advanced echocardiography providers perform at least 50 studies per year. We recommend 100 ultrasound examinations per year, 50 of which are CCUS examinations and 50 ACCE examinations (including 20 TEE examinations of ongoing competence in TEE is desired) for maintenance of certification, in line with SCCM recommendations [9]. We also recommend ongoing education in ultrasound, which includes at least 10 h of CME credits annually or their equivalents, or other ultrasound-related activities in CCUS and ACCE [9]. As standards at this time remain elusive, it is likely that they will continue to evolve to meet demands. If certification becomes a part of CCUS credentialing, existing certification for the ASCeXAM and PTEeXAM occur on a 10-year cycle requiring periodic follow-up.

Program Infrastructure

Program Director

Ultimately a director of a CCUS program serves as advocate for a program and implementation of ultrasound in the ICU. Though little has been published on this topic, the director ultimately supervises primary program objectives. He is responsible for interacting with other specialties using ultrasound, overseeing quality assurance, and introduces novel technology to the critical care environment. The following are areas where a director and other members of an ultrasound program may invest time, though this is not an exclusive list (Chap. 2).

Management of Equipment and Practical Material Needs

A director is a key stakeholder in management of an effective ultrasound fleet. This involves both ongoing maintenance and new procurement. Since the success of a program depends on utility of the technology, a director of an ultrasound program should be assured the equipment is performing adequately at least every week by a personal visit or subsidiary, and verify whether consumables important for machine operation, such as gel and appropriate cleaning materials, are adequate. This is important, particularly if a machine needs to be taken out of service for an easily missed, potential patient hazard such as a cracked transducer housing or battery failure. A director also should be centrally involved in new ultrasound equipment purchases for the ICU as this person will bring to the table an intimate knowledge of ultrasound use and ongoing needs important for machine selection. In this sense a director should also advocate for responsible billing of ultrasound services.

Supervision of Ultrasound Use Including Image Archiving

Image archiving is also important in program administration from the standpoint of appropriate documentation, education, and quality assurance. A director can directly or indirectly supervise the archiving of images from ultrasound devices. Management of the archive gives the director a comprehensive perspective of departmental ultrasound use and needs. In addition image review can highlight areas of individual or group education, as well as areas to improve ultrasound use that could be rectified with protocols for machine use or new equipment. A well-managed archive facilitates credentialing of staff and trainees for their future program, and justifies ongoing use to administration.

Coordination of Quality Assurance Activities

The Program Director is accountable for the overall conduct of ultrasound activities in the ICU and therefore has a vested interest in coordinating quality assurance activities. These activities are detailed in section "Quality Assurance" below.

Structuring of Ultrasound Education in the ICU

A director does not need to be the unit expert on ultrasound however should be familiar with all equipment and technological processes involved in the typical ICU ultrasound workflow as the director will often be called upon to remedy problems. Organized education facilitates a common knowledge base and dialogue within the department on ultrasound, and helps maintain a minimum standard for ultrasound services (Chaps. 5 and 6).

Representation of Program to Other Institutional Structures Both Administrative and Clinical

This includes interaction with other imaging specialties that are both primarily decision-makers at the bedside (Emergency Medicine, Inpatient Medicine) and diagnostic (Diagnostic Radiology, Neurophysiology). As an advocate for the program, it is essential that the director speaks on behalf of the program to extradepartmental entities when interdepartment discussions are necessary for advice, collaboration, or issue resolution. In addition the director works with department entities on accounting for program activities and requests for departmental support. This is essential in defining the role the program plays within the medical center.

Research Protocol Implementation

The director or designates may also play a role in assurance of clinically responsible research in line with institutional ethical protocols, and also does not endanger patients, the program, or its equipment. In this role the director may coordinate use of machines in research balancing existing knowledge on research topics, safe utilization, and support of ICU staff pursuing scientific questions.

Equipment

The capabilities of ultrasound machines assigned to an ICU depend on available support, needs of the ICU, and practitioner ability to utilize resources well. We summarized recommendations on ultrasound equipment for ICU in Table 27.5. See Chapter 12–Ultrasound Equipment and Purchase.

A machine should facilitate documentation of ultrasound activities with image recording and patient identifiers. It should also be portable and maneuverable at the ICU bedside even in congested situations. A battery is not always included in some higher end machines, but this is useful for moving the machines in cramped or rapidly changing quarters. Since a machine may see every room in the ICU regularly, easy device sanitization is also required. A rapid startup time is also an asset in the ICU.

Table 27.5 Suggested machine capabilities based on basic and advanced applications

Categories	Basic equipment	Advanced equipment
General machine attributes	1. General clinical use US machine capable of 2D imaging	1. Advanced US machine capable of diagnostic imaging accuracy (devices marketed for diagnostic imaging specialties)
	2. Ability to store patient specific imaging with identifiers	2. Wireless image transmission
	3. Standard output file formats for offline visualization	3. DICOM format output
	4. Battery that lasts ≥30 min	
	5. Maneuverability at ICU bedside	
	6. Sanitizable for infectious exposures	
	7. Rapid startup time < 2 min	
Cardiac ultrasound	1. Low-frequency phased array probe	1. Additional smaller phased array probes
	2. Color flow and pulsed-wave Doppler	2. Transesophageal echocardiography probe
	3. M-mode	3. Pedoff Doppler probe
		4. Continuous wave Doppler
		5. Echocardiography post-processing software
		6. EKG leads
Airway, pulmonary, and vascular or drainage procedural ultrasound	1. Linear array transducer with ~8–11 MHz center frequency, ~3–5 cm face length	1. High frequency linear array probe with >12 MHz center frequency, "hockey stick" or standard linear array
	2. Color flow and pulsed-wave Doppler (procedural)	2. Microconvex array probe
		3. Power Doppler (procedural)

(continued)

Table 27.5 (continued)

Categories	Basic equipment	Advanced equipment
Abdominal ultrasound	1. Curvilinear transducer with low center frequency	1. Microconvex array probe
		2. Power Doppler
Neurological ultrasound	1. Low-frequency phased array probe	1. Transcranial Doppler apparatus
	2. Linear array transducer with face length < 4 cm for eye	2. Microconvex array probe
	3. Ability to adjust US transmission power	
Regional anesthesia	1. Linear array transducer with ~8–11 MHz center frequency, ~3–5 cm face length	1. High frequency linear array probe with >12 MHz center frequency, "hockey stick" or standard linear array
		2. Linear array transducer with face length > 4 cm
		3. Microconvex array probe

Details of what each core application entails are included in section "Ultrasound Knowledge"
Both focused cardiac ultrasound and advanced critical care echocardiography may include use of transesophageal echocardiography in addition to transthoracic echocardiography

Advanced machine capabilities include advanced quantitative metrics useful for documentation and research. Wireless image transmission and DICOM format output also facilitate transfer of information to data storage systems and simplify ultrasound workflow.

With regard to cardiac imaging, a low-frequency phased array transducer is essential for echocardiography and most devices leverage rapid framerate 2D and Doppler-based imaging at the expense of image resolution to optimize images through the cardiac cycle. As practitioners expand their ultrasound acumen, advanced echocardiographic measures may require specialized equipment such as an array of smaller echocardiographic probes for difficult imaging. Additional applications require special probes such as transesophageal or Pedoff probes. Accurate characterization of systole and diastole for echocardiographic analysis benefits from ECG tracing. Finally, advanced post-processing may be helpful for quantitative assessment for clinical and research purposes.

Airway, pulmonary, and procedural ultrasound may seem disparate applications but benefit from similar probes. Visualization of the pleural line, trachea, as well as procedural applications both benefit from accurate near-field visualization of surface structures less than a centimeter below the surface. A linear array probe is well suited for these purposes. Advanced applications in these arenas also require similar probes. A high frequency linear array enhances near-field visualization further, and in particular a "hockey-stick" style transducer can be used for submental or light pressure assessments of the airway in addition to difficult peripheral access. A microconvex array can be used to visualize near-field structures in a fan-like sector if imaging windows are limited. This may be helpful in small or contracted patients for both pulmonary and vascular applications. Doppler functions are useful for procedural applications for identifying vessels to puncture in the case of vascular access, and to avoid in the case of paracentesis and pericardiocentesis. Color Doppler functions may also be useful in pleural ultrasound for characterization of pleural effusion.

Though abdominal imaging can be performed using a phased array transducer, a low center frequency curvilinear array is a mainstay of abdominal imaging due to its large face and low-frequency imaging which optimizes deep structure resolution at the expense of framerate. At times the size of a large curvilinear may preclude imaging of a small patient. In these cases a smaller curvilinear probe or a microconvex array are useful. Power Doppler is also useful in this population for imaging perfusion of organ vessel beds where vascular flow occurs in multiple directions relative to the probe simultaneously and direction effects are minimized by the modality.

Regional anesthesia is similar to procedural ultrasound with regard to requiring good near-field imaging with a linear or microconvex array. However given that the majority of these procedures are performed with long-axis needle visualization, transducer face length is an important consideration as inappropriate transducer sizing can limit needle excursion for the procedure. Therefore a variety of long and short, low and high frequency linear probes are useful. In addition curvilinear probes are useful for long-axis insertion in areas limited by imaging window size.

These recommendations also do not speak to the number of devices a unit may require. Indeed, this is primarily based on utilization and is not predictable based on strict unit characteristics. As such, procurement of an ultrasound fleet is usually piecemeal based upon demand from clinical services and caregivers. One important consideration is whether a machine's use should be distributed geographically across multiple units. This introduces additional issues in machine availability and is likely not helpful for an ICU environment.

Equipment management should incorporate regular assessment of ultrasound devices by the director or designates. These assessments should verify safety and readiness of the equipment for use with patients including clearing infectious and electrical hazards.

Data Management

Components for ultrasound documentation recommended by the American Institute of Ultrasound in Medicine include:

1. Patient's name and other identifying information (usually date of birth and medical record number)
2. Facility information
3. Date of examination
4. Image orientation when appropriate
5. In addition, worksheet-based formats may also include exam type, clinically relevant information, examination requested, name of clinical provider if applicable

As such, responsible image recording may be limited by workflow complexity at the bedside and a concerted effort is required unit-wide to ensure responsible image accounting. Measures to improve accounting may include mandatory report states within the machine requiring operator login, barcode readers, and reminders to clinical staff to appropriately document studies. Importantly imaging studies for procedures require an image visualizing needle placement within the target of interest.

Imaging data should be treated as protected health information and stored within protected institutional data systems. In particular name-identifiable patient images are easily disseminated and have at times made their way to medical textbooks, so practitioners should be extremely cautious about transferring files. If possible, corruption resistant storage systems with data duplication (such as mirrored servers or Redundant Array of Independent Disks [RAID] storage systems) are advisable. Ultimately, because the data includes protected health information it should be optimally maintained on a hospital-based protected system.

An appropriate indexing system includes patient identifiers, study type and indication, and should also incorporate operator identifiers for the purpose of training, quality assurance, and credentialing. A number of solutions for this range between directory-based cataloging of images, media management software allowing multiple attributes to be attached to images for further analysis, and radiology file management software that usually provides a comprehensive solution including mass file transfer from devices (Chaps. 17 and 18).

Quality Assurance

Periodic review of program activities and images is fundamental to ensuring good care delivery with ultrasound. A process of quality assurance review should be supervised by the program director but may take form in multiple ways. Involved parties should naturally involve ultrasound operators and other skilled providers. These providers may include individuals from within the critical care division as well as imaging experts from other disciplines such as radiology, cardiology, and vascular imaging, among others. Targets for review should include second read verification of ultrasound interpretation by novices, periodic review of selected images from credentialed providers, and interesting cases for which a second read is useful.

Meetings should be conducted with regularity dependent on volume of studies to review and personnel availability. Review can be performed in large group meetings with other imaging specialists, or in smaller settings on a one-to-one basis as long as a documentable process for reviewed studies is in place (Chap. 16).

Conclusion

Establishing an ultrasound program in the critical care setting should facilitate provision of ultrasound services in the unique environment of the ICU. Such a process is similar to other examples in the emergency medicine and inpatient medicine settings, with particular attention towards advanced cardiac and pulmonary imaging. With ongoing ultrasound development, more nuances pertaining to ultrasound use in the ICU will likely develop. Thoughtful construction of a program will allow for adaptation of new modalities and further evolution of ultrasound within critical care medicine.

Pitfalls

1. Failure to establish proper infrastructure can significantly limit ICU ultrasound program development and growth.
2. Lack of proper data management can lead to improper storage of sensitive information and inability to perform quality assurance reviews.
3. An inadequate number of ultrasound machines, especially if shared across multiple locations or units can lead to lack of availability when need is critical.
4. Not paying attention to intradepartmental and facility needs which could be addressed by or raised by ultrasound may limit program support and growth.
5. Not tracking programs directors time and resource utilization may make it harder to prove the need for support to administration.

Key Recommendations

1. Quality assurance and improvement should be planned for and set up whenever an ultrasound program in an ICU is being considered.
2. Plan for ultrasound utilization and the number of machines required to limit unavailability.
3. Work with administration to maintain program support and funding.
4. Pay attention to the needs of the department, program and hospital to expand upon programs utility and support.

References

1. American Medical Association. Privileging for Ultrasound Imaging.;H-230.960 (Res. 802, I-99; Reaffirmed: Sub. Res. 108, A-00; Reaffirmed: CMS Rep. 6, A-10).
2. Critical Care Medicine. Critical Care Medicine: echocardiography in intensive care medicine. Crit Care Med. 2007;35(8)(Suppl):S123–S307.
3. Critical Care Medicine. Critical Care Medicine: focused applications of ultrasound in critical care medicine. Crit Care Med. 2007;35(5)(Suppl):309–433.
4. Mayo PH, Beaulieu Y, Doelken P, et al. American College of Chest Physicians/la Societe de reanimation de langue Francaise statement on competence in critical care ultrasonography. Chest. 2009;135(4):1050–60. doi:10.1378/chest.08-2305.
5. Price S, Via G, Sloth E, et al. Echocardiography practice, training and accreditation in the intensive care: document for the World Interactive Network Focused on Critical Ultrasound (WINFOCUS). Cardiovasc Ultrasound. 2008;6:49. doi:10.1186/1476-7120-6-49.

6. Expert Round Table on Ultrasound in ICU. International expert statement on training standards for critical care ultrasonography. Intensive Care Med. 2011;37(7):1077–83. doi:10.1007/s00134-011-2246-9; 10.1007/s00134-011-2246-9.

7. Expert Round Table on Echocardiography in ICU. International consensus statement on training standards for advanced critical care echocardiography. Intensive Care Med. 2014;40(5):654–66. doi:10.1007/s00134-014-3228-5.

8. Fagley RE, Haney MF, Beraud AS, et al. Critical care basic ultrasound learning goals for American anesthesiology critical care trainees: recommendations from an expert group. Anesth Analg. 2015;120(5):1041–53. doi:10.1213/ANE.0000000000000652.

9. Pustavoitau A, Blaivas M, Brown SM, et al. Recommendations for Achieving and Maintaining Competence and Credentialing in Critical Care Ultrasound with Focused Cardiac Ultrasound and Advanced Critical Care Echocardiography. http://journals.lww.com/ccmjournal/Documents/Critical%20Care%20Ultrasound.pdf. Accessed 15 Feb 2015.

10. American College of Emergency Physicians. Emergency ultrasound guidelines. Ann Emerg Med. 2009;53(4):550–70. doi:10.1016/j.annemergmed.2008.12.013; 10.1016/j.annemergmed.2008.12.013.

11. Cahalan MK, Abel M, Goldman M, et al. American Society of Echocardiography and Society of Cardiovascular Anesthesiologists task force guidelines for training in perioperative echocardiography. Anesth Analg. 2002;94(6):1384–8.

Chapter 28
Primary Care

Apostololos P. Dallas

Objectives

- Introduce the unique challenges in implementing a primary care office-based ultrasound program
- Review physician educational needs required to establish a program
- Promote a pattern of education that produces a gradual acceptance of primary care US
- Suggest a method for computing return-on-investment for US machine purchases
- Discuss barriers and pitfalls in managing a primary care program

Introduction

While clinical ultrasonography, variously termed bedside ultrasonography, hand-held ultrasonography, portable ultrasonography, and point-of-care ultrasonography, has found many clinical uses and early acceptance as a valuable tool in emergency medicine, critical care, anesthesia, surgery, obstetrics, and gynecology, the specialties of internal medicine and family medicine, in general, have only recently begun to utilize this tool. Hospital use of point-of-care ultrasonography is quickly gaining traction. However, clinical ultrasonography in the primary care office setting, with its unique challenges, has yet to attain common let alone, generalized use. Literature supporting use of ultrasound in the primary care office setting is scarce and

A.P. Dallas, MD, FACP, CHCP
Department of Internal Medicine, Virginia Tech Carilion School of Medicine and Research Institute, Roanoke, VA, USA
e-mail: apdallas@carilionclinic.org

© Springer International Publishing AG 2018
V. S. Tayal et al. (eds.), *Ultrasound Program Management*,
https://doi.org/10.1007/978-3-319-63143-1_28

concerns about appropriate use remain. In this chapter, we will describe experiences at a medical school affiliated internal medicine office-based practice as an example and perhaps a model for developing, maintaining, and managing a clinical ultrasound program in the primary care office setting.

Needs Assessment

Since the material in this management book is not easily researched, found in textbooks or referenced, practical experience of primary care US, gained over years of championing outpatient US in the primary care setting will be shared in this chapter.

The outpatient physician–patient interaction is often one that contains a good deal of uncertainty. Diagnoses and therapeutic decisions surrounding those diagnoses are often arrived over a period of several visits, labs and imaging ordered sequentially and not concurrently as in the hospital medicine. An ambulatory clinic-based physician may need to be comfortable with diagnostic uncertainty from visit to visit, prior to diagnostic certainty, if that actually ever happens. So the advent of point-of-care ultrasound can buttress physician decisions. Just as in inpatient settings where the use of ultrasound can change physician decisions, pilot studies have shown the clinical impact of ultrasound in the ambulatory setting can be significant. In one study, medical decisions were reinforced in 76% of patients and changed in 40% of patient encounters based on the use of ultrasound devices [1]. While this study was conducted in 2006, over a decade has elapsed and primary care has still lagged behind in US usage. Noncardiac point-of-care ultrasound by nonradiologist physicians is not widespread in primary care. In one study evaluating Medicare Part B Physician Supplier Procedure Master files, in 2009 alone, utilization rates of 425 Medicare noncardiac ultrasound examinations per 1000 beneficiaries showed that only 11% were performed by primary care physicians [2]. From 2004 to 2009, there was relatively little growth in utilization rates among primary care physicians. A limitation of the study was that it could not account for the possible ultrasound use in informal, non-billed manners. While the American Medical Association has declared that each medical specialty should define its own requirement in training in ultrasound [3] and other national organizations, emergency medicine for instance, have promulgated guidelines for US training and use, internal medicine and family medicine organizations have remained silent in this regard. The members of these organizations have voiced their desire to be taught. In 2011, the American College of Physicians (ACP) Clinical Skills committee reviewed feedback from participants in the previous national meeting. Five out of the top 11 most requested topics for educational needs were ultrasound based, echocardiography, abdominal ultrasound, vascular ultrasound, etc. The ACP has responded by offering more ultrasound education at both national and state meetings.

Other ambulatory setting practices have been evaluated with respect to US attitudes and utilization. Geriatricians in South Carolina were surveyed to determine their willingness to adopt the technology and willingness to educate physicians and medical students and to identify hurdles for implementation in the clinical and educational environment [4]. Most physicians (92.8%) had heard of bedside portable US and 21.4% had previous formal training. Only one out of 18 physicians felt comfortable using the machine and none felt ready to instruct other medical staff or students. Most of the participating group (71–85%) expressed an interest in learning this new skill. Sports medicine physicians are recognizing the utility of ultrasound for their specialty beyond the musculoskeletal system and are advocating expansion of its use in the athlete to diagnose pulmonary, cardiac, solid organ, intra-abdominal, and eye injuries [5]. Limited abdominal ultrasound has been used to follow splenomegaly in athletes with mononucleosis and to determine regression of splenomegaly prior to returning to competition [6].

In the family practice setting, a group of general practitioners were able to perform assessments of left ventricular function that were comparable to cardiologist examinations after only minimal training [7]. Another study, looking at rural family physicians, showed that abdominal aortic aneurysm screening can be safely performed in the office [8]. This screening test can be completed with the time constraints of a busy family practice office visit, with a mean time to screen of 212 seconds (95% CI 194–230). Military family physicians in the clinic setting, inpatient wards and potentially military-deployed settings found pocket-sized devices easy to use, valuable in discerning a diagnosis and were not prohibitively time consuming [9]. In fact, although not measured, physicians felt it actually decreased the overall time required to make a diagnosis. In addition, patients were perceived by participants to have been satisfied with the use of the device.

Practical Considerations

The author's experience, in a comprehensive hospital and outpatient system comprising over 80 outpatient practices and 8 hospitals, the largest, an 826 bed tertiary care center in Southwest Virginia, may be illustrative. At Virginia Tech Carilion School of Medicine (VTC), a recent expansion in clinical departments, residency and fellowship educational programs and an increase in patient demand led to novel approaches in delivering care and teaching learners. In this setting of educational and clinical growth, the Internal Medicine outpatient department served a vital role in educating students, internal medicine residents, and physician colleagues in continuing medical education activities.

In 2006, Carilion Clinic Continuing Medical Education (CME) began offering some of the first courses in portable US for critical care. Because of their significant expertise, the faculty teaching in these local courses were invited to plan and teach courses at national critical care conferences. Since one of the co-chairs of these local conferences is an internal medicine physician, the natural progression was to develop and offer conferences to address the US needs of hospitalists and eventually primary care doctors. Since their inception, over 700 clinicians have received CME training in portable ultrasonography.

To complement their education, starting in 2010 the first year medical students began a 4 year longitudinal US curriculum. In 2014 this curriculum included US-guided procedure didactics and model-based hands-on experience. The CME US offerings as well as the students' experience with US lead to resident interest and in 2011, the Internal Medicine Residency program began requiring internal medicine interns to attend a 24 hour US Boot Camp. This camp involved the standard physics, knobs, echo, abdomen, and vascular US instruction as well as US-guided procedure training. In addition to this Camp experience, lectures and hands-on US sessions were conducted throughout the year on musculoskeletal, small parts, sinuses, lymph nodes, and other lumps and bumps.

Our internal medicine clinic's use of ultrasound began in the above environment and seemed to be a natural organic growth of US from the inpatient to the outpatient setting. Some experiences became lessons that were key in establishing and managing this program.

Early accepters of disruptive technology often find challenges others may not face. Our earliest efforts to incorporate US in clinical ambulatory medicine met with skepticism. Some physicians reported, in CME evaluations, that US was exciting but doubted its widespread application. Others recognized the need to learn it, as students and residents would be trained beyond the supervisor's ability to supervise or teach the learners. The following lessons were learned:

1. A physician champion must be identified. This should be an internist with either expertise in US or a desire to learn US. The physician champion would be the communicator of all issues dealing with US acting as a bridge between the clinicians, administrators, and other learners. This person should be prepared to meet resistance when advocating for US in the primary care setting. While we have several US machines in our internal medicine clinics, other family medicine clinics have had more difficult times convincing administration that these machines were necessary and this despite disseminating literature touting US in the ambulatory setting. The physician champion should have a ready supply of references to support US. Using some of the ones in this book could prove fruitful. An "elevator talk," a standard two minute, 6 sentence explanation of the utility of US, should be available to the champion. This talk can serve as an enthusiasm-generating micro-educational interlude that can be delivered even as an elevator is traveling between floors. Physicians have precious little time and to be able to expose them to some new information quickly is welcomed and much appreciated.

2. The physician champion must then enlist the support of a champion in hospital administration. Mutual understanding of clinical issues (patient care, physician workload, etc.) and administrative issues (budgetary constraints, staffing concerns, etc.) should guide this relationship. It is helpful that the administrator have some clinical background such as nursing for instance. Often, the reason our CME

attendees expressed their inability to learn and practice US was not being able to convince an administrator to purchase an US machine. This is the basis for including a lecture entitled, "Selling the machine to your administrator" in our CME US conferences. We designate this lecture to be delivered by an administrator champion. Buy-in by this administrator to deliver the talk usually signifies acceptance of US as a key modality in any particular setting, hospital or ambulatory.

Key elements to share with administration include return-on-investment, hospital admissions saved, and patient outcomes. While robust data on reimbursement is limited in the ambulatory setting, there is information from other settings. Implementing a novel point-of-care ultrasound billing and reimbursement program in an emergency department resulted in a 45% increase in faculty participation in billing for patient exams [10]. The number of ultrasound billable examinations increased 5.1-fold and net profits realized by the ED ultrasound program was approximately $350,000 in one year. In another study, cost modeling for handheld US (HHU) vs physical examination in patients referred for transthoracic echocardiography revealed that HHU cost $644.43 vs %707.44 for physical examination when considering all the downstream testing and overall costs comparing the two [11]. In another study, evaluating bedside ultrasound and community-based paracentesis in a palliative care service, half of the scans being performed at home, resulted in less time spent at the local hospital while not affecting complication rates [12]. And lastly, patient outcomes can be improved in the outpatient setting with US use. Ultrasound guidance for diagnosis and treatment of shoulder impingement resulted in better outcomes in shoulder function, physician global assessment, and visual analog pain scores [13].

A return-on-investment calculation would include cost of machine and accessories compared against number of diagnostic and US-assisted procedures done. One should figure out the reimbursement per US use, tabulate this over a time period, and calculate when the machine will have paid for itself. The clinic needs to be careful as reimbursement guidelines are constantly changing and several carriers are now requiring extra training, certification, and/or accreditation in order to reimburse for limited US in the clinic environment.

3. With the initiation and supervision of the physician champion and with input from the ambulatory physicians in the clinic, a broad US curriculum should be established. Initially this should include topics that will drive a simple message about the utility of US in the primary care setting. Our initial lectures, entitled "Ultrasound: what you can do in your office on Monday" included topics like carpal tunnel syndrome. A simple US measuring technique can be just as accurate at defining carpal tunnel syndrome as expensive referral for advanced testing with nerve conduction velocities [14, 15]. In-office diagnosis of temporal arteritis always interests the general internist and the data is so compelling. The finding of a bilateral halo sign from edema around the temporal artery has a specificity of 100% when compared to temporal artery biopsy [15]. Other topics that challenge physicians to rethink how they might use ultrasound in the clinical setting include differentiating Baker's cyst from deep venous thrombosis, treating meralgia paresthetica, diagnosis sinusitis, evaluating the eye and the temporal mandibular

joint, performing US-guided arthrocentesis and injections. These are common conditions encountered by clinicians and to define how US helps in caring for patients with these diagnoses may spark interest in other US applications.

The next series of lectures and hands-on centered around musculoskeletal US, lymph nodes, and lumps and bumps. While in the inpatient setting, cardiac, abdominal, and vascular US may be more helpful, musculoskeletal complaints in the outpatient setting are more common and drive US [16, 17]. One case that I often share when discussing lymph node evaluation was of a 75-year-old gentleman with new axillary nodes of several weeks duration. An ultrasound in the clinic on his initial visit revealed images consistent with metastatic disease. He had a biopsy that afternoon and his chemotherapeutic regimen started 3 days later for his lymphoma. He still remains impressed by the rapidity of his diagnosis and treatment.

In order to respect the time constraints clinicians have, the didactic portions of the education for US for colleagues should be electronically distributed prior to the hands-on sessions, which we recommend conducting at the least disruptive times of the day, perhaps during lunch or before clinic starts, whichever the majority of clinicians prefer. New learners should be given immediate responsibilities to teach others. These task will compel the learner to learn better, as to teach is to learn twice. Teachers often prepare better, practice more and perhaps, dreading the appearance of being a novice in front of junior learners, may become quicker facile practitioners with US.

4. Ultrasound machines should be placed in the most visible areas of the clinic. Theft concerns aside, the machines should be in a place where nonusers can see others taking the machines with them into patient encounters, a hallway, perhaps, and not locked up in a special room. This will remind them that their partners are using the machine and may act as an incentive to learn US imaging themselves, passive peer pressure serving as an effective impetus.

5. The physician champion and supporting physician experts should make themselves available to their partners for quick consultations, to share interesting cases and images and to act as sounding boards for quality technique and assurance. Two recent cases highlight helpfulness as a bridge to learning. Twice in the past year, one of our internists was consulted by hand specialists to perform US evaluations of a damaged transposed ulnar nerve with ulnar neuropathy in one and a possible flexor pollicis longus rupture in another. Both patients had hardware which precluded MRI. In both cases, the US helped define the damage and guided the hand surgeons to a much less invasive procedure in one and better surgical planning in the other. Needless to say, this consultation of a generalist to help a specialized surgeon was both gratifying to the internist and edifying to colleagues with which he shared the cases. Another case of being available concerned a retired internist who presented with jaw claudication. An ultrasound done in the clinic revealed bilateral halo signs with skip areas of involvement classical for temporal arteritis. The patient was started that day on steroids, felt great within a week and continues to be impressed with how US has changed medicine in the few years since his retirement.

6. Finally, to revisit the issue of reimbursement, the challenges of paying for physician and technical components of US remain. Our experience suggests that billing personal need consistent education and supervision to incorporate systems for appropriate billing. While this may seem laborious for the physician champion, regular reminders to the billing department, technology services, and the administrative champion can help to keep this issue from languishing.

Pitfalls

1. Inertia—The first challenge that must be addressed is the nascent inertia in changing established practice patterns in physicians. The standard way of practicing becomes ingrained and is difficult to change. Educating physicians with didactics and hands-on sessions, as discussed already, may be helpful. However, skills demonstrated to learners will not translate into competency or performance in those learners unless accompanied by consistent exposure to and practice of new techniques. Through our US CME courses we've noticed physicians returning to take introductory courses and even intermediate courses several times. When queried about this, the learners reported that since their offices had not purchased machines, they had no opportunity to practice and their knowledge had diminished to the point they needed refresher courses. So, readily available US machines in the office setting will encourage new learners to practice. While machine availability is necessary, it is not sufficient. Machines can remain unused if supervision is not available to remind learners of techniques, ranging from turning the machine on, to image acquisition and optimization, to image storage and retrieval. Contact between learners and teachers, and access to quick helpful feedback can address this challenge.
2. Education—in the relatively new expansion of US in the outpatient setting, local teachers with experience in US and expertise in teaching may be few and far between. Teaching the teacher programs are key in growing the base of primary care US teachers. Continued exposure and interest in US will remedy this situation, but will take some time. Although it doesn't solve all issues, the problem of availability of local resources can be addressed with internet learning [18]. Learners still value hands-on scanning sessions, small-group formats, and video-clip examples and view them as the most effective methods to learn ultrasound [19].
3. Time—Physicians report that the time pressure in the outpatient setting limits their desire to add even a few minutes to patient encounters by utilizing primary care US. Patient time constraints have limited some opportunities to perform US as well. This is one of the hardest hurdles to overcome but the utility of US may trump the extra time cost.
4. Cost—Costs associated with primary care US are not insignificant. In one study, the top 8 purchasers of compact ultrasound systems did not include primary care outpatient-based clinics [16]. The costs of machines can be managed

through return-on-investment calculations and represent relatively hard numbers. The absolute cost of portable US machines has decreased markedly and several cost less than $10,000 now. The opportunity costs of physician CME travel to learn US and lost productivity in the learning phase, as a result of slower patient encounters, slower US machine use, may be more difficult to quantify. Certainly, e-learning can be less expensive in some regards but still requires a commitment of time on the physician's part. Much available e-content is free and even visuomotor and visuospatial skills necessary to create diagnostic images can be as effectively taught via web as in classroom-based programs [20]. Closely associated with costs of machines and costs of learning is reimbursement for US use. This is moving target. Payers are changing their reimbursement requirements and payers in various states have instituted rules governing reimbursement based on office accreditation and physician certification. In addition to documenting in the patient record, storing images for diagnostic and procedural US, checking with local and state policies for reimbursement is paramount.
5. Quality Assurance—Challenges revolving around competence of physicians and quality assurance have yet to make it to the forefront in discussions.

Key Recommendations

1. Identify a physician champion who will educate colleagues about ultrasound, its utility, ease of use, ability to help in diagnosis and decision-making and patient satisfaction.
2. Identify an administrative champion who can coordinate information for return-on-investment calculations and business plan determinations.
3. Define a longitudinal educational curriculum, first with easy to learn techniques involving commonly seen outpatient patient complaints (carpal tunnel, lumps and bumps) then to more complex skills (musculoskeletal, cardiac US, abdominal US, etc.)
4. Provide educational interludes on a regular basis, during less busy clinic times such as lunch breaks, to include didactics and hands-on practice sessions.
5. The physician champion should identify other physicians interested in US and cultivate their enthusiasm to lead and teach.
6. Provide new physician learners responsibilities for teaching students, residents, and staff quickly in order to motivate them to practice and improve skills.
7. Make US machines readily available so that infrequent users will actually be reminded of their presence and will easily notice when others are taking machines in and out of patient encounters.

8. Enlist the support of billing and reimbursement experts in your institution to maximize revenue that can support machine use and further purchases.
9. Physician users should make themselves available to colleagues to help demonstrate primary care US utility in their colleagues' patients.

References

1. Croft LM, Wl D, Golman ME. A pilot study of the clinical impact of hand-carried cardiac ultrasound in the medical clinic. Echocardiography. 2006;23(6):439–46.
2. Levin DC, Rao VM, Parker L, Frangos AJ. Noncardiac point-of-care ultrasound by Nonradiologist physicians: how widespread is it? J Am Coll Radiol. 2011;8:772–5.
3. Weinreb JC, Wilcox PA. How do training, education, and experience affect quality in radiology? J Am Coll Radiol. 2004;1:510–5.
4. Leone AF, Schumacher SM, Krothis DE, Eleazer GP. Geriatricians' Interest to Learn Bedside Portable Ultrasound (GEBUS) for Application in the Clinical Practice and in Education. JAMDA 2012; 13;308.e7–308.e10.
5. Berkoff DJ, English J, Theodoro D. Sports medicine ultrasound(US) beyond the musculoskeletal system: use in the abdomen, solid organs, lung, heart and eye. Br J Sports Med. 2015;49:161–5.
6. Hosey RG, Kriss V, Uhl TL, et al. Ultrasonographic evaluation of splenic enlargement in athletes with acute infectious mononucleosis. Br J Sports Med. 2008;42:974–7.
7. Mjolstad OC, Snare SR, Folkvord L, et al. Assessment of left ventricular function by GPs using pocket-sized ultrasound. Fam Pract. 2012;29(5):534–40.
8. Blois, B. Office-based ultrasound screening for abdominal aortic aneurysm. Can Fam Physician 2011;58:e 172–8.
9. Bornemann MAJ, Bornemann G. Military family physicians' perceptions of a pocket point-of-care ultrasound device in clinical practice. Mil Med. 2014;79:1474–7.
10. Akhikari MD, Amini R, Stolz L, et al. Implementation of a novel point-of-care ultrasound billing reimbursement program: fiscal impact. Am J of Emerg Med. 2014;32:592–5.
11. Mehta M, Jacobson T, Peters D, et al. Handheld ultrasound versus physical examination in patients referred for transthoracic echocardiography for a suspected cardiac condition. J Am Coll Cardiol Img. 2014;7(10):983–90.
12. Landers A, Ryan B. The use of bedside ultrasound and community based paracentesis in a palliative care service. J Prim Health Care. 2014;6(2):148–51.
13. El Miedany YM, Aty SA, Ashour S. Ultrasonography versus nerve conduction study in patients with carpal tunnel syndrome: substantive or complementary tests? Rheumatology. 2004;43(7):887–95.
14. Ziswiler HR, Reichenbach S, Vogelin E, Bachmann LM, Villiger PM, Juni P. Diagnostic value of sonography in patients with suspected carpal tunnel syndrome. Arthritis Rheum. 2005;52(1):304–11.
15. Arida A, Kyprianou M, Kanakis M, Sfikakis P. The diagnostic role of ultrasonography-derived edema of the temporal artery wall in giant cell arteritis: a second metanalysis. BMC Musculoskelet Disord. 2010;11:44–7.
16. McGahan JP, Pozniak MA, Cronan J, et al. Handheld ultrasound: threat or opportunity? Appl Radiol. 2015;3:20–5.
17. Spencer JK, Adler RS. Utility of portable ultrasound in a community in Ghana. J Ultrasound Med. 2008;27:1735–43.

18. PLatz D, Goldflam K, Mennicke M, et al. Comparison of web versus classroom-based basic ultrasonographic and EFAST training in 2 Euporean hospitals. AEM. 2010;56:660–7.
19. C. Cartier R, Skinner C, Laselle B. Perceived Effectiveness of Teaching Methods for Point of Care Ultrasound. J Emerg Med 2014;47:86–91.
20. Bowra J, Dawson M, Goudie A, and Mallin M. Sounding out the future of ultrasound education. Ultrasound 2014;1–5. C. Cartier R, Skinner C, Laselle B. Perceived Effectiveness of Teaching Methods for Point of Care Ultrasound. J Emerg Med 2014;47:86–91.

ACEP US Guidelines

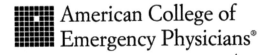

American College of
Emergency Physicians®

ADVANCING EMERGENCY CARE ____/_

POLICY
STATEMENT

Approved June 2016

Ultrasound Guidelines: Emergency, Point-of-Care, and Clinical Ultrasound Guidelines in Medicine

Revised and approved by the
ACEP Board of Directors with
current title June 2016

Revised and approved by the
ACEP Board of Directors
October 2008

Originally approved by the
ACEP Board of Directors
June 2001

© Springer International Publishing AG 2018
V. S. Tayal et al. (eds.), *Ultrasound Program Management*,
https://doi.org/10.1007/978-3-319-63143-1

Section 1 - Introduction

Ultrasound (US) has become an integral modality in emergency care in the United States during the last two decades. Since the last update of these guidelines in 2008, US use has expanded throughout clinical medicine and established itself as a standard in the clinical evaluation of the emergency patient. There is a wide breadth of recognized emergency US applications offering advanced diagnostic and therapeutic capability benefit to patients across the globe. With its low capital, space, energy, and cost of training requirements, US can be brought to the bedside anywhere a clinician can go, directly or remotely. The use of US in emergency care has contributed to improvement in quality and value, specifically in regards to procedural safety, timeliness of care, diagnostic accuracy, and cost reduction. In a medical world full of technological options, US fulfills the concept of "staged imaging" where the use of US first can answer important clinical questions accurately without the expense, time or side effects of advanced imaging or invasive procedures.

Emergency physicians have taken the leadership role for the establishment and education of bedside, clinical, point-of-care US use by clinicians in the United States and around the world. Ultrasonography has spread throughout all levels of medical education, integrated into medical school curricula, through residency, to postgraduate education of physicians, and extended to other providers such as nursing, advanced practice professionals, and prehospital providers. US curricula in undergraduate medical education is growing exponentially due to the leadership and advocacy of emergency physicians. US in emergency medicine (EM) residency training has now been codified in the Accreditation Council for Graduate Medical Education (ACGME) Next Accreditation System (NAS). Emergency US specialists have created the foundation of a subspecialty of ultrasonography that provides the expertise for establishing clinical practice, educating across the educational spectrum, and researching the wide range of applications of ultrasonography. Within healthcare institutions and healthcare systems, emergency physicians are now leading institutional clinical US programs that have used this guideline as a format for multidisciplinary programs.

US imaging and information systems have become more sophisticated and digital over the last decade allowing emergency US examinations to have versatility, mobility and integration. US hardware for emergency care has become more modular, smaller, and powerful, ranging from smartphone size to slim, cart-based systems dedicated to the emergency medicine market. US hardware has evolved to allow on-machine reporting, wireless connectivity and electronic medical record (EMR) and picture archiving and communication system (PACS) integration. A new software entity, US management systems, was created to provide administrative functionality and the integration of US images into electronic records. Emergency physician expertise was integral in the development of these hardware and software advances.

These guidelines reflect the evolution and changes in the evolving world of emergency medicine and the growth of US practice. Themes of universality of practice, educational innovation, core credentialing, quality improvement, and value highlight this new edition of the guidelines. The ultimate mission of providing excellent patient care will be enhanced by emergency physicians and other clinicians being empowered with the use of US.

Section 2- Scope of Practice

Emergency Ultrasound (EUS) is the medical use of US technology for the bedside evaluation of acute or critical medical conditions.[1] It is utilized for diagnosis of any emergency condition, resuscitation of the acutely ill, critically ill or injured, guidance of procedures, monitoring of certain pathologic states and as an adjunct to therapy. EUS examinations are typically performed, interpreted, and integrated into care by emergency physicians or those under the supervision of emergency physicians in the setting of the emergency department (ED) or a non-ED emergency setting such as hospital unit, out-of-hospital, battlefield, space, urgent care, clinic, or remote or other settings. It may be performed as a single examination, repeated due to clinical need or deterioration, or used for monitoring of physiologic or pathologic changes.

Emergency US is synonymous with the terms clinical, bedside, point-of-care, focused, and physician performed, but is part of a larger field of clinical ultrasonography. In this document, EUS refers to US performed by emergency physicians or clinicians in the emergency setting, while clinical ultrasonography refers to a multidisciplinary field of US use by clinicians at the point-of-care.[2] Table 1 summarizes relevant US definitions in EUS.

Other medical specialties may wish to use this document if they perform EUS in the manner described above. However, guidelines which apply to US examinations or procedures performed by consultants, especially consultative imaging in US laboratories or departments, or in a different setting may not be applicable to emergency physicians.

Emergency US is an emergency medicine procedure, and should not be considered in conflict with exclusive "imaging" contracts that may be in place with consultative US practices. In addition, emergency US should be reimbursed as a separate billable procedure.[3] (See Section 6- Value and Reimbursement) EUS is a separate entity distinct from the physical examination that adds anatomic, functional, and physiologic information to the care of the acutely-ill patient.[4] It provides clinically significant data not obtainable by inspection, palpation, auscultation, or other components of the physical examination.[5] US used in this clinical context is also not equivalent to use in the training of medical students and other clinicians in training looking to improve their understanding of anatomic and physiologic relationships of organ systems.

EUS can be classified into the following functional clinical categories:

1. *Resuscitative*: US use as directly related to an acute resuscitation
2. *Diagnostic*: US utilized in an emergent diagnostic imaging capacity
3. *Symptom or sign-based*: US used in a clinical pathway based upon the patient's symptom or sign (eg, shortness of breath)
4. *Procedure guidance*: US used as an aid to guide a procedure
5. *Therapeutic and Monitoring*: US use in therapeutics or in physiological monitoring

Within these broad functional categories of use, 12 core emergency US applications have been identified as Trauma, Pregnancy, Cardiac /Hemodynamic assessment, Abdominal aorta, Airway/Thoracic, Biliary, Urinary Tract, Deep Vein Thrombosis (DVT), Soft-tissue/Musculoskeletal (MSK), Ocular, Bowel, and Procedural Guidance. Evidence for these core applications may be found in Appendix 1. The criteria for inclusion for core are widespread use, significant evidence base, uniqueness in diagnosis or decision-making, importance in primary emergency diagnosis and patient care, or technological advance.

Alternatively, symptom and sign based US pathways, such as Shock or Dyspnea, may be considered an integrated application based on the skills required in the pathway. In such pathways, applications may be mixed and utilized in a format and order that maximizes medical decision-making, outcomes, efficiency and patient safety tailored to the setting, resources, and patient characteristics. See Figure 1.

Emergency physicians should have basic education in US physics, instrumentation procedural guidance, *and FAST* as part of EM practice. It is not mandatory that every clinician performing emergency US examinations utilize or be expert in each core application, but it is understood that each core application is incorporated into common emergency US practice nationwide. The descriptions of these examinations may be found in the ACEP policy, Emergency Ultrasound Imaging Criteria Compendium.[6] Many other

US applications or advanced uses of these applications may be used by emergency physicians. Their non-inclusion as a core application does not diminish their importance in practice nor imply that emergency physicians are unable to use them in daily patient care.

Each EUS application represents a clinical bedside skill that can be of great advantage in a variety of emergency patient care settings. In classifying an emergency US a single application may appear in more than one category and clinical setting. For example a focused cardiac US may be utilized to identify a pericardial effusion in the diagnosis of an enlarged heart on chest x-ray. The focused cardiac US may be utilized in a cardiac resuscitation setting to differentiate true pulseless electrical activity from profound hypovolemia. The focused cardiac US can be used to monitor the heart during resuscitation in response to fluids or medications. If the patient is in cardiac tamponade, the cardiac US can also be used to guide the procedure of pericardiocentesis In addition, the same focused cardiac study can be combined with one or more additional emergency US types, such as the focused abdominal, the focused aortic or the focused chest US, into a clinical algorithm and used to evaluate a presenting symptom complex. Examples of this would be the evaluation of patients with undifferentiated non-traumatic shock or the focused assessment with sonography in trauma (FAST), or extended FAST examination in the patient presenting with traumatic injury. See Figure 1.

Ultrasound guided procedures provide safety to a wide variety of procedures from vascular access (eg, central venous access) to drainage procedures (eg, thoracentesis pericardiocentesis, paracentesis, arthrocentesis) to localizations procedure like US guided nerve blocks. These procedures may provide additional benefits by increasing patient safety and treating pain without the side-effects of systemic opiates FAST as required procedure.

Other US applications are performed by emergency physicians, and may be integrated depending on the setting, training, and needs of that particular ED or EM group. Table 2 lists other emergency US applications.

Other settings or populations

Pediatrics. US is a particularly advantageous diagnostic tool in the management of pediatric patients, in whom radiation exposure is a significant concern. EUS applications such as musculoskeletal evaluation for certain fractures (rib, forearm, skull), and lung for pneumonia may be more advantageous in children than in adults due to patient size and density.[7] US can be associated with increased procedural success and patient safety, and decreased length of stay.[8,9] While most US modalities in the pediatric arena are the same as in adult patients (the EFAST exam for trauma, procedural guidance), other modalities are unique to the pediatric population such as in suspected pyloric stenosis and intussusception, or in the child with hip pain or a limp).[10-12] Mostly recently, EUS has been formally incorporated into Pediatric EM fellowship training.[13-14]

Critical care. EUS core applications are being integrated into cardiopulmonary and non-invasive hemodynamic monitoring into critical care scenarios.[15-16] Dual-trained physicians in emergency medicine and critical care are leading the application, education, and research of US for critically ill patients, and have significant leadership in advancing US concepts in multidisciplinary critical care practice. Advanced cardiopulmonary US application are being integrated into critical care practice.

Prehospital. There is increasing evidence that US has an increasing role in out-of-hospital emergency care.[17-18] Challenges to the widespread implementation of out-of-hospital US include significant training and equipment requirements, and the need for careful physician oversight and quality assurance. Studies focusing on patient outcomes need to be conducted to further define the role of out-of-hospital US and to identify settings where the benefit to the patient justifies the investment of resources necessary to implement such a program.[19]

International arena including field, remote, rural, global public health and disaster situations. US has become the primary initial imaging modality in disaster care.[20-24] US can direct and optimize patient care in domestic and international natural disasters such as tsunami, hurricane, famine or man-made disasters such as battlefield or refugee camps. US provides effective advanced diagnostic technology in remote geographies such as rural areas, developing countries, or small villages which share the common characteristics of limited technology (ie, x-ray, CT, MRI), unreliable electrical supplies, and minimally trained health care providers. US use in outer space is unique as the main imaging modality for space exploration and missions.[25-26] Ultrasound has also been used in remote settings such as international exploration, mountain base camps, and cruise ships.[27] The increasing portability of US machines with increasing image resolution has expanded the use of emergent imaging in such settings. See ACEP linked resources at www.globalsono.org

Military and tactical. The military has embraced the utilization of US technology in austere battlefield environments.[28-29] It is now routine for combat support hospitals as well as forward surgical teams to deploy with next generation portable ultrasonography equipment. Clinical ultrasonography is often used to inform decisions on mobilization of casualties to higher echelons of care and justify use of limited resources.

Within the last decade, emergency physicians at academic military medical centers have expanded ultrasonography training to clinical personnel who practice in close proximity to the point of injury, such as combat medics, special operations forces, and advanced practice professionals.[30] The overarching goal of these training programs is to create a generation of competent clinical sonologists capable of practicing "good medicine in bad places." The military is pursuing telemedicine-enabled US applications, automated US interpretation capabilities, and extension of clinical ultrasonography in additional areas of operation, such as critical care air evacuation platforms.[3]

Section 3 – Training and Proficiency
There is an evolving spectrum of training in clinical US from undergraduate medical education through post-graduate training, where skills are introduced, applications are learned, core concepts are reinforced and new applications and ideas evolve in the life-long practice of US in emergency medicine.[32-33]

Competency and Curriculum Recommendations
Competency in EUS requires the progressive development and application of increasingly sophisticated knowledge and psychomotor skills for an expanding number of EUS applications. This development parallels the performance of any EUS exam.

The ACEP definition of US competency includes the following components. First, the clinician needs to recognize the indications and contraindications for the EUS exam. Next, the clinician must be able to acquire adequate images. This begins with an understanding of basic US physics, translated into the skills needed to operate the US system correctly (knobology), while performing exam protocols on patients presenting with different conditions and body habitus. Simultaneous with image acquisition, the clinician needs to interpret the imaging by distinguishing between normal anatomy, common variants, as well as a range of pathology from obvious to subtle. Finally, the clinician must be able to integrate EUS exam findings into individual patient care plans and management. Ultimately, effective integration includes knowledge of each particular exam accuracy, as well as proper documentation, quality assurance, and EUS reimbursement. See ACEP linked resources at www.sonoguide.com

An EUS curriculum requires considerable faculty expertise, dedicated faculty time and resources, and departmental support. These updated guidelines continue to provide the learning objectives (See Appendix 2), educational methods, and assessment measures for any EUS residency or practice-based curriculum. As part of today's effort to reinvent medical education, all educators are now faced with the challenge of creating curricula that provide for individualized learning yet result in the standardized outcomes such as those outlined in current residency milestones.[34]

Innovative Educational Methods and Assessment Measures
As a supplement to traditional EUS education already described in previous guidelines, recent online and technological innovation is providing additional individualized educational methods and standardized assessment measures to meet this challenge.[32, 35-36] Free open access medical (FOAM) education podcasts and narrated lectures provide the opportunity to create the flipped EUS classroom.[37-40] For the trainee, asynchronous learning provides the opportunity to repeatedly review required knowledge on demand and at their own pace. For educators, less time may be spent providing recurring EUS didactics, and more time dedicated to higher level tasks such as teaching psychomotor skills and integration of exam findings into patient and ED management. Both EUS faculty and trainees together may identify potential FOAM resources. However, EUS faculty must now take the new role of FOAM curator. New online resources must be carefully reviewed to ensure that each effectively teaches the objectives in these guidelines before being introduced into an EUS curriculum.

Similar to knowledge learning, there are new educational methods to teach the required psychomotor skills of EUS. The primary educational method continues to be small group hands-on training in the ED with EUS faculty, followed by supervised examination performance with timely quality assurance review. Simulation is currently playing an increasingly important role as both an EUS educational method and assessment measure.[36] Numerous investigators have demonstrated that simulation results in equivalent image acquisition, interpretation, and operator confidence in comparison to traditional hands-on training.[41-42] US simulators provide the opportunity for deliberate practice of a new skill in a safe environment prior to actual clinical performance. The use of simulation for deliberate practice improves the success rate of invasive procedures and reduces patient complications.[43-44] Additionally, simulation has the potential to expose trainees to a wider spectrum of pathology and common variants than typically encountered during an EUS rotation. Blended learning created by the flipped classroom, live instructor training, and simulation provide the opportunity for self-directed learning, deliberate practice and mastery learning.[45-47]

Simulation also provides a valid assessment measure of each component of EUS competency. Appropriately designed cases assess a trainee's ability to recognize indications, demonstrate image acquisition and interpretation, as well as apply EUS findings to patient and ED management.[42] These proven benefits and the reduction in direct faculty time justify the cost of a high fidelity US simulator. Furthermore, costs may be shared across departments.

Documenting Experience and Demonstrating Proficiency
Traditional number benchmarks for procedural training in medical education provide a convenient method for documenting the performance of a reasonable number of exams needed for a trainee to develop competency.[48-49] However, learning curves vary by trainee and application.[49] Individuals learn required knowledge and psychomotor skills at their own pace. Supervision, opportunities to practice different applications and encounter pathology also differ across departments.
Therefore, in addition to set number benchmarks individualized assessment methods need to be utilized. Recommended methods include the following: real time supervision during clinical EUS, weekly QA teaching sessions and image review, ongoing QA exam feedback, standardized knowledge assessments,

small group Observed Structured Clinical Examinations (OSCEs), one-on-one standardized direct observation tools (SDOTs), simulation assessments and other focused educational tools.[36] Ideally these assessment measures are completed both at the beginning and the end of a training period. Initial assessment measures identify each trainee's unique needs, providing the opportunity to modify a local curriculum as needed to create more individualized learning plans. Final assessment measures demonstrate current trainee competency and future learning needs, as well as identify opportunities for improvement in local EUS education.

Trainees should complete a benchmark of 25-50 quality-reviewed exams in a particular application. It is acknowledged that the training curve may level out below or above this recommended threshold, and that learning is a lifelong process with improvements beyond initial training. Previously learned psychomotor skills are often applicable to new applications. For example, experience with FAST provides a springboard to learning resuscitation, genitourinary, and transabdominal pelvic EUS.

Overall EUS trainees should complete a benchmark of 150-300 total EUS exams depending on the number of applications being utilized. For example, an academic department regularly performing greater than six applications may require residents to complete more than 150 exams, while a community ED with practicing physicians just beginning to incorporate EUS with FAST and vascular access should require less.

If different modalities such as endovaginal technique are being used for an application, the minimum may need to include a substantial experience in that technique. We would recommend a minimum of 10 examinations in the other technique (eg, endocavitary for early pregnancy) with the assumption that educational goals of anatomic, pathophysiology, and abnormal states are identified with all technqiues taught.

Procedural US applications require fewer exams given prior knowledge, psychomotor skills, and clinical experience with traditional blind technique. Trainees should complete five quality reviewed US-guided procedure examinations or a learning module on an US-guided procedures task trainer.

Training exams need to include patients with different conditions and body types. Exams may be completed in different settings including clinical and educational patients in the ED, live models at EUS courses, utilizing US simulators, and in other clinical environments. Abnormal or positive scans should be included in a significant number of training exams used to meet credentialing requirements. Image review or simulation may be utilized for training examinations in addition to patient encounters when adequate pathology is not available for the specific application. In-person supervision is optimal during introductory education but is not required for residency or credentialing examinations after initial didactic training.

During benchmark completion, all EUS exams should be quality reviewed for technique and accuracy by EUS faculty. Alternatively, an EUS training portfolio of exam images and results may be compared to other diagnostic studies and clinical outcomes in departments where EUS faculty are not yet available. After initial training, continued quality assurance of EUS exams is recommended for a proportion (5-10%) of ongoing exams to document continued competency.

Recently, several secure online quality assurance workflow systems have become commercially available (See Section 5- Quality and US Management). Current systems greatly enhance trainee feedback by providing for more timely review of still images and video loops, customized application and feedback forms, typed and voice feedback, as well as storage and export of data within a relational database.

Training Pathways

There are two recommended pathways for clinicians to become proficient in EUS. See Figure 2. The majority of emergency physicians today receive EUS training as part of an ACGME-approved EM residency. A second practice-based pathway is provided for practicing EM physicians and other EM clinicians who did not receive EUS training through completion of an EM residency program.

These updated EUS guidelines continue to provide the learning objectives, educational methods and assessment measures for either pathway. Learning objectives for each application are described in Appendix 2.

Residency Based Pathway

EUS has been considered a fundamental component of emergency medicine training for over two decades.[50-52] The ACGME mandates procedural competency in EUS for all EM residents as it is a "skill integral to the practice of Emergency Medicine" as defined by the 2013 Model of the Clinical Practice of EM.[53] The ACGME and the American Board of Emergency Medicine (ABEM) recently defined twenty-three sub competency milestones for emergency medicine residency training.[34] Patient Care Milestone twelve (12) describes the sequential learning process for EUS and should be considered a guideline in addition to other assessment methods mentioned in this guideline. Appendix 3 provides recommendations for EM residency EUS education.

Upon completion of residency training, emergency medicine residents should be provided with a standardized EM Resident EUS credentialing letter. For the EUS faculty, ED Director or Chairperson at the graduate's new institution, this letter provides a detailed description of the EUS training curriculum completed, including the number of quality reviewed training exams completed by application and overall, and performance on SDOTs and simulation assessments.

Practice Based Pathway

For practicing emergency medicine (EM) attendings who completed residency without specific EUS training, a comprehensive course, series of short courses, or preceptorship is recommended. Shorter courses covering single or a combination of applications may provide initial or supplementary training. As part of pre-course preparation, EUS faculty must consider the unique learning needs of the participating trainees. The course curriculum should include trainee-appropriate learning objectives, educational methods and assessment measures as outlined by these guidelines. If not completed previously, then introductory training on US physics and knobology is required prior to training in individual applications. Pre-course and post-course online learning may be utilized to reduce the course time spent on traditional didactics and facilitate later review. Small group hands-on instruction with EUS faculty on models, simulators, and task trainers provides experience in image acquisition, interpretation, and integration of EUS exam findings into patient care. See Appendix 4.

Preceptorships typically lasting 1-2 weeks at an institution with an active EUS education program have also been utilized successfully to train practicing physicians. Each preceptorship needs to begin with a discussion of the trainees unique educational needs, hospital credentialing goals as well as financial support for faculty teaching time. Then the practicing physician participates in an appropriately tailored curriculum typically in parallel with ongoing student, resident, fellow and other educational programming.

Similar to an EM Resident EUS credentialing letter, course and preceptorship certificates should include a description of the specific topics and applications reviewed, total number of training exams completed with expert supervision, performance on other course assessment measures such as SDOTs or simulation cases, as well as the number of CME hours earned. These certificates are then given to local EUS faculty or ED Director/Chairperson to document training.

Advanced Practice Providers, Nursing, Paramedics, and other EM clinicians

In many practice environments, EUS faculty often provide clinical US training to other to non-physician staff including Advanced Practice Professionals, Nurses, Paramedics, Military Medics and Disaster Response Team members. The recommendations in these guidelines should be utilized by EUS faculty when providing such training programs. Pre-course preparation needs to include discussions with staff leadership to define role-specific learning needs and applications to be utilized. Introductory US physics, knobology, and relevant anatomy and pathophysiology are required prior to training in targeted applications.

For Advanced Practice Providers and other clinicians practicing in rural and austere environments where direct EUS trained EM physician oversight is not available, EUS training needs to adhere to the recommendations in these guidelines. Specifically, comprehensive didactics and skills training, as well as minimum benchmarks need to be completed prior to independent EUS utilization. Beyond this initial training, EUS faculty are needed to provide ongoing quality assurance review. Telemedicine may provide the opportunity for real time patient assessment, assistance with image acquisition, and immediate review of patient images.

Ongoing Education As with all aspects of emergency medicine ongoing education is required regardless of training pathway. The amount of education needed depends on the number of applications being performed, frequency of utilization, the local practice of the individual clinician and other developments in EUS and EM. Individual EUS credentialed physicians should continue their education with a focus on US activities as part of their overall educational activities. Educational sessions that integrate US into the practice of EM are encouraged, and do not have to be didactic in nature, but may be participatory or online. Recommended EUS educational activities include conference attendance, online educational activities, preceptorships, teaching, research, hands-on training, program administration, quality assurance, image review, in-service examinations, textbook and journal readings, as well as morbidity and mortality conferences inclusive of US cases. US quality improvement is an example of an activity that may be used for completion of the required ABEM Assessment of Practice Performance activities.

Fellowship Training

Fellowships provide the advanced training needed to create future leaders in evolving areas of medicine such as clinical US. This advanced training produces experts in clinical US and is not required for the routine utilization of EUS.

An EUS fellowship provides a unique, focused, and mentored opportunity to develop and apply a deeper comprehension of advanced principles, techniques, applications, and interpretative findings. Knowledge and skills are continually reinforced as the fellow learns to effectively educate new trainees in EUS, as well as clinicians in other specialties, and practice environments. A methodical review of landmark and current literature, as well as participation in ongoing research, creates the ability to critically appraise and ultimately generate the evidence needed for continued improvements in patient care through clinical US. Furthermore, fellowship provides practical experience in EUS program management including quality assurance review, medical legal documentation, image archiving, reimbursement, equipment maintenance, and other administrative duties of an EUS program director.

Recommendation for fellowship content, site qualifications, criteria for fellowship directors, and minimum graduation criteria for fellows have been published by national EUS leadership and ACEP Emergency Ultrasound Fellowship Guidelines.[54-55] Each fellowship program's structure and curriculum will vary slightly based on local institution and department resources. At all fellowship programs, mentorship and networking are fundamental to a fellow's and program's ultimate success. Both require significant EUS faculty time for regular individual instruction as well as participation in the clinical US community locally and nationally. Hence, institution and department leadership support is essential to ensuring an appropriate number of EUS faculty, each provided with adequate non-clinical time.

For the department, a fellowship speeds the development of an EUS program. Fellowships improve EM resident training resulting in increased performance of EUS examinations.[56] Furthermore, a fellowship training program may have a significant positive impact on overall EUS utilization, timely quality assurance review, faculty credentialing, billing revenue, and compliance with documentation.[57] For an institution, an EUS fellowship provides a valuable resource for other specialties just beginning clinical US programs. Collaborating with EUS faculty and fellows, clinicians from other departments are often able to more rapidly educate staff and create effective clinical US programs.

US in Undergraduate Medical Education

Emergency Medicine has again taken a lead role in efforts to improve Undergraduate Medical Education (UME) through the early integration of clinical US.[58-62] During the preclinical years, US has been demonstrated to be an effective educational method to reinforce student understanding of anatomy, physical examination skills, pathology and bedside diagnostic skills.[63-68] During the clinical years, students are then better able to utilize US for clinical diagnosis and on specific rotations. US exposure in UME can provide a solid knowledge base for individuals to build upon and later utilize as US is integrated into their clinical training.

Integrating US into UME

Integration of US into pre-clinical UME often begins with medical student and faculty interest. By working closely with a medical school's curriculum committee, US may then be incorporated as a novel educational method to enhance learning within existing preclinical courses. Athough dedicated US specific curriculum time is not often available in UME, considerable clinical US faculty time and expertise is still required for effective integration of US into existing medical school courses. Widespread clinical US utilization by different specialties within a medical school's teaching hospitals, and education within Graduate Medical Education programs, provides initial faculty expertise, teaching space, and US equipment. Ongoing education then requires local departmental and medical school leadership support, as well as continued organized collaboration between faculty from participating specialties.

Innovative educational methods again provide the opportunity for clinical US faculty to focus on small group hands-on instruction as described in the innovative education section.[60,64,69-70]

Many academic departments that currently offer clinical rotations within Emergency Medicine already include an introduction to EUS as a workshop, or a set number of EUS shifts. Dedicated EUS elective rotations provide an additional opportunity for medical students interested in Emergency Medicine and other specialties utilizing clinical US to participate in an EUS rotation adapted to their level of training and unique career interests. See Appendix 5 for recommendations for EUS and Clinical US medical school rotations.

US in UME continuing into Clinical US in GME

UME US experience should prepare new physicians to more rapidly utilize clinical US to improve patient care during graduate medical education (GME) training. Medical students today therefore should graduate with a basic understanding of US physics, machine operation, and common exam protocols such as US guided vascular access. Medical students matriculating from a school with an integrated US curriculum, as well as those completing an elective clinical US rotation, should be provided with a supporting letter similar in regards to didactics, hands-on training, and performed examinations. Although all trainees need to complete the EUS residency milestones, trainees with basic proficiency in clinical US from UME training may progress more rapidly and ultimately achieve higher levels of EUS expertise during GME.

Additionally, these residents may provide considerable EUS program support as peer-to-peer instructors, residency college leaders, investigators and potentially future fellows.

Section 4 – Credentialing and Privileging

Implementing a transparent, high quality, verifiable and efficient credentialing system is an integral component of an emergency US program. An emergency US director, along with the department leadership, should oversee policies and guidelines pertaining to emergency US. The department should follow the specialty- specific guidelines set forth within this document for their credentialing and privileging process.

Pertaining to clinician performed US, the American Medical Association (AMA) House of Delegates in 1999 passed a resolution (AMA HR. 802) recommending hospitals' credentialing committees follow specialty-specific guidelines for hospital credentialing decisions related to US use by clinicians.[71] This resolution affirms that US imaging is within the scope of practice of appropriately trained physician specialists and provides clear support for hospital credentialing committees to grant emergency US (EUS) privileging based on the specialty-specific guidelines contained within this document without the need to seek approval from other departments. Furthermore, HR 802 states that opposition that is clearly based on financial motivation meets criteria to file an ethical complaint to the AMA.

The provision of clinical privileges in EM is governed by the rules and regulations of the department and institution for which privileges are sought. The EM Chairperson or Medical Director or his/her designate (eg, emergency US director) is responsible for the assessment of clinical US privileges of emergency physicians. When a physician applies for appointment or reappointment to the medical staff and for clinical privileges, including renewal, addition, or rescission of privileges, the reappraisal process must include assessment of current competence. The EM leadership will, with the input of department members, determine the means by which each emergency physician will maintain competence and skills and the mechanism by which each physician is monitored.

EM departments should list emergency US within their core emergency medicine privileges as a single separate privilege for "Emergency US" or US applications can be bundled into an "US core" and added directly to the core privileges. EM should take responsibility to designate which core applications it will use, and then track its emergency physicians in each of those core applications. To help integrate physicians of different levels of sonographic competency (graduating residents, practicing physicians, fellows and others), it is recommended that the department of emergency medicine create a credentialing system that gathers data on individual physicians, which is then communicated in an organized fashion at predetermined thresholds with the institution-wide credentialing committee. This system focuses supervision and approval at the department level where education, training, and practice performance is centered prior to institutional final review. As new core applications are adopted, they should be granted by an internal credentialing system within the department of emergency medicine.

Eligible providers to be considered for privileging in emergency ultrasonography include emergency physicians or other providers who complete the necessary training as specified in this document via residency training or practice based training (see Section 3 - Training and Proficiency). After completing either pathway, these skills should be considered a core privilege with no requirement except consistent utilization. At institutions that have not made EUS a core privilege, submission of 5-10% of the initial requirement for any EUS application is sufficient to demonstrate continued proficiency.

Sonographer certification or emergency US certification by external entities is not an expected, obligatory or encouraged requirement for emergency US credentialing.[72] Physicians with advanced US training or responsibilities may be acknowledged with a separate hospital credential if desired.

Regarding recredentialing or credentialing at a new health institution or system, ACEP recommends that once initial training in residency or by practice pathway is completed, credentialing committees recognize that training as a core privilege, and ask for proof of recent updates or a short period of supervision prior to granting full privileges.

In addition to meeting the requirements for ongoing clinical practice set forth in this document, physicians should also be assessed for competence through the CQI program at their institution. (See Section 5-Quality and US Management) The Joint Commission (TJC) in 2008 implemented a new standard mandating detailed evaluation of practitioners' professional performance as part of the process of granting and maintaining practice privileges within a healthcare organization.[73] This standard includes processes including the Ongoing Professional Practice Evaluation (OPPE) and the Focused Professional Practice Evaluation (FPPE). Specific to FPPE and US credentialing, for infrequently performed US examinations, FPPE monitoring can be performed on a pre-determined number of examinations (ie, review of the diagnoses made on the first 10 or 20 of a particular US examination). The FPPE process should: 1. Be clearly defined and documented with specific criteria and a monitoring plan; 2. Be of fixed duration; and 3. Have predetermined measures or conditions for acceptable performance. OPPE can incorporate EUS quality improvement processes. US directors should follow these guidelines when setting up their credentialing and privileging processes.

Section 5 – Quality and US Management
In order to ensure quality, facilitate education, and satisfy credentialing pathways, a plan for an emergency US quality assurance (QA) and improvement program should be in place. This plan should be integrated into the overall ED operations. The facets of such a program are listed below. Programs should strive for meeting these criteria, and may seek accreditation through the Clinical Ultrasound Accreditation Program (CUAP).[74]

Emergency US Director
The emergency US director is a board-eligible or certified emergency physician who has been given administrative oversight over the emergency US program from the EM Chairperson, director or group. This may be a single or group of physicians, depending on size, locations, and coverage of the group. Specific responsibilities of an US director and associates may include:

- Developing and ensuring compliance to overall program goals: educational, clinical, financial, and academic.
- Selection of appropriate US machine for clinical care setting and developing and monitoring maintenance care plan to ensure quality and cleanliness
- Designing and managing an appropriate credentialing and privileging program for physicians, residents, or advanced practice providers (APP) or other type of providers within the group and/or academic facility.
- Designing and implementing in-house and/or out-sourced educational programs for all providers involved in the credentialing program.
- Monitoring and documenting individual physician privileges, educational experiences, and US scans,
- Developing, maintaining, and improving an adequate QA process in which physician scans are reviewed for quality in a timely manner and from which feedback is generated.

The emergency US director must be credentialed as an emergency physician and maintain privileges for emergency US applications. If less than two years in the position of US director, it is recommended that the director have either: 1) graduated from an emergency US fellowship, 2) participated in an emergency US management course, or 3) completed an emergency US preceptorship or mini-fellowship. If part of a multihospital group, consideration of local US directors with support from overall system US director. Institutional and departmental support should be provided for the administrative components listed above.

Supervision of US Training and Examinations

Ultrasound programs in clinical specialties have a continuing and exponential educational component encompassing traditionally graduate and post-graduate medical training, but now undergraduate, APP, prehospital, remote, and other trainees are seeking training. Policies regarding the supervision and responsibility of these US examinations should be clear. (See Sections 2, 3, and 4)

US Documentation

Emergency US is different from consultative US in other specialties as the emergency physician not only performs but also interprets the US examination. In a typical hospital ED practice, US findings are immediately interpreted, and should be communicated to other physicians and services by written reports in the ED medical record. Emergency US documentation reflects the nature of the exam, which is focused, goal-directed, and performed at the bedside contemporaneously with clinical care. This documentation may be preliminary and brief in a manner reflecting the presence or absence of the relevant findings. Documentation as dictated by regulatory and payor entities may require more extensive reporting including indication, technique, findings, and impression. Although EMRs are quickly becoming the norm, documentation may be handwritten, transcribed, templated, or computerized. Regardless of the documentation system, US reports should be available to providers to ensure timely availability of interpretations for consultant and health care team review.[75] Ideally, EMR systems should utilize effective documentation tools to make reporting efficient and accurate.

During out-of-hospital, remote, disaster, and other scenarios, US findings may be communicated by other methods within the setting constraints. Incidental findings should be communicated to the patient or follow-up provider. Discharge instructions should reflect any specific issues regarding US findings in the context of the ED diagnosis. Hard copy (paper, film, video) or digital US images are typically saved within the ED or hospital archival systems. Digital archival with corresponding documentation is optimal and recommended.[76] Finally, documentation of emergency US procedures should result in appropriate reimbursement for services provided.[77-78] (See Section 6 – Value and Reimbursement)

Quality Improvement Process

Quality improvement (QI) systems are an essential part of any US program. The objective of the QI process is to evaluate the images for technical competence, the interpretations for clinical accuracy, and to provide feedback to improve physician performance.

Parameters to be evaluated might include image resolution, anatomic definition, and other image quality acquisition aspects such as gain, depth, orientation, and focus. In addition, the QI system should compare the impression from the emergency US interpretation to patient outcome measures such as consultative US, other imaging modalities, surgical procedures, or patient clinical outcome.

The QI system design should strive to provide timely feedback to physicians. Balancing quality of review with provision of timely feedback is a key part of QA process design. Any system design should have a data storage component that enables data and image recall.

A process for patient callback should be in place and may be incorporated into the ED's process for calling patients back. Callbacks should occur when the initial image interpretation, upon QA review, may have been questionable, inappropriate and of clinical significance. In all cases, the imaging physician is informed of the callback and appropriate counseling/training is provided.

Due to the necessities of credentialing, it is prudent to expect that all images obtained prior to a provider attaining levels sufficient for credentialing should be reviewed.

Once providers are credentialed, programs should strive to sample a significant number of images from each provider that ensures continued competency. Due to the varieties of practice settings the percentage of scans undergoing quality assurance should be determined by the US director and should strive to protect patient safety and maintain competency. While this number can vary, a goal of 10% may be reasonable, adjusted for the experience of the providers and newness of the US application in that department.

The general data flow in the QA system is as follows:
1. Images obtained by the imaging provider should be archived, ideally on a digital system. These images may be still images or video clips, and should be representative of the US findings.
2. Clinical indications and US interpretations are documented on an electronic or paper record by the imaging provider.
3. These images and data are then reviewed by the US director or his/her designee.
4. Reviewers evaluate images for accuracy and technical quality and submit the reviews back to the imaging provider.
5. Emergency US studies are archived and available for future review should they be needed.

QA systems currently in place range from thermal images and log books to complete digital solutions. Finding the system that works best for each institution will depend on multiple factors, such as machine type, administrative and financial support, and physician compliance. Current digital management systems offer significant advantages to QA workflow and are recommended.

US QA may also contribute to the ED's local and national QI processes. US QA activities may be included in professional practice evaluation, practice performance, and other quality improvement activities. Measures such as performance of a FAST exam in high acuity trauma, detection of pregnancy location, use of US for internal jugular vein central line cannulation may be the initial logical elements to an overall quality plan. In addition, US QA databases may contribute to a registry regarding patient care and clinical outcomes.

US programs that include multiple educational levels and various types of providers should implement processes to integrate QA into the education process as well as the departmental or institutional quality framework. Technology allowing remote guidance and review may be integrated into the US QA system.

US Machines, Safety, and Maintenance
Dedicated US machines located in the ED for use at all times by emergency physicians are essential. Machines should be chosen to handle the rigors of the multi-user, multi-location practice environment of the ED.[72] Other issues that should be addressed regarding emergency US equipment include: regular in-service of personnel using the equipment and appropriate transducer care, stocking and storage of supplies, adequate cleaning of external and internal transducers with respect to infection control, maintenance of US machines by clinical engineering or a designated maintenance team, and efficient communication of equipment issues. Ultrasound providers should follow common ED US safety practices including ALARA, probe decontamination, and machine maintenance.

Risk Management
US can be an excellent risk reduction tool through 1) increasing diagnostic certainty, 2) shortening time to definitive therapy, and 3) decreasing complications from procedures that carry an inherent risk for complications.[80] An important step to managing risk is ensuring that physicians are properly trained and

credentialed according to national guidelines such as those set by ACEP. Proper quality assurance and improvement programs should be in place to identify and correct substandard practice. The greatest risk in regards to emergency US is lack of its use in appropriate cases.

The standard of care for emergency US is the performance and interpretation of US by a credentialed emergency physician within the limits of the clinical scenario. Physicians performing US imaging in other specialties or in different settings have different goals, scopes of practice, and documentation requirements, and consequently should not be compared to emergency US. As emergency US is a standard emergency medicine procedure, it is included in any definition of the practice of emergency medicine with regards to insurance and risk management.

Section 6 – Value and Reimbursement
Value in health care has been defined as outcomes that matter to patients relative to cost.[81] The value of clinical US is maximized when time spent by the clinician prevents costly imaging, invasive therapeutics, unnecessary consultations and produces accessible real-time results for the patient and the health care system.

Value is added to the medical system when US imaging increases patient health or decreases the cost to achieve that same level of patient heath. Clinical US contributes to patient health in several ways:
1. Improving patient safety by reducing medical errors during procedures
2. Increasing patient satisfaction
3. Improving departmental resource utilization
4. Eliminating costly or invasive procedures
5. Improved Clinical Decision Making

Reimbursement for US derives from Current Procedural Terminology (CPT) codes and their respective relative value units (RVUs). The reimbursements for US are calculated on work performed by entities within the healthcare system, with some going to physicians and some going to hospital entities.[3] The current system assumes a similar workflow for all US. The evolution of clinician-performed or clinical US has changed the workflow for many clinicians.

The current workflow for clinical US differs widely from the historical workflow. While consultative US centers on providing a work product for the interpreting physician, clinical US centers on the patient. The clinician evaluating the patient utilizes US at the patient's bedside to answer a focused question or guide an invasive procedure. The bedside physician takes over tasks that are attributed to the hospital's practice expense such as bringing the unit to the bedside, obtaining US images, and archiving images for the medical record. Figure 3 shows the workflow in the model of clinical US.

In addition to workflow differences, clinical bedside US has low expenses related to capital equipment, physical plant and supplies. The US machine is a less expensive mobile unit located in the ED and moved to the patient's bedside. Hospitals are turning to lower cost archiving alternatives to PACS, US management systems (also known as middleware or workflow solutions,) or cloud based software solutions which allow readily accessible digitally archived images.

CPT values physician work (wRVU) required for common emergency US at approximately 40% of the global RVU (total professional plus total technical). Active emergency US programs allow the hospital to bill technical fees which support the cost of the machine, supplies, and arriving/quality assurance software.

Efficiencies gained by incorporating bedside US imaging in the care of emergency medicine patients can produce an overall cost savings to the health care system. Clinical point-of-care ultrasound may provide significant benefits by reducing the needs for hospitalization, improved diagnosis and improved outcomes. With these benefits, shared savings should be attributed appropriately to the entity which affected the change.

A more detailed calculation of work depends on the specific clinical system organization and division of labor/resources. Future alternative payment structures such as value based purchasing, bundled payments, or accountable care organizations (ACOs) should appropriately factor the resources, efficiency and value of clinical based US into the value and reimbursement of emergency medical care.

Section 7- Clinical US Leadership in Healthcare Systems
Increasingly, many specialties have an interest in utilizing US in their clinical practice across diverse patient care settings. Consequently, there is a need for direction, leadership, and administrative oversight for hospital systems to efficiently deliver this technology in an organized and coordinated manner. Emergency physicians by nature have a broad scope of practice and interact with essentially all specialties and are thus uniquely positioned to take this role. Specifically, healthcare and hospital systems should:
   1) consider clinical, point-of-care ultrasonography separate from consultative imaging and
   2) use these guidelines for design of institutional clinical US programs, and
   3) strongly consider experienced emergency physician US leaders for system leadership in clinical, point-of-care ultrasonography.

There are many approaches to institutional oversight of multidisciplinary US programs including consensus from major utilizers, the formation of a governing body such as a clinical US steering committee or the creation of the position of an institutional clinical US director, who has a broad understanding of all the uses of clinical US. Specific items to consider which require leadership and coordination include policy development, equipment purchase, training and education, competency assessment and credentialing, quality assurance, and value/reimbursement.

Inherently, there will be a large number of requests for point-of-care US equipment. There may be significant advantages to standardizing or coordinating hardware and software when possible so that providers may share equipment across departments. This standardization may allow purchasing and cost saving advantages due to bulk deals and offers advantages in training and machine familiarity (eg, resuscitation areas). Standardization may have some negative effects with vendor exclusivity in regards to advancement in technologies and feature availability which may benefit individual settings.

In academic and community centers there will be a need for educating all levels of trainees. Ideally, education for each individual specialty should come from within that specialty. In the situation where education is needed, but there are no leaders within a specific specialty, then the training may fall to the director or committee as described above. In these cases, the director should work with the leadership within each specific specialty to make sure the training meets the specific need of that department. "Train the trainer" programs should be encouraged. It is crucial to develop multiple leaders within the hospital to meet the ever-increasing educational needs. Once these leaders are established it will be useful to have the committee or director to oversee and coordinate to make sure the education is consistent across specialties, and that resources and work effort are shared and not duplicated.

Credentialing for each specialty should follow national guidelines and be specialty specific.[71] However if national training guidelines for specialties do not exist, the director or committee should work to create general credentialing guidelines based on the ACEP structure, that are flexible enough to work with each specialty to meet their needs for specific applications.

Quality assurance should be organized and runs within a department; however, frequently, there are not leaders with the time, qualifications, and/or interest in providing this service and need. In these cases, the director or committee should develop a plan to meet this need. Institutions must provide appropriate resources to system-wide Clinical US programs to allow efficient operations including hardware (US machines) and software such as US management programs. (See Section 5 –Quality and US Management)

Clinical US in hospital and health care systems can be coordinated with successful initiation, maturation, and continual operation of a well-developed plan led by knowledgeable physicians with point-of-care experience. Coordination of specialties, equipment, software, education, quality review, and reimbursement are essential elements of such programs.

Section 8- Future Issues
Recent technological advances have improved access and overall US imaging. Wireless transducers, handheld systems and app based imaging connected via smart device are all reality.[82-85] These enhancements represent novel and exciting forms of US technology that expand the availability of US to new clinical settings due to increased portability and relative affordability. These new devices are currently being evaluated in a variety of clinical settings and more diverse situations that had not previously been possible.

Telesonography is a rapidly developing model which allows transfer of US images and video from remote locations to obtain consultation and treatment recommendations.[80,86] Recent advances in US and informatics allow remote experts to direct on-site less experienced ultrasonographers to obtain and interpret images that can impact patient care in real-time. An expert US mentor could potentially guide distant untrained health care providers geographically dispersed over multiple locations around the world. This paradigm may be utilized across all applications including procedural assistance. The practice of remote telesonography has the potential to improve quality of care in underserved communities in both domestic and international settings.

The automation of clinical US is yet another developing arena. Several companies have announced plans to build automated diagnostic protocols such as B-line detection in lung US and echocardiographic parameter assessment. These automated protocols may become the great equalizers by allowing a relative novice access to the same diagnostic information others have spent years training to attain. Finally, transducer technology will continue to change, including high resolution transducers that optimize sonographic windows, integrated probe/machine devices, and devices that use existing and new computer connections. Continuous advancements will allow clinicians to utilize US technology more and more and to limit inherent limitations and obstacles to use.

Other health care providers are also now realizing the utility of clinical US in their daily practice. Advanced practice professionals, nurses, emergency medical service personnel and others recognize the potential in their practice settings and desire to learn appropriate applications. Emergency physicians will continue to work with our colleagues at local, regional and national levels to help educate and establish appropriate training and practice standards for the safety of our patients. Leadership, supervision, and collaboration with other point-of-care specialists will continue to be critical to assure the safe, effective use of clinical US.

Advanced users of US in emergency, clinical, and point-of-care US have been creating a subspecialty of expert ultrasonographers who provide education, research, and advanced clinical practice with US. In addition, quality programs such as the Clinical Ultrasound Accreditation Program will provide leadership to EDs who can meet the criteria in this document.

As emergency US moves forward, continued high quality research in the field needs to occur. Future methodological improvements focused on patient outcomes are crucial for the advancement of point-of-care US within academic medicine. Multi-center studies producing higher level of evidence will allow the continued growth and appropriate use of US in emergency care. The future, while undeniably bright still requires much effort on the part of us all.

Section 9 – Conclusion

ACEP endorses the following statements on the use of emergency clinical, point-of-care US:

1. Emergency point-of-care ultrasound performed, interpreted, and integrated into clinical care by emergency physicians is a fundamental skill in the practice of emergency medicine.
2. The scope of practice of emergency US can be classified into categories of resuscitation, diagnostic, symptom or sign-based, procedural guidance, and monitoring/therapeutics in which a variety of emergency US applications exists, including the core applications of trauma, pregnancy, abdominal aorta, cardiac/HD assessment, biliary, urinary tract, deep venous thrombosis, thoracic-airway, soft-tissue/musculoskeletal, ocular, bowel and procedural guidance.
3. Training and proficiency requirements should include didactic, experiential and integrative components as described within this document.
4. Emergency US training in emergency medicine residency programs should be fully integrated into the curriculum and patient care experience.
5. Emergency US should be considered a core credential for emergency physicians undergoing privileging in modern healthcare systems without need for external certification.
6. US QA and management require appropriate resources including physician direction, dedicated US machines, digital US management systems, and resources for QA.
7. Healthcare clinical point-of-care ultrasound programs optimally led by emergency physicians should be supported with resources for leadership, quality improvement, training, hardware and software acquisition and maintenance.
8. Emergency US is an independent procedure that should be reimbursed and valued, independent of the ED history, physical examination, and medical decision-making.
9. Emergency physicians with advanced US expertise should contribute leadership in clinical ultrasonography at the departmental, institutional, system, national, and international level.
10. Evolving technological, educational, and practice advancements may provide new approaches and efficiencies, modalities in the care of the emergent patient.

Table 1. Relevant Ultrasound Definitions

Resuscitative	US use directly related to a resuscitation
Diagnostic	US utilized a diagnostic imaging capacity
Symptom or sign-based	US used in a clinical pathway based upon the patient's symptoms or sign (eg, shortness of breath)
Therapeutic and Monitoring	US use in therapeutics or physiological monitoring
Procedural guidance	US used as an aid to guide a procedure

Consultative Ultrasound	A written or electronic request for an US examination & interpretation for which the patient is transported to a laboratory or imaging department outside of the clinical setting.
Emergency Ultrasound	Performed and interpreted by the provider as an emergency procedure and directly integrated into the care of the patient

Clinical Ultrasound	US used in the clinical setting, distinct from the physical examination, that adds anatomic, functional and physiologic information to the care of the acutely ill patient.
Educational Ultrasound	US performed in a non-clinical setting by medical students or other clinician trainees to enhance physical examination skills. Exams usually performed on cadavers or live models.

Table 2. Other emergency ultrasound applications (adjunct or emerging)

Advanced Echo
Transesophageal Echo
Adnexal Pathology
Testicular
Transcranial Doppler
Vascular
Contrast Studies
ENT
Infectious Disease

Figure 1. ACEP 2016 Emergency US Guidelines Scope of Practice

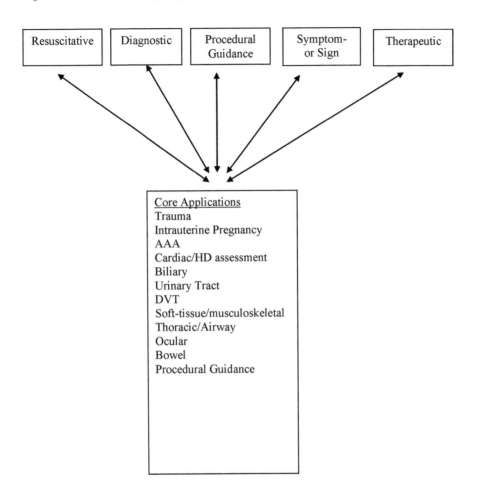

Figure 2. Pathways for emergency ultrasound training, credentialing, and incorporation
of new applications

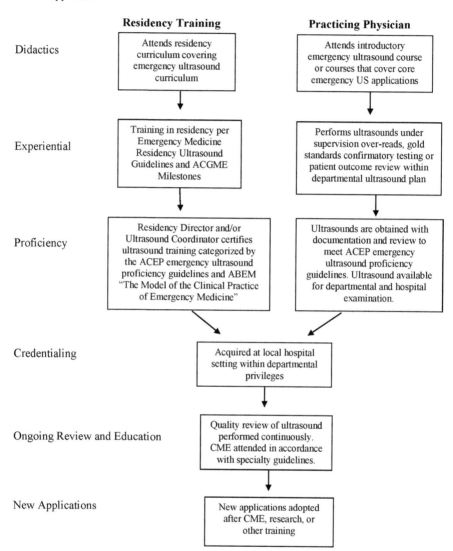

Figure 3 – Clinical Ultrasound Workflow

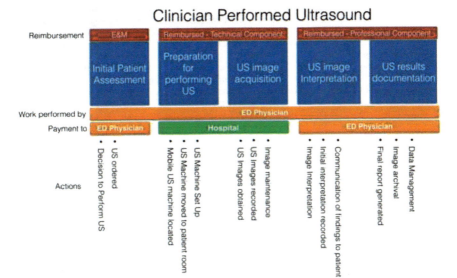

Appendix 1. Evidence for Core Emergency Ultrasound Applications
Trauma
The use of US in trauma patient is typically for the detection of abnormal fluid or air collection in the torso. This application applies to both blunt and penetrating trauma in all ages. Perhaps the first bedside US technique studied in the hands of non-radiologists was the focused assessment with sonography in trauma (FAST) examination. First demonstrated in Europe and by surgeons, the technique was later adopted by emergency physicians.[87] In one early prospective study, FAST was 90% sensitive and 99% specific in detecting peritoneal bleeding in blunt trauma, and 91% sensitive and 100% specific in penetrating trauma.[88] A retrospective review of patients with penetrating thoracic trauma demonstrated 100% sensitivity for the detection of pericardial effusion and more rapid diagnosis and management when US was employed in their assessment.[89] Recently, a prospective randomized controlled study assessed 262 blunt trauma patients managed using the FAST exam as a diagnostic adjunct vs. no FAST exam. Patients randomized to the FAST exam group had more rapid disposition to the operating room, required fewer CT scans, and incurred shorter hospitalizations, fewer complications, and lower charges than those in whom the FAST was not performed.[90] During the last decade, pneumothorax has been added to the FAST exam as the EFAST examination.[91] FAST examination also may have an effect on the utilization of ionizing radiation tests.[92]

Pregnancy
Use of emergency US in pelvic disorders centers on the detection of intrauterine pregnancy (IUP), detection of ectopic pregnancy, detection of fetal heart rate in all stages of pregnancy, dating of the pregnancy, and detection of significant free fluid. Bedside pelvic US during the first trimester of pregnancy can be used to exclude ectopic pregnancy by demonstrating an intrauterine pregnancy. Studies of EP-performed US in this setting have demonstrated sensitivity of 76-90% and specificity of 88-92% for the detection of ectopic pregnancy.[77-78,93-94] In one study, EPs were able to detect an intrauterine pregnancy in 70% of patients with suspected ectopic pregnancy (first trimester pregnancy with abdominal pain or vaginal bleeding).[93] When intrauterine fetal anatomy was visualized at the bedside, ectopic pregnancy was ruled out with a negative predictive value of essentially 100%. When bedside US evaluation was incorporated into a clinical algorithm for the evaluation of patients with suspected ectopic pregnancy, the incidence of discharged patients returning with ruptured ectopic pregnancy was significantly reduced.[95] Pelvic US by emergency physicians also save resources including length of stay and consultative imaging.[96]

Abdominal Aortic Aneurysm (AAA)
The use of emergency US of the aorta is mainly for the detection of AAA, though aortic dissection may occasionally be detected. Although CT scan and MRI often serve as the criterion standard for AAA assessment, US is frequently used by radiology departments as a screening modality as well. In the ED, bedside US demonstrates excellent test characteristics when used by emergency physicians to evaluate patients with suspected AAA. One study of 68 ED patients with suspected AAA demonstrated sensitivity, specificity, positive and negative predictive values of 100%.[97] In another, 125 patients were assessed by EPs. Sensitivity was 100%, specificity 98%, positive predictive value 93% and negative predictive value 100% in this study.[98] In both studies, CT scan, radiology US, MRI, and operative findings served as a combined criterion standard.

Emergent Echocardiography and Hemodynamic Assessment
Emergent cardiac US can be used to assess for pericardial effusion and tamponade, cardiac activity, a global assessment of contractility, and the detection of central venous volume status. One early study of bedside echocardiography by EPs demonstrated 100% sensitivity for the detection of pericardial effusion in the setting of penetrating chest trauma. In this series, patients evaluated with US were diagnosed and treated more rapidly when US was employed in their assessment.[89,99] Test characteristics of EP-performed

echocardiography (when compared to expert over-read of images) for effusion include sensitivity of 96-100%, specificity 98-100%, positive predictive value 93-100% and negative predictive value 99-100%. The prognostic value of EP-performed bedside echocardiography has been well-established.[100] In one study of 173 patients in cardiac arrest, cardiac standstill on US was 100% predictive of mortality, regardless of electrical rhythm (positive predictive value of 100%).[101] US has been incorporated into the resuscitation of the critically ill and arrest patient. In the assessment of patients with undifferentiated hypotension, EP assessment of cardiac contractility correlated well and has improved diagnostic accuracy (R=0.84).[102-104] Emergent cardiac US has expanded to the use of heart failure and dyspnea.[105-106] In addition hemodynamic assessment with US for preload, cardiac function, and afterload has become an accepted diagnostic and monitoring tool.[107-116]

Hepatobiliary System

The use of emergency US for hepatobiliary disease has centered on biliary inflammation and biliary obstruction. Although many sonographic criteria for acute cholecystitis exist (including gallstones, thickened gallbladder wall, pericholecystic fluid, sonographic Murphy's sign, and common bile duct dilatation), gallstones are present in 95-99% of acute cholecystitis cases.[117] This finding is quite accessible to the EP using bedside US, and may be placed into the context of an individual patient's clinical picture (presence of fever, tenderness, laboratory evaluation, etc.). The test characteristics for gallstone detection by bedside US are: sensitivity 90-96%, specificity 88-96%, positive predictive value 88-99% and negative predictive value 73-96%.[118-121] A retrospective review of 1252 cases of suspected cholecystitis demonstrated that bedside emergency physician US vs radiology US evaluation decreased length of stay by 7% (22 minutes) overall, and up to 15% (52 minutes) when patients were evaluated during evening or nighttime hours.[122]

Urinary Tract

The use of emergency US in the urinary tract is for detection of hydronephrosis and bladder status. The detection of hydronephrosis on bedside US, when combined with urinalysis and clinical assessment, may be helpful in differentiating patients with acute renal colic.[123-124] Bedside renal US by experienced EPs has demonstrated sensitivity of 75-87% and specificity of 82-89% when compared with CT scan.[125-126] Urinary tract US has also been shown similar to radiology US and CT imaging for imaging for patients with suspected renal colic.[127]

Deep Vein Thrombosis

The use of emergency US for detection of DVT has centered on the use of multilevel compression US on proximal veins, especially in the lower extremity.[128-129] A number of ED studies have examined the test characteristics of EP-performed limited venous compression sonography for the evaluation of DVT. A recent systematic review of six studies, (with a total of 132 DVTs in 936 patients) found a pooled sensitivity and specificity of 95% and 96%, respectively.[41,130] One study demonstrated more rapid disposition for patients undergoing bedside US for DVT assessment compared with radiology department DVT assessment (95 vs. 225 minutes).[131]

Soft tissue/musculoskeletal

The use of emergency US in soft-tissue has focused on soft-tissue infection, foreign bodies, and cutaneous masses. Although a host of musculoskeletal applications of bedside US have been studied by EPs, among the most common and best described is the assessment of cellulitis and abscess at the bedside. Ultrasound has been shown to improve the clinical assessment of patients with cellulitis and possible abscess in several studies.[132] In one study of 105 patients with suspected abscess, US demonstrated sensitivity of 98%, specificity 88%, positive predictive value 93% and negative predictive value 97% compared with needle aspiration.[132-133] Another study demonstrated that bedside US altered the management of patients with cellulitis (and no clinically obvious abscess) in 56% of cases.[134] These patients were found to have abscesses or require surgical evaluations which were not evident on clinical examination alone. Fractures have been identified in series and prospective studies with good accuracy.[135-136] Tendons injuries and joint effusions have been studied with excellent clarity.[137-139]

Thoracic-Airway

The use of emergency US in the thorax has been for the detection of pleural effusion and pneumothorax, interstitial and inflammatory disorders.[140-144] Bedside US for the evaluation of thoracic disorders was described in the 1990s in European critical care settings. Since then, emergency physicians have utilized the technology for the detection of pneumothorax and other acute pathology. In the setting of blunt thoracic trauma, EP-performed US demonstrated sensitivity of 92-98%, specificity 99%, positive predictive value 96-98% and negative predictive value 99% compared with CT scan or air release during chest tube placement.[145] In the last decade, tracheal and airway assessment and endotracheal guidance has been studied with US. Recent cardiac resuscitation guidelines have included tracheal US as an alternative confirmatory test in cardiac arrest.[146-152]

Ocular

The use of emergency US in the eye has described for the detection of posterior chamber and orbital pathology. Specifically US has been described to detect retinal detachment, vitreous hemorrhage, and dislocations or disruptions of structures.[153-156] In addition the structures posterior to the globe such as the optic nerve sheath diameter may be a reflection of other disease in the central nervous system.

Bowel

Abdominal US can aid in the diagnosis a wide array of bowel pathology. Appendicitis is the most common surgical emergency of the abdomen and has traditionally been diagnosed by CT; however trained emergency physicians have been capable of diagnosing appendicitis with point-of-care US with 60-96% sensitivity and 68-98% specificity.[157-171] Emergency US has been shown to decrease radiation exposure and length of stay.[9] Ultrasound for ileus and small bowel obstruction has been performed for decades. It has been shown to be more sensitive and specific for obstruction than x-ray, and can be performed accurately by emergency providers.[172-174] Pneumoperitoneum can be also diagnosed by US with high sensitivity and specificity, and due to its availability and speed, has been proposed as a screening tool in the acute abdomen. In some countries, US is the first line imaging modality for the diagnosis of diverticulitis.[175-176] With proper training and experience, emergency providers can use this tool to facilitate diagnosis of diverticulitis.[177] Ultrasound can give quick information about abdominal wall masses and suspected hernias, even aiding in the classification of hernias.[178-181] In addition, it can be performed dynamically and facilitate the reduction of hernias in real-time.[178-181] Ultrasound plays a particularly important role in the pediatric population, and is the initial diagnostic method of choice for both intussusception and pyloric stenosis. Studies have shown that emergency providers with limited training can effectively diagnose these conditions.[182-183]

Procedural Guidance

Ultrasound guidance has been studied as a useful adjunct to many common ED procedures, including venous access, thoracentesis, paracentesis, joint aspiration, and others.[137,184-185] Studies since the early 1990s have demonstrated the efficacy of US guidance for central venous cannulation, and the use of this technology has been advocated by the United States Agency for Healthcare Research and Quality as one of the top 11 means of increasing patient safety in the United States.[186] Recently, and randomized controlled study of 201 patients undergoing central venous cannulation demonstrated higher success rates with dynamic US guidance (98% success) when compared with static US guidance (82%) or landmark-based methods (64%).[136]

Appendix 2. Emergency Ultrasound Learning Objectives
Listed below are recommended learning objectives for a comprehensive EUS clinician curriculum, rotation, or series of training courses. For detailed indications, limitations, protocols, documentation requirements, and other important details for each application, please refer to the ACEP Emergency Ultrasound Imaging Criteria Compendium.[5]

Introduction
- Distinguish between consultative, clinical, point of care, and emergency ultrasound (EUS).
- Recognize primary EUS applications.
- Discuss support for EUS from key organizations including ACEP, AMA, ABEM, SAEM, and AIUM.
- Describe ACEP recommendations training and credentialing in EUS.

Physics & Instrumentation
- Explain ultrasound physics relevant to EUS:
  Piezoelectric effect
  Frequency
  Resolution
  Attenuation
  Echogenicity
  Doppler including pulse wave, color and power
- Operate the EUS system as needed to obtain and interpret images adequate for clinical decision making including:
  Image mode
  Gain
  Time gain compensation
  Focus
  Probe types
- Recognize common ultrasound artifacts including:
  Reverberation
  Side lobe
  Mirror
  Shadowing
  Enhancement
  Ring-down

Trauma
- Describe the indications, clinical algorithm, and limitations of EUS in blunt and penetrating thoracoabdominal trauma.
- Perform the EUS protocol for Trauma.
- Identify relevant US anatomy including the pleura, diaphragm, inferior vena cava, pericardium, liver, spleen, kidneys, bladder, prostate and uterus.
- Recognize pathologic findings and pitfalls in the evaluation of pneumothorax, hemothorax, hemopericardium, cardiac activity, volume status, and hemoperitoneum.
- Integrate Trauma EUS findings into individual patient, departmental, and disaster management.

First-Trimester Pregnancy
- Describe the indications, clinical algorithm, and limitations of EUS in first-trimester pregnancy pain and bleeding.

- Understand the utility of quantitative B-HCG in the evaluation of first-trimester pregnancy pain and bleeding.
- Perform EUS protocols for transabdominal and transvaginal views as needed, including fetal heart rate and gestational age measurement techniques.
- Identify relevant US anatomy including the cervix, uterus, adnexa, bladder and cul-de-sac.
- Recognize the relevant findings and pitfalls when evaluating for intrauterine and ectopic pregnancy:
  - Early embryonic structures including the gestational sac, yolk sac, fetal pole, and heart
  - Location of embryonic structures in pelvis
  - Embryonic demise
  - Molar pregnancy
  - Findings of ectopic pregnancy including pseudogestational sac, free fluid, and adnexal masses
- Integrate First Trimester Pregnancy EUS findings into individual patient and departmental management.

Abdominal Aorta
- Describe indications, clinical algorithm, and limitations of EUS in the evaluation of aortic pathology.
- Perform EUS protocols to evaluate the abdominal aorta including measurement techniques.
- Identify relevant US anatomy including the aorta with major branches, inferior vena cava, and vertebral bodies.
- Recognize pathologic findings and pitfalls when evaluating for aortic aneurysm and dissection.
- Integrate Aorta EUS findings into individual patient and departmental management.

Echocardiography and HD Assessment
- Describe the indications and limitations of emergency echocardiography.
- Perform standard echocardiography windows (subcostal, parasternal, and apical) and planes (four chamber, long and short axis).
- Identify relevant US anatomy including pericardium, cardiac chambers, valves, aorta and inferior vena cava.
- Estimate qualitative left ventricular function and central venous pressure to guide HD assessment of patient.
- Recognize cardiac arrest, pericardial effusions with or without tamponade, and dilation of the aortic root or the descending aorta.
- Integrate Emergency echocardiography findings into individual patient and departmental management.

Biliary Tract
- Describe the indications and limitations of EUS of the biliary tract.
- Perform EUS protocols to evaluate the biliary tract.
- Identify relevant US anatomy including the gallbladder, portal triad, inferior vena cava, and liver.
- Recognize the relevant findings and pitfalls when evaluating for cholelithiasis and cholecystitis.
- Integrate EUS of the biliary tract into individual patient and departmental management.

Urinary Tract
- Describe the indications and limitations of EUS of the urinary tract.
- Perform EUS protocols to evaluate the urinary tract.
- Identify relevant US anatomy including the renal cortex, renal pelvis, ureter, bladder, liver, and spleen.

- Recognize the relevant findings and pitfalls when evaluating for hydronephrosis, renal calculi, renal masses, and bladder volume.
- Integrate EUS of the urinary tract into individual patient and departmental management.

Deep Vein Thrombosis
- Describe the indications and limitations of EUS for the detection of deep venous thrombosis.
- Perform EUS protocols for the detection of deep venous thrombosis of the upper and lower extremities including:
  – Vessel identification
  – Compression
  – Doppler imaging of respiratory variation and augmentation.
- Identify relevant US anatomy of the upper and lower extremities including the deep venous and arterial systems, major nerves, and lymph nodes.
- Recognize the relevant findings and pitfalls when evaluating for deep venous thrombosis.
- Integrate EUS for deep venous thrombosis into individual patient and departmental management.

Soft Tissue & Musculoskeletal
- Describe the indications and limitations of soft tissue and musculoskeletal EUS.
- Perform EUS protocols for the evaluation of soft tissue and musculoskeletal pathology.
- Identify relevant US anatomy including:
  – Skin
  – Adipose
  – Fascia
  – Muscle
  – Tendons and Ligaments
  – Muscles
  – Lymph Nodes
  – Bones and Joints
- Recognize the relevant findings and pitfalls when evaluating the following:
  – Soft tissue infections: Abscess versus cellulitis
  – Subcutaneous fluid collection identification
  – Foreign body location and removal
  – Tendon injury (laceration, rupture)
  – Fractures
  – Joint identification
- Integrate soft tissue and musculoskeletal EUS findings into individual patient and departmental management.

Thoracic -Airway
- Describe the indications and limitations Thoracic EUS
- Perform EUS protocols for the detection of:
  – Pneumothorax
  – Pleural Effusion
  – Alveolar Interstitial Syndromes
- Identify relevant US anatomy of thoracic structures.
- Recognize the relevant findings and pitfalls when evaluating for thoracic pathology

- Recognize the sonographic findings of tracheal and esophageal anatomy, especially in regards to EM procedures
- Integrate thoracic EUS findings into individual patient and departmental management.

Ocular
- Describe the indications and limitations of ocular EUS.
- Perform EUS protocols for the detection of vitreous hemorrhage, retinal detachment, and other pathology.
- Identify relevant US anatomy of the globe and orbital structures.
- Recognize the relevant findings and pitfalls when evaluating for ocular pathology.
- Integrate ocular EUS into individual patient and departmental management.

Procedural Guidance
- Describe the indications and limitations when using US guidance for bedside procedures.
- Perform EUS protocols for procedural guidance including both transverse and longitudinal approaches when appropriate. These procedures may include:
  - Vascular access: Central and peripheral
  - Confirmation of endotracheal intubation
  - Pericardiocentesis
  - Paracentesis
  - Thoracentesis
  - Foreign body detection removal
  - Bladder aspiration
  - Arthrocentesis
  - Pacemaker placement and capture
  - Abscess identification and drainage
- Identify relevant US anatomy for each particular procedure.
- Recognize the relevant findings and pitfalls when performing EUS for procedural guidance.
- Integrate EUS for procedural guidance into individual patient and departmental management.

Bowel
- Describe the indications and limitations of Bowel EUS
- Perform EUS protocols when for the detection of:
  - Appendicitis
  - Bowel Obstruction
  - Pneumoperitoneum
  - Diverticulitis
  - Hernia
  - Pediatric Intussception and Pyloric Stenosis
- Identify relevant US anatomy of bowel structures.
- Recognize the relevant findings and pitfalls when evaluating for bowel pathology
- Integrate bowel EUS findings into individual patient and departmental management.

Appendix 3. Recommendations for an EM Residency EUS Education Program

Successful EUS Residency Education in accordance with these guidelines requires significant departmental and institutional support. The purpose of these additional recommendations is to delineate the scope of resources required to facilitate the rapid development and maintenance of EUS Residency Education programs. Application of these recommendations is dependent on EM Residency size, current and planned EUS utilization, and institutional capabilities.

EUS Faculty:

1. EUS Director: At least one full time EM attending faculty with sufficient EUS program coordination expertise. Sufficient non-clinical time for planning and conducting all EUS program activities is essential to ensuring adequate resident training.
2. EUS Faculty: At least one additional full time EM attending faculty member committed to actively developing EUS program expertise. Sufficient non-clinical time for conducting EUS program activities is essential to ensuring adequate resident training. The number of dedicated EUS faculty needed is dependent on the size of the residency and quality of the training program provided.
3. Credentialed EUS Faculty: To adequately supervise and educate residents in EUS, a minimum of fifty percent of Core Faculty members at all EM residency programs need to be credentialed in EUS. For example, if a program has 12 core faculty, then 6 need to be credentialed in EUS. May be inclusive of the EUS Director and Faculty.

Equipment and Materials:

1. EUS systems with appropriate transducers and imaging capabilities readily available for immediate resident clinical use 24/7.
2. EUS online or print text reference resources readily available in the ED.
3. Recent and landmark EUS literature as well as opportunities to participate in local quality improvement and research projects need to be provided to residents and core US faculty.

Educational Program Activities:

1. Initial EUS Training: Didactic and hands on instruction in EUS physics, machine use, and at least one springboard application such as the Trauma exam need to be provided early in residency as a half or full day course.
2. Annual EUS Rotations: Two week rotation in the first year to learn basic EUS knowledge and skills, followed by at least one week in each subsequent year to reinforce learning and acquire more advanced skills. One rotation without continued learning within the EM residency curriculum is inadequate. For each trainee, a minimum of 80 hours of dedicated EUS rotation time is recommended during an EM residency.
3. Suggested rotation educational methods and assessment measures:
   a. Orientation: Begin rotation with a baseline EUS skills assessment to identify trainee's unique learning needs. Follow with hands on small group instruction in the ED focusing on machine operation, exam protocols, image optimization and interpretation, documentation, as well as integration of EUS findings into daily clinical practice.
   b. Daily supervised scanning shifts with EUS faculty in the ED to provide opportunities for both proctored and semi-independent image acquisition and interpretation. All training exams are submitted for timely quality assurance review.
   c. Weekly Academic Day:
      i. Quality Assurance Review session during which a portion of current trainee's EUS exams are discussed, focusing on challenging cases, pathology, and integration into daily patient and ED management.

      ii.   Simulation cases and review of image libraries for additional exposure to less common pathology.

      iii.   Journal club including a discussion of a recent or landmark EUS literature, an online narrated didactic or live lecture, or chapter review.

      iv.   Hands on small group instruction in the ED focusing on current trainees learning needs identified during QA Review or scanning shifts.

    d. End the rotation with a final assessment of EUS knowledge utilizing a standardized exam such as the ACEP US Online Exams, as well as an additional EUS skill assessment.

    e. Provide a timely end of EUS rotation assessment of knowledge and skills to each resident. Additionally, provide trainees with continued opportunities to evaluate the EUS program itself.

4.   Achieving EUS exam requirements: Completion of set number procedural benchmarks documents adequate experience to develop proficiency. Additional assessment measures described in these guidelines are needed to ensure EUS competency such as participation in QA sessions, SDOT's, OSCE's, and simulation assessments.

5.   Ongoing Quality Assurance System: Digital archiving system for EUS exam images and interpretations for timely quality assurance review and trainee feedback on individual exams.

    a. All trainee exams need to be reviewed by EUS faculty until minimum benchmarks are achieved. After this, a proportion of trainee exams need to be reviewed on an ongoing basis throughout residency.

    b. Timely exam feedback must be provided to trainees during and between EUS rotations. Trainees need ready access to individual exam feedback and total exams completed by application and overall.

6.   Integrated EUS training in the residency curriculum: Learning needs to be reinforced during quarterly or biannual EUS workshops comprised of EUS didactics and hands on instruction. An additional 20 hours of dedicated EUS learning between rotations is recommended during a 3 or 4 year residency.

Appendix 4. Recommendations for an EUS Course

Successful training courses in EUS require significant advance planning and resource commitment. Each course requires a curriculum designed by the course director that includes a local trainee needs assessment, learning objectives, educational methods, and assessment measures. The learning objectives for any EUS Course or rotation are listed in Appendix 2. Important considerations are discussed below:

1. Faculty: Course director must be an emergency ultrasound faculty physician. The course director will recruit other clinicians already credentialed in EUS to assist with knowledge learning, skills training, and trainee assessment. A faculty planning meeting is needed during curriculum development. Additionally, a meeting immediately prior to the course provides all faculty with an understanding of the setup and curriculum.

2. Site and Set Up: The ideal course site includes a large didactic room as well as separate rooms or areas for scanning stations. Private areas for endovaginal US are required.
    a. Ultrasound Stations: Appropriate machines and transducers are necessary. The student to instructor ratio should be no higher than 5 to 1 to ensure appropriate skills training.
    b. Ultrasound Models: Image acquisition protocols may be learned on normal live models. Image interpretation requires the incorporation of patients with known pathologic findings, simulators, or incorporation of image libraries.
        i.   Pathology models may include otherwise healthy paid or volunteer persons with pericardial effusions, cholelithiasis, aortic aneurysms and chronic ambulatory peritoneal dialysis patients.
        ii. Full informed consent should be obtained from all models and a signed waiver of responsibility is recommended. If an undiagnosed finding is discovered in a model, then the Course Director must appropriately notify the model and ensure appropriate follow up.

3. Knowledge Learning:
    a. An introductory course for trainees must include instruction in basic US physics, machine operation, and a small number of initial EUS applications to be clinically utilized. Suggested initial applications include Trauma Ultrasound, Central and Peripheral Venous Access, and Abdominal Aortic Aneurysm Ultrasound. However, the initial applications will vary by local site as determined by a pre-course needs assessment completed by the course director and local trainee leadership.
        i.   A half day introductory course is appropriate for a single applications. Longer courses are required for additional applications. Shorter, repeated courses, supplemented by routine, quality assured, EUS performance during clinical work, are more likely to improve learning and utilization.
    b. Pre and post course educational materials must be provided to reinforce course learning. Suggested sources of information include course director approved online narrated lectures, podcasts, websites, traditional textbooks, didactic syllabi, and journal articles.
        i.   Utilization of the flipped classroom provides the opportunity for more focused didactics reviewing key concepts and answering trainee questions at the course. Focused didactics provide the opportunity for increased skill training.
        ii. Frequent rotations between didactics and skills training sessions improve trainee and faculty engagement.

4. Skills Training:
    a. The technical laboratory is an integral component of any ultrasound course.
        iii. Based on the needs assessment, appropriate and specific learning objectives need to be defined for each station.

        iv. Trainees should be deliberately assigned to small groups not necessarily including immediate peers to create more focused learning teams.
        v.   For trainees with prior EUS experience, an initial skills assessment with an SDOT or simulator will help to ensure that trainee specific instruction is provided.
        vi. Instructors should work to maximize the time that the transducer is the trainee's' hands, avoid over teaching of advanced concepts beyond the trainees needs, encourage questions, and consistently engage each trainee.

Appendix 5. EUS and CUS Training for Medical Students

EUS Training during an one month EM Rotation:
General EM clerkships should include an introduction to EUS that may entail a single dedicated emergency US shift with direct faculty supervision, a one-day EUS course, or simply case-by-case incorporation of EUS into patient care in the ED. Students should strive to become familiar with a single emergency US application such as the FAST exam, and should be exposed to additional EUS exams over the course of the clerkship. EUS literature and selected textbook chapters should be made available for student review.

Dedicated EUS rotation recommendations:
1. Emergency US rotations begins with instruction in Physics/Instrumentation, followed by select applications such as FAST, Aorta, Renal, Biliary Cardiac, Procedures, Pelvic (including endovaginal US), Deep Venous Thrombosis, and Skin/Soft Tissue/Musculoskeletal.
2. Didactic education should be delivered in electronic, preferably online, format in an attempt to maximize hands-on education in the clinical area. Course directors may choose to utilize the emergency US didactic materials available on the ACEP Web site.
3. Assessment should include an online pre-test including still image/video interpretation and case-based applications of EUS. To assess their progress, students will complete the test again at the end of the rotation.
4. Each student should obtain approximately 100 scans over the course of a 4-week rotation, or approximately 75 scans over the course of a 2-week rotation. Dedicated shifts may include evenings or weekends to maximize exposure to pathology and interesting emergency US cases. Students should generate personal log of EUS exams on which to build during their postgraduate education.
5. All student-performed scans should be directly supervised by EUS credentialed faculty or recorded for subsequent quality assurance review with the rotation director.
6. Students should complete the reading of one EUS text or viewing of an online curriculum over the course of the rotation. In addition, students should identify a current publication relevant to EUS and discuss their findings with the rotation director.

Additional Opportunities for CUS Training in Undergraduate Medical Education:
Additionally, opportunities abound for EUS directors to get involved in medical student education at the various levels of medical school training. With the advent of more US in the various specialties, this preparation in medical school can benefit students with interests outside of emergency medicine.

EUS directors could consider incorporating US into.
1. Gross anatomy course highlighting common US anatomy (eg, FAST exam during study of the abdomen, heart)
2. Physiology course highlighting doppler, M mode, and basic waveform analysis.
3. Pathology course highlighting common pathologies such as fluid in potential spaces, depressed cardiac function, cellulitis, abscess, retinal detachment or other commonly seen pathologies in the ED.
4. Introduction to Clinical Medicine course highlighting US guided vascular access.
5. Ultrasound in the physical exam. Although US use in clinical practice is a diagnostic test that warrants a generated report, it can be used to teach components of the physical exam. For example teaching the traditional cardiac auscultation can be augmented with cardiac images of the heart.
6. Ultrasound training before clinical rotations. Some schools have developed short clinical skills time before rotations where US can be implemented to help student learners see how US is used in that particular field.

7. Ultrasound electives in the 4th year can include a longitudinal program where US lectures, hands on, and journal club can be incorporated into a course.

The future of US in medical education is still being built. It seems like there are early adopters trying to implement US yet there is still a lack of consensus if or how US should be optimally applied in medical education. The key component is finding an US champion to spearhead US into the undergraduate medical education framework. From there, getting students involved through an US interest group can improve the impact through direct feedback and student motivation. The two methods of a top down administrative implementation of US in medical education is the best method, yet warrants buy in from the dean and the curriculum committee. A bottom up approach through student interest, electives and extracurricular exposure takes longer but can still impact student competence in US. The next 5-10 years are sure to bring more clarity to this topic as US continues to expand.

References

1. Heller MB, Mandavia D, Tayal VS, et al. Residency training in emergency ultrasound: fulfilling the mandate. Acad Emerg Med. 2002;9:835-9.
2. ACR-SPR-SRU Practice Parameter for Performing and Interpreting Diagnostic Ultrasound Examinations. 2014. Accessed May 13, 2016 at https://www.acr.org/~/media/13B896B9F4844E3082E7D7ED66AFC148.pdf
3. ACEP Emergency Ultrasound Section. Emergency Ultrasound Coding and Reimbursement Document. 2009. Accessed June 6, 2016 at https://www.acep.org/Clinical---Practice-Management/Emergency-Ultrasound-Coding-and-Reimbursement-Update---2009/
4. Geria RN, Raio CC, Tayal V. Point-of-care ultrasound: not a stethoscope-a separate clinical entity. J Ultrasound Med. 2015;34:172-3.
5. American College of Emergency Physicians. Definition of Clinical Ultrasonography [policy statement]. Approved January 2014. Accessed May 13, 2016 at https://www.acep.org/clinical---practice-management/definition-of-clinical-ultrasonography/
6. American College of Emergency Physicians. Emergency Ultrasound Imaging Criteria Compendium [policy statement]. Approved October 2014. Accessed May 13, 2016 at https://www.acep.org/clinical---practice-management/emergency-ultrasound-imaging-criteria-compendium
7. Shah VP, Tunik MG, Tsung JW. Prospective evaluation of point-of-care ultrasonography for the diagnosis of pneumonia in children and young adults. JAMA Pediatr. 2013;167:119-25.
8. Gallagher RA, Levy J, Vieira RL, et al. Ultrasound assistance for central venous catheter placement in a pediatric emergency department improves placement success rates. Acad Emerg Med. 2014;21:981-6.
9. Elikashvili I, Tay ET, Tsung JW. The effect of point-of-care ultrasonography on emergency department length of stay and computed tomography utilization in children with suspected appendicitis. Acad Emerg Med. 2014;21:163-70.
10. Bartocci M, Fabrizi G, Valente I, et al. Intussusception in childhood: role of sonography on diagnosis and treatment. J Ultrasound. 2015;18:205-11.
11. Plumb J, Mallin M, Bolte RG. The role of ultrasound in the emergency department evaluation of the acutely painful pediatric hip. Pediatr Emerg Care. 2015;31:54-8; quiz 9-61.
12. Deanehan J, Gallagher R, Vieira R, et al. Bedside hip ultrasonography in the pediatric emergency department: a tool to guide management in patients presenting with limp. Pediatr Emerg Care. 2014;30:285-7.
13. Marin JR, Lewiss RE, AAP, et al. Point-of-care ultrasonography by pediatric emergency medicine physicians. Pediatrics. 2015;135(4):e1113-22.
14. Vieira RL, Hsu D, Nagler J, et al. Pediatric emergency medicine fellow training in ultrasound: consensus educational guidelines. Acad Emerg Med. 2013;20:300-6.
15. Zieleskiewicz L, Muller L, Lakhal K, et al. Point-of-care ultrasound in intensive care units: assessment of 1073 procedures in a multicentric, prospective, observational study. Intensive Care Med. 2015;41:1638-47.
16. Gallard E, Redonnet JP, Bourcier JE, et al. Diagnostic performance of cardiopulmonary ultrasound performed by the emergency physician in the management of acute dyspnea. Am J Emerg. Med. 2015;33:352-8.
17. Nelson BP, Sanghvi A. Out of hospital point of care ultrasound: current use models and future directions. Eur J Trauma Emerg Surg. 2015.
18. Press GM, Miller SK, Hassan IA, et al. Evaluation of a training curriculum for prehospital trauma ultrasound. J Emerg Med. 2013;45:856-64.
19. Taylor J, McLaughlin K, McRae A, et al. Use of prehospital ultrasound in North America: a survey of emergency medical services medical directors. BMC Emerg Med. 2014;14:6.

20. Shorter M, Macias DJ. Portable handheld ultrasound in austere environments: use in the Haiti disaster. Prehosp Disaster Med. 2012;27:172-7.
21. Zhou J, Huang J, Wu H, et al. Screening ultrasonography of 2,204 patients with blunt abdominal trauma in the Wenchuan earthquake. J Trauma Acute Care Surg. 2012;73:890-4.
22. Zhang S, Zhu D, Wan Z, et al. Utility of point-of-care ultrasound in acute management triage of earthquake injury. Am J Emerg Med. 2014;32:92-5.
23. Raja AS, Propper BW, Vandenberg SL, et al. Imaging utilization during explosive multiple casualty incidents. J Trauma. 2010;68:1421-4.
24. Shah S, Dalal A, Smith RM, et al. Impact of portable ultrasound in trauma care after the Haitian earthquake of 2010. Am J Emerg Med. 2010;28:970-1.
25. Kirkpatrick AW, Campbell MR, Novinkov OL, et al. Blunt trauma and operative care in microgravity: a review of microgravity physiology and surgical investigations with implications for critical care and operative treatment in space. J Am Coll Surg. 1997;184:441-53.
26. Campbell MR, Billica RD, Johnston SL, et al. Performance of advanced trauma life support procedures in microgravity. Aviat Space Environ Med. 2002;73:907-12.
27. Nelson BP, Sanghvi A. Out of hospital point of care ultrasound: current use models and future directions. Eur J Trauma Emerg Surg. 2016;42:139-50.
28. Russell TC, Crawford PF. Ultrasound in the austere environment: a review of the history, indications, and specifications. Mil Med. 2013;178:21-8.
29. Rozanski TA, Edmondson JM, Jones SB. Ultrasonography in a forward-deployed military hospital. Mil Med. 2005;170:99-102.
30. Morgan AR, Vasios WN, Hubler DA, et al. Special operator level clinical ultrasound: an experience in application and training. J Spec Oper Med. 2010;10:16-21.
31. Strode CA, Rubal BJ, Gerhardt RT, et al. Satellite and mobile wireless transmission of focused assessment with sonography in trauma. Acad Emerg Med. 2003;10:1411-4.
32. American College of Emergency Physicians. Emergency Ultrasound Guidelines [policy statement]. Ann Emerg Med. 2009;53:550-70.
33. American College of Emergency Physicians. Emergency Ultrasound Guidelines-2001. Ann Emerg Med. 2001;38:470-81.
34. Beeson MS, Carter WA, Christopher TA, et al. The development of the emergency medicine milestones. Acad Emerg Med. 2013;20:724-9.
35. American College of Emergency Physicians. Use of Ultrasound Imaging by Emergency Physicians. Ann Emerg Med. 2001;38:469-70.
36. Lewiss RE, Hoffmann B, Beaulieu Y, et al. Point-of-care ultrasound education: the increasing role of simulation and multimedia resources. J Ultrasound Med. 2014;33:27-32.
37. Thoma B, Joshi N, Trueger NS, et al. Five strategies to effectively use online resources in emergency medicine. Ann Emerg Med. 2014;64:392-5.
38. Scott KR, Hsu CH, Johnson NJ, et al. Integration of social media in emergency medicine residency curriculum. Ann Emerg Med. 2014;64:396-404.
39. American College of Emergency Physicians. Sonoguide. Accessed June 3, 2016 at http://www.sonoguide.com)
40. AEUS Narrated Lecture Series. SAEM, 2015. Accessed June 3, 2016 at: http://community.saem.org/blogs/matt-fields/2014/09/07/aeus-narrated-lecture-series
41. Knudson MM, Sisley AC. Training residents using simulation technology: experience with ultrasound for trauma. J Trauma. 2000;48:659-65.
42. Damewood S, Jeanmonod D, Cadigan B. Comparison of a multimedia simulator to a human model for teaching FAST exam image interpretation and image acquisition. Acad Emerg Med. 2011;18:413-9.
43. Barsuk JH, McGaghie WC, Cohen ER,. Simulation-based mastery learning reduces complications during central venous catheter insertion in a medical intensive care unit. Crit Care Med. 2009;37:2697-701.

44.   Barsuk JH, Cohen ER, Vozenilek JA,. Simulation-based education with mastery learning improves paracentesis skills. J Grad Med Educ. 2012;4:23-7.
45.   Mendiratta-Lala M, Williams T, de Quadros N, et al. The use of a simulation center to improve resident proficiency in performing ultrasound-guided procedures. Acad Radiol. 2010;17:535-40.
46.   Sekiguchi H, Bhagra A, Gajic O, et al. A general Critical Care Ultrasonography workshop: results of a novel Web-based learning program combined with simulation-based hands-on training. J Crit Care. 2013;28:217.e7-12.
47.   Ericsson KA. Acquisition and maintenance of medical expertise: a perspective from the expert-performance approach with deliberate practice. Acad Med. 2015;90:1471-86.
48.   Lewiss RE, Pearl M, Nomura JT, et al. CORD-AEUS: consensus document for the emergency ultrasound milestone project. Acad Emerg Med. 2013;20:740-5.
49.   Blehar DJ, Barton B, Gaspari RJ. Learning curves in emergency ultrasound education. Acad Emerg Med. 2015;22:574-82.
50.   Mateer J, Plummer D, Heller M, et al. Model Curriculum for Physician Training in Emergency Ultrasonography. Ann Emerg Med. 1994;23:95-102.
51.   Strauss R. US is an embedded requirement for EM Residencies. Atlanta, Georgia: SAEM meeting; 2001.
52.   Akhtar S, Theodoro D, Gaspari R, et al. Resident training in emergency ultrasound: consensus recommendations from the 2008 Council of Emergency Medicine Residency Directors Conference. Acad Emerg Med. 2009;16 Suppl 2:S32-6.
53.   Counselman FL, Borenstein MA, Chisholm CD, et al. The 2013 Model of the Clinical Practice of Emergency Medicine. Acad Emerg Med. 2014;21:574-98.
54.   Emergency Ultrasound Fellowship Guidelines - An Information Paper. July 2011. Accessed May 13, 2016, at http://www.acep.org/workarea/DownloadAsset.aspx?id=80954
55.   Lewiss RE, Tayal VS, Hoffmann B, et al. The core content of clinical ultrasonography fellowship training. Acad Emerg Med. 2014;21:456-61.
56.   Adhikari S, Raio C, Morrison D, et al. Do emergency ultrasound fellowship programs impact emergency medicine residents' ultrasound education? J Ultrasound Med. 2014;33:999-1004.
57.   Adhikari S, Fiorello A. Emergency ultrasound fellowship training: a novel team-based approach. J Ultrasound Med. 2014;33:1821-6.
58.   Hoppmann R, Cook T, Hunt P, et al. Ultrasound in medical education: a vertical curriculum at the University of South Carolina School of Medicine. J S C Med Assoc. 2006;102:330-4.
59.   Cook T, Hunt P, Hoppman R. Emergency medicine leads the way for training medical students in clinician-based ultrasound: a radical paradigm shift in patient imaging. Acad Emerg Med. 2007;14:558-61.
60.   Fox JC, Chiem AT, Rooney KP, et al. Web-based lectures, peer instruction and ultrasound-integrated medical education. Med Educ. 2012;46:1109-10.
61.   Dreher SM, DePhilip R, Bahner D. Ultrasound exposure during gross anatomy. J Emerg Med. 2014;46:231-40.
62.   Bahner DP, Jasne A, Boore S, et al. The ultrasound challenge: a novel approach to medical student ultrasound education. J Ultrasound Med. 2012;31:2013-6.
63.   Hall MK, Mirjalili SA, Moore CL, et al. The student's dilemma, liver edition: incorporating the sonographer's language into clinical anatomy education. Anat Sci Educ. 2015;8:283-8.
64.   Ahn JS, French AJ, Thiessen ME, et al. Training peer instructors for a combined ultrasound/physical exam curriculum. Teach Learn Med. 2014;26:292-5.
65.   Swamy M, Searle RF. Anatomy teaching with portable ultrasound to medical students. BMC Med Educ 2012;12:99.
66.   Fodor D, Badea R, Poanta L, et al. The use of ultrasonography in learning clinical examination - a pilot study involving third year medical students. Med Ultrasound. 2012;14:177-81.

67. Decara JM, Kirkpatrick JN, Spencer KT, et al. Use of hand-carried ultrasound devices to augment the accuracy of medical student bedside cardiac diagnoses. J Am Soc Echocardiogr. 2005;18:257-63.

68. Arger PH, Schultz SM, Sehgal CM, et al. Teaching medical students diagnostic sonography. J Ultrasound Med. 2005;24:1365-9.

69. Knobe M, Münker R, Sellei RM, et al. Peer teaching: a randomised controlled trial using student-teachers to teach musculoskeletal ultrasound. Med Educ. 2010;44:148-55.

70. Jeppesen KM, Bahner DP. Teaching bedside sonography using peer mentoring: a prospective randomized trial. J Ultrasound Med. 2012;31:455-9.

71. American Medical Association. H-230.960 Privileging for Ultrasound Imaging. Accessed May 13, 2016, at https://www.ama-assn.org/ssl3/ecomm/PolicyFinderForm.pl?site=www.ama-assn.org&uri=/resources/html/PolicyFinder/policyfiles/HnE/H-230.960.HTM

72. American College of Emergency Physicians. Emergency Ultrasound Certification by External Entities [policy statement]. Approved June 2014. Accessed June 7, 2016 at https://www.acep.org/clinical---practice-management/emergency-ultrasound-certification-by-external-entities/

73. OPPE and FPPE: Tools to help make privileging decisions. The Joint Commission, 2013. Accessed December 20, 2015, at http://www.jointcommission.org/jc_physician_blog/oppe_fppe_tools_privileging_decisions/

74. American College of Emergency Physicians. Clinical Ultrasound Accreditation Program. 2015. Accessed June 7, 2016, at http://www.acep.org/CUAP

75. American College of Emergency Physicians. Emergency Ultrasound Standard Reporting Guidelines. Accessed June 7, 2016 at https://www.acep.org/membership/sections/emergency-ultrasound-section/standard-reporting-guidelines.

76. American College of Emergency Physicians. Emergency Ultrasound: Workflow White Paper. 2013. Accessed June 7, 2016 at https://www.acep.org/uploadedFiles/ACEP/memberCenter/SectionsofMembership/ultra/Workflow%20White%20Paper.pdf

77. Mandavia DP, Aragona J, Childs J, et al. Prospective evaluation of standardized ultrasound training for emergency physicians. Acad Emerg Med. 1999;6:382.

78. Stein JC, Wang R, Adler N, et al. Emergency physician ultrasonography for evaluating patients at risk for ectopic pregnancy: a meta-analysis. Ann Emerg Med. 2010;56:674-83.

79. Ideal Ultrasound Machine Features for the EM and Critical Care Environment. 2008. Accessed May 13, 2016 at http://www.acep.org/Clinical---Practice-Management/Ideal-Ultrasound-Machine-Features-for-the-Emergency-Medicine-and-Critical-Care-Environment-2008/)

80. Sutherland JE, Sutphin D, Redican K, et al. Telesonography: foundations and future directions. J Ultrasound Med. 2011;30:517-22.

81. Labovitz AJ, Noble VE, Bierig M, et al. Focused cardiac ultrasound in the emergent setting: a consensus statement of the American Society of Echocardiography and American College of Emergency Physicians. J Am Soc Echocardiogr. 2010;23:1225-30.

82. Sonosite iViz. 2016. Accessed March 30, 2016, at http://www.sonosite.com/sonosite-iviz.

83. Philips Lumify. Accessed March 30, 2016, at http://www.lumify.philips.com/web/.

84. Acuson Siemens Freestyle Ultrasound System. Siemens. Accessed March 30, 2016, at http://www.healthcare.siemens.com/ultrasound/ultrasound-point-of-care/acuson-freestyle-ultrasound-machine.

85. VScan portfolio. Accessed March 30, 2016, at http://www3.gehealthcare.com/en/products/categories/ultrasound/vscan_portfolio.

86. Sutherland JE, Sutphin HD, Rawlins F, et al. A comparison of telesonography with standard ultrasound care in a rural Dominican clinic. J Telemed Telecare. 2009;15:191-5.

87. Hoffmann R, Pohlemann T, Wippermann B, et al. [Management of sonography in blunt abdominal trauma]. Unfallchirurg. 1989;92:471-6.

88. Ma OJ, Mateer JR, Ogata M, et al. Prospective analysis of a rapid trauma ultrasound examination performed by emergency physicians. J Trauma. 1995;38:879-85.

89. Plummer D, Brunnette D, Asinger R,et al. Emergency Department Echocardiography Improves Outcome in Penetrating Cardiac Injury. Ann Emerg Med. 1992;21:709-12.

90. Melniker LA, Leibner E, McKenney MG, et al. Randomized controlled clinical trial of point-of-care, limited ultrasonography for trauma in the emergency department: the first sonography outcomes assessment program trial. Ann Emerg Med. 2006;48:227-35.

91. Nandipati KC, Allamaneni S, Kakarla R, et al. Extended focused assessment with sonography for trauma (EFAST) in the diagnosis of pneumothorax: experience at a community based level I trauma center. Injury. 2011;42:511-4.

92. Sheng AY, Dalziel P, Liteplo AS, et al. Focused Assessment with Sonography in Trauma and Abdominal Computed Tomography Utilization in Adult Trauma Patients: Trends over the Last Decade. Emerg Med Int. 2013;2013:678380.

93. Durham B. Emergency medicine physicians saving time with ultrasound. Am J Emerg Med. 1996;14:309-13.

94. Jang TB, Ruggeri W, Dyne P, et al. Learning curve of emergency physicians using emergency bedside sonography for symptomatic first-trimester pregnancy. J Ultrasound Med. 2010;29:1423-8.

95. Mateer JR, Valley VT, Aiman EJ, et al. Outcome analysis of a protocol including bedside endovaginal sonography in patients at risk for ectopic pregnancy. Ann Emerg Med. 1996;27:283-9.

96. Panebianco NL, Shofer F, Fields JM, et al. The utility of transvaginal ultrasound in the ED evaluation of complications of first trimester pregnancy. Am J Emerg Med. 2015;33:743-8.

97. Kuhn M, Bonnin RL, Davey MJ, et al. Emergency department ultrasound scanning for abdominal aortic aneurysm: accessible, accurate, and advantageous. Ann Emerg Med. 2000;36:219-23.

98. Tayal VS, Graf CD, Gibbs, MA. Prospective Study of Accuracy and Outcome of Emergency Ultrasound for Abdominal Aortic Aneurysm over Two Years. Acad Emerg Med. 2003;10:867-71.

99. Goodman A, Perera P, Mailhot T, et al. The role of bedside ultrasound in the diagnosis of pericardial effusion and cardiac tamponade. J Emerg Trauma Shock. 2012;5:72-5.

100. Mandavia D, Hoffner R, Mahaney K, et al. Bedside Echocardiography by Emergency Physicians. Ann Emerg Med. 2001;38:377-82.

101. Blaivas M, Fox J. Outcome in cardiac arrest patients found to have cardiac standstill on the bedside emergency department echocardiogram. Acad Emerg Med. 2001;8:616-21.

102. Moore CL, Rose GA, Tayal VS, et al. Determination of Left Ventricular Function by Emergency Physician Echocardiography of Hypotensive Patients. Acad Emerg Med. 2002;9(3):186-93.

103. Jones AE, Tayal VS, Sullivan DM, et al. Randomized, controlled trial of immediate versus delayed goal-directed ultrasound to identify the cause of nontraumatic hypotension in emergency department patients. Crit Care Med. 2004;32:1703-8.

104. Volpicelli G, Lamorte A, Tullio M, et al. Point-of-care multiorgan ultrasonography for the evaluation of undifferentiated hypotension in the emergency department. Intensive Care Med. 2013;39:1290-8.

105. Anderson KL, Jenq KY, Fields JM, et al. Diagnosing heart failure among acutely dyspneic patients with cardiac, inferior vena cava, and lung ultrasonography. Am J Emerg Med. 2013;31:1208-14.

106. Russell FM, Ehrman RR, Cosby K, et al. Diagnosing acute heart failure in patients with undifferentiated dyspnea: a lung and cardiac ultrasound (LuCUS) protocol. Acad Emerg Med. 2015;22:182-91.

107. Kanji HD, McCallum J, Sirounis D,et al. Limited echocardiography-guided therapy in subacute shock is associated with change in management and improved outcomes. J Crit Care. 2014;29:700-5.

108. Nagdev AD, Merchant RC, Tirado-Gonzalez A, et al. Emergency department bedside ultrasonographic measurement of the caval index for noninvasive determination of low central venous pressure. Ann Emerg Med. 2010;55:290-5.

109. Machare-Delgado E, Decaro M, Marik PE. Inferior vena cava variation compared to pulse contour analysis as predictors of fluid responsiveness: a prospective cohort study. J Intensive Care Med. 2011;26:116-24.

110. Barbier C, Loubières Y, Schmit C, et al. Respiratory changes in inferior vena cava diameter are helpful in predicting fluid responsiveness in ventilated septic patients. Intensive Care Med. 2004;30:1740-6.

111. Blehar DJ, Glazier S, Gaspari RJ. Correlation of corrected flow time in the carotid artery with changes in intravascular volume status. J Crit Care. 2014;29:486-8.

112. Lichtenstein DA, Mezière GA, Lagoueyte JF, et al. A-lines and B-lines: lung ultrasound as a bedside tool for predicting pulmonary artery occlusion pressure in the critically ill. Chest. 2009;136:1014-20.

113. Dinh VA, Ko HS, Rao R, et al. Measuring cardiac index with a focused cardiac ultrasound examination in the ED. Am J Emerg Med. 2012;30:1845-51.

114. Weekes AJ, Thacker G, Troha D, et al. Diagnostic Accuracy of Right Ventricular Dysfunction Markers in Normotensive Emergency Department Patients With Acute Pulmonary Embolism. Ann Emerg Med. 2016. Mar 11. pii: S0196-0644(16)00037-8. doi: 10.1016/j.annemergmed.2016.01.027. [Epub ahead of print]

115. Weekes AJ, Reddy A, Lewis MR, et al. E-point septal separation compared to fractional shortening measurements of systolic function in emergency department patients: prospective randomized study. J Ultrasound Med 2012.31:1891-7.

116. Weekes AJ, Tassone HM, Babcock A, et al. Comparison of serial qualitative and quantitative assessments of caval index and left ventricular systolic function during early fluid resuscitation of hypotensive emergency department patients. Acad Emerg Med. 2011;18:912-21.

117. Villar J, Summers SM, Menchine MD, et al. The Absence of Gallstones on Point-of-Care Ultrasound Rules Out Acute Cholecystitis. J Emerg Med. 2015;49:475-80.

118. Kendall JL, Shimp RJ. Performance and Interpretation of Limited Right Upper Quadrant Ultrasound by Emergency Physicians. J Emerg Med. 2001;21(1)7-13.

119. Miller AH, Pepe PE, Brockman CR, et al. ED ultrasound in hepatobiliary disease. J Emerg Med. 2006;30:69-74.

120. Ross M, Brown M, McLaughlin K, et al. Emergency physician-performed ultrasound to diagnose cholelithiasis: a systematic review. Acad Emerg Med. 2011;18:227-35.

121. Summers SM, Scruggs W, Menchine MD, et al. A prospective evaluation of emergency department bedside ultrasonography for the detection of acute cholecystitis. Ann Emerg Med. 2010;56:114-22.

122. Blaivas M, Harwood RA, Lambert MJ. Decreasing Length of Stay with Emergency Department Gallbladder Ultrasonography. Acad Emerg Med. 1999;6:541.

123. Fields JM, Fischer JI, Anderson KL, et al. The ability of renal ultrasound and ureteral jet evaluation to predict 30-day outcomes in patients with suspected nephrolithiasis. Am J Emerg Med. 2015;33:1402-6.

124. Ng C, Tsung JW. Avoiding Computed Tomography Scans By Using Point-Of-Care Ultrasound When Evaluating Suspected Pediatric Renal Colic. J Emerg Med. 2015;49:165-71.

125. Rosen CL, Brown DFM, Sagarin M, et al. Ultrasonography by Emergency Physicians in Detecting Hydronephrosis in Patients with Suspected Ureteral Colic. Acad Emerg Med. 1996;3:541.

126. Gaspari RJ, Horst K. Emergency ultrasound and urinalysis in the evaluation of flank pain. Acad Emerg Med. 2005;12:1180-4.

127. Smith-Bindman R, Aubin C, Bailitz J, et al. Ultrasonography versus computed tomography for suspected nephrolithiasis. N Engl J Med. 2014;371:1100-10.

128. Pomero F, Dentali F, Borretta V, et al. Accuracy of emergency physician-performed ultrasonography in the diagnosis of deep-vein thrombosis: a systematic review and meta-analysis. Thromb Haemost. 2013;109:137-45.

129. Jang T, Docherty M, Aubin C, et al. Resident-Performed Compression Ultrasonography for the Detection of Proximal Deep Vein Thrombosis: Fast And Accurate. Acad Emerg Med. 2004;4:319-22.
130. Burnside PR, Brown MD, Kline JA. Systematic review of emergency physician-performed ultrasonography for lower-extremity deep vein thrombosis. Acad Emerg Med. 2008;15:493-8.
131. Theodoro D, Blaivas M, Duggal S, et al. Real-time B-mode ultrasound in the ED saves time in the diagnosis of deep vein thrombosis (DVT). Am J Emerg Med. 2004;22:197-200.
132. Adhikari S, Blaivas M. Utility of bedside sonography to distinguish soft tissue abnormalities from joint effusions in the emergency department. J Ultrasound Med. 2010;29:519-26.
133. Squire BT, Fox JC, Anderson C. ABSCESS: applied bedside sonography for convenient evaluation of superficial soft tissue infections. Acad Emerg Med. 2005;12:601-6.
134. Tayal VS, Hasan N, Norton HJ, et al. The effect of soft-tissue ultrasound on the management of cellulitis in the emergency department. Acad Emerg Med. 2006;13:384-8.
135. Marshburn TH, Legome E, Sargsyan A, et al. Goal-directed ultrasound in the detection of long-bone fractures. J Trauma. 2004;57:329-32.
136. O'Malley P, Tayal VS. Use of emergency musculoskeletal sonography in diagnosis of an open fracture of the hand. J Ultrasound Med. 2007;26:679-82.
137. Roy S, Dewitz A, Paul I. Ultrasound-assisted ankle arthrocentesis. Am J Emerg Med. 1999;17:300-1.
138. Freeman K, Dewitz A, Baker WE. Ultrasound-guided hip arthrocentesis in the ED. Am J Emerg Med. 2007;25:80-6.
139. Nesselroade RD, Nickels LC. Ultrasound diagnosis of bilateral quadriceps tendon rupture after statin use. West J Emerg Med. 2010;11:306-9.
140. Tayal VS, Nicks BA, Norton HJ. Emergency ultrasound evaluation of symptomatic nontraumatic pleural effusions. Am J Emerg Med. 2006;24:782-6.
141. Volpicelli G, Zanobetti M. Lung ultrasound and pulmonary consolidations. Am J Emerg Med. 2015;33:1307-8.
142. Volpicelli G, Boero E, Sverzellati N, et al. Semi-quantification of pneumothorax volume by lung ultrasound. Intensive Care Med. 2014;40:1460-7.
143. Volpicelli G. Point-of-care lung ultrasound. Praxis (Bern 1994). 2014;103:711-6.
144. Volpicelli G. Interpreting lung ultrasound B-lines in acute respiratory failure. Chest. 2014;146:e230.
145. Blaivas M, Lyon M, Duggal S. A prospective comparison of supine chest radiography and bedside ultrasound for the diagnosis of traumatic pneumothorax. Acad Emerg Med. 2005;12:844-9.
146. Karacabey S, Sanrı E, Gencer EG, et al. Tracheal ultrasonography and ultrasonographic lung sliding for confirming endotracheal tube placement: Faster? Reliable? Am J Emerg Med. 2016. Jan 26. pii: S0735-6757(16)00037-1. doi: 10.1016/j.ajem.2016.01.027. [Epub ahead of print]
147. Siddiqui N, Arzola C, Friedman Z, et al. Ultrasound Improves Cricothyrotomy Success in Cadavers with Poorly Defined Neck Anatomy: A Randomized Control Trial. Anesthesiology. 2015;123:1033-41.
148. Gottlieb M, Bailitz J. Can Transtracheal Ultrasonography Be Used to Verify Endotracheal Tube Placement? Ann Emerg Med. 2015;66:394-5.
149. Gottlieb M, Bailitz JM, Christian E, et al. Accuracy of a novel ultrasound technique for confirmation of endotracheal intubation by expert and novice emergency physicians. West J Emerg Med. 2014;15:834-9.
150. Tessaro MO, Arroyo AC, Haines LE, et al. Inflating the endotracheal tube cuff with saline to confirm correct depth using bedside ultrasonography. CJEM. 2015;17:94-8.
151. Li Y, Wang J, Wei X. Confirmation of endotracheal tube depth using ultrasound in adults. Can J Anaesth. 2015;62:832.
152. Das SK, Choupoo NS, Haldar R, et al. Transtracheal ultrasound for verification of endotracheal tube placement: a systematic review and meta-analysis. Can J Anaesth. 2015;62:413-23.

153. Vrablik ME, Snead GR, Minnigan HJ, et al. The diagnostic accuracy of bedside ocular ultrasonography for the diagnosis of retinal detachment: a systematic review and meta-analysis. Ann Emerg Med. 2015;65:199-203.e1.
154. Tayal VS, Neulander M, Norton HJ, et al. Emergency department sonographic measurement of optic nerve sheath diameter to detect findings of increased intracranial pressure in adult head injury patients. Ann Emerg Med. 2007;49:508-14.
155. Kilker BA, Holst JM, Hoffmann B. Bedside ocular ultrasound in the emergency department. Eur J Emerg Med. 2014;21:246-53.
156. Blaivas M. Bedside emergency department ultrasonography in the evaluation of ocular pathology. Acad Emerg Med. 2000;7:947-50.
157. Mallin M, Craven P, Ockerse P, et al. Diagnosis of appendicitis by bedside ultrasound in the ED. Am J Emerg Med. 2015;33:430-2.
158. Zeidan BS, Wasser T, Nicholas GG. Ultrasonography in the diagnosis of acute appendicitis. J R Coll Surg Edinb. 1997;42:24-6.
159. West W, Brady-West D, McDonald A, et al. Ultrasound and white blood cell counts in suspected acute appendicitis. West Indian Med J. 2006;55:100-2.
160. Terasawa T, Hartling L, Cramer K, Klassen T. Diagnostic Accuracy of Ultrasound and Computed Tomography for Emergency Department Diagnosis of Appendicitis: A Systematic Review. 2nd International EM Conference 2003.
161. Terasawa T, Blackmore CB, Bent S, et al. Systematic review: Computed tomography and ultrasonography to detect acute appendicitis in adults and adolescents. Ann Intern Med. 2004;141:537-46.
162. Tayal VS, Bullard M, Swanson DR, et al. ED endovaginal pelvic ultrasound in nonpregnant women with right lower quadrant pain. Am J Emerg Med. 2008;26:81-5.
163. Sivitz AB, Cohen SG, Tejani C. Evaluation of acute appendicitis by pediatric emergency physician sonography. Ann Emerg Med. 2014;64:358-64.e4.
164. Puylaert JB, Rutgers PH, Lalisang RI, et al. A prospective study ultrasonongraphy in the diagnosis of appendicitis. N Engl J Med. 1987;317:666-9.
165. Poortman P, Lohle PNM, Schoemaker CMC, et al. Comparison of CT and sonography in the diagnosis of acute appendicitis. AJR Am J Roentgenol. 2003;181:1355-9.
166. Oshita R, Hunt M, Fox J, et al. A retrospective analysis of the use of bedside ultrasonography in the diagnosis of acute appendicitis. Ann Emerg Med. 2004;44:S112.
167. O'Malley M, Wilson S. Ultrasonography and computed tomography of appendicitis and diverticulitis. Sem Roentgenol. 2001;36:138-47.
168. Nelson M, Chiricolo G, Raio C, et al. Can emergency physicians positively predict acute appendicitis on focused right lower quadrant ultrasound? Ann Emerg Med. 2005;46:27-8.
169. Min YG, Lee CC, Bae Y, et al. Accuracy of sonography performed by emergency medicine residents for the diagnosis of acute appendicitis. Ann Emerg Med. 2004;44:S60.
170. Lam SH, Grippo A, Kerwin C, et al. Bedside ultrasonography as an adjunct to routine evaluation of acute appendicitis in the emergency department. West J Emerg Med. 2014;15:808-15.
171. Garcia-Pena BM, Taylor GA, Fishman SJ, et al. Costs and Effectiveness of Ultrasonography and Limted Computed Tomography for Diagnosing Appendicitis in Children. Pediatrics. 2000;106:672-6.
172. Hollerweger A, Rieger S, Mayr N, et al. Strangulating closed-loop obstruction: Sonographic signs. Ultraschall Med. 2015 Apr 15. [Epub ahead of print]
173. Hollerweger A, Wüstner M, Dirks K. Bowel obstruction: Sonographic evaluation. Ultraschall Med. 2015;36:216-35; quiz 36-8.
174. Jang TB, Schindler D, Kaji AH. Predictive value of signs and symptoms for small bowel obstruction in patients with prior surgery. Emerg Med J. 2012;29:769-70.
175. Hefny AF, Corr P, Abu-Zidan FM. The role of ultrasound in the management of intestinal obstruction. J Emerg Trauma Shock. 2012;5:84-6.

176. Chen S-C, Wang H-P, Chen W-J, et al. Selective use of ultrasonography for the detection of pneumoperitoneum. Acad Emerg Med. 2002;9:643-5.
177. Baker JB, Mandavia D, Swadron SP. Diagnosis of diverticulitis by bedside ultrasound in the emergency department. J Emerg Med. 2006;30:327-9.
178. Siadecki SD, Frasure SE, Saul T, Lewiss RE. Diagnosis and reduction of a hernia by bedside ultrasound: a case report. J Emerg Med 2014;47:169-71.
179. Nazeer SR, Dewbre H, Miller AH. Ultrasound-assisted paracentesis performed by emergency physicians vs the traditional technique: a prospective, randomized study. Am J Emerg Med. 2005;23:363-7.
180. Robinson P, Hensor E, Lansdown MJ, et al. Inguinofemoral hernia: accuracy of sonography in patients with indeterminate clinical features. AJR Am J Roentgenol. 2006;187:1168-78.
181. Rettenbacher T, Hollerweger A, Macheiner P, et al. Abdominal wall hernias: cross-sectional imaging signs of incarceration determined with sonography. AJR Am J Roentgenol. 2001;177:1061-6.
182. Sivitz AB, Tejani C, Cohen SG. Evaluation of hypertrophic pyloric stenosis by pediatric emergency physician sonography. Acad Emerg Med. 2013;20:646-51.
183. Malcom GE, Raio CC, Del Rios M, et al. Feasibility of emergency physician diagnosis of hypertrophic pyloric stenosis using point-of-care ultrasound: a multi-center case series. J Emerg Med. 2009;37:283-6.
184. Leung J, Duffy M, Finckh A. Real-time ultrasonographically-guided internal jugular vein catheterization in the emergency department increases success rates and reduces complications: a randomized, prospective study. Ann Emerg Med. 2006;48:540-7.
185. Doniger SJ, Ishimine P, Fox JC, et al. Randomized controlled trial of ultrasound-guided peripheral intravenous catheter placement versus traditional techniques in difficult-access pediatric patients. Pediatr Emerg Care. 2009;25:154-9.
186. Agency for Healthcare Research and Quality. Evidence Report/Technology Assessment: Number 43. Making Health Care Safer. A Critical Analysis of Patient Safety Practices: Summary. Accessed May 13, 2016 at http://archive.ahrq.gov/clinic/ptsafety/pdf/ptsafety.pdf

ACEP Emergency US Imaging Criteria Compendium

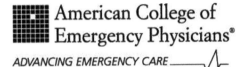

Developed by the
following members of
ACEP's Emergency
Ultrasound Section:

John L. Kendall, MD,
FACEP, Chair of Policy
Development;
David P. Bahner, MD,
RDMS, FACEP;
Michael Blaivas, MD,
FACEP;
Gavin Budhram, MD;
Anthony J. Dean, MD;
J. Christian Fox, MD,
RDMS, FACEP;
Stephen Hoffenberg, MD,
FACEP;
Brooks Laselle, MD;
Chris Moore, MD, RDMS,
RDCS, FACEP;
Gary Quick, MD, FACEP;
Christopher C. Raio, MD,
MBA, FACEP;
Cliff Rice, MD;
Paul R. Sierzenski, MD,
RDMS, FACEP;
Vivek S. Tayal, MD,
FACEP

POLICY STATEMENT

Approved by the ACEP
Board of Directors
October 2014

Emergency Ultrasound Imaging Criteria Compendium

- Aorta
- Cardiac
- Kidney and Bladder
- Lung and Pleura
- Ocular
- Pelvic
- Right Upper Quadrant
- Soft tissue/Musculoskeletal
- Trauma
- Ultrasound-Guided Procedures
- Venous Thrombosis

© Springer International Publishing AG 2018
V. S. Tayal et al. (eds.), *Ultrasound Program Management*,
https://doi.org/10.1007/978-3-319-63143-1

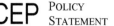

ACEP Emergency Ultrasound Imaging Criteria:
Aorta

1. Introduction
   The American College of Emergency Physicians (ACEP) has developed these criteria to assist
   practitioners performing emergency ultrasound studies (EUS) of the abdomen and retroperitoneum in
   patients suspected of having an acute abdominal aortic aneurysm (AAA).

   Ultrasound has been shown to accurately identify both aneurysmal and normal abdominal aortas. In
   most cases, EUS is used to identify or exclude the presence of infrarenal AAA. In some cases, EUS of
   the abdominal aorta can also identify the presence of suprarenal AAA or of distal dissection. If
   thoracic aortic aneurysm or proximal dissection is suspected, these may be detected using
   transthoracic techniques or may require additional diagnostic modalities. Patients in whom AAA is
   identified also need to be assessed for free intraperitoneal fluid.

   EUS evaluation of the aorta occurs in conjunction with other EUS applications and other imaging and
   laboratory tests. It is a clinically focused examination, which, in conjunction with historical and
   laboratory information, provides additional data for decision-making. It attempts to answer specific
   questions about a particular patient's condition. While other tests may provide information that is
   more detailed than EUS, have greater anatomic specificity, or identify alternative diagnoses, EUS is
   non-invasive, is rapidly deployed and does not entail removal of the patient from the resuscitation
   area. Further, EUS avoids the delays, costs, specialized technical personnel, the administration of
   contrast agents and the biohazardous potential of radiation. These advantages make EUS a valuable
   addition to available diagnostic resources in the care of patients with time-sensitive or emergency
   conditions such as acute AAA.

2. Indications/Limitations
   a. Primary
      i. The rapid evaluation of the abdominal aorta from the diaphragmatic hiatus to the aortic
         bifurcation for evidence of aneurysm.

   b. Extended
      i. Abdominal aortic dissection
      ii. Thoracic aortic dissection
      iii. Intraperitoneal free fluid in the event that AAA is identified
      iv. Iliac, splenic, and other abdominal artery aneurysms

   c. Contraindications
      i. There are no absolute contraindications to EUS of the abdominal aorta. There may be relative
         contraindications based on the patient's clinical situation.

   d. Limitations
      i. EUS of the aorta is a single component of the overall and ongoing resuscitation. Since it is a
         focused examination, EUS does not identify all abnormalities or diseases of the aorta. EUS,
         like other tests, does not replace clinical judgment and should be interpreted in the context of
         the entire clinical picture. If the findings of the EUS are equivocal additional diagnostic
         testing may be indicated.
      ii. Examination of the aorta may be technically limited by
          1. Obese habitus
          2. Bowel gas
          3. Abdominal tenderness

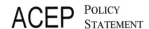

4. Abdominal dressings
e. Pitfalls
 i. While most aneurysms are fusiform, extending over several centimeters of aorta, saccular aneurysms are confined to a short focal section of the aorta, making them easily overlooked. This may be avoided by methodical, systematic real-time scanning through all tissue planes in both transverse and longitudinal sections.
 ii. When bowel gas or other technical factors prevent a complete systematic real-time scan in orthogonal planes, these limitations should be identified and documented. Such limitations may mandate further evaluation by alternative methods, as clinically indicated.
 iii. A small aneurysm does not preclude rupture. A patient with symptoms consistent with acute AAA and an aortic diameter greater than 3.0 cm should undergo further diagnostic evaluation.
 iv. The absence of free intraperitoneal fluid does not rule out acute AAA as most acute AAAs presenting to the ED do not have free peritoneal fluid.
 v. The presence of retroperitoneal hemorrhage cannot be reliably identified by EUS.
 vi. If an AAA is identified, it still may not be the cause of a patient's symptoms.
 vii. The presence of free intraperitoneal fluid with an AAA, does not necessarily mean that the aneurysm is the source of the fluid.
 viii. Oblique or angled cuts exaggerate the true aortic diameter. Scanning planes should be obtained that are either exactly aligned with, or at exact right angles to, the main axis of the vessel.
 ix. Off-plane longitudinal images and transverse images not obtained at the level of maximal dilatation will underestimate the true diameter of the vessel.
 x. With a tortuous or ectatic aorta "longitudinal" and "transverse" views should be obtained with respect to the axis of the vessel in order to avoid artifactual exaggeration of the aortic diameter.
 xi. Large para-aortic nodes may be confused with the aorta and/or AAA. They usually occur anterior to the aorta, but may be posterior, displacing the aorta away from the vertebral body. They can be distinguished by an irregular nodular shape, identifiable in real-time. If color flow Doppler is utilized, nodes will not demonstrate high-velocity luminal flow.
 xii. Longstanding thrombus within an AAA may become calcified and mistaken for bowel outside the aorta, thereby obscuring the aortic walls and preventing recognition of the aneurysm. Gain should be adjusted so that blood within the lumen of the vessel appears anechoic (ie, black).

3. Qualifications and Responsibilities of the Clinician Performing the Examination
EUS of the aorta provides information that is the basis of immediate decisions about further evaluation, management, and therapeutic interventions. Because of its direct bearing on patient care, the rendering of a diagnosis by EUS represents the practice of medicine, and therefore is the responsibility of the treating physician.

Due to the time-critical and dynamic nature of acute AAA, emergent interventions may be mandated by the diagnostic findings of EUS of the aorta. For this reason, EUS of the aorta should occur as soon as the clinical decision is made to evaluate the patient with ultrasound.

Physicians of a variety of medical specialties may perform EUS of the aorta. Training should be in accordance with specialty or organization specific guidelines. Physicians should render a diagnostic interpretation in a time frame consistent with the management of acute AAA, as outlined above.

4. Specifications for Individual Examinations

a. <u>General</u> – Simultaneously with other aspects of resuscitation, ultrasound images are obtained demonstrating the abdominal aorta from the diaphragmatic hiatus to the bifurcation.

b. <u>Technique</u>
   i. Identification. The aorta is most easily identified and most accurately measured in the transverse plane. The transverse image of the vertebral body is identified. In this plane, the normal aorta is a circular, hypoechoic structure identified adjacent to the left anterior surface of the vertebral body.
   ii. Real-time scanning technique.
      1. <u>Overview</u>. The abdominal aorta extends from the diaphragmatic hiatus to the bifurcation. The surface anatomy corresponding to these points are the xiphoid process and the umbilicus. If possible, the probe is held at right angles to the skin and slid from the xiphoid process inferiorly to the umbilicus, providing real-time systematic scanning through all planes from the diaphragm to the bifurcation. The probe is then rotated 90 degrees and images are obtained in the longitudinal plane by rocking or sliding the probe from side-to-side.

      2. <u>Details of technique</u>. In the subxiphoid region, the liver often provides a sonographic window. A cooperative patient may be asked to take a deep breath, which augments this window by lowering the diaphragm and liver margin. Frequently, gas in the transverse colon obscures the midsection of the aorta in a roughly 5-centimeter band inferior to the margin of the liver. This may preclude an uninterrupted and/or complete visualization of the aorta. In order to circumvent the gas-filled transverse colon, it may be necessary to use a fanning technique in the windows above and below this sonographic obstacle. Alternatively, applying downward constant pressure with the probe, in conjunction with peristalsis, may dissipate bowel gas.

      After a systematic real-time scan in transverse plane, the aorta should be scanned longitudinally. In this view, abnormalities in the lateral walls may be missed, but focal abnormalities in the anterior or posterior walls and absence of normal tapering are more easily appreciated.

      3. <u>Additional windows</u>. If bowel gas and/or truncal obesity interfere with visualization of the aorta in the anterior midline, the emergency physician should use any probe position that affords windows of the aorta. In particular, two additional windows can be used. First, in the right midaxillary line intercostal views using the liver as an acoustic window may provide alternate images of the aorta. To optimize this approach, the patient may be placed in a left decubitus position. On this view, the aorta will appear to be lying "deep" to the inferior vena cava. Second, the distal aorta can sometimes be visualized with the probe placed in a left paraumbilical region.

      Evaluation of the ascending aorta, aortic arch, and descending aorta for dissection or aneurysm can be performed using parasternal and suprasternal windows. These are discussed in the "Cardiac" criteria.

      4. <u>Measurements</u>. The aorta (and other abdominal arteries) are measured from the outside margin of the wall on one side to the outside margin of the other wall. In most instances, the anterior and posterior walls are usually more sharply defined, so an antero-posterior measurement is most precise. However, since many AAAs have larger side-to-side than antero-posterior diameters, measurements are obtained in both directions when possible.

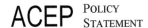

The maximum aortic diameter should be measured in both transverse and longitudinal planes.

5. <u>Additional technical considerations.</u> – If an AAA is identified, evaluation of the peritoneal cavity for free fluid (using the approach of the Focused Assessment by Sonography in Trauma) should be made.

5. <u>Documentation</u>
In performing EUS of the aorta, images are interpreted by the treating physician as they are acquired and are used to guide contemporaneous clinical decisions. Such interpretations should be documented in the medical record. Documentation should include the indication for the procedure, a description of the organs or structures identified and an interpretation of the findings. Images should be stored as a part of the medical record and done so in accordance with facility policy requirements. Given the often emergent nature of such ultrasound examinations, the timely delivery of care should not be delayed by archiving ultrasound images.

6. <u>Equipment Specifications</u>
Curvilinear abdominal or phased array ultrasound probes can be utilized. A 2.0 – 5.0 MHz multi-frequency transducer is ideal. The lower end of this frequency range may be needed in larger patients, while the higher frequency will give more detail in those with low body mass index. Both portable and cart-based ultrasound machines may be used.

7. <u>Quality Control and Improvements, Safety, Infection Control and Patient Education</u>
Policies and procedures related to quality, safety, infection control and patient education should be developed in accordance with specialty or organizational guidelines. Specific institutional guidelines may be developed to correspond with such guidelines

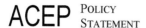

ACEP Emergency Ultrasound Imaging Criteria:
Cardiac

1. Introduction
    The American College of Emergency Physicians (ACEP) has developed these criteria to assist
    practitioners performing emergency ultrasound studies (EUS) of the heart in patients suspected of
    having emergent conditions where cardiac imaging may influence diagnosis or therapy.

    The primary applications of cardiac EUS are in the diagnosis or exclusion of pericardial effusion,
    cardiac tamponade and the evaluation of gross cardiac function. Increasingly, evaluation of the right
    ventricle and aortic root are considered integral parts of focused cardiac EUS, and evaluation of the
    inferior vena cava for fluid status may be considered part of the cardiac exam. Cardiac EUS is an
    integral component of patient evaluation and/or resuscitation. It is a clinically focused examination,
    which, in conjunction with historical and laboratory information, provides additional data for
    decision-making. It attempts to answer specific questions about a particular patient's condition. Other
    diagnostic or therapeutic interventions may take precedence or may proceed simultaneously with the
    cardiac EUS evaluation. While other tests may provide information that is more detailed than EUS,
    have greater anatomic specificity, or identify alternative diagnoses, EUS is non-invasive, is rapidly
    deployed and does not entail removal of the patient from the resuscitation area. Further, EUS avoids
    the delays, costs, specialized technical personnel, the administration of contrast agents and the
    biohazardous potential of radiation. These advantages make EUS a valuable addition to available
    diagnostic resources in the care of patients with time-sensitive or emergency conditions such as acute
    cardiac disease. In addition, cardiac EUS is an integral component of the trauma EUS evaluation.

2. Indications/ Limitations
    a. Primary
        i. Detection of pericardial effusion and/or tamponade
        ii. Evaluation of gross cardiac activity in the setting of cardiopulmonary resuscitation
        iii. Evaluation of global left ventricular systolic function

    b. Extended
        i. Gross estimation of intravascular volume status and cardiac preload.
        ii. Identification of acute right ventricular dysfunction and/or acute pulmonary hypertension in
            the setting of acute and unexplained chest pain, dyspnea, or hemodynamic instability.
        iii. Identification of proximal aortic dissection or thoracic aortic aneurysm.
        iv. Procedural guidance of pericardiocentesis, pacemaker wire placement and capture.

    c. Contraindications
    There are no absolute contraindications to cardiac EUS. There may be relative contraindications
    based on specific features of the patient's clinical situation.

    d. Limitations
        i. Cardiac EUS is a single component of the overall and ongoing evaluation. Since it is a
            focused examination EUS does not identify all abnormalities or diseases of the heart. EUS,
            like other tests, does not replace clinical judgment and should be interpreted in the context of
            the entire clinical picture. If the findings of the EUS are equivocal additional diagnostic
            testing may be indicated.
        ii. Cardiac ultrasound is capable of identifying many conditions beyond the primary and
            extended EUS applications listed above. These include but are not limited to: assessment of
            focal wall motion abnormalities, diastolic dysfunction, valvular abnormalities,intracardiac
            thrombus or mass, ventricular aneurysm, septal defects, aortic dissection, hypertrophic

cardiomyopathy. While these conditions may be discovered when performing cardiac EUS, they are typically outside of the scope of focused cardiac EUS and should typically undergo appropriate consultant-performed imaging for confirmation or follow-up.

   iii. Cardiac EUS is technically limited by:
1. Abnormalities of the bony thorax
2. Pulmonary hyperinflation
3. Massive obesity
4. The patient's inability to cooperate with the exam
5. Subcutaneous emphysema

e. Pitfalls
   i. When technical factors prevent an adequate examination, these limitations should be identified and documented. As usual in emergency practice, such limitations may mandate further evaluation by alternative methods, as clinically indicated.
   ii. The measured size of a pericardial effusion should be interpreted in the context of the patient's clinical situation. A small rapidly forming effusion can cause tamponade, while extremely large slowly forming effusions may be tolerated with minimal symptoms.
   iii. Clotted hemopericardium may be isoechoic with the myocardium or hyperechoic, so that it can be overlooked if the examining physician is expecting the anechoic of most effusions.
   iv. Sonographic evidence of cardiac standstill should be interpreted in the context of the entire clinical picture.
   v. Cardiac EUS may reveal sonographic evidence of right ventricular strain in cases of massive pulmonary embolus sufficient to cause hemodynamic instability. However, a cardiac EUS may not demonstrate the findings of right ventricular strain and a normal EUS does not exclude pulmonary embolism.
   vi. Evidence of right ventricular strain may be due to causes other than pulmonary embolus. These include acute right ventricular infarct, pulmonic stenosis, and chronic pulmonary hypertension.
   vii. Small or loculated pericardial effusions may be overlooked. As with other EUS, the heart should be scanned through multiple tissue planes in two orthogonal directions.
   viii. Pleural effusions may be mistaken for pericardial fluid. Evaluation of other areas of the chest usually reveals their characteristic shape and location.
   ix. Occasionally, hypoechoic epicardial fat pads may be mistaken for pericardial fluid. Epicardial fat usually demonstrates some internal echoing, is not distributed evenly in the pericardial space, and moves with epicardial motion.
   x. The descending aorta may be mistaken for a posterior effusion. This can be resolved by rotating the probe into a transverse plane.

3. Qualifications and Responsibilities of the Clinician Performing the Examination

Cardiac EUS provides information that is the basis of immediate decisions about further evaluation, management, and therapeutic interventions. Because of its direct bearing on patient care, the rendering of a diagnosis by cardiac EUS represents the practice of medicine, and therefore is the responsibility of the treating physician.

Due to the time-critical and dynamic nature of cardiac disease, emergent interventions may be mandated by the diagnostic findings of EUS examination. For this reason, cardiac EUS should be performed as soon as the clinical decision is made that the patient needs a sonographic evaluation.

Physicians of a variety of medical specialties may perform focused cardiac ultrasound. Training should be in accordance with specialty or organization-specific guidelines. Physicians should render a

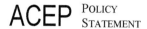

diagnostic interpretation in a time frame consistent with the management of acute cardiac disease, as outlined above.

4. Specifications for Individual Examinations
    a. <u>General</u> - Images are obtained and interpreted in real time without removing the patient from the clinical care area. Images are ideally obtained in a left-semi-decubitus position, although the clinical situation often limits the patient to lying supine. Images may be captured for documentation and/or quality review. Recording of moving images, either in video or cine loops, may provide more information than is possible with still cardiac EUS images. However, capturing moving images may be impractical in the course of caring for the acutely ill patient.

    b. <u>Technique</u>
        i. Overview
           Both patient habitus and underlying pathological conditions affect the accessibility of the heart to sonographic evaluation. For example, patients with causes of pulmonary hyperinflation (eg, emphysema or intubation) are likely to have poor parasternal windows, while patients with abdominal distension or pain may have an inaccessible subcostal window. For this reason, familiarity in evaluating the heart from a number of cardiac windows and planes increases the likelihood of successful EUS performance and interpretation.

        ii. Orientation
            Cardiologists have traditionally used an alternate image orientation convention from general ultrasound and other EUS applications. In this cardiology convention, the probe indicator corresponds to the right side of the screen as it is viewed, rather than the left of the screen for a general or EUS convention. Since reversing the screen for certain images and/or parts of an EUS exam can be time-consuming and confusing, especially under the emergent conditions typical of cardiac EUS, most emergency physicians have adopted the convention of not adjusting the screen orientation. Throughout this document, this EUS convention will be followed to obtain the views described, and the emergency physician will not need to reverse the orientation of the screen. The approximate orientation of the probe marker in the various classic cardiac views is described in terms of a clock face where 12 o'clock is directed to the head, 6 o'clock is directed to the feet, 9 o'clock is directed to the patient's right, and so on.

        iii. The primary cardiac views
             Throughout the following discussion "windows" refer to locations that typically afford sonographic access to the heart. Conversely, "views" refer to cardinal imaging planes of the heart, defined by specific structures that they demonstrate. In the following discussion, typical surface anatomical locations are described for the cardiac windows, but these are subject to significant individual variation based on the location and lie of the heart. The emergency physician should focus on identifying the key features of the primary cardiac views, regardless of the window where the probe needs to be positioned to obtain them.

             1. Subcostal four-chamber view (subxiphoid)
                This view is obtained by placing the probe just under the rib cage or xiphoid process with the transducer directed towards the patient's left shoulder and the probe marker directed towards the patient's right (9-o'clock). The liver is used as a sonographic window. The heart lies immediately behind the sternum, so that it is necessary, in a supine patient, to direct the probe in a plane that is almost parallel with the horizontal plane of the stretcher.

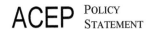

This requires firm downward pressure, especially in patients with a protuberant abdomen. Structures imaged in the subcostal four-chamber view include the right atrium, tricuspid valve, right ventricle, left atrium and left ventricle. The pericardial spaces should be examined both anterior and posterior to the heart. By scanning inferiorly, the inferior vena cava may also be visualized as it drains into the right atrium. This can help with orientation, as well as giving information about the patient's preload and intravascular volume status.

2. Parasternal long axis view
   This view is typically obtained using the third, fourth, and fifth intercostal spaces, immediately to the left of the patient's sternum. Structures imaged on this view include the pericardial spaces (anterior and posterior), the right ventricle, the septum, the left atrium and left ventricular inflow tract, the left ventricle in long axis, the left ventricular outflow tract, the aortic valve, and the aortic root.

   The probe marker is directed to the patient's left hip (approximately 4-o'clock). In this view the aortic outflow and left atrium will be on the right side of the screen as it is viewed and the cardiac apex will be on the left side of the screen.

   Alternately, the probe may be directed to the patient's *right* shoulder (approximately 10-o'clock). This will provide a view that is reversed 180 degrees from that seen in cardiology texts, but is consistent with orientation in the rest of emergency ultrasound, with the apex (a leftward structure) on the right side of the screen as it is viewed. In this probe position the orientation will appear very similar to the subcostal view, only slightly higher so that the aortic outflow tract is seen instead of the right atrium.

3. Parasternal short axis view
   This view is obtained by directing the marker in an approximately 8-o'clock direction. By rocking the probe in these interspaces, images can be obtained from the apex of the left ventricle inferiorly up to the aortic root superiorly. Intervening structures which can be identified, all in cross-section, include the entire left ventricular cavity, the right ventricle, the papillary muscles, the mitral valve, the aortic outflow tract, the aortic valve, the aortic root and the left atrium. The view at and immediately below the mitral valve may be particularly helpful for determining overall left ventricular systolic function.

4. Apical four-chamber view
   This view is obtained by placing the probe at the point of maximal impulse (PMI) as determined by physical exam. Normally this is in the fifth intercostal space and inferior to the nipple, however this location is subject to great individual variation. The probe is directed up along the axis of the heart toward the right shoulder, with the marker oriented towards the patient's right or 9-o'clock, which is towards the ceiling in a supine patient. The apex of the heart is at the center of the image with the septum coursing vertically in the center of the screen. The left ventricle and left atrium will be on the right side of the screen, and the right ventricle and atrium will be on the left side of the screen. This view demonstrates both the mitral and tricuspid valves and gives a clear view of the relative volumes of the two ventricular cavities, the motions of their free walls, and the interventricular septum.

iv. Secondary cardiac views
   1. Subxiphoid short axis view
      This view is obtained by placing the probe in the same location as the subxiphoid four-
      chamber view, but rotating the probe marker 90 degrees clockwise into a cephalad
      direction at 12-o'clock. This provides a short axis view of the right and left ventricles.
      With side to side rocking motion, a longitudinal view of the inferior vena cava emptying
      into the right atrium can be seen.

   2. Venous windows
      The inferior vena cava (IVC) may be traced by following hepatic veins in a subcostal
      window. Comparing the maximal IVC diameter in exhalation with the minimal IVC
      diameter in inhalation may provide a qualitative estimate of preload. Collapse of 50 -
      99% is normal; complete collapse may indicate volume depletion and <50% collapse may
      indicate volume overload, pericardial tamponade and/or right ventricular failure.

   3. Suprasternal notch view
      This view is obtained by placing the probe in the suprasternal notch, directed inferiorly
      into the mediastinum. The marker is usually directed obliquely between the patient's
      right and anterior since this is the plane followed by the aortic arch as it crosses from
      right anterior to left posterior of the mediastinum. A bolster under the patient's shoulders
      with the neck in full extension will facilitate this view used to visualize the aortic arch
      and great vessels.

   4. Apical two chamber view
      This view is obtained by rotating the probe clockwise 90 degrees from the apical four
      chamber view, so that the probe marker is directed in a cephalad direction or 12-o'clock.
      This allows visualization of the anterior and inferior left ventricular walls as well as the
      mitral and aortic valves. This view is infrequently utilized in the cardiac EUS.

v. Relationship of the cardiac views
   Several of the cardiac views provide images of the same planes of the heart from different
   angles. This is true of the following pairs of views: the parasternal long axis and apical two-
   chamber views; the apical four-chamber and sub-xiphoid four-chamber views; and the
   parasternal short axis and the subxiphoid short axis views.

c. Key components of the cardiac EUS evaluation
   i. Evaluation of pericardial effusion. Pericardial effusion usually appears as an anechoic or
      hypoechoic fluid collection within the pericardial space. With inflammatory, infectious,
      malignant or hemorrhagic etiologies, this fluid may have a more complex echogenicity. Fluid
      tends to collect dependently, but may be seen in any portion of the pericardium. Very small
      amounts of pericardial fluid can be considered physiologic and are seen in normal
      individuals. A widely used system classifies effusions as none, small (< 10 mm in diastole,
      often non-circumferential), moderate (circumferential, no part greater than 10 mm in width in

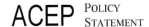

diastole), large (10-20 mm in width), and very large (>20 mm and/or evidence of tamponade physiology).

ii. Echocardiographic evidence of tamponade. Diastolic collapse of any chamber in the presence of moderate or large effusion is indicative of tamponade. Hemodynamic instability with a moderate or large pericardial effusion, even without identifiable diastolic collapse, is suspicious for tamponade physiology. A dilated non-collapsible IVC in the presence of pericardial effusion is also suspicious for tamponade physiology.

iii. Evaluation of gross cardiac motion in the setting of cardiopulmonary resuscitation. Terminal cardiac dysfunction typically progresses through global ventricular hypokinesis, incomplete systolic valve closure, absence of valve motion, absence of ventricular motion, and finally culminating in intracardiac gel-like densities. The lack of mechanical cardiac activity, or true cardiac standstill, demonstrated by EUS has the gravest of prognoses. The decision to terminate resuscitative efforts should be made on clinical grounds in conjunction with the sonographic findings.

iv. Evaluation of global cardiac function. Published investigations demonstrate that emergency physicians with relatively limited training and experience can accurately estimate cardiac ejection fraction. Left ventricular systolic function is typically graded as normal (EF>50%), moderately depressed (EF 30-50%), or severely depressed (EF<30%).

5. Documentation

In performing EUS of the heart, images are interpreted by the treating physician as they are acquired and are used to guide contemporaneous clinical decisions. Such interpretations should be documented in the medical record. Documentation should include the indication for the procedure, a description of the organs or structures identified and an interpretation of the findings. Images should be stored as a part of the medical record and done so in accordance with facility policy requirements. Given the often emergent nature of such ultrasound examinations, the timely delivery of care should not be delayed by archiving ultrasound images.

6. Equipment Specifications

A phased array cardiac transducer is optimal, since it facilitates scanning through the narrow intercostal windows, and is capable of high frame rates, which provide better resolution of rapidly moving cardiac structures. If this is not available, a 2-5 MHz general-purpose curved array abdominal probe, preferably with a small footprint, will suffice. The cardiac presets available on most equipment may be activated to optimize cardiac images. Doppler capability may be helpful in certain extended emergency echo indications but is not routinely used for the primary cardiac EUS indications. Both portable and cart-based ultrasound machines may be used, depending on the location and setting of the examination.

7. Quality Control and Improvements, Safety, Infection Control and Patient Education

Policies and procedures related to quality, safety, infection control and patient education should be developed in accordance with specialty or organizational guidelines. Specific institutional guidelines may be developed to correspond with such guidelines.

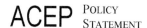

ACEP Emergency Ultrasound Imaging Criteria
Kidney and Bladder

1. Introduction
    The American College of Emergency Physicians (ACEP) has developed these criteria to assist
    practitioners performing emergency ultrasound studies (EUS) of the kidneys and bladder in patients
    suspected of having diseases involving the urinary tract.

    Emergency ultrasound of the kidneys and urinary tract may identify both normal and pathological
    conditions. The primary indications for this application of EUS are in the evaluation of obstructive
    uropathy and acute urinary retention. The evaluation of perirenal structures and the peritoneum for
    perirenal fluid is considered in the criteria for trauma EUS.

    EUS of the kidneys and urinary tract occurs as a component of the overall clinical evaluation of a
    patient with possible urinary tract disease. It is a clinically focused examination, which, in
    conjunction with historical and laboratory information, provides additional data for decision-making.
    It attempts to answer specific questions about a particular patient's condition. While other tests may
    provide information that is more detailed than EUS, have greater anatomic specificity, or identify
    alternative diagnoses, EUS is non-invasive, is rapidly deployed and does not entail removal of the
    patient from the resuscitation area. Further, EUS avoids the delays, costs, specialized technical
    personnel, the administration of contrast agents and the biohazardous potential of radiation. These
    advantages make EUS a valuable addition to available diagnostic resources in the care of patients
    with time-sensitive or emergency conditions such as acute renal colic and urinary retention.

2. Indications/Limitations
    a. Primary
        i.   The rapid evaluation of the urinary tract for sonographic evidence of obstructive uropathy
             and/or urinary retention in a patient with clinical findings suggestive of these diseases.

    b. Extended
        i.   Causes of obstructive uropathy
        ii.   Causes of acute hematuria
        iii. Causes of acute renal failure
        iv.   Infections and abscesses of the kidneys
        v.   Renal cysts and masses
        vi.   Gross bladder and prostate abnormalities
        vii. Renal trauma

    c. Contraindications: No absolute contraindications exist. Contraindications are relative, based on
        specific features of the patient's clinical condition.

    d. Limitations
        i.   EUS of the kidney and urinary tract is a single component of the overall and ongoing
             evaluation. Since it is a focused examination EUS does not identify all abnormalities or
             diseases of the urinary tract. EUS, like other tests, does not replace clinical judgment and
             should be interpreted in the context of the entire clinical picture. If the findings of the EUS
             are equivocal, additional diagnostic testing may be indicated.
        ii. Examination of the kidneys and collecting system may be technically limited by:
             1. Patient habitus including obesity, paucity of subcutaneous fat, narrow intercostal spaces
             2. Bowel gas
             3. Abdominal or rib tenderness

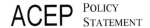

          4. An empty bladder

  e. Pitfalls

      i. When bowel gas or other technical factors prevent a complete real-time scan through all tissue planes, the limitations of the examination should be identified and documented. As is customary in emergency practice, such limitations may mandate further evaluation by alternative methods, as clinically indicated.

      ii. Hydronephrosis may be mimicked by several normal and abnormal conditions including dilated renal vasculature, renal sinus cysts, and bladder distension. Medullary pyramids may mimic hydronephrosis, especially in young patients.

      iii. Presence of obstruction may be masked by dehydration.

      iv. Absence of hydronephrosis does not rule out a ureteral stone. Many ureteral stones, especially small ones, do not cause hydronephrosis.

      v. Patients with an acutely symptomatic abdominal aortic aneurysm may present with symptoms suggestive of acute renal colic.

      vi. Both kidneys should be imaged in order to identify the presence of either unilateral kidney or bilateral disease processes.

      vii. The bladder should be imaged as part of EUS of the kidney and urinary tract. Many indications of this EUS exam are caused by conditions identifiable in the bladder.

      viii. Variations of renal anatomy are not uncommon and may be mistaken for pathologic conditions. These include reduplicated collection systems, unilateral, bipartite, ectopic and horse-shoe kidney.

      ix. Renal stones smaller than 3 mm are usually not identified by current sonographic equipment. Renal stones of all sizes may be missed and are usually identified by the shadowing they cause as their echogenicity is similar to that of surrounding renal sinus fat.

3. <u>Qualifications and Responsibilities of the Clinician Performing the Examination</u>
EUS of the kidneys and urinary tract provides information upon which immediate decisions for further evaluation, management and interventions are based. Rendering a diagnosis by EUS impacts patient care directly and qualifies as the practice of medicine. Therefore, performing and interpreting EUS is the responsibility of the treating physician.

Due to the time-critical and dynamic nature of many conditions of renal pathology, emergency interventions may be undertaken based upon findings of the EUS exam. For this reason, EUS should occur as soon as the clinical decision is made that the patient needs a sonographic exam.

Physicians of a variety of medical specialties may perform renal ultrasound examinations. Training should be in accordance with specialty or organization specific guidelines. Physicians should render a diagnostic interpretation in a time frame consistent with the management of acute renal pathology, as outlined above.

4. <u>Specifications for Individual Examinations</u>

  a. <u>General.</u> An attempt should be made to image both kidneys and the bladder in patients with suspected renal tract pathology undergoing EUS. In addition, hydronephrosis and urinary retention are frequently unsuspected causes of abdominal pain and may be recognized in the course of other abdominal or retroperitoneal EUS examinations.

  b. <u>Technique</u>

      i. <u>Identification.</u> The kidneys are more easily identified in their longitudinal axis. They are paired structures that lie oblique to every anatomic plane and at different levels on each side. Their inferior poles are anterior and lateral to their superior poles. Both hila are also directed

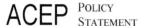

obliquely. Orientation is defined with respect to the axes of the organ of interest (longitudinal, transverse, and oblique), rather than standardized anatomic planes (sagittal, coronal, oblique and transverse). The long axis of the kidney approximates the intercostal spaces and longitudinal scans may be facilitated by placing the transducer plane parallel to the intercostal space. By convention, the probe indicator is always toward the head or the vertebral end of the rib on both the right and left sides. Transverse views of the kidneys are therefore usually also transverse to the ribs, resulting in prominent rib shadows that may make visualizing the kidneys more difficult unless a small footprint or phased array probe is available. Transverse views are obtained on both sides by rotating the probe 90 degrees counter-clockwise from the plane of the longitudinal axis.

ii. Real-time scanning technique

1. Overview. The kidneys are retroperitoneal in location and are usually above the costal margin of the flanks in the region of the costovertebral angle. A general-purpose curved array abdominal probe with a frequency range of between 2.0 -5.0 MHz is generally used. A small footprint or phased array probe may facilitate scanning between the ribs, but may require several windows in the longitudinal plane if the kidney is long, or superficial. Images of both kidneys should be obtained in the longitudinal and transverse planes for purposes of comparison and to exclude absence of either kidney. The bladder should be imaged to assess for volume, evidence of distal ureteral obstruction and for calculi. As with other EUS exams, the organs of interest are scanned in real-time through all tissue planes in at least two orthogonal directions.

2. Details of technique. The right kidney may be visualized with an anterior subcostal approach using the liver as a sonographic window. Imaging may be facilitated by having the patient in the left lateral decubitus position or prone. Asking the patient to take and hold a deep breath may serve to extend the liver window so that it includes the inferior pole of the kidney. Despite these techniques, parts or the entire kidney may not be seen in this view due to interposed loops of bowel, in which case the kidney should be imaged using an intercostal approach in the right flank between the anterior axillary line and midline posteriorly. For this approach, the patient can be placed in the decubitus position with a bolster under the lower side with the arm of the upper side fully abducted, thus spreading the intercostal spaces. Separate views of the superior and inferior poles are often required to adequately image the entire kidney in its longitudinal plane. To obtain transverse images, the transducer is rotated 90 ° counter-clockwise from the longitudinal plane. Once in the transverse plane, the transducer can be moved superiorly and medially, or inferiorly and laterally to locate the renal hilum. Images cephalad to the hilum represent the superior pole and those caudad represent the inferior pole. The left kidney lacks the hepatic window, necessitating an intercostal approach similar to the one described above for the right flank.

The bladder is imaged from top to bottom and from side to side, in transverse and sagittal planes, respectively. While a full bladder facilitates bladder scanning, distension may be a cause of artifactual hydronephrosis and is therefore to be avoided in scanning the kidneys. Ideally, the bladder is scanned prior to voiding (and again post-void, if outlet obstruction is a consideration), and kidney scanning performed after voiding. Such ideal conditions are rarely met with the exigencies of EUS and emergency care.

3. Key components of the examination. The kidneys should be studied for abnormalities of the renal sinus and parenchyma. Under normal circumstances, the renal collecting system contains no urine, so that the renal sinus is a homogeneously hyperechoic structure. A

distended bladder can cause mild hydronephrosis in normal healthy adults. Several classifications of hydronephrosis have been suggested. One that is easily applied and widely utilized is Mild or Grade I (any hydronephrosis up to Grade II), Moderate or Grade II (the calices are confluent resulting in a "bear's paw" appearance), or Severe or Grade III (the hydronephrosis is sufficiently extensive to cause effacement of the renal parenchyma). Other abnormalities identified including cysts, masses and bladder abnormalities may require additional diagnostic evaluation. Measurements may be made of the dimensions of abnormal findings and the length and width of the kidneys. Such measurements are rarely relevant in the EUS examination.

5. Documentation
    In performing EUS of the kidneys and urinary tract, images are interpreted by the treating physician as they are acquired and are used to guide contemporaneous clinical decisions. Such interpretations should be documented in the medical record. Documentation should include the indication for the procedure, a description of the organs or structures identified and an interpretation of the findings. Images should be stored as a part of the medical record and done so in accordance with facility policy requirements. Given the often emergent nature of such ultrasound examinations, the timely delivery of care should not be delayed by archiving ultrasound images.

6. Equipment Specifications
    A curved array abdominal transducer with a frequency range of between 2.0 -5.0 MHz is generally used. A small footprint or phased array probe may facilitate scanning between the ribs. A higher frequency 5.0-7.0 MHz transducer may give better resolution in children and smaller adults. Both portable and cart-based ultrasound machines may be used, depending upon the location of the patient and the setting of the examination.

7. Quality Control and Improvements, Safety, Infection Control and Patient Education
    Policies and procedures related to quality, safety, infection control and patient education should be developed in accordance with specialty or organizational guidelines. Specific institutional guidelines may be developed to correspond with such guidelines

Emergency Ultrasound Imaging Criteria Compendium
Lung and Pleura

1. Introduction
   The American College of Emergency Physicians (ACEP) has developed these criteria to assist practitioners performing emergency ultrasound (EUS) studies of the chest to rule out pneumothorax and abnormal collections of pleural fluid.

   Ultrasound has been shown to be helpful in the diagnosis of acute pneumothorax and is particularly sensitive for ruling out the presence of pneumothorax and pleural effusion. The ultrasound evaluation for pneumothorax examines the apposition of visceral and parietal pleura. The ultrasound evaluation for pleural effusion or hemothorax seeks to identify abnormal collections of pleural fluid. Extended applications for thoracic ultrasound include the diagnosis of abnormal interstitial lung water. Recent literature has shown that ultrasound is both sensitive and specific for interstitial lung fluid caused by congestive heart failure, volume overload, acute respiratory distress syndrome (ARDS), interstitial lung disease, and a variety of other diseases. Advantages of thoracic ultrasound are rapid deployment in critically ill patients with immediate diagnostic information without the need to transport or transfer the patient, the ability to perform the exam with portable ultrasound machines in remote or difficult clinical situations, and the ability to integrate the exam with sonographic evaluation of multiple organ systems. It is important to understand that thoracic ultrasound is a part of the resuscitative effort and is an emergent procedure. Other procedures may take precedence or may proceed simultaneously. It is not a comprehensive imaging test such as computerized tomography. The judicious use of ultrasound can add to the rapid, non-invasive, and dynamic evaluation of the critical patient.

2. Indications/Limitations
   a. Primary
      i. Acute pneumothorax
      ii. Abnormal collections of pleural fluid

   b. Extended
      i. Interstitial lung fluid caused by CHF and other conditions
      ii. Pneumonia
      iii. Pulmonary fibrosis

   c. Contraindications
      i. Known, tension pneumothorax requiring emergent intervention

   d. Relative Contraindications
      i. Significant pain in the area to be scanned
      ii. Open wounds or dressings in area to be scanned

   e. Limitations
      i. Morbidly obese patients can present so much adipose tissue that adequate imaging with ultrasound is technically difficult
      ii. While bedside thoracic ultrasound is more sensitive to diagnose pleural effusion than chest X-ray, the performance of the exam is dependent on the skill level of the sonologist

   f. Pitfalls

     i. Absence of pleural sliding is not 100% specific for pneumothorax, as prior pleurodesis, pleural scarring, lung contusions, bronchial obstruction, and advanced bullous emphysema, may result in absence of lung sliding.

     ii. The presence of pleural sliding only excludes pneumothorax immediately under the transducer. It does not rule out the presence of pneumothorax in other parts of the chest.

     iii. Thoracic ultrasound does not exclude the presence of a pulmonary embolism

     iv. The presence of B-lines posteriorly in the supine patient may be a normal finding.

     v. The presence of interstitial lung fluid on bedside thoracic ultrasound can be caused by many disease processes. Sonographic information should be correlated with history, physical exam, and with other clinical findings.

     vi. Motion of the transducer with respect to the patient's chest wall may give the impression of pleural motion, resulting in failure to identify pneumothorax.

3. Qualifications and Responsibilities of the Clinician Performing the Examination

Chest EUS is the basis of immediate decisions concerning further evaluation, management, and therapeutic interventions. Because of its direct bearing on patient care, the rendering of a diagnosis by chest EUS represents the practice of medicine, and therefore is the responsibility of the treating physician.

Due to the time-critical and dynamic nature of many causes of chest pathology, emergency interventions may be undertaken based upon findings of the EUS exam. For this reason, EUS should occur as soon as the clinical decision is made that the patient needs a sonographic exam.

Personnel that may perform EUS of the chest include physicians of multiple specialties, ultrasound technologists, physician extenders, and emergency medical personnel. Training should be in accordance with specialty or organization specific guidelines.

4. Specifications for Individual Examinations

    a. General - Chest EUS is performed simultaneously with other aspects of resuscitation. The transducer is placed systematically in each of the appropriate windows based on the clinical scenario. The ultrasound images are interpreted in real-time as the exam is being performed. If possible, images may be retained for purposes of documentation, quality assurance, or teaching.

    b. Technique. Overview. The chest ultrasound examination requires little patient preparation except for positioning in the bed at an ergonomic height for the examiner. Multiple areas of the chest are scanned. A generous amount of ultrasound gel is helpful, as wide areas of the chest are evaluated. In the absence of pleural adhesions, a pneumothorax typically occurs in the most anterior aspect of the chest in a supine patient. Conversely, pleural effusions or hemothoraces tend to accumulate posteriorly in the costophrenic sulci. When evaluating a patient for pulmonary edema, the patient is often in a semi-recumbent or upright position. Experienced sonologists often perform lung and pleural exams with the transducer parallel to the ribs, but for most emergency sonologists, an orientation perpendicular to the ribs facilitates identification of the pleural line, immediately deep to the ribs, which are useful landmarks recognizable in older children and adults by distal shadowing. When evaluating the lung bases via the liver and spleen, the sonologist should identify the solid organ below the diaphragm, and the thoracic cavity superior to the diaphragm, indirectly recognizable by mirror artifact of liver (on the right) and spleen (on the left).

    c. Pathologic findings

      i. Pneumothorax

        1. Anterior chest. In a trauma patient on a backboard, the anterior chest will be the most sensitive area to identify a pneumothorax. In this window, a linear array transducer is

ideal, with the focal zone set at the pleural line. However, a curvilinear or phased array transducer may also be used, using their high frequency range, and with adjustment of the focal zone. The transducer is placed in the mid-clavicular line, immediately inferior to the clavicles, and the orientation marker is directed cephalad in a sagittal plane. Two ribs, with distal shadowing should be identified. The pleural line beneath the ribs should be identified. The physician should evaluate for pleural sliding or shimmering as the patient breathes, indicating that the lung is expanded with the visceral and parietal pleura directly apposed. Other findings that exclude pneumothorax under the transducer include "lung pulse" (motion of visceral pleura and lung in time with cardiac motion) and the presence of B-lines (see below). The absence of any of these findings is highly suggestive of the presence of a pneumothorax. Conversely, the presence of the "leading edge" or "lung point" sign (created by the site of transition between expanded and collapsed lung) is pathognomonic of the *presence* of pneumothorax. Each interspace in the mid-clavicular line should be systematically evaluated to the level of the diaphragm on both sides. At each interspace, the sonologist should anchor the probe to the patient's chest wall using his/her examining hand, in order to minimize chest wall motion, which can be mistaken for lung sliding. The movement of the pericardium should not be mistaken for either pleural sliding or the lung-point sign in the left chest. In most cases, the probe should be placed more laterally when examining the left chest in the region of the heart.

2. Lateral chest. The technique for examining the lateral chest is identical to the anterior chest, except the physician will examine each interspace in the mid-axillary line.

3. Posterior thorax. The technique for examining the posterior thorax is identical to the anterior chest, except the physician will examine each interspace on the patient's back. The patient is examined sitting up if possible. Ultrasound waves do not penetrate the scapulae, so these should be abducted by asking the patient to grasp the contralateral shoulder with each hand.

4. Abbreviated exam. In critical situations, an ultrasound exam of the entire chest may not be feasible. In such circumstances, the evaluation may be limited to a single location on each anterior hemothorax. This two-point exam may identify large pneumothoraces, but miss a smaller pneumothorax.

5. M-Mode evaluation. M-Mode can be used to help identify or to document the presence of a pneumothorax. The M-mode sampling bar is placed in the middle of the intercostal space and the resulting M-Mode tracing is evaluated over time. In the normal patient a linear pattern superficial to the pleural line is in sharp distinction to the granular pattern deep to it (the "seashore sign"). With pneumothorax, there is a horizontal linear pattern above and below the pleural line ("stratosphere sign" or "barcode sign").

ii. Pleural effusion
1. Evaluation of right lung base in the supine patient. Similar to the evaluation of fluid in Morrison's Pouch, the physician can rapidly identify fluid above the diaphragm. Typically, a curvilinear or phased array probe is placed in an intercostal space around the nipple line in the coronal plane or parallel with the ribs, with the orientation marker directed cephalad. Following the identification of the kidney, liver, and diaphragm, the examiner angles or rocks the probe to evaluate above the diaphragm, using the liver as the acoustic window. Free fluid in the hemithorax will be identified as an anechoic or black area above the diaphragm. The examiner may also identify consolidated lung

sitting in large pleural effusions. The examiner should be aware that B-mode ultrasound is preferred to identify the presence of pleural effusion and hemothorax.

2. Evaluation of left lung base in the supine patient. Similar to the evaluation of free abdominal fluid in the left flank, the physician can rapidly identify fluid above the left diaphragm. Typically, a curvilinear or phased array probe is placed in an intercostal space around the mid-axillary line in the coronal plane or parallel with the ribs, with the orientation marker directed cephalad. Following the identification of the spleen, liver, and diaphragm, the examiner angles or rocks the probe to evaluate above the diaphragm, using the spleen as the acoustic window. Free fluid in the hemithorax will be identified as an anechoic or black area above the diaphragm. The examiner may also identify consolidated lung sitting in large pleural effusions. This view is often more challenging secondary to the relatively smaller size of the spleen compared to the liver.

3. Evaluation in the upright patient can be performed by placing the transducer on the midscapular line in a sagittal orientation, and sliding it from the level of the liver (on the right) or the spleen (on the left) in a cephalad direction until the diaphragm and costophrenic sulcus are identified. In the normal patient, this will be recognized by the presence of pleural sliding. Abnormal fluid collections (effusion, hemothorax, empyema, etc.) appear anechoic or hypoechoic.

4. Large pleural effusions. Occasionally, a large fluid collection may be identified during the evaluation of the pleura on the anterior chest wall.

5. E-FAST. During trauma scenarios, many clinicians now include evaluation of the pleural spaces for hemothorax during the E-FAST exam. The technique is as described above for "Evaluation of the lung bases in the supine patient" (see 7.f.vi.1 above and 7.f.vi.2 above).

iii. Interstitial lung fluid
1. Undifferentiated dyspnea. There is a substantial body of literature supporting the use of ultrasound for the differentiation of intrinsic lung disease and pulmonary edema states as a cause of acute dyspnea. The ultrasound finding of relevance is the presence of widespread B-lines. These are fine reverberation artifacts that extend from the pleural line to the far field. (Traditionally, depth is set at 15 cm.) These represent accumulation of fluid within the pulmonary interstitium. Many qualitative and quantitative methods have been described to assess B-lines. One of the most widely used divides the anteriolateral thorax into eight zones. In each hemithorax, the four zones are defined approximately by the anterior axillary line (anterior and posterior) and the nipple line (superior and inferior). Scattered B-lines may be normal in the more posterior areas of lung in the supine patient, but are abnormal if found anteriorly. In general, the greater the number of rib spaces with B-lines, and the more anterior in distribution, the more specific the finding for abnormal increased interstitial lung water. If the B-lines are unilateral or more localized, a focal process such as pneumonitis is more likely. Bilateral and extensive B-lines are more likely to be due to a more generalized process such as volume overload, heart failure, or ARDS. In infants and children, the differential diagnosis of B-lines is different from that in adults, and is the subject of ongoing elucidation. In extreme cases, the B-lines can become confluent, giving the appearance of a swinging curtain of artifact. A recent consensus conference has endorsed the use of "B-lines" to apply to the variety of terms used in the early literature on the topic including "comet tail artifacts", and "lung rockets". Ideally a small footprint curvilinear transducer is used with the focus

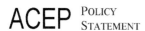

at, or slightly below the pleural line and a 12 to 15 cm depth of field (greater depth also allows easier recognition of consolidations). If such a transducer is not available, a curved array abdominal transducer or a phased array transducer can be used. Linear array transducers (ideal for the assessment of pneumothorax) are suboptimal due to their limited depth of field. If possible, artifact-reduction technologies such as multibeam processing and tissue harmonic imaging should be turned off. The transducer should be oriented in the sagittal plane to identify two ribs and the pleural line immediately beneath the ribs. Scattered comet tail artifacts that dissipate in the far field are caused by minor irregularities in the visceral pleura are referred to as "Z-lines," and have no clinical significance. They can be distinguished from B-lines, which are multiple and do not diminish in the far-field.

5. Documentation

In performing EUS of the lung and pleural spaces, images are interpreted by the treating physician as they are acquired and are used to guide contemporaneous clinical decisions. Such interpretations should be documented in the medical record. Documentation should include the indication for the procedure, a description of the organs or structures identified and an interpretation of the findings. Images should be stored as a part of the medical record and done so in accordance with facility policy requirements. Given the often emergent nature of such ultrasound examinations, the timely delivery of care should not be delayed by archiving ultrasound images.

6. Equipment Specifications

A linear array transducer with a frequency range of 5.0 to 12.0 MHz will allow the sonologist to image the superficial pleura and its artifacts. A curvilinear or phased array probe with a low frequency range of 2.0 – 5.0 MHz can be used for the evaluation of pleural effusion and B-lines. Both portable and cart-based ultrasound machines may be used, depending on the location and setting of the examination.

7. Quality Control and Improvements, Safety, Infection Control, and Patient Education

Policies and procedures related to quality, safety, infection control, and patient concerns should be developed in accordance with specialty or organizational guidelines. Specific institutional guidelines may be developed to correspond with such guidelines.

ACEP POLICY
STATEMENT

ACEP Emergency Ultrasound Imaging Criteria:
Ocular

1. Introduction
   The American College of Emergency Physicians (ACEP) has developed these criteria to assist practitioners performing emergency ultrasound (EUS) studies of the eye to evaluate for traumatic and non-traumatic findings.

   The use of EUS of the eye has been used for the detection of posterior chamber and orbital pathology. Specifically, ultrasound has been described to detect retinal detachment, vitreous hemorrhage, and dislocations or disruptions of structures. In addition, the structures posterior to the globe such as the optic nerve sheath diameter may be a reflection of other disease in the central nervous system.

   EUS evaluation of the eye occurs in conjunction with other EUS applications and other imaging and laboratory tests. It is a clinically focused examination, which, in conjunction with historical and laboratory information, provides additional data for decision-making. It attempts to answer specific questions about a particular patient's condition. While other tests may provide information that is more detailed than EUS, have greater anatomic specificity, or identify alternative diagnoses, EUS is non-invasive, is rapidly deployed and does not entail removal of the patient from the resuscitation area. Further, EUS avoids the delays, costs, specialized technical personnel, the administration of contrast agents and the biohazardous potential of radiation. These advantages make EUS a valuable addition to available diagnostic resources in the care of patients with time-sensitive or emergency conditions such as ocular complaints.

2. Indications/Limitations
   a. Primary
      i. Retinal detachment (RD) with or without vitreous detachment

   b. Extended
      i. Intracranial pressure indirectly via optic nerve sheath diameter measurement
      ii. Vitreous hemorrhage
      iii. Lens dislocation
      iv. Intraocular foreign body
      v. Globe rupture
      vi. Retrobulbar hemorrhage
      vii. Central retinal artery/vein occlusion
      viii. Subretinal hemorrhage
      ix. Posterior vitreous detachment (PVD)
      x. Direct and consensual light reflex

   c. Limitations
      i. Patient's inability to tolerate exam secondary to eye pain

   d. Relative Contraindications
      i. Open ocular trauma with leaking aqueous or vitreous humor; globe rupture. This risk may be minimized with the use of a Tegaderm and copious gel over the closed eyelid.
      ii. Periorbital wounds

   e. Pitfalls
      i. Missed pathology due to visualization in only one plane or neglecting to utilize kinetic echography to visualize all quadrants and contents of the globe.

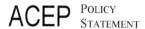

    ii. Applying too much pressure in a patient with suspected globe rupture or intraocular foreign body. In these patients a Tegaderm may be placed over the closed eyelid and copious gel applied. Scanning may then proceed using minimal or no applied pressure.

    iii. Failure to differentiate retinal detachment from other pathologies such as chronic vitreous hemorrhage, PVD, or fibrinous vitreous bands.

3. Qualifications and Responsibilities of the Clinician Performing the Examination

Ocular EUS is the basis of immediate decisions concerning further evaluation, management, and therapeutic interventions. Because of its direct bearing on patient care, the rendering of a diagnosis by ocular EUS represent the practice of medicine, and therefore is the responsibility of the treating physician.

Due to the time-critical and dynamic nature of many causes of ocular pathology, emergency interventions may be undertaken based upon findings of the EUS exam. For this reason, EUS should occur as soon as the clinical decision is made that the patient needs a sonographic exam.

Physicians of a variety of medical specialties may perform ocular ultrasound. Training should be in accordance with specialty or organization specific guidelines. Physicians should render a diagnostic interpretation in a time frame consistent with the management of ocular disease, as outlined above.

4. Specifications for Individual Examinations

    a. General – The eye is examined systematically in real time in all quadrants and in at least two orthogonal directions. Evaluation of the eye for evidence of other pathologies such as lens dislocation or vitreous hemorrhage, as described in "Extended Indications," are then performed based on the clinical situation and the physician's sonographic experience. The ultrasound images are interpreted in real-time as the exam is being performed. Images may be captured for archiving and/or quality review.

    b. Technique

        i. Identification

            1. Anterior chamber. The anterior chamber of the eye is the smaller of the two chambers. It appears in the near field and is bounded posteriorly by the iris and lens.

            2. Iris. In a transverse section, the iris is usually seen as 2 horizontal hyperechoic lines flanking the lens. In a longitudinal plane, the iris is donut-shaped, hyperechoic, and changes size when light is applied.

            3. Lens. Due to its density and composition, the lens is difficult to completely visualize. Usually only the anterior and posterior surfaces, represented by two gently curved inverse arcs between the horizonal lines of the iris, can be seen. Reverberation artifact may also be seen extending posteriorly from the lens.

            4. Posterior chamber. The posterior chamber of the eye is the larger of the two chambers. It is located directly posterior to the iris and lens, and should be completely anechoic and without internal echoes in the absence of pathology.

        ii. Real-time scanning technique

            1. Overview. The ocular examination can be performed at the patient's bedside and requires little patient preparation except for positioning in the bed (supine or 20 degrees of head elevation), and a 5-12 MHz probe. If intraocular foreign body or globe rupture/perforation are suspected, a Tegaderm may first be placed over the closed lid and then a generous amount of sterile ultrasound gel applied. After the exam, the Tegaderm is gently removed and the need to wipe gel away from the eye is negated. Both eyes are insonated. The examiner should rest the examining hand on the patient's forehead or face to avoid unnecessary pressure on the globe. Typically the examination is begun on the

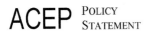

affected side and scanning is performed in two planes while and the patient is asked to move their eyes in all 4 directions. This serves two purposes: 1) all quadrants may be assessed and 2) identification of certain pathologies, such as retinal detachment and vitreous hemorrhage are easier since they move with eye movement (kinetic echography).

iii. Key components of the exam. Both eyes are systematically scanned in all quadrants as described above.

1. Traumatized eye. Evaluation of the traumatized eye with ultrasound is especially helpful when swelling limits direct visualization and evaluation of the eye and surrounding structures. The contours of the posterior chamber should be perfectly circular, and particular attention is paid to the posterior surface of the posterior chamber for evidence of retinal detachment. The vitreous is examined for hemorrhage or foreign bodies. Attention should also be paid to the retrobulbar space for hemorrhage and assessment of optic nerve edema. Direct and consensual light reflex of the iris may be checked with light applied to the closed eyelid of the traumatized eye as well as the unaffected eye.

2. Non-traumatized eye. Evaluation of the non-traumatized eye is a useful adjunct to the physical exam and slit lamp exam, especially with complaints of sudden onset vision loss. Attention is again paid to the posterior chamber for evidence of vitreous detachment with or without accompanying retinal detachment or hemorrhage. If the examiner is sufficiently skilled, color and power Doppler can be used to examine blood flow if central retinal artery/vein occlusion is suspected.

iv. Pathologic findings

1. Fibrinous vitreous bands. Usually an asymptomatic bilateral finding that occurs increasingly with age, these bands are also associated with diabetic retinopathy, sickle cells, prematurity, or previous vitreous hemorrhage. Bands appear as multiple hyperechoic mobile fibers in the posterior chamber that move with eye movement. Gain setting must usually be significantly increased to see fibrinous bands.

2. Retinal detachment. A brightly echogenic line separated from the posterior globe and tethered to optic nerve is indicative of RD. This should move as the eye is taken through range of motion. Depending on the cause of the detachment, other findings such as posterior vitreous detachment, vitreous hemorrhage, or subretinal hemorrhage may also be present. RD should be easily seen at normal gain levels.

3. Vitreous hemorrhage. The sonographic appearance of vitreous hemorrhage depends on the quantity and age of the hemorrhage. A small amount of fresh hemorrhage will appear as hyperechoic flecks that move with eye movement. A greater amount of blood will tend to layer along the posterior surface of the eye and also moves with eye movement. As blood ages, it tends to coalesce as string-like bands in the posterior chamber that move with eye movement.

4. Posterior vitreous detachment. PVD occurs increasingly with age and is usually an asymptomatic process but sometimes presents with photopsia. PVD is usually seen at higher gain levels and appears as a single, delicate string-like membrane that is detached from the posterior globe and moves with eye movement. It is thinner and less echogenic than an RD and notably, should *not* be tethered to the optic nerve. PVD can become more symptomatic when it causes a tear in the retina resulting in hemorrhage and a retinal detachment.

5. Subretinal hemorrhage. Appears as a shifting fluid collection along the posterior globe that is slightly more echoic than the vitreous body, and separated from it by the brightly echogenic retina.

6. Lens dislocation. Bedside ultrasound suggests a lens dislocation when the position of the lens in the affected eye to the relative position in the unaffected eye is disrupted and out of place.

7. Foreign body. Bedside ultrasound suggests an orbital foreign body when hyperechoic

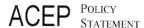

foreign material is appreciated in the globe when scanning in two planes. Thin-slice CT has a slightly higher sensitivity for intraocular foreign bodies, mainly because intraocular air introduced with the foreign body can hinder the view of deeper structures and pathology. All foreign bodies will appear hyperechoic with varying posterior artifact based on the composition of the foreign body itself (Metal and glass tend to produce reverberation artifact. Wood, gravel, and plastic are hyperechoic with a trailing shadow.)

8. Globe rupture. Ultrasound suggests globe rupture when the depth of the affected globe is shallow relative to the unaffected side. The globe typically loses the perfectly circular contour and vitreous hemorrhage is commonly seen in the posterior chamber. The scan is performed using a thick layer of sterile gel to avoid direct contact between probe and eyelid.

9. Retrobulbar hemorrhage. Usually appears as a hypoechoic fluid collection posterior to the globe.

10. Optic nerve edema. The intra-orbital subarachnoid space is distensible and subject to the same pressure shifts as the intracranial compartment which contains the optic nerve. In an axis perpendicular to the optic nerve 3mm behind the globe, the optic nerve sheath diameter is measured. The optic nerve should be aligned directly opposite the probe but the optic nerve sheath diameter width measured perpendicular to the vertical axis of the scanning plane. A mean optic nerve sheath diameter of < = 5mm has been suggested as the upper limits of normal in an adult with concern for increased ICP. This measurement shows high negative predictive value.

11. Central retinal artery occlusion. Ocular ultrasound suggests occlusion to the central retinal artery or vein when there is loss of color flow along the posterior globe or overlying the optic nerve (the retinal artery and vein run within the optic nerve sheath). Power Doppler should be used if color flow is not evident, and both arterial and venous waveforms should be documented in pulse Doppler mode.

12. Light response. It is possible to assess the pupil for direct and consensual light response through a closed or edematous eyelid. The iris is usually visualized in a long axis by moving the transducer to the top of the orbit in a transverse plane and fanning inferiorly while asking the patient to look at their feet. Light is then applied to either closed eyelid and the iris assessed for constriction. Measurements of pupil constriction can also be formally obtained with this method.

5. Documentation

In performing EUS of the eye, images are interpreted by the treating physician as they are acquired and are used to guide contemporaneous clinical decisions. Documentation of the ocular EUS should be incorporated into the medical record. Documentation should include the indication for the procedure, the views obtained, a description of the organs or structures identified and an interpretation of the findings. Images should be stored as a part of the medical record and in accordance with facility policy requirements. Given the often emergent nature of such ultrasound examinations, the timely delivery of care should not be delayed by archiving ultrasound images.

6. Equipment Specifications

A high frequency linear array probe with a frequency range of 8 to 14 MHz is ideal, as this range will allow the sonographer to image the globe in detail. An endocavitary transducer with similar frequency range can also be used, and allows a sector field of view for better imaging of the retrobulbar space. B-mode imaging is preferred to avoid exposure of the eye to higher power outputs. Color-flow and Doppler modes may be used for focused evaluations of the optic nerve and retina but these examinations should be minimized.

7. Quality Control and Improvements, Safety, Infection Control, and Patient Education

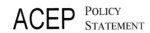

POLICY
STATEMENT

Policies and procedures related to quality, safety, infection control, and patient concerns should be developed in accordance with specialty or organizational guidelines. Specific institutional guidelines may be developed to correspond with such guidelines

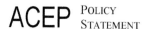

Proposed ACEP Emergency Ultrasound Imaging Criteria
Pelvic

1. Introduction

    The American College of Emergency Physicians (ACEP) has developed these criteria to assist practitioners performing emergency ultrasound studies (EUS) of the pelvis in emergency patients to evaluate for evidence of acute pathology including ectopic pregnancy, ovarian cysts and tubo-ovarian abscess.

    First trimester pregnancy complications such as abdominal pain and vaginal bleeding are common presenting complaints. Ultrasound finding of a clear intrauterine pregnancy, in many instances, minimizes the possibility of ectopic pregnancy and can decrease throughput time and decrease morbidity. The scope of practice for pelvic ultrasound will vary depending on individual experience, comfort/skill level and departmental policies. However, some centers may choose to evaluate the ovaries and seek to identify tubo-ovarian abscess, fibroids, and pelvic masses.

    EUS of the pelvis occurs as a component of the overall clinical examination of a patient presenting with symptoms related to the pelvic area. It is a clinical focused examination, which, in conjunction with historical and laboratory information, provides additional data for decision-making. It attempts to answer specific questions about a particular patient's condition. Other diagnostic tests may provide more detailed information than EUS, show greater anatomic detail, or identify alternative diagnoses. However, EUS is non-invasive, rapidly deployed, allows the patient to remain under a physician's direct care, and avoids delays, costs, specialized technical personnel, and bio-hazardous potentials of radiation and contrast agents. These advantages make it a valuable addition to the diagnostic resources available to the physician caring for patients with time-sensitive or emergency conditions such as ectopic pregnancy and other causes of acute pelvic pain.

2. Indications/Limitations:
    a. Primary
        i. To evaluate for the presence of intrauterine pregnancy, minimizing the likelihood of an ectopic pregnancy when modifying factors such as infertility treatment are not present.

    b. Extended
        i. Ovarian cysts
        ii. Fibroids
        iii. Tubo-ovarian abscess
        iv. Ruling out ovarian torsion by ruling out cyst or mass
        v. Identifying suspected ectopic pregnancy

    c. Limitations
        i. Infertility patients or others with specifically known risk factors for heterotopic pregnancy.
        ii. Assessing pelvic sonographic anatomy after vaginal-rectal surgery
        iii. Evaluation of fetal health outside of fetal heart rate determination

    d. Pitfalls
        i. Ovarian torsion evaluation in the presence of ovarian, para-ovarian, tubal or para-tubal mass
        ii. Ovarian mass evaluation for presence of malignancy versus benign mass

iii.　Interstitial pregnancy

3.　Presence of ovarian torsion due to a mass or cyst in first trimester patient with identified first
trimester intrauterine pregnancyQualifications and Responsibilities of the Clinician Performing the
Examination

Pelvic EUS provides information that is the basis of immediate decisions concerning further
evaluation, management, and therapeutic interventions. Because of the direct bearing on patient care,
the rendering of a diagnosis by EUS represents the practice of medicine, and therefore is the
responsibility of the treating physician.

Due to the time-critical and dynamic nature of ectopic pregnancy and other pathologic conditions of
the pelvis, emergency interventions may be mandated by the diagnostic findings of the EUS of the
pelvis. For this reason, EUS of the pelvis should occur as soon as the clinical decision is made that the
patient needs a sonographic evaluation.

Physicians of a variety of medical specialties may perform EUS of the pelvis. Training should be in
accordance with specialty or organizational specific guidelines. Physicians should render a diagnostic
interpretation in a time frame consistent with the management of acute presentations related to the
pelvic area, as outlined above.

4.　Specifications for Individual Examinations
　　a.　General – Organs and structures evaluated by pelvic EUS are scanned systematically in real time
　　　　through all tissue planes in at least two orthogonal directions. The primary focus of the pelvic
　　　　EUS is the identification on an intrauterine pregnancy. Pelvic sonographic evaluations for other
　　　　pelvic pathology, as described in "Extended Indications," are performed based on the clinical
　　　　situation and appropriate physician's sonographic experience.

　　b.　Technique
　　　　i.　Identification
　　　　　　1.　Uterus. The uterus should be examined in at least two planes, the short- and long-axis, to
　　　　　　　　avoid missing important findings that may lie off midline or outside the endometrial
　　　　　　　　canal, such as an interstitial pregnancy or fibroids. The uterus should be traced from the
　　　　　　　　fundus to the cervix, confirming that it is actually the uterus that is being scanned rather
　　　　　　　　than a gestational reaction from a large ectopic pregnancy. Fibroids, which can cause
　　　　　　　　significant pain and even bleeding, should be noted. A pregnancy located less than 5 to 7
　　　　　　　　mm (exact minimum normal distance varies from reference to reference) from the edge
　　　　　　　　of the myometrium is concerning for being an interstitial ectopic pregnancy.
　　　　　　2.　Cul-de-sac. The cul-de-sac or pouch of Douglas may contain small to moderate amounts
　　　　　　　　of fluid in the normal female pelvis depending on her point in the menstrual cycle. Large
　　　　　　　　amounts of fluid are abnormal but may not be tied to significant pathology. When an
　　　　　　　　ectopic pregnancy is of concern, a significant amount of fluid in the pouch of Douglas
　　　　　　　　raises the concern for rupture. Echogenic fluid in the pelvis may be consistent with either
　　　　　　　　pus or blood.
　　　　　　3.　Ovaries. Each ovary should also be scanned in at least two planes, short- and long-axis.
　　　　　　　　This technique should enable visualization of possible masses juxtaposed to the ovary as
　　　　　　　　well as cysts located on the periphery of an ovary. In the first trimester patient with pain
　　　　　　　　evaluating the ovaries may identify an unexpected cause for pain. For instance, ovarian
　　　　　　　　masses, cysts, or ovarian torsion may be the etiology of a patient's pain.
　　　　　　4.　Fallopian tubes. The normal fallopian tube can be visualized as it originates from the
　　　　　　　　cornua of the uterus. Visualization can be limited by significant bowel gas or enhanced
　　　　　　　　when distended by fluid such as in hyrosalpinx or tubo-ovarian abscess.

ii. Real-time scanning technique

1. Overview. The pelvic ultrasound examination can be performed at the patient's bedside and when possible, immediately following the pelvic examination portion of the physical examination to limit the time a patient spends in the lithotomy position. A chaperone should also be present for all endovaginal examinations. In most instances, the transabdominal portion of the ultrasound exam should precede the transvaginal component as information regarding bladder fullness, position of the uterus, and anatomic variations can be appreciated. As well, in a certain percentage of patients, an intrauterine pregnancy will be documented, thereby minimizing the need to perform the endovaginal ultrasound exam.

2. Transabdominal. The patient lies supine on the examination table. The transducer is placed on the lower abdomen just above the symphysis pubis and the pelvic organs are examined through a window of the distended bladder. Bladder filling is ideal when the bladder dome is just above the uterine fundus. Under distention limits visualization of the uterus and other pelvic organs. Images are obtained in sagittal and transverse planes. To optimally image the uterus, the transducer is aligned with the long axis of the uterus, which is often angled right or left of the midline cervix. The ovaries and adnexa are best seen by sliding the transducer to the contralateral side and angling back toward the ovary of interest. The transabdominal technique provides the best overview of the pelvis.

3. Transvaginal. For the transvaginal examination, optimal imaging is achieved with an empty bladder. Two possible patient positions will facilitate endovaginal scanning. In the first, the patient is supine on a stretcher or bed with her legs flexed. Folded sheets or pads are placed under her buttocks to elevate her pelvis above the examination table to allow room for transducer movement. Alternatively, the patient may be scanned on a pelvic examination table with her feet in stirrups. The probe may be placed in the vagina by the patient or the examiner. The uterus is examined entirely in two planes. When in the sagittal plane, the examiner sweeps the transducer laterally to each side to visualize the uterus in its entirety, because it is often deviated to one side. The transducer is then rotated 90 degrees counterclockwise to obtain a coronal view. The transducer can then be angled anteriorly, posteriorly, and to each side to obtain a full assessment of the uterus.

After the sagittal and coronal planes of the uterus have been fully interrogated, other structures in the pelvis can be visualized, such as the cul-de-sac, fallopian tubes, and ovaries. The cul-de-sac is posterior to the uterus and the ovaries are located lateral to the uterus and usually lie anterior to the internal iliac veins and medial to the external iliac vessels.

5. Documentation

In performing EUS of the pelvis, images are interpreted by the treating physician as they are acquired and are used to guide contemporaneous clinical decisions. Such interpretations should be documented in the medical record. Documentation should include the indication for the procedure, a description of the organs or structures identified and an interpretation of the findings. Images should be stored as part of the medical record and done so in accordance with facility policy requirements. Given the often emergent nature of such ultrasound examinations, the timely delivery of care should not be delayed by archiving ultrasound images.

6. Equipment specifications

A curved linear array abdominal transducer with a range of approximately 3.0 to 5.0 MHz as well as an endovaginal transducer with an approximate range of 6.0 to 10.0 MHz range is used for pelvic

ACEP POLICY
STATEMENT

ultrasound. Color or power Doppler and pulsed wave Doppler are critical if an assessment of blood flow will be made. Both portable and cart-based ultrasound machines may be used, depending on the location and setting of the examination. There is no indication to interrogate the fetus with pulsed wave Doppler, therefore avoiding high-energy ultrasound in early pregnancy. Further, all pelvic ultrasound studies should be kept to a reasonably limited amount of time when sensitive tissue such as the fetus is involved.

7. Quality Control and Improvements, Safety, Infection Control, and Patient Education
   Policies and procedures related to quality, safety, infection control, and patient education should be developed in accordance with specialty or organizational guidelines. Specific institutional guidelines may be developed to correspond with such guidelines

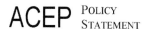

ACEP Emergency Ultrasound Imaging Criteria:
Right Upper Quadrant

1. Introduction
    The American College of Emergency Physicians (ACEP) has developed these criteria to assist
    practitioners performing emergent ultrasound (EUS) studies of the right upper quadrant (RUQ) in
    patients suspected of having acute biliary disease.

    Abdominal pain is a common presenting complaint in the emergency department. Biliary disease is
    frequently a consideration among the possible etiologies. In many cases, EUS of the RUQ may be
    diagnostic for biliary disease, may exclude biliary disease, or may identify alternative causes of the
    patient's symptoms. If biliary disease is identified, EUS also guides disposition by helping to
    distinguish emergent, urgent, and expectant conditions.

    EUS of the RUQ occurs as a component of the overall clinical evaluation of a patient with abdominal
    pain. It is a clinically focused examination, which, in conjunction with historical and laboratory
    information, provides additional data for decision-making. It attempts to answer specific questions
    about a particular patient's condition. While other tests may provide information that is more detailed
    than EUS, have greater anatomic specificity, or identify alternative diagnoses, EUS is non-invasive, is
    rapidly deployed and does not entail removal of the patient from the resuscitation area. Further, EUS
    avoids the delays, costs, specialized technical personnel, the administration of contrast agents and the
    biohazardous potential of radiation. These advantages make EUS a valuable addition to available
    diagnostic resources in the care of patients with time-sensitive or emergency conditions such as acute
    biliary colic or cholecystitis, as well as other causes of abdominal pain.

2. Indications/Limitations
    a. Primary
        i. Identification of cholelithiasis

    b. Extended
        i.   Cholecystitis
        ii.   Common bile duct abnormalities, including dilatation and choledocholithiasis
        iii. Liver abnormalities, including tumors, abscesses, intrahepatic cholestasis, pneumobilia,
              hepatomegaly
        iv.   Portal vein abnormalities
        v.   Abnormalities of the pancreas
        vi.   Other gallbladder abnormalities, including tumors
        vii. Unexplained jaundice
        viii. Ascites

    c. Contraindications
        i. There are no absolute contraindications to RUQ EUS. There may be relative
            contraindications based on specific features of the patient's clinical situation.

    d. Limitations
        i. EUS of the RUQ is a single component of the overall and ongoing evaluation. Since it is a
            focused examination, EUS does not identify all abnormalities or diseases of the RUQ. EUS,
            like other tests, does not replace clinical judgment and should be interpreted in the context of
            the entire clinical picture. If the findings of the EUS are equivocal, additional diagnostic
            testing may be indicated.
        ii. The primary focus of RUQ EUS is to identify or exclude gallstones. Other entities, including

hepatic tumors, abnormalities of the pancreas or abnormalities of the portal system would not usually be identified by a limited and focused exam.
  iii. Examination of the RUQ may be technically limited by:
       1. Obese habitus Bowel gas
       2. Abdominal tenderness

  e. Pitfalls
     i. When bowel gas or other technical factors prevent an adequate examination, these limitations should be identified and documented. As usual in emergency practice, such limitations may mandate further evaluation by alternative methods.
     ii. Failure to identify the gallbladder may occur with chronic cholecystitis particularly when filled with stones, or, in the rare instances of gallbladder agenesis. Failure to identify the gallbladder should warrant additional diagnostic imaging.
     iii. The gallbladder may be confused with other fluid filled structures including the portal vein, the inferior vena cava, and hepatic or renal cysts or loculated collections of fluid. These can be more accurately identified with careful scanning in multiple planes.
     iv. Measurement of posterior gallbladder wall thickness may be inaccurate due to layered gallstones, acoustic enhancement from bile, and closely apposed loops of bowel. Consequently, measurement of gallbladder wall thickness should be made on the anterior wall, adjacent to the hepatic parenchyma.
     v. Small gallstones may be overlooked or mistaken for gas in an adjacent loop of bowel. In questionable cases, gain settings should be optimized, the area should be scanned in several planes, and the patient should be repositioned to check for the mobility of gallstones.
     vi. Gas in loops of bowel adjacent to the posterior wall of the gallbladder may be mistaken for stones. Intraluminal gas can be distinguished by noting peristalsis and specifically identifying the bowel wall. Stones are characterized by anechoic shadowing and movement with patient repositioning.
     vii. Small stones in the gallbladder neck may easily be overlooked or mistaken for lateral cystic shadowing artifact (edge shadows). It may be necessary to image this area in several planes to avoid this pitfall.
     viii. Common bile duct stones may only be identified by the shadowing they cause.
     ix. Cholesterol stones are often small, less echogenic, may float, and may demonstrate comet tail artifacts.
     x. Pneumobilia and emphysematous cholecystitis are subtle findings and may produce increased echogenicity and comet–tail artifact caused by gas in the biliary tree and gallbladder wall.
     xi. Polyps may be mistaken for gallstones. The former are non-mobile, do not shadow, and are adjacent and attached to the inner gallbladder wall.
     xii. Gallbladder wall thickening may not represent biliary pathology, but may be physiological, as in the post-prandial state, or with non-surgical conditions such as hypoproteinemia and congestive heart failure.
     xiii. The presence of gallstones or other findings consistent with cholecystitis does not rule out the presence of other life-threatening causes of epigastric pain such as aortic aneurysm or myocardial infarction.
     xiv. Except for emergency physicians with extensive experience in EUS, evaluations of the liver, pancreas and Doppler examination of the portal venous system are not part of the normal scope of EUS of the RUQ.

3. Qualifications and Responsibilities of the Clinician Performing the Examination
   EUS of the RUQ provides information that is the basis of immediate decisions concerning further evaluation, management, and therapeutic interventions. Because of its direct bearing on patient care, the rendering of a diagnosis by RUQ EUS represent the practice of medicine, and therefore is the

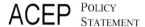

responsibility of the treating physician.

Due to the time-critical and dynamic nature of many causes of abdominal pain and biliary pathology, emergency interventions may be undertaken based upon findings of the EUS exam. For this reason, EUS should occur as soon as the clinical decision is made that the patient needs a sonographic exam. Physicians of a variety of medical specialties may perform biliary ultrasound. Training should be in accordance with specialty or organization specific guidelines. Physicians should render a diagnostic interpretation in a time frame consistent with the management of acute biliary disease, as outlined above.

4. Specifications for Individual Examinations
    a. General –Organs and structures evaluated in the RUQ are scanned systematically in real time through all tissue planes in at least two orthogonal directions. The primary focus of the biliary EUS examination is the identification of gallstones. Evaluation of the gallbladder for evidence of cholecystitis and examination of the liver and biliary tree, as described in "Extended Indications," are performed based on the clinical situation and the emergency physician's ultrasound experience.
    b. Technique
        i. Identification
            1. Gallbladder. The normal gallbladder is highly variable in size, shape, axis, and location. It may contain folds and septations, and may lie anywhere between the midline and the midaxillary line. The axis and location of the porta hepatis are also highly variable. Orientation of images of the gallbladder and common bile duct are conventionally defined with respect to their axes as longitudinal, transverse, and oblique, rather than standardized anatomic planes such as sagittal, coronal, oblique and transverse.

            In most cases, the gallbladder lies immediately posterior to the inferior margin of the liver in the mid-clavicular line. In some patients, the fundus may extend several centimeters below the costal margin; in others, the gallbladder may be high in the hilum of the liver, almost completely surrounded by hepatic parenchyma. In order to avoid confusing it with fluid-filled tubular structures, the entire extent of the gallbladder should be scanned in its long and short axes.

            2. Common bile duct. It is usually located by following the neck of the gallbladder to the portal triad where it can be found in conjunction with the portal vein and the hepatic artery. The use of color Doppler helps identify vascular structures from the common bile duct.

        ii. Real-time scanning technique
            1. Overview: A general-purpose curved array abdominal probe with a frequency range of 2.0-5.0 MHz is generally used. A small footprint or phased array probe may facilitate scanning between the ribs. As with other EUS, the organs of interest are scanned methodically through all tissue planes in at least two orthogonal directions.

            2. In most patients, the inferior margin of the liver provides a sonographic window for the gallbladder below the costal margin. In many cases, this window can be augmented by asking the patient to take and hold a deep breath. It may also be helpful to place the patient in a left decubitus position. The transducer is placed high in the epigastrium with the indicator in a cephalad orientation. The probe is swept laterally while being held immediately adjacent to the costal margin. The liver margin should be maintained within the field of view on the screen.

3. In patients whose liver margin cannot be visualized below the costal margin, an intercostal approach is necessary. In order to minimize rib shadowing, the transducer is oriented with the plane of the probe parallel to the intercostal space and the indicator directed toward the vertebral end of the rib. This plane is about 45 degrees counter-clockwise from the long axis of the patient's body. The probe is swept laterally from the sternal border to the midaxillary line until the gallbladder is located.

4. When the gallbladder has been located, its long and short axes are identified. In the long axis, images are obtained, by convention, with the gallbladder neck on the left of the screen, and the fundus on the right. The gallbladder is scanned systematically through all tissue planes in both long and short axis views. In many patients, a combination of subcostal and intercostal windows allow for views of the gallbladder from multiple directions and may help identify small stones, resolving artifacts, and examining the gall bladder neck.

5. The common bile duct is most easily located sonographically by finding and identifying the portal vein and hepatic artery, which comprise the portal triad. Several techniques can be used to locate the common bile duct in addition to anatomic location. These include tracking the hepatic artery from the celiac axis, tracking the portal vein from the confluence of the splenic and superior mesenteric veins, and following the portal vessels in the liver to the hepatic hilum. In a transverse view of the portal triad, the common bile duct and hepatic artery are typically seen anterior to the portal vein. The common bile duct is usually more lateral than the hepatic artery or more to the left on the screen. It can also be distinguished by its absence of a color flow Doppler signal if this modality is employed.

iii. Key components of the exam. The gallbladder is systematically scanned with particular attention to the neck. For patients with low-lying gallbladder, the fundus may be obscured by gas-filled colon. Decubitus positioning or inhalation may help provide adequate windows in this situation. The principal abnormal finding is gallstones that are echogenic with distal shadowing. Measurement of wall thickness, if performed, is made on the anterior wall between the lumen and the hepatic parenchyma. Measurements of gallbladder size are rarely helpful in EUS, although gross increases in transverse diameter or overall size may be evidence of cholecystitis and hydrops, respectively. A qualitative assessment of the wall and pericholecystic regions should also be made, looking for mural irregularity, breakdown of the normal trilaminar mural structure, and fluid collections.

The common bile duct, like other tubular structures, is most accurately measured when imaged in a transverse plane. It is most reliable to measure the intraluminal diameter (inside wall to inside wall). Anatomically, it is preferable to measure the common bile at its largest diameter, which typically occurs extra-hepatic ally. Identification of the common bile duct in this location is best achieved with long axis visualization, rather than the transverse orientation. Becoming facile with imaging in both planes is a key element to successful measurements of the common bile duct. Evaluation of the common bile duct may reveal shadowing suggesting stones and/or comet-tail artifact suggesting pneumobilia. The question of such findings would warrant additional diagnostic testing.

iv. Pathologic findings
1. Cholelithiasis - Gallstones are often mobile (move with patient positioning) and usually cause shadowing. Optimization of gain, frequency and focal zone settings may be necessary to identify small gallstones and to differentiate their shadows from those of

adjacent bowel gas.

2. Cholecystitis - This diagnosis is based on the entire clinical picture in addition to the findings of the EUS. The following sonographic findings support the diagnosis of cholecystitis.
    a. Thickened, irregular, or heterogeneously echogenic gallbladder wall is measured along the anterior surface. Thickness greater than 3 millimeters is considered abnormal.
    b. Pericholecystic fluid may appear as hypo- or an-echoic regions seen along the anterior surface of the gallbladder within the hepatic parenchyma and suggests acute cholecystitis.
    c. A Sonographic Murphy's sign is tenderness reproducing the patient's abdominal pain elicited by probe compression directly on the gallbladder, combined with the absence of similar tenderness when it is compressed elsewhere.
    d. Increased transverse gallbladder diameter greater than 5 cm may be evidence of cholecystitis.
3. Common bile duct dilatation - The normal upper limit of common bile duct diameter has been described as 3 mm, although several studies have demonstrated increasing diameter with aging in patients without evidence of biliary disease. For this reason, many authorities consider that the normal common bile duct may increase by 1 mm for every decade of age.
4. Pathologic findings of the liver and other structures are beyond the scope of the EUS.

5. Documentation
    In performing EUS of the RUQ, images are interpreted by the treating physician as they are acquired and are used to guide contemporaneous clinical decisions. Documentation of the RUQ EUS should be incorporated into the medical record. Documentation should include the indication for the procedure, the views obtained, a description of the organs or structures identified and an interpretation of the findings. Images should be stored as a part of the medical record and in accordance with facility policy requirements. Given the often emergent nature of such ultrasound examinations, the timely delivery of care should not be delayed by archiving ultrasound images.

6. Equipment Specifications
    A curvilinear abdominal transducer with frequencies of 2.0-5 .0 MHz is appropriate. A small footprint curved array probe or phased array probe facilitates intercostal scanning. Both portable and cart-based ultrasound machines may be used, depending on the location and setting of the examination.

7. Quality Control and Improvements, Safety, Infection Control and Patient Education
    Policies and procedures related to quality, safety, infection control and patient education should be developed in accordance with specialty or organizational guidelines. Specific institutional guidelines may be developed to correspond with such guidelines.

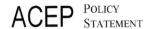

ACEP Emergency Ultrasound Imaging Criteria:
Soft tissue/Musculoskeletal

1. Introduction

   The American College of Emergency Physicians (ACEP) has developed these criteria to assist practitioners performing emergency ultrasound (EUS) studies of soft tissue and musculoskeletal systems (ST-MSK).

   Ultrasound allows the practitioner to rapidly assess patients for pathology that is difficult or impractical to assess by other means. Primarily, ultrasound can aid in the classification of soft tissue infection, localization of foreign bodies (FB), detection of joint effusions and guidance of arthrocentesis. Secondarily, ultrasound can aid in the diagnosis of deep space infection, guidance of foreign body removal, fracture detection and reduction, and evaluation for ligament and tendon pathology. It is a clinically focused examination, which, in conjunction with history, physical examination and other imaging, provides important data for decision-making and patient care.

2. Indications/Limitations
   a. Primary
      i. Soft tissue: sonographic evaluation of
         1. Cellulitis versus abscess
         2. Foreign bodies
      ii. Musculoskeletal
         1. Evaluation of joint effusion
         2. Guidance of arthrocentesis

   b. Extended
      i. Soft tissue
         1. Identification of deep space infection
         2. Guidance of foreign body removal
      ii. Musculoskeletal
         1. Fracture detection and reduction
         2. Identification of tendon/ligament injury
         3. Diagnosis of tenosynovitis

   c. Contraindications
      i. Need for immediate operative management

   d. Relative contraindications
      i. Significant pain or open wounds over the area to be scanned

   e. Limitations
      i. Ultrasound does not replace clinical judgment, especially when emergent surgical procedures are indicated.

   f. Pitfalls
      i. Soft tissue
         1. Infection
            a. Early in the infectious course, classic sonographic findings of soft tissue infection may not be present.
            b. Deep space infections may be difficult to detect secondary to inadequate penetration with higher frequency transducers and settings.

      c. Abscesses typically have variable internal densities and consistencies, so sonographic appearance can also be variable.

      d. The appearance of cellulitis is indistinguishable from sterile edematous tissue. In these scenarios, sonographic findings should be interpreted in the context of the clinical history.

  2. Foreign body identification

      a. Small FBs (< 2 mm) may be difficult to detect and require careful and methodical examination.

      b. Superficial foreign bodies can also be difficult to detect since they are not typically located within the optimal focal zone of the sonographic window.

      c. Confined spaces, such as web interspaces, can be difficult to image due to the contours of the transducer.

      d. FBs adjacent to bone can be difficult to detect. Sonographers typically use shadowing or other artifacts as an important visual cue for presence of FB, and these may be obscured by closely adjacent bone.

      e. Other echogenic material in the skin, such as air, scar tissue, ossified cartilage and keratin plugs, may produce false positive findings.

      f. Although ultrasound is sensitive for the presence of a FB, this sensitivity does not reach 100%. Ultrasound cannot definitively rule-out the presence of a FB.

  3. Foreign body localization and removal – see 'Ultrasound Guided Procedures" criteria.

ii. Musculoskeletal

  1. Ultrasound has been shown to be highly accurate in the detection of long bone fractures. Certain fractures may be difficult to detect, including:

      a. non-displaced fractures

      b. small avulsion fractures

      c. fractures involving

         i. articular surfaces

        ii. intertrochanteric regions

       iii. hands and feet

  2. Joint effusions are occasionally difficult to detect if they are:

      a. very small in size

      b. early in an infectious course

  3. Ligaments and Tendons require careful and methodical evaluation since:

      a. incomplete lacerations may be difficult to visualize

      b. anisotropy may lead to misinterpretation of the sonographic images

      c. early in the infectious course, the typical sonographic findings of tenosynovitis may not be present

3. <u>Qualifications and Responsibilities of the Clinician Performing the Examination</u>

ST-MSK EUS is the basis of immediate decisions concerning further evaluation, management, and therapeutic interventions. Because of its direct bearing on patient care, the rendering of a diagnosis by ST-MSK EUS represents the practice of medicine, and therefore is the responsibility of the treating physician.

Due to the time-critical and dynamic nature of many causes of soft tissue-MSK pathology, interventions may be undertaken based upon findings of the EUS exam. For this reason, EUS should occur as soon as the clinical decision is made that the patient needs a sonographic exam.

Physicians of a variety of medical specialties may perform ST-MSK ultrasound. Training should be in accordance with specialty or organization specific guidelines. Physicians should render a

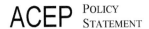

diagnostic interpretation in a time frame consistent with the management of ST-MSK disease, as outlined above.

4. Specifications for Individual Examinations
   a. General. The ST-MSK examination can be performed at the patient's bedside and requires little patient preparation except for positioning in the bed and control of significant pain in the scanning area if present. The ultrasound probe is placed over the area of interest and imaging is performed in both sagittal and transverse planes. The probe should be initially placed at the primary window and then be tilted, rocked and rotated to allow for real-time imaging of the area(s) involved. This may take more time with difficult windows, challenging patients or other patient priorities. Interpretation should be done at the bedside immediately with performance of the real-time examination. Comparison to the contralateral "normal" side and dynamic imaging are both critical in ST-MSK sonography.
   b. Technique
      i. Identification
         1. Dermal layer. Most superficial echogenic structure encountered (deep to the stand-off pad if one is being used).
         2. Subcutaneous fat. Located deep to the dermis, this is a relatively hypoechoic layer with a reticular pattern of interspersed echogenic connective tissue.
         3. Muscle tissue. Hypoechoic striated tissue typically found in bundles.
         4. Tendons/ligaments. Hyperechoic tissue with a fibrillar appearance in the long axis. Tendons can be observed to move as the corresponding joints are passively flexed and extended. Ligaments may be more difficult to visualize at ninety degrees to the ultrasound beam and therefore may appear more hypoechoic.
         5. Blood vessels. Anechoic with a circular profile when observed in a short-axis.
         6. Bones. Bony cortices are brightly echogenic with posterior shadowing. Typically only the most superficial surface of the bone will be visible.
         7. Nerves. Typically hyperechoic and fibrillar in the long axis and with a honeycomb appearance in a short axis, nerves may be confused for tendons. Nerves usually do not move significantly with joint movement, and are localized in relation to vascular structures.
      ii. Real-time scanning technique
         1. Overview. A high frequency linear or hockey stick transducer is typically employed for ST-MSK ultrasound. This enables high-resolution imaging but typically limits depth of penetration to a few centimeters. Imaging may be improved with certain devices such as stand-off pads or water bath to place the item of interest central in the focal zone. The items of interest should be scanned *methodically* in 2 orthogonal planes.
         2. Soft tissue. The transducer is generally first dragged over an area of normal skin adjacent to the area of interest. As the transducer moves closer to the area of interest, the sonographer will carefully assess for signs of cellulitis, abscess, or cutaneous foreign body. Of particular note, when interrogating a soft tissue abscess, the application of gentle pressure will often elicit movement within the abscess cavity and liquid contents are displaced.
         3. Bones. Ultrasound is very useful for the detection of fractures and to help guide fracture reduction. In most instances, a high frequency linear array is used to evaluate bone for the presence of a fracture; however, depending on the depth of bone being visualized, a lower frequency probe may be necessary to assure adequate tissue penetration. The probe is placed in the long axis over the bone in question to visualize the hyperechoic bony cortex. The sonographer then slides the probe along the length of the bone looking for interruptions, step-offs, and angulations of the

cortex. The same technique can than be repeated in the short axis to acquire more information. In some instances, a comparison of the contralateral bone may be helpful.

4. Joint effusions: Due to the unique anatomy of individual joints, the scanning technique is variable. In general, the probe is placed in the long axis over the bone proximal or distal to the joint in question in order to visualize the hyperechoic bony cortex. Keeping the cortex in view, the probe is slid toward the joint space looking for the presence of an anechoice/hypoechoic collection representing a joint effusion. In every instance, the contralateral joint should be used for comparison. It is generally accepted that an effusion exists if there is at least a 2mm difference in the amount of fluid present in the affected joint when compared to the contralateral joint.

5. Tendons/ligaments: Ultrasound is useful for the detection of tendon and ligamentous lacerations, ruptures, and tenosynovitis. In most instances, a high frequency linear array transducer is used to evaluate the structure of interest. In addition, superficial tendons or ligaments may be better visualized with the use of a standoff or water bath technique. Visualized in long axis, tendons and ligaments appear hyperechoic and fibrillar, and move as the corresponding joint is ranged. Disruption is most easily seen in the long axis. If infection is suspected, the sonographer should assess for fluid collections surrounding the tendon, which can be seen in either axis.

iii. Key components of the exam

1. Soft tissue. The normal/unaffected skin should be scanned prior to scanning the suspected infectious region. This comparison may aid in the recognition of subtle findings suggestive of soft tissue infection. In the assessment for abscess, the sonographer should remember that different internal densities of the abscess will lead to different echogenicities in the sonographic window. Gentle pressure should be applied to elicit movement within the abscess cavity, confirming the presence of pus. Foreign bodies can be difficult to locate, but several techniques improve visualization: scanning slow and methodically, imaging in multiple planes (to detect obliquely oriented objects), utilizing a standoff pad or water bath technique for superficial objects and ideally, imaging the foreign body directly perpendicular or parallel to its long axis. Familiarity with adjacent anatomic structures will allow the discernment of foreign bodies from muscle, nerve, fascia, tendon, blood vessels, bone and subcutaneous air.

2. Bones. The identification of small bone fractures is relatively uncomplicated given the high resolution and shallow field of view of the linear transducer. When used to assess progress in fracture reduction, ultrasound coupling gel may make reduction difficult by making the surfaces slippery. The gel should be wiped away with a towel before further attempts at reduction. When examining for femur fractures, a curvilinear transducer is helpful to obtain the depth necessary for imaging deep to the thick quadriceps muscles.

3. Joint effusions. Knowledge of the sonoanatomy of the individual joints is of the utmost importance. In most instances, a high frequency linear array is used; however, in deeper joints (ie, hip, shoulder) a lower frequency probe may be needed to assure adequate tissue penetration

4. Tendons/ligaments. Tendons should be imaged from multiple angles to minimize the effect of anisotropy. This sonographic artifact is usually hypoechoic and triangular, and mimics a disruption in the tendon or ligament, but will correct as the transducer is moved and the beam strikes the structure at 90 degrees. Tendons may also be easily identified by ranging the accompanying joint and observing for movement of the tendon.

iv. Pathologic findings

1. <u>Cellulitis.</u> Sonographic findings suggestive of cellulitis are non-specific but include tissue thickening, increased echogenicity of the subcutaneous tissue and reticular regions of hypoechoic edema which may yield a cobblestone-like appearance. Differentiating bands of edematous fluid from irregular collections of pus can be difficult.

2. <u>Abscess.</u> A subcutaneous abscess may have a variety of appearances. In general a hyperechoic rim of edematous tissue surrounds an elliptical or spherical-shaped, hypo-echoic fluid-filled cavity which demonstrates posterior acoustic enhancement. At times, however, an abscess can be irregularly shaped, lack a clear surrounding rim and demonstrate variable degrees of internal echogenicity due to purulent material, debris, septae or gas. Color flow Doppler can help confirm the absence of flow within the cavity and may reveal a region of hyperemia surrounding the abscess. Pressure applied over the infected region may reveal mobility of the purulent material within the cavity, helping to confirm its liquid nature. Prior to drainage of an abscess, recognition of surrounding anatomic structures (blood vessels, muscles, tendons, nerves) is essential.

3. <u>Foreign bodies.</u> All foreign bodies appear hyperechoic but will display variable degrees of artifact. Metal and glass tend to produce reverberation artifact. Wood, gravel, and plastic are hyperechoic with a trailing shadow. Substances that have been present in the body longer than 24 hours typically have a small amount of surrounding inflammatory fluid, which appears as an anechoic halo surrounding the hyperechoic material.

4. <u>Foreign body localization and removal.</u> See "Ultrasound Guided Procedures" criteria.

5. <u>Deep space infections.</u> In order to assure adequate tissue penetration a lower frequency transducer may be needed. The diagnosis of necrotizing fasciitis with ultrasound has not been studied systematically and thus ultrasound should not be utilized to exclude this diagnosis. A number of sonographic findings suggestive of this disease have been described including thickening of the subcutaneous fascia, a fluid layer > 4 mm adjacent to deep fascia and subcutaneous gas.

6. <u>Joint effusions.</u> Joint effusions are easily seen by ultrasound as hypoechoic fluid collections in the joint space. The transducer is dragged along the long axis of the bone towards the articular surface. There, a V-shaped depression will be seen that is formed by the articular surface of the connecting bone. If an effusion is present this space will be filled by hypoechoic fluid collection. The precise location of the largest fluid collection may then be easily marked for aspiration.

7. <u>Arthrocentesis.</u> A joint effusion may be aspirated using static or dynamic visualization techniques.
   a. Static – The ultrasonographer visualizes the joint effusion and marks the overlying skin in two distinct planes noting the depth of the fluid as well as the optimal angle of entry. The probe is then removed, and the joint tapped using standard technique.
   b. Dynamic – The sonographer obtains a view of the joint effusion and under direct visualization uses the ultrasound to guide ther needle into the most readily accessible fluid collection. This may be done in short or long axis depending on the site and sonographer preference.

8. <u>Fractures.</u>
   a. Small bone fractures: Ultrasound may be helpful in the identification of small fractures, or those not easily or practically imaged with conventional radiography. These include facial fractures, rib fractures, and nasal bone fractures. The sonographer typically first identifies the hyperechoic bony cortex. Then, the transducer is dragged along the surface of the bone in both orthogonal

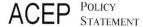

planes as the continuity of the cortex is carefully assessed. Since the window depth of a high frequency transducer is 1-5 cm, fractures displaced by as little as a few millimeters will typically be obvious.

b. Long bone fractures: Ultrasound is also helpful in the identification of long bony fractures. This includes use in austere environments such as the wilderness or battlefield. It may also be useful for a quick femoral survey in the hypotensive trauma patient when other sources of bleeding are not immediately obvious and bleeding into the femoral compartment is suspected. In this setting, a curvilinear transducer is helpful to obtain the depth necessary for imaging deep to the thick quadriceps muscles.

9. <u>Fracture reduction.</u> Ultrasound is helpful in fracture reduction when other imaging is impractical. This is most evident during procedural sedation when quick radiographs cannot be obtained to assess the success of the procedure. The bone is intermittently assessed along sagittal, coronal, and axial planes for adequacy of reduction as the clinician attempts to bring the cortices into alignment.

10. <u>Tendon/ligament lacerations and ruptures.</u> The ultrasound probe is placed in the longitudinal and transverse planes over the structure of interest in an attempt to visualize partial and complete tears. Partial tears will appear as hypoechoic areas within the normal fibrillar tendon architecture, while complete lacerations and ruptures will extend through the entire length of the tendon in question. Active and passive range of motion of the tendon can help to assist in the presence or absence of pathology; scanning the contralateral body part for comparison may be useful as well.

11. <u>Tenosynovotis.</u> The ultrasound probe is placed in the longitudinal and transverse planes over the tendon in question in order to assess for the presence of an anechoic/hyoechoic area around the tendon representing a collection of fluid suggesting infection. In addition, infected tendons may demonstrate enlargement when compared to the contralateral side.

5. Documentation

In performing ST-MSK EUS, images are interpreted by the treating physician as they are acquired and are used to guide contemporaneous clinical decisions. Documentation of the ST-MSK EUS should be incorporated into the medical record. Documentation should include the indication for the procedure, the views obtained, a description of the organs or structures identified and an interpretation of the findings. Images should be stored as a part of the medical record and in accordance with facility policy requirements. Given the often emergent nature of such ultrasound examinations, the timely delivery of care should not be delayed by archiving ultrasound images.

6. Equipment Specifications

Most of the applications described in this section involve superficial structures. Thus optimal visualization occurs with linear ultrasound transducers at frequencies of 8.0-12.0 MHz. Occasionally a curvilinear or phased array transducer of 3.5-5.0 MHz will be necessary to evaluate deeper structures such as in cases of suspected hip effusion/septic hip joint or deep space abscess. Endocavitary probes can be used to identify abscess formation in areas such as the oropharynx. Both portable and cart-based ultrasound machines may be used, depending on the location and setting of the examination.

7. Quality Control and Improvements, Safety, Infection Control, and Patient Education

Policies and procedures related to quality, safety, infection control, and patient concerns should be developed in accordance with specialty or organizational guidelines. Specific institutional guidelines may be developed to correspond with such guidelines.

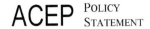

ACEP Emergency Ultrasound Imaging Criteria:
Trauma

1. Introduction
   The American College of Emergency Physicians (ACEP) has developed these criteria to assist
   practitioners who are performing emergency ultrasound studies (EUS) of the torso of the injured
   patient and commonly referred to as the Focused Assessment by Sonography in Trauma (FAST)
   exam.

   Trauma EUS is used to evaluate the peritoneal, pericardial or pleural spaces in anatomically
   dependent areas by combining several separate focused ultrasound examinations of the chest, heart,
   abdomen and pelvis. Since a variety of formats and content have been advocated for the FAST exam,
   and because this document considers some applications of trauma ultrasonography that are beyond
   the scope of the FAST, this document will refer to such examinations as "Emergency Ultrasound
   (EUS) in Trauma," or "Trauma EUS."

   The primary indication for this application is to identify pathologic collections of free fluid or air
   released from injured organs or structures. Trauma EUS is performed at the bedside to assess for
   hemopericardium, hemothorax, hemoperitoneum or other abnormal fluids such as urine or bile, or
   pneumothorax. Free fluid is a marker of injury, not the injury itself. Since certain important traumatic
   conditions such as hollow viscus injury, mesenteric vascular injury, and diaphragmatic rupture may
   cause minimal hemorrhage, they can be easily be overlooked by trauma EUS. Trauma EUS also may
   not differentiate between different types of pathological fluid such as urine and blood. These
   characteristics of trauma EUS have implications for management of patients in whom these injuries
   are a consideration. Pneumothorax may be mimicked by lack of respiratory effort, mainstem
   intubation, adhesed or pleurodesed lung, or pleural masses (see "Lung and Pleura" criteria).

   Trauma EUS is performed as an integral component of trauma resuscitation. Other diagnostic or
   therapeutic interventions may take precedence or may proceed simultaneously with the EUS
   evaluation. It is a clinically focused examination, which, in conjunction with historical and laboratory
   information, provides additional data for decision-making. It attempts to answer specific questions
   about a particular patient's condition. While other tests may provide information that is more detailed
   than EUS, have greater anatomic specificity, or identify alternative diagnoses, EUS is non-invasive, is
   rapidly deployed and does not entail removal of the patient from the resuscitation area. Further, EUS
   avoids the delays, costs, specialized technical personnel, the administration of contrast agents and the
   biohazardous potential of radiation. These advantages make EUS a valuable addition to available
   diagnostic resources in the care of patients with time-sensitive or emergency conditions such as acute
   thoracic and abdominal trauma.

   Trauma EUS is well suited to mass casualty situations where it can be used to rapidly triage multiple
   victims. It can be performed on the patient with spinal immobilization and with portable equipment,
   allowing it to be used in remote or difficult clinical situations such as aeromedical transport,
   wilderness rescue, expeditions, battlefield settings, and space flight. Finally, serial trauma EUS exams
   can be repeated as frequently as is clinically indicated. These advantages make it a valuable addition
   to diagnostic resources available in the care of patients with the time-sensitive and/or emergent
   conditions associated with torso trauma.

2. Indications/Limitations
   a. Primary
      i. To rapidly evaluate the torso for evidence of traumatic free fluid or pathologic air suggestive
         of injury in the peritoneal, pericardial, and pleural cavities.

ACEP POLICY
STATEMENT   *Page 42 of 55*

b. Extended
   i. Solid organ injury
   ii. Triage of multiple or mass casualties

c. Contraindications
   i. There are no absolute contraindications to trauma EUS. There may be relative contraindications based on specific features of the patient's clinical situation, eg, extensive abdominal or chest wall trauma.
   ii. The need for immediate laparotomy is often considered a contraindication to trauma EUS; however, even in this circumstance, EUS evaluation for pericardial tamponade or pneumothorax may be indicated prior to transfer to the operating room.

d. Limitations
   i. Trauma EUS is a single component of the overall and ongoing resuscitation. Since it is a focused examination, EUS does not identify all abnormalities resulting from truncal trauma. EUS, like other tests, does not replace clinical judgment and should be interpreted in the context of the entire clinical picture. If the findings of the EUS are equivocal, additional diagnostic testing may be indicated.
   ii. EUS in trauma is technically limited by:
       1. Bowel gas
       2. Obesity
       3. Subcutaneous emphysema
   iii. Trauma EUS is likely to be less accurate in the following settings:
       1. Pediatric patients
       2. Patients with other reasons for free fluid such as prior diagnostic peritoneal lavage, ascites, ruptured ovarian cyst, pelvic inflammatory processes

e. Pitfalls
   i. When bowel gas or other technical factors prevent a complete or adequate exam, these limitations should be identified and documented. As usual in emergency practice, such limitations may mandate further evaluation by alternative methods, as clinically indicated.
   ii. Most studies show that peritoneal free fluid is not identified by EUS until at least 500 ml is present. Thus, a negative exam does not preclude early or slowly bleeding injuries.
   iii. Some injuries may not give rise to free fluid and may therefore easily be missed by trauma EUS. These include contained solid organ injuries, mesenteric vascular injuries, hollow viscus injuries, and diaphragmatic injuries.
   iv. Non-traumatic fluid collections such as ascites, or pleural and pericardial effusions, which are due to antecedent medical conditions, may be mistakenly ascribed to trauma. Credible history and associated clinical findings, as well as the sonographic features of the free fluid may suggest such conditions.
   v. Trauma EUS does not specifically identify most solid organ injuries.
   vi. EUS does not identify retroperitoneal hemorrhage.
   vii. A negative trauma EUS is not accurate in excluding intra-abdominal injury after isolated penetrating trauma.
   viii. Blood clots form rapidly in the peritoneum. Clotted blood has sonographic qualities similar to soft tissue, and may be overlooked.
   ix. Perinephric fat may be mistaken for hemoperitoneum.
   x. Fluid in the stomach or bowel may be mistaken for hemoperitoneum.
   xi. Small hemothoraces may be missed in the supine position.
   xii. In the evaluation of the pericardium, epicardial fat pads, pericardial cysts, and the descending aorta have been mistaken for free fluid.

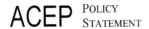

xiii. Patients with peritoneal or pleural adhesions with significant hemorrhage may not develop free fluid in the normal locations.
xiv. In the suprapubic view, posterior acoustic enhancement caused by the bladder can result in pelvic free fluid being overlooked. Gain settings should be adjusted accordingly.

3. Qualifications and Responsibilities of the Clinician Performing the Examination
Trauma EUS provides information that is the basis of immediate decisions about further evaluation, management, and therapeutic interventions. Because of its direct bearing on patient care, the rendering of a diagnosis by trauma ultrasound represents the practice of medicine, and therefore is the responsibility of the treating physician.

Due to the time-critical and dynamic nature of traumatic injury, emergent interventions may be mandated by the diagnostic findings of EUS examination. For this reason, trauma EUS should be performed as soon as possible (usually minutes) following the decision that the patient needs a sonographic evaluation.

Physicians of a variety of medical specialties may perform the FAST examination. Training should be in accordance with specialty or organization specific guidelines. Physicians should render a diagnostic interpretation in a time frame consistent with the management of acute traumatic injury, as outlined above.

4. Specifications for Individual Examinations
    a. General Trauma EUS is performed simultaneously with other aspects of resuscitation. The transducer is placed systematically in each of 4 general regions with known windows to the peritoneum, pericardium and pleural spaces for detection of fluid and other sonographic abnormalities. The precise location of these regions varies from patient to patient, and is only used as a means to the real goal of identifying specific potential spaces where pathological collections of free fluid are known to collect. The transducer is placed in each of the regions consecutively and then tilted, rocked and rotated to allow for real-time imaging of the underlying potential space(s). The ultrasound images obtained are interpreted in real-time as the exam is being performed. If possible, images may be retained for purposes of documentation, quality assurance, or teaching.

    b. Technique
        i.   Overview. The trauma EUS exam evaluates 4 general regions or "views" for free fluid in defined potential spaces. The order in which the regions are examined may be determined by clinical factors such as the mechanism of injury or external evidence of trauma. Since scientific investigations have shown that the single most likely site for free fluid to be identified is the right upper quadrant, many practitioners start with this view, and then progress in a clockwise rotation through the sub-xiphoid, left upper quadrant, and suprapubic views. As with other EUS, the potential spaces being examined should be scanned methodically in real-time through all tissue planes. If possible, they should be evaluated in at least two orthogonal directions. Identification of the potential spaces in a single still image or plane is likely to result in early injuries, or those with small volumes of free fluid, being overlooked.

        ii. Real-time scanning technique
            1. The right flank. Also known as the perihepatic view, Morison's pouch view or right upper quadrant view. Four potential spaces for the accumulation of free fluid are examined in this region (listed in a cephalad to caudad direction): the pleural space, the

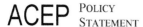

subphrenic space, the hepatorenal space (Morison's pouch), and the inferior pole of the kidney, which is a continuation of the right paracolic gutter.

In this region, the liver usually provides a sonographic window for all four potential spaces. If the liver margin is sufficiently low, the probe can be placed in a subcostal location in the mid-clavicular line. Cooperative patients may facilitate this by being asked to "take a deep breath and hold" while the four potential spaces are examined. In the majority of patients the liver does not afford an adequate window with a subcostal probe position, so an intercostal approach is necessary. In order to minimize rib shadowing, the transducer should be placed in an intercostal space in a location between the mid-clavicular and posterior axillary lines, with the plane of the probe parallel with the ribs. This plane is about 45 degrees counter-clockwise from the long axis of the patient's body. The probe indicator, by convention, is always directed toward the head (the vertebral end) of the rib. By angling the probe superiorly, the subhepatic space and the right pleural space may be visualized for fluid. Abnormal fluid collections in the pleural space are visualized as anechoic or hypoechoic collections above the diaphragm.

Angling inferiorly allows visualization of Morison's pouch and may show the inferior pole of the right kidney. In many patients, bowel gas is interposed between the liver and the inferior pole of the kidney, necessitating a more posterior approach to visualize this space.

Gain settings should be adjusted so that the diaphragm and renal sinus fat appear white, and known hypoechoic structures (such as the inferior vena cava, gallbladder, or renal vein) appear black.

2. The pericardial view. Also known as the subcostal or subxiphoid view. To examine the pericardium, the liver in the epigastric region is most commonly used as a sonographic window to the heart. The heart lies immediately behind the sternum, so that it is necessary, in a supine patient, to direct the probe in a direction toward the left shoulder that is almost parallel with the horizontal plane of the stretcher. This requires firm downward pressure, especially in patients with a protuberant abdomen, in order to obtain a view posterior to the sternum ("under" the sternum) in the supine patient. Both sagittal and transverse planes may be used. Many find the transverse plane easier, especially in obese patients, since it requires slightly less compression of the abdominal wall to obtain adequate views. The potential space of the pericardial sac is examined for fluid both inferiorly (between the diaphragmatic surface and the inferior myocardium) and posteriorly. Slight angulation in a caudal direction when the probe is held in a transverse orientation allows visualization of the IVC and hepatic veins including their normal respiratory variability. In some patients, a subxiphoid view is not possible due to anterior abdominal trauma, or body habitus. In this case, other routinely used cardiac windows such as the parasternal or apical four-chamber views may be used. These are described in the "Cardiac" criteria.

3. Left flank. In this view, also known as the perisplenic or left upper quadrant view, four potential spaces are sonographically explored, analogous to the right upper quadrant view. These four spaces are: the pleural space, the subphrenic space, the splenorenal space, and the inferior pole of the kidney, which is a continuation of the left paracolic gutter. This view can make some use of the spleen as a sonographic window, but, being so much smaller, it provides a much more limited window than the liver on the right. For this reason the posterior intercostal approach described for the right upper quadrant is

utilized extensively in the left upper quadrant. In order to avoid the gas filled splenic flexure and descending colon it is usually necessary to place the probe on the posterior axillary line or even more posteriorly. As is the case on the right side, the probe indicator, by convention, is always directed toward the head (the vertebral end) of the rib. This requires that, on the left, the probe is rotated approximately 45 degrees clockwise from the long axis of the patient's body. Angulation superiorly allows visualization of the left pleural space. As on the right, the pleural spaces are investigated for evidence of hemothorax by looking for anechoic or hypoechoic collections above the diaphragm. In order to visualize the inferior pole of the left kidney and the superior extent of the left paracolic gutter, it is usually necessary to move the probe one to three rib spaces in a caudal direction. In each rib space, the probe is systematically swept through all planes in a search for free fluid.

4. Pelvic. Also known as the suprapubic view, retrovesical, and rectovesical view (in the male), and the retrouterine, rectouterine, and pouch of Douglas view (in the female). This space is the most dependent peritoneal space in the supine position. A full bladder is ideal to visualize the potential spaces in the pelvis, but adequate views can often be obtained with a partly filled bladder. When the bladder is empty, large volumes of anechoic or hypoechoic free fluid may still be seen, however it is not possible to reliably rule out the presence of smaller amounts of free fluid. The probe is placed in the transverse plane immediately cephalad to the pubic bone. This maximizes the sonographic window afforded by the bladder. The probe is rocked from inferior to the dome of the bladder in a systematic manner through all tissue planes. The probe may be rotated 90 degrees counter-clockwise into the sagittal plane for additional visualization of the bladder and pelvic peritoneum.

   Gain settings usually need to be decreased in this view to account for the posterior acoustic enhancement caused by the fluid-filled bladder.

5. Anterior pleural (Bilateral). In non-collapsed lung, the anterior visceral and parietal pleura are intimately apposed, and slide past one another during respiration. Absence of identifiable pleural sliding is indicative of separation of the parietal–visceral pleural interface by interposed gas, ie, pneumothorax. In the supine position, the anterior pleura are examined by placing the probe in a sagittal plane in the rib interspaces between the clavicle and diaphragm. The approximate midclavicular line is used on both sides. It is necessary to adjust frequency, depth, focus and gain settings to optimally image these superficial structures. This exam is discussed in more detail in the "Lung and Pleura" criteria.

iii. Additional windows
   1. Paracolic gutters. These potential spaces are anatomically continuous with the hepatorenal and splenorenal spaces. Windows inferior to the level of kidneys and next to the iliac crests may reveal bowel surrounded by fluid.

iv. Other considerations
   Trendelenburg and sitting position may increase the sensitivity of the ultrasound exam for abnormal fluid in the right upper quadrant and pelvis, respectively. Serial trauma EUS may be performed in response to changes in the patient's condition, to check for the development of previously undetectable volumes of free fluid or for purposes of ongoing monitoring, as indicated clinically.

5. Documentation

In performing trauma EUS exams, images are interpreted by the treating physician as they are acquired and are used to guide contemporaneous clinical decisions. Such interpretations should be documented in the medical record. Documentation should include the indication for the procedure, a description of the organs or structures identified and an interpretation of the findings. Images should be stored as a part of the medical record and done so in accordance with facility policy requirements. Given the often emergent nature of such ultrasound examinations, the timely delivery of care should not be delayed by archiving ultrasound images.

6. Equipment Specifications

Generally, a curvilinear abdominal or phased array cardiac ultrasound probe at frequencies of 2.0-5.0 MHz with a mean of 3.5 MHz will be used for an adult and 5.0 MHz for children and smaller adults. A small footprint may facilitate scanning between the ribs. A depth of field of up to 25 cm may be required in order to adequately visualize deeper structures in the right upper quadrant in large patients. A linear probe or curvilinear probe with frequencies of 7.0 MHz and above would be optimal for visualizing the near field of pleural line. Both portable and cart-based ultrasound machines may be used, depending on the location and setting of the examination.

7. Quality Control and Improvements, Safety, Infection Control and Patient Education

Policies and procedures related to quality, safety, infection control and patient education should be developed in accordance with specialty or organizational guidelines. Specific institutional guidelines may be developed to correspond with such guidelines.

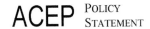

POLICY
STATEMENT

ACEP Emergency Ultrasound Imaging Criteria:
Ultrasound-Guided Procedures

1. Introduction
   The American College of Emergency Physicians (ACEP) has developed these criteria to assist practitioners utilizing emergency ultrasound (EUS) to facilitate the performance of procedures in the emergency patient.

   Ultrasound has been shown to be helpful in determining patency of vascular structures and with the placement of central lines as well as peripheral lines. The Agency for Healthcare Research and Quality highlighted ultrasound-guided central lines as a key intervention that should be implemented immediately into twenty-first century patient care. This focus on patient safety will promote procedural ultrasound as it enables trained operators toward a "one stick" standard. These ultrasound examinations are performed at the bedside to identify vascular anatomy and guide direct visualization and cannulation of vessels.

   Additional procedural applications for ultrasound include assessing for potential abscess formation and to drain fluid collections that accumulate pathologically; confirming fracture reduction and endotracheal tube placement; assessing bladder volume and directing aspiration; guiding nerve blocks and arthrocentesis; and facilitating lumbar puncture or pacemaker placement.

   The advantages of procedural ultrasound include, improved patient safety, decreased procedural attempts, and decreased time to perform many procedures in patients whom the technique would otherwise be difficult. It is important to recognize that procedural ultrasound is a method to identify relevant anatomy and pathology before proceeding with invasive procedures while aiding the accurate execution and minimizing procedural complications. Procedural ultrasound is an adjunct to emergency care.

2. Indications/Limitations
   a. Primary
      i. Vascular access
         1. To identify central venous structures, their relative location and their patency in facilitating placement of central venous catheters.
         2. To identify peripheral venous structures, their relative location and patency in facilitating placement of peripheral venous access.
         3. To identify arterial structures, their relative location and flow characteristics in facilitating placement of arterial lines.

   b. Extended
      i. To evaluate for and/or drain with ultrasound guidance or localization:
         1. soft tissue abscess
         2. peritonsillar abscess
         3. pericardial effusion (pericardiocentesis)
         4. pleural effusion (thoracentesis)
         5. peritoneal fluid (paracentesis)
         6. joint effusion (arthrocentesis)
         7. cerebrospinal fluid (lumbar puncture)
      ii. To evaluate for and localize with ultrasound:
         1. soft tissue foreign bodies
         2. pacemaker placement and capture

         3. fracture reduction
         4. endotracheal tube placement
      iii. Ultrasound-guided nerve blocks

   c. Limitations
      i. Procedural ultrasound is an adjunct to care. No modality is absolutely accurate. Procedural ultrasound should be interpreted and utilized in the context of the entire clinical picture.
      ii. Procedural ultrasound may be technically limited by:
         1. obese habitus
         2. subcutaneous air
         3. anomalous anatomy/prior surgical changes

   d. Pitfalls
      i. Needle localization and its associated artifact must be visualized before proceeding with any procedure. The short axis transverse approach allows only a cross section of the needle to be visualized by the ultrasound beam and may lead to errors in depth perception of the needle. The long axis orientation allows the operator to trace the entire path and angle of the needle from the entry site at the skin and is preferred when this transducer orientation is possible.
      ii. It is important to identify a vessel by multiple means before attempting cannulation. The difference between veins and arteries can be determined by compressibility (veins compress), shape (arteries tend to be circular in transverse view, with muscular walls) and flow dynamics if Doppler is available and/or utilized.
      iii. Many times abnormal structures can be compared to adjacent tissue or to the other normal side. If questions persist about the sonographic appearance of a structure, another imaging modality may be warranted.

3. Qualifications and Responsibilities of the Clinician Performing the Examination
Physicians of a variety of medical specialties may perform procedural ultrasound. Training should be in accordance with specialty or organization specific guidelines.

4. Specifications for Individual Examinations
   a. General – Ultrasound can be used systematically during the pre scan to localize the relevant anatomy in orthogonal planes before executing the procedure in a sterile manner with sterile probe covers and real-time assessment. All invasive procedures should employ standard sterile techniques to diminish the risk of infection. A high frequency ultrasound probe is placed over the anatomy of interest in both sagittal and transverse planes. The probe should be initially placed at the primary window and then be fanned, rocked and rotated to allow for real-time imaging of the area(s) involved. This may take more time with difficult windows, challenging patients or other patient priorities. Interpretation should be done at the bedside immediately with performance of the real-time examination.

   b. Procedural ultrasound techniques- Ultrasound guidance or ultrasound-assisted procedures can be performed using either of two accepted techniques:
      i. Ultrasound Assisted: Anatomic structures are identified and an insertion position is identified with ultrasound. The procedure is carried out without the use of real time ultrasound guidance.
      ii. Real-Time: The ultrasound transducer is placed in a sterile covering and the key components of the procedure are performed with simultaneous ultrasound visualization during the procedure (eg, using ultrasound to visualize a needle entering a vessel)

   c. Procedural ultrasound examinations

     i. Internal jugular vein
    ii. Femoral vein
   iii. Subclavian vein
   iv. External jugular vein
    v. Brachial and cephalic veins
   vi. Arterial cannulation

  d. Additional Procedures
     i. Soft tissue abscess drainage
    ii. Peritonsillar abscess drainage
   iii. Pericardiocentesis
   iv. Pleurocentesis
    v. Paracentesis
   vi. Arthrocentesis
   vii. Lumbar puncture
  viii. Fracture reduction
   ix. Endotracheal tube confirmation
    x. Bladder volume assessment-suprapubic aspiration
   xi. Nerve blocks

5. Documentation
Procedural ultrasound requires documentation of the ultrasound assisted procedure. Documentation should include the indication for the procedure, a description of the organs or structures identified and an interpretation of the findings. Images should be stored as a part of the medical record and in accordance with facility policy requirements. Given the often emergent nature of such ultrasound examinations, the timely delivery of care should not be delayed by archiving ultrasound images.

6. Equipment Specifications
Multiple probes can be used, yet high frequency (7.0-12.0 MHz) linear array transducers work best to image superficial and vascular structures. Microconvex endoluminal probes can be used to identify abscess formation in areas such as the oropharynx. Portable and cart-based ultrasound machines may be used, depending on the location and setting of the examination.

7. Quality Control and Improvements, Safety, Infection Control and Patient Education
Policies and procedures related to quality, safety, infection control and patient education should be developed in accordance with specialty or organizational guidelines. Specific institutional guidelines may be developed to correspond with such guidelines.

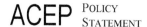

ACEP Emergency Ultrasound Imaging Criteria:
Venous Thrombosis

1. Introduction

   The American College of Emergency Physicians (ACEP) has developed these criteria to assist practitioners performing emergency ultrasound studies (EUS) of the venous system in the evaluation of venous thrombosis.

   The primary application of venous EUS is in evaluation of deep venous thrombosis (DVT) of the proximal lower extremities. Lower extremity venous EUS differs in two fundamental aspects from the "Duplex" evaluation performed in a vascular laboratory. First, its anatomic focus is limited to two specific regions of the proximal deep venous system. Second, its sonographic technique consists primarily of dynamic evaluation of venous compressibility in real time. This approach to lower extremity proximal venous EUS is often referred to as limited compression ultrasonography (LCU). Since B-mode (gray-scale) equipment is widely available, and because substantial scientific evidence supports the use of limited compression ultrasonography, this guideline is focused on the evaluation of proximal lower extremity DVT using this technique. It is recognized that many emergency physicians have access to equipment with color flow and Doppler capabilities, and are experienced in its use. It is likely that they will augment their venous EUS with this technology.

   Lower extremity venous EUS is performed and interpreted in the context of the entire clinical picture. It is a clinically focused examination, which, in conjunction with historical and laboratory information, provides additional data for decision-making. It attempts to answer specific questions about a particular patient's condition. EUS of the lower extremities does not identify all abnormalities or diseases of the deep venous system. If the findings of lower extremity venous EUS exam are equivocal, further imaging or testing may be needed.

2. Indications/Limitations
   a. Primary
      i. Evaluation for acute proximal DVT in the lower extremities.

   b. Extended
      i. Chronic DVT
      ii. Distal DVT
      iii. Superficial venous thrombosis
      iv. Diagnosis of other causes of lower extremity pain and swelling under consideration in the evaluation of DVT such as cellulitis, abscess, muscle hematoma, fasciitis, and Baker's cyst
      v. Upper extremity venous thrombosis

   c. Contraindications
      i. Known, acute proximal DVT. If an ultrasound examination would not have any bearing on clinical decision-making, it should not be performed.
      ii. Other contraindications are relative, based on specific features of the patient's clinical condition.

   d. Limitations
      i. EUS of the lower extremity deep venous system is a single component of the overall and ongoing evaluation. Since it is a focused examination EUS does not identify all abnormalities or diseases of the lower extremity veins. EUS, like other tests, does not replace clinical judgment and should be interpreted in the context of the entire clinical picture. If the findings of the EUS are equivocal, additional diagnostic testing may be indicatedA prior history of

DVT may limit the utility of LCU. The chronic effects of DVT are highly variable in extent, location, timing and morphology. A completely normal venous EUS exam is likely to exclude both acute and chronic DVT. However, the interpretation of abnormal findings in patients with a history of prior DVT may be outside the scope of a lower extremity venous EUS examination.

ii. Examination can be limited by:
1. Obesity
2. Local factors such as tenderness, sores, open wounds, or injuries
3. The patient's ability to cooperate with the exam

e. Pitfalls
i. A non-compressible vein may be mistaken for an artery, leading to a false negative result.
ii. An artery may be mistaken for a non-compressible vein, leading to a false positive result.
iii. Large superficial veins may be mistaken for deep veins. This pitfall is more likely in obese patients and those with occlusive DVT causing distension in the collateral superficial veins. Depending on the compressibility of the vein, this can lead to both false positive and false negative results.
iv. While thrombus may be directly visualized on examination, it is frequently isoechoic to unclotted blood and failure to see echogenic clot should not be used to exclude the diagnosis of DVT. This is especially problematic in obese patients due to the depth of some venous structures and resultant decrease in image clarity.
v. Inguinal lymphadenopathy may be mistaken for a non-compressible common femoral vein.
vi. Failure to arrange for repeat venous evaluation in patients with suspicion for isolated calf or distal DVT.
vii. Failure to consider the possibility of iliac or inferior vena cava obstruction as a cause for lower extremity pain or swelling. While color flow and Doppler techniques may identify the presence of these conditions, they are beyond the usual scope of the EUS exam.
viii. A negative scan for a lower extremity DVT does not rule out the presence of pulmonary embolism.
ix. Not recognizing that the superficial femoral vein is part of the deep venous system. This sometimes confusing terminology has resulted in some authorities referring to the superficial femoral vein as simply the femoral vein.
x. Failing to recognize that a proximal greater saphenous vein thrombus, that is seen approaching the common femoral vein, will readily seed the common femoral vein and poses a significant risk and should be treated like a DVT.

3. Qualifications and Responsibilities of the Clinician Performing the Examination
Limited compression ultrasound of the venous system provides information that is the basis of immediate decisions concerning the patient's evaluation, management, and therapy. Because of its direct bearing on patient care, the rendering of a diagnosis by venous EUS represents the practice of medicine, and therefore is the responsibility of the treating physician.

Due to the potential for life-threatening complications arising from acute DVT, emergent interventions may be mandated by the diagnostic findings of the EUS exam. For this reason, the EUS exam should occur as soon as the clinical decision is made that the patient needs a sonographic evaluation.

Physicians of a variety of medical specialties may perform a lower extremity LCU. Training should be in accordance with specialty or organization specific guidelines. Physicians should render a

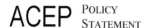

POLICY
STATEMENT

diagnostic interpretation in a time frame consistent with the management of acute DVT, as outlined above.

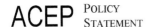

4. Specifications for Individual Examinations

 a. General. Emergency ultrasound for the diagnosis of DVT evaluates for compressibility of the lower extremity deep venous system with specific attention directed towards key sections of the common femoral, femoral, deep femoral and popliteal veins. These sections constitute two short regions of the lower extremity, the inguinal region and popliteal fossa.

 b. Technique

   i. Identification of veins. For the purposes of lower extremity EUS, the proximal deep veins of the lower extremity are those in which thrombus poses a significant risk of pulmonary embolization. These include the common femoral, femoral (formerly superficial femoral vein), and popliteal veins. It is important to note that the superficial femoral vein is part of the deep system, not the superficial system as the name suggests. The deep femoral vein is easily overlooked, but much like the proximal greater saphenous vein it readily seeds thrombus into the common femoral vein. Therefore, it should be assessed for compression as part of the proximal region.

   In the distal leg, the popliteal vein is formed by the confluence of the anterior and posterior tibial veins with the peroneal vein approximately 4-8 cm distal to the popliteal crease. Continuing proximally, the popliteal vein becomes the superficial femoral vein as it passes through the adductor canal approximately 8-12 cm proximal to the popliteal crease. The femoral vein joins the deep femoral vein to form the common femoral vein approximately 5-7 cm below the inguinal ligament. Prior to passing under the inguinal ligament to form the external iliac vein, the common femoral is joined by the great saphenous vein (a superficial vein) merging from the medial thigh. In relation to the companion arteries, the popliteal vein is superficial to the artery. The common femoral vein lies medial to the artery only in the region immediately inferior to the inguinal ligament. The vein abruptly runs posterior to the artery distal to the inguinal region.

   ii. Compression. The sonographic evaluation is performed by compressing the vein directly under the transducer while watching for complete apposition of the anterior and posterior walls. If complete compression is not attained with sufficient pressure to cause arterial deformation, obstructing thrombus is likely to be present.

   iii. Patient positioning. To facilitate the identification of the veins and test for compression, they need to be distended. This is accomplished by placing the lower extremities in a position of dependency preferably by placing the patient on a flat stretcher in reverse Trendelenberg. If the patient is on a gurney where this is not possible, the patient should be placed semi-sitting with 30 degrees of hip flexion.

   iv. Transducer. A linear array vascular probe with a frequency of 6 – 10 MHz and width of approximately 50 mm is often ideal. Narrower transducers may make it harder to localize the veins and to apply uniform compression. For larger patients, a lower frequency or even an abdominal probe will facilitate greater tissue penetration.

   v. Real-time scanning technique.

     1. The common femoral vein, saphenous vein inflow, deep femoral and femoral vein region. Gel is applied to the groin and medial thigh for a distance about 10 centimeters distal to the inguinal crease. Filling of the common femoral vein might be augmented by placing a small bolster under the knee resulting in slight (about 10 degrees) hip flexion. Mild external rotation of the hip (30 degrees) may also be helpful. The vein and artery may have almost any relationship with one another, although the vein is frequently seen

posterior to the artery. Distinction of the two vessels may therefore depend on size (the vein is usually larger), shape (the vein is more ovoid) and compressibility. If color-flow or Doppler is utilized characteristic arterial or venous signals can help with differentiation.

Compressive evaluation of the vessel commences at the highest view obtainable at the inguinal ligament. Angling superiorly, a short section of the distal common iliac vein might be scanned. Systematic scanning commences at the level of the inflow of the greater saphenous vein into the common femoral vein, applying compression every centimeter. Compression should be continued through the bifurcation of the common femoral vein into its femoral and deep femoral veins and approximately 2 cm beyond, since branch points are particularly susceptible to thrombosis. If difficulty is encountered in following the common femoral vein to the bifurcation, or in clearly identifying the two branching vessels, techniques to optimize the angle of interrogation should be used. In equivocal cases, comparison with the contralateral side may be helpful.

2. The popliteal vein. The patient can be placed in either a prone or decubitus position. In the latter case, the knee is flexed 10 – 30 degrees, and the side of the leg being examined should be down. If the patient is prone, placing a bolster under the ankle to flex the knee to about 15 degrees facilitates filling of the popliteal vein. Again, reverse Trendelenberg positioning promotes venous filling. Gel is applied from about 12 centimeters superior, to 5 centimeters inferior to the popliteal crease. The vein usually lies superficial to the artery. Both vessels lie superficial to the bony structures, which can be used as landmarks to anticipate the depth of the vessels. If difficulty is encountered in identifying the terminal branches of the popliteal vein, it is possible that the patient has one of the common variants of venous anatomy. In the absence of clear anatomic identification of the termination of the popliteal vein, the major venous structures should be imaged to approximately 7 centimeters below the popliteal crease. In equivocal cases, comparison with the contralateral side may be helpful. The popliteal vein should be compressed just into the proximal distal branches to catch any calf thrombus about to seed the popliteal vein.

vi. Additional components of the exam.
1. The femoral vein. As noted previously, this vein is not a primary focus of the standard lower extremity EUS evaluation, other than its proximal portion. In cases where there is a high suspicion of DVT and an otherwise normal exam of the common femoral and popliteal veins, the femoral vein may also be evaluated more extensively.
2. Color flow and Doppler. Color flow and Doppler assessment may be used to localize the vessels, although the use of this technology is beyond the scope of the standard EUS exam. Additionally, data suggest color and power Doppler adds little in ruling out DVT.

vii. Gray scale identification of clot. While thrombus may be hyperechoic, and thus directly visualized on exam, it is also frequently isoechoic to unclotted blood. Consequently, failure to see echogenic clot should not be used to exclude the diagnosis of DVT.

5. Documentation
In performing venous EUS, images are interpreted by the treating physician as they are acquired and are used to guide contemporaneous clinical decisions. Image documentation should be incorporated into the medical record. Documentation should include the indication for the procedure, the views obtained, a description of the structures identified and an interpretation of the findings. Limitations of the exam, and impediments to performing a complete exam should be noted. The written report of the

ACEP POLICY STATEMENT

venous EUS should document the presence of complete, partial or absent collapse in each vein examined. Images should be stored as a part of the medical record and done so in accordance with facility policy requirements. Since the LCU exam is a dynamic test, repeated multiple times over the lengths of the common femoral vein and popliteal vein, it is not practical in the emergency setting to obtain a still image record of each site evaluated with and without compression. If still image records are obtained for documentation, one or more representative images of each vein, reflecting the key findings with and without compression, should be recorded.

6. Equipment Specifications

A linear array vascular probe with a frequency of 6.0 – 10.0 MHz and width of 6 – 8 cm is often ideal. Narrower transducers may make it harder to localize the veins and to apply uniform compression. For larger patients, a lower frequency or even an abdominal probe will facilitate greater tissue penetration. Color or power Doppler capabilities may be of assistance in localizing venous structures. Both portable and cart-based ultrasound machines may be used, depending on the location and setting of the examination.

7. Quality Control and Improvements, Safety, Infection Control and Patient Education

Policies and procedures related to quality, safety, infection control and patient education should be developed in accordance with specialty or organizational guidelines. Specific institutional guidelines may be developed to correspond with such guidelines.

ACEP Emergency Ultrasound Fellowship Guidelines 2011

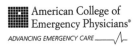

American College of
Emergency Physicians®
ADVANCING EMERGENCY CARE ____/___

Emergency Ultrasound Fellowship Guidelines
an Information Paper

A Consensus Document Developed by the
ACEP Emergency Ultrasound Section

July 2011

© Springer International Publishing AG 2018   551
V. S. Tayal et al. (eds.), *Ultrasound Program Management*,
https://doi.org/10.1007/978-3-319-63143-1

Emergency Ultrasound Fellowship Guidelines
Information Paper

Index

I.   Introduction:

The American College of Emergency Physicians (ACEP), Emergency Ultrasound Section has been the primary organization representing emergency physicians who perform ultrasound in their practice. Since 1996, ACEP's Ultrasound Section has established policies and guidelines that have become a voice for the specialty.

The Emergency Ultrasound Fellowship Guidelines are a consensus document that will serve to assist departments and individuals who seek training in programs that offer innovative post-residency training in emergency ultrasound. As the numbers of emergency ultrasound fellowships proliferate, we believe these guidelines will serve to assist potential fellows, fellowship directors, and emergency physicians who seek the expertise of such graduates. A large number of emergency ultrasound fellowships now operating follow different curricula, use different teaching methods, and have fellowship directors with varying training backgrounds. The Emergency Ultrasound Fellowship Guidelines submitted are an attempt to assure quality education in emergency ultrasound fellowships. The outline includes minimum equipment, resources, support required, and minimum types of ultrasound applications that must be taught in order to have an emergency ultrasound fellowship. This revision reflects the growth of the subspecialty and the ever increasing number of ultrasound applications performed in the emergency department.

These guidelines are not a substitute for, nor are intended to replace any hospital medical staff application and/or privileging process. The Emergency Ultrasound Fellowship Guidelines are not policy or mandates from any legislative, judicial, or regulatory body, or ACEP.

II.   Site Qualification Requirements:

1. The ultrasound machine(s) utilized for fellowship training must be owned or controlled by the emergency department (ED) and must be available on a 24 hour/7 days per week basis.

2. The ultrasound machine utilized by the fellow must be able to perform endovaginal ultrasound, linear ultrasound, and cardiac and abdominal ultrasound applications with high quality. At least three ultrasound transducers (probe) types must be available at all times: linear, endovaginal/endocavity

and either curved linear for abdomen and separate one (microconvex or phased array) for cardiac or microconvex that can be used for both abdominal and cardiac.

3. Hospital credentialing must be available and formal diagnostic reports that appear as part of the patient medical record must be issued by the emergency physicians in the department.

4. At least one other emergency medicine faculty aside from the fellowship director must be hospital credentialed for emergency ultrasound at the primary facility for all of the applications listed.

5. Quality assurance (QA) review of all ultrasound examinations performed by the emergency ultrasound fellow(s) must be documented.

6. A quality assurance log of all ultrasound examinations performed in the ED should be maintained by the ultrasound director for the ED.

7. The type of emergency ultrasound examinations taught and performed at the primary fellowship site should at a minimum be consistent with the most current ACEP Emergency Ultrasound Guidelines http://www.acep.org/WorkArea/DownloadAsset.aspx?id=32878. The program, ideally would model its content after any consensus curriculum set forth by ACEP and the Society for Academic Emergency Medicine (SAEM).

8. All teaching for emergency ultrasound applications must be available from the fellowship director or other faculty members with credentials in emergency ultrasound and designated by the fellowship director. All aspects of emergency ultrasound education should take place under the auspices of the emergency ultrasound fellowship faculty. It is understood that supplemental education outside the department may take place especially for advanced or novel applications, however, this time should be minimal and only supplemental to the basis of the fellowship

9. The emergency ultrasound fellow should not work more than 20 clinical hours per week (seeing patients in the ED/urgent care/fast track/triage, etc. as the attending or other), the remainder of the time should be academic/research hours.

10. The emergency ultrasound fellow should be a full time equivalent employee of the group or ED where he or she is enrolled in the fellowship. The fellowship should be at least 12 consecutive months.

11. Video (dynamic media) quality assurance is considered ideal for all ultrasound examinations utilized for teaching of fellow(s). It is understood that this form of QA is not possible for all departments and still image quality assurance is an acceptable alternative.

12. Emergency ultrasound fellows should have at least five scanning (on average) shift equivalents per month. A scanning shift is a shift that a fellow is not working clinically and spends the majority of the scanning shift scanning patients in the ED directly with the fellowship director or other credentialed faculty member intimately involved in the education of ultrasound within the department. The fellowship director or said designee must be present for a majority of scans during that shift in order to give appropriate hands on training to the ultrasound fellow. This close supervision is integral to the fellows' education early in the fellowship year and this time should be reduced as the director feels that such intense supervision becomes low yield for the fellow. As the fellowship progresses, scanning shifts may be substituted for scanning shift equivalents that might include research, administrative or teaching activities at the discretion and under the mentorship of the fellowship director or faculty designee.

13. A formal evaluative feedback process should exist, and the fellowship director and fellow should meet at least three times during the year. This evaluation should be both of the fellow by the fellowship director, and of the fellowship by the fellow.

2

III. Minimum Criteria to be a Fellowship Director:

1. If not fellowship trained, the director should have at least three years of ultrasound use in clinical practice after residency training.

2. A fellowship-trained person should not direct a fellowship for one year following completion of their fellowship. A fellowship-trained physician should not start a new program from the ground up for at least two years post fellowship.

3. Publish at least three peer reviewed emergency ultrasound articles in Medline indexed journals.

4. At least two of the above mentioned publications must be original ultrasound research with the emergency ultrasound director as first author on one of them.

5. The third ultrasound publication can be a review article for a Medline indexed journal.

6. The emergency ultrasound fellowship director must utilize all of the clinical ultrasound applications listed in the most recent ACEP Emergency Ultrasound Guidelines http://www.acep.org/WorkArea/DownloadAsset.aspx?id=32878 and have experience in more advanced applications.

7. The emergency ultrasound fellowship director must have at least four regional and national abstract research presentations at meetings conducted by organizations such as ACEP, SAEM, American Institute of Ultrasound in Medicine (AIUM) or similar meetings over a three-year period, or must be intimately involved in advancing emergency ultrasound by actively participating or leading one of the previously mentioned nationally recognized organizations in regard to emergency ultrasound.

8. The fellowship director should have a record of excellence in teaching. This ability can be demonstrated by teaching awards, consistently favorable evaluations by residents and/or fellows, or the like.

9. The criteria to be a fellowship director are intended to be used for emergency ultrasound fellowship guidelines only, and are not intended to be standards for teaching residents. These criteria should not affect resident teaching programs.

IV. Fellowship Minimum Criteria for Graduation:

1. A minimum of 1000 ultrasound examinations must be performed by the emergency ultrasound fellow per year by him or herself. Quality assurance review of other's ultrasound examinations or observing actual ultrasound examinations performed by others will not count toward this number. T This number serves more as a minimum guide as it is understood that with more hands-on experience one becomes more proficient. It is preferable however to utilize an objective tool to assure competence in all aspects of emergency ultrasound upon completion of the fellowship program. Supplemental written and practical exams might be considered.

2. The emergency ultrasound fellow should design at least one research project to be submitted to the home site institutional review board and start on it during the course of the fellowship.

3. At least one abstract should be submitted with the fellow's name as first author and presenter to a national meeting such as ACEP, SAEM, or AIUM during their fellowship.

4. The emergency ultrasound fellow should be involved with at least one other ultrasound research project (does not have to be one he/she designed and implemented from the ground up) during their fellowship for which publication is planned with the fellow as an author.

3

5. The emergency ultrasound fellow must be involved with the various admistrative and quality assurance duties involving emergency ultrasound. Such duties include but are not limited to internal billing audits, interdepartmental meetings, and monitoring the credentialing process of colleagues.

6. The emergency ultrasound fellow must prepare and deliver lectures on at least four separate topics on the basic emergency ultrasound applications to their department (residents and faculty). The emergency ultrasound fellow should be encouraged to prepare and deliver at least one lecture on an advanced or novel application.

7. The emergency ultrasound fellow must show at least 20 hours per month of hands-on teaching of residents and/or other faculty in bedside emergency ultrasound. This includes but is not limited to didactic lectures, bedside teaching, research involvement of residents or faculty, and QA education.

8. The emergency ultrasound fellow must attend one national emergency ultrasound organization meeting during the year.

Suggested Reporting Guidelines 2011

Emergency Ultrasound Standard Reporting Guidelines

October 2011

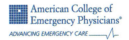

American College of
Emergency Physicians®
ADVANCING EMERGENCY CARE

© Springer International Publishing AG 2018   557
V. S. Tayal et al. (eds.), *Ultrasound Program Management*,
https://doi.org/10.1007/978-3-319-63143-1

Emergency Ultrasound Standard Reporting Guidelines: Introduction and Statement of Purpose
Developed by members of the ACEP Emergency Ultrasound Section

These guidelines represent the product of a working group that was formed based on discussions at the Industry Roundtable subcommittee of the American College of Emergency Physicians (ACEP) Ultrasound Section. The impetus for these guidelines emerged from discussions with emergency ultrasound leaders and industry, both ultrasound manufacturers and electronic medical record (EMR) companies that indicated a need for a more structured method to report and communicate the findings of point-of-care (POC) emergency ultrasound (EUS).

This document serves as a resource to clinicians with a wide range of experience, and as such may contain fields or terms that may not be appropriate in all situations or by all clinicians. It is important to note that these guidelines **in no way represent required elements of reporting**. In fact, in general these guidelines err on the side of including more fields than may be used by most emergency physicians, and it is expected that many fields may remain unused depending on the situations. The elements that are **BOLDED** represent the core emergency ACEP views, findings and interpretations for each application.

The purpose of these guidelines is to define fields that may be helpful for POC EUS in a consistent order, with consistent definitions, and in a method that may be easily coded into electronic communications and computer databases. The goal of this document is to accurately report the findings that commonly result from an ultrasound performed by a clinician in the emergency department and to avoid confusion with reports generated by other specialties.

We hope to eventually use these guidelines to work with existing reporting structures such as DICOM and initiatives through the Integrated Health Enterprise (IHE) to develop consistent non-proprietary methods of reporting and communicating POC EUS examination findings.

Exams included in this draft:
- FAST
- Focused Abdominal Aorta
- Focused Pelvic Ultrasound
  - Obstetrical
  - Non-obstetrical
- Focused Biliary
- Focused Renal/ Urinary Tract
- Focused Thoracic
- Focused Lower Extremity Venous
- Focused Cardiac (Echo)
- Focused Soft Tissue/MSK
- Focused Ocular

In development:
Ultrasound guided procedures
Testicular
Symptom based (hypotension, dyspnea, abdominal pain, chest pain)

FORMAT

All diagnostic examinations should include:
- Patient/exam demographics
- Indications for examination
- Views
- Findings
- Interpretation
- Quality assurance

The first and last portions should be consistent across exam types and are presented here.

Patient/ exam demographics:

Patient name: _____
Patient gender: ☐ M ☐ F
DOB: ___ / ___ / ___
MR#: _____
Bar Code/Patient Identifier:_____
Hospital Name:_____
Date and time of exam: ___ / ___ / ___
Exam type:
      ☐ Diagnostic
      ☐ Educational
      ☐ Procedural
Clinical category:
      ☐ Resuscitative
      ☐ Symptom based
      ☐ Therapeutic
      ☐ Unknown/other
☐ Initial exam
☐ Repeat exam
Primary person obtaining/ interpreting images: _____
Secondary person obtaining/ interpreting images: _____
Additional person(s) obtaining/ interpreting images: _____

Quality assurance:

Suggested Quality Assurance Grading Scale

	1	2	3	4	5
Grading Scale Definitions	No recognizable structures, no objective data can be gathered	Minimally recognizable structures but insufficient for diagnosis	Minimal criteria met for diagnosis, recognizable structures but with some technical or other flaws	Minimal criteria met for diagnosis, all structures imaged well and diagnosis easily supported	Minimal criteria met for diagnosis, all structures imaged with excellent image quality and diagnosis completely supported

Image quality   1   2   3   4   5
Accuracy of interpretation of images as presented   TP   TN   FP   FN
Accuracy of interpretation of images as compared to
gold standard (ie, CT, operative report)   TP   TN   FP   FN

       Comments: _____

FAST EXAM

The elements that are **BOLDED** *represent the core emergency ACEP views, findings and interpretations for each application.*

Patient/ exam demographics:

Patient name: _____
Patient gender: ☐ M ☐ F
DOB: ___ / ___ / ___
MR#: _____
Bar Code/Patient Identifier:_____
Hospital Name:_____
Date and time of exam: ___ / ___ / ___
Exam type:
      ☐ Diagnostic
      ☐ Educational
      ☐ Procedural

Clinical category:
      ☐ Resuscitative
      ☐ Symptom based
      ☐ Therapeutic
      ☐ Unknown/ other
☐ Initial exam
☐ Repeat exam

Primary person obtaining/ interpreting images: _____
Secondary person obtaining/ interpreting images: _____
Additional person(s) obtaining/ interpreting images: _____

Indication(s) for exam:

☐ blunt trauma	☐ tachycardia
☐ penetrating trauma	☐ dyspnea
☐ abdominal pain	☐ altered mental status
☐ chest pain	☐ pregnancy
☐ hypotension	☐ educational
☐ other: _____	

Views:

Hepatorenal	☐ **adequate**	☐ **limited**	☐ **not obtained**
Perisplenic	☐ **adequate**	☐ **limited**	☐ **not obtained**
Suprapubic	☐ **adequate**	☐ **limited**	☐ **not obtained**
Pericardial	☐ **adequate**	☐ **limited**	☐ **not obtained**
R thorax for fluid	☐ **adequate**	☐ **limited**	☐ **not obtained**
R thorax for lung sliding	☐ **adequate**	☐ **limited**	☐ **not obtained**
L thorax for fluid	☐ **adequate**	☐ **limited**	☐ **not obtained**
L thorax for lung sliding	☐ **adequate**	☐ **limited**	☐ **not obtained**
	☐ other: _____		

Findings:

Hepatorenal free fluid:	☐ **absent**	☐ **present**	☐ **indeterminate**
Perisplenic free fluid:	☐ **absent**	☐ **present**	☐ **indeterminate**
Suprapubic free fluid:	☐ **absent**	☐ **present**	☐ **indeterminate**
Right thoracic fluid:	☐ **present**	☐ **absent**	☐ **indeterminate**
Right lung sliding	☐ **present**	☐ **absent**	☐ **indeterminate**

lung point sign	❏ **yes**	❏ **no**	
Left thoracic fluid:	❏ **present**	❏ **absent**	❏ **indeterminate**
Left lung sliding:	❏ **present**	❏ **absent**	❏ **indeterminate**
lung point sign	❏ **yes**	❏ **no**	
Pericardial effusion:	❏ **present**	❏ **absent**	❏ **indeterminate**
size if present ❏ **small**	❏ **moderate**	❏ **large**	
	❏ **present size not specified**		
❏ other: _____			

Interpretation:

Peritoneal free fluid:	❏ **present**	❏ **absent**	❏ **indeterminate**
Pericardial effusion:	❏ **present**	❏ **absent**	❏ **indeterminate**
Right thoracic fluid:	❏ **present**	❏ **absent**	❏ **indeterminate**
Left thoracic fluid:	❏ **present**	❏ **absent**	❏ **indeterminate**
Right lung pneumothorax:	❏ **present**	❏ **absent**	❏ **indeterminate**
Left lung pneumothorax:	❏ **present**	❏ **absent**	❏ **indeterminate**
	❏ **other:** _____		

Quality assurance:

Suggested Quality Assurance Grading Scale

	1	2	3	4	5
Grading Scale Definitions	No recognizable structures, no objective data can be gathered	Minimally recognizable structures but insufficient for diagnosis	Minimal criteria met for diagnosis, recognizable structures but with some technical or other flaws	Minimal criteria met for diagnosis, all structures imaged well and diagnosis easily supported	Minimal criteria met for diagnosis, all structures imaged with excellent image quality and diagnosis completely supported

Image quality   1   2   3   4   5

Accuracy of interpretation of images as presented   TP   TN   FP   FN

Accuracy of interpretation of images as compared to gold standard (ie, CT, operative report)   TP   TN   FP   FN

Comments: _____

FOCUSED ABDOMINAL AORTA

The elements that are **BOLDED** *represent the core emergency ACEP views, findings and interpretations for each application.*

Patient/ exam demographics:

Patient name: _____
Patient gender: ☐ M ☐ F
DOB: ___ / ___ / ___
MR#: _____
Bar Code/Patient Identifier: _____
Hospital Name: _____
Date and time of exam: ___ / ___ / ___
Exam type:
    ☐ Diagnostic
    ☐ Educational
    ☐ Procedural

Clinical category:
    ☐ Resuscitative
    ☐ Symptom based
    ☐ Therapeutic
    ☐ Unknown/ other
☐ Initial exam
☐ Repeat exam

Primary person obtaining/ interpreting images: _____
Secondary person obtaining/ interpreting images: _____
Additional person(s) obtaining/ interpreting images: _____

Indication(s) for exam:

☐ abdominal pain   ☐ syncope
☐ chest pain   ☐ hypotension
☐ back pain   ☐ tachycardia
☐ flank pain   ☐ educational
☐ pulsatile abdominal mass
☐ other: _____

Views:

Proximal Transverse view:	☐ **complete**	☐ **inadequate**
Distal Transverse view	☐ **complete**	☐ **inadequate**
Sagittal view:	☐ **complete**	☐ **inadequate**
Celiac artery:	☐ visualized	☐ not visualized
Bifurcation:	☐ **visualized**	☐ **not visualized**

Findings:

Aneurysm: ☐ **present**   ☐ **absent**   ☐ **indeterminate**
    If present: ☐ suprarenal   ☐ infrarenal   ☐ both   ☐ iliac
Maximal aortic diameter: ____cm
☐ other: _____

Interpretation:

Sonographic Evidence for Aneurysm: ☐ **present**   ☐ **absent**   ☐ **indeterminate**
    If present: ____ **cm transverse diameter**
☐ other: _____

Quality assurance:

Suggested Quality Assurance Grading Scale

	1	2	3	4	5
Grading Scale Definitions	No recognizable structures, no objective data can be gathered	Minimally recognizable structures but insufficient for diagnosis	Minimal criteria met for diagnosis, recognizable structures but with some technical or other flaws	Minimal criteria met for diagnosis, all structures imaged well and diagnosis easily supported	Minimal criteria met for diagnosis, all structures imaged with excellent image quality and diagnosis completely supported

Image quality   1   2   3   4   5
Accuracy of interpretation of images as presented   TP   TN   FP   FN
Accuracy of interpretation of images as compared to
gold standard (ie, CT, operative report)   TP   TN   FP   FN

Comments: _____

FOCUSED OBSTETRICAL PELVIC ULTRASOUND

The elements that are **BOLDED** *represent the core emergency ACEP views, findings and interpretations for each application.*

Patient/ exam demographics:

Patient name: _____
Patient gender: ☐ M ☐ F
DOB: ___ / ___ / ___
MR#: _____
Bar Code/Patient Identifier:_____
Hospital Name:_____
Date and time of exam: ___ / ___ / ___
Exam type:
    ☐ Diagnostic
    ☐ Educational
    ☐ Procedural

Clinical category:
    ☐ Resuscitative
    ☐ Symptom based
    ☐ Therapeutic
    ☐ Unknown/ other
☐ Initial exam
☐ Repeat exam

Primary person obtaining/ interpreting images: _____
Secondary person obtaining/ interpreting images: _____
Additional person(s) obtaining/ interpreting images: _____

Indication(s) for exam:

☐ qualitative (urine) hCG positive   ☐ back pain
☐ quantitative hCG positive   ☐ vaginal bleeding
    Level: _____
☐ pregnant by patient history   ☐ syncope
☐ abdominal pain   ☐ hypotension
☐ pelvic pain   ☐ trauma
☐ other: _____   ☐ educational

Views obtained:

Transabdominal sagittal	☐ **adequate**	☐ **limited**	☐ **not obtained**
Transabdominal transverse	☐ **adequate**	☐ **limited**	☐ **not obtained**
Endovaginal sagittal	☐ **adequate**	☐ **limited**	☐ **not obtained**
Endovaginal coronal	☐ **adequate**	☐ **limited**	☐ **not obtained**
Cul-de-sac	☐ adequate	☐ limited	☐ not obtained
Left adnexa	☐ adequate	☐ limited	☐ not obtained
Right adnexa	☐ adequate	☐ limited	☐ not obtained
Hepatorenal space	☐ adequate	☐ limited	☐ not obtained

☐ other: _____

Findings:

Uterus: ☐ anteverted   ☐ retroverted   ☐ indeterminate
Cul-de-sac   ☐ fluid present   ☐ no significant fluid   ☐ indeterminate
    If fluid present: ☐ small   ☐ moderate   ☐ large
    ☐ amount not specified

Intrauterine Pregnancy: ❏ **present**   ❏ **absent**   ❏ **indeterminate**
          If present: ❏ **Yolk sac**
                          Yolk sac diameter: ____mm
                ❏ **Fetal pole**
                          Measurement: ____mm
                ❏ **Fetal heart**
                          FHR: ____bpm
                ❏ **Fetal motion**
                ☐ Double decidual sign
                ☐ Gestational sac
                          Diameter: ____mm

    For IUP:
        Location: ☐ fundus   ☐ eccentric   ☐ indeterminate
        Myometrial mantle: ☐ adequate   ☐ inadequate   ☐ indeterminate
           Minimal thickness: _____mm
        Crown-rump-length: _____mm
        Biparietal diameter: _____mm
            Gestational age: ___w ___d
☐ other: _____

    For No IUP
        Intrauterine contents: ☐ indeterminate
                         ☐ empty/endometrial stripe
                         ☐ non-specific endometrial fluid collection
                         ☐ heterogenous endometrial material
                         ☐ molar pregnancy
☐ other: _____

        R adnexa: ☐ no significant abnormality
                         ☐ ovarian cyst
                              ☐Diameter:____mm
                              ☐Simple   ☐complex
                         ☐ ovarian mass
                         ☐ indeterminate
☐ other: _____

        L adnexa: ☐ no significant abnormality
                         ☐ ovarian cyst
                              ☐Diameter:____mm
                              ☐Simple   ☐complex
                         ☐ ovarian mass
                         ☐ indeterminate
☐ other: _____

        Hepatorenal space fluid: ☐ absent   ☐ present   ☐ indeterminate
☐ other: _____

<u>Interpretation:</u>
             ❏ **no definitive intrauterine pregnancy**
             ❏ **intrauterine pregnancy**
             ❏ **live intrauterine pregnancy**
             ❏ **indeterminate**
             ☐ abnormal intrauterine pregnancy
             ❏ **molar pregnancy**
             ☐ fetal demise

☐ definite ectopic
☐ simple ovarian cyst
☐ complex ovarian cyst
☐ adnexal mass
☐ free pelvic fluid
☐ free intraperitoneal fluid
☐ other: _____

Quality assurance:

Suggested Quality Assurance Grading Scale

	1	2	3	4	5
Grading Scale Definitions	No recognizable structures, no objective data can be gathered	Minimally recognizable structures but insufficient for diagnosis	Minimal criteria met for diagnosis, recognizable structures but with some technical or other flaws	Minimal criteria met for diagnosis, all structures imaged well and diagnosis easily supported	Minimal criteria met for diagnosis, all structures imaged with excellent image quality and diagnosis completely supported

Image quality   1   2   3   4   5
Accuracy of interpretation of images as presented   TP   TN   FP   FN
Accuracy of interpretation of images as compared to
gold standard (ie, CT, operative report)   TP   TN   FP   FN

Comments: _____

.

FOCUSED Non-Obstetric PELVIC ULTRASOUND

Patient/ exam demographics:

Patient name: _____

Patient gender: ☐ M ☐ F

DOB: ___ / ___ / ___

MR#: _____

Bar Code/Patient Identifier:_____

Hospital Name:_____

Date and time of exam: ___ / ___ / ___

Exam type:
- ☐ Diagnostic
- ☐ Educational
- ☐ Procedural

Clinical category:
- ☐ Resuscitative
- ☐ Symptom based
- ☐ Therapeutic
- ☐ Unknown/ other

☐ Initial exam

☐ Repeat exam

Primary person obtaining/ interpreting images: _____

Secondary person obtaining/ interpreting images: _____

Additional person(s) obtaining/ interpreting images: _____

Indication(s) for exam:

☐ qualitative (urine) hCG negative	☐ vaginal bleeding
☐ quantitative hCG negative	☐ syncope
☐ abdominal pain	☐ hypotension
☐ pelvic pain	☐ trauma
☐ back pain	☐ educational
☐ other: _____	

Views obtained:

Transabdominal sagittal	☐ adequate	☐ limited	☐ not obtained
Transabdominal transverse	☐ adequate	☐ limited	☐ not obtained
Endovaginal sagittal	☐ adequate	☐ limited	☐ not obtained
Endovaginal coronal	☐ adequate	☐ limited	☐ not obtained
Cul-de-sac	☐ adequate	☐ limited	☐ not obtained
Left adnexa	☐ adequate	☐ limited	☐ not obtained
Right adnexa	☐ adequate	☐ limited	☐ not obtained
Hepatorenal space	☐ adequate	☐ limited	☐ not obtained
	☐ other: _____		

Findings:

Uterus: ☐ anteverted   ☐ retroverted   ☐ indeterminate

Endometrium: ☐ empty endometrial stripe

Endometrial stripe max thickness: ____mm

☐ heterogenous material in endometrium

☐ uterine fibroid present

Measurement: ____mm

Cul-de-sac: ☐ fluid present☐ no significant fluid ☐ indeterminate
  If fluid present: ☐ small ☐ moderate ☐ large
           ☐ amount not specified
           ☐ simple ☐ complex
  R adnexa:
    ovarian size: ☐ normal ☐ enlarged ☐ indeterminate
          length: ____mm width: ____mm height: ____mm
          volume: ____ ml
          ☐ ovarian cyst
            ☐Diameter:____mm
            ☐Simple   ☐complex
    Color flow: ☐ present ☐absent ☐ indeterminate ☐ not obtained
    Spectral flow: ☐ present ☐absent ☐ indeterminate ☐ not obtained
          Resistive index: ____
          ☐ ovarian mass
          ☐ indeterminate
 L adnexa:
    ovarian size: ☐ normal ☐ enlarged ☐ indeterminate
          length: ____mm width: ____mm height: ____mm
          volume: ____ ml
          ☐ ovarian cyst
            ☐Diameter:____mm
            ☐Simple   ☐complex
    Color flow: ☐ present ☐absent ☐ indeterminate ☐ not obtained
    Spectral flow: ☐ present ☐absent ☐ indeterminate ☐ not obtained
          Resistive index: ____
          ☐ ovarian mass
          ☐ indeterminate
☐ other: _____

Interpretation:
  ☐ No sonographic evidence of gynecological pathology.
  ☐ ovarian cyst: ☐simple ☐complex
  ☐ sonographic evidence suggestive of ovarian torsion
  ☐ adnexal mass
  ☐ fibroid(s)
  ☐ sonographic evidence of abnormal free fluid in the pelvis
☐ other: _____

Quality assurance:

Suggested Quality Assurance Grading Scale

	1	2	3	4	5
Grading Scale Definitions	No recognizable structures, no objective data can be gathered	Minimally recognizable structures but insufficient for diagnosis	Minimal criteria met for diagnosis, recognizable structures but with some technical or other flaws	Minimal criteria met for diagnosis, all structures imaged well and diagnosis easily supported	Minimal criteria met for diagnosis, all structures imaged with excellent image quality and diagnosis completely supported

Image quality	1	2	3	4	5				
Accuracy of interpretation of images as presented						TP	TN	FP	FN
Accuracy of interpretation of images as compared to gold standard (ie, CT, operative report)						TP	TN	FP	FN

Comments: _____

FOCUSED BILIARY

The elements that are **BOLDED** *represent the core emergency ACEP views, findings and interpretations for each application.*

Patient/ exam demographics:

Patient name: _____
Patient gender: ☐ M ☐ F
DOB: ___ / ___ / ___
MR#: _____
Bar Code/Patient Identifier:_____
Hospital Name:_____
Date and time of exam: ___ / ___ / ___
Exam type:
       ☐ Diagnostic
       ☐ Educational
       ☐ Procedural

Clinical category:
       ☐ Resuscitative
       ☐ Symptom based
       ☐ Therapeutic
       ☐ Unknown/ other
☐ Initial exam
☐ Repeat exam

Primary person obtaining/ interpreting images: _____
Secondary person obtaining/ interpreting images: _____
Additional person(s) obtaining/ interpreting images: _____

Indication(s) for exam:

       ☐ abnormal labs   ☐ pancreatitis
       ☐ abdominal pain   ☐ fever
       ☐ jaundice   ☐ educational
       ☐ other: _____

Views obtained:

Gallbladder long axis:	**☐ adequate**	**☐ limited**	**☐ not obtained**
Gallbladder short axis:	**☐ adequate**	**☐ limited**	**☐ not obtained**
Common bile duct:	☐ adequate	☐ limited	☐ not obtained
Main lobar fissure:	☐visualized	☐not visualized	
Portal vein:	☐visualized	☐not visualized	

Findings:

Gallstone(s):	**☐ present**	**☐ absent**	**☐ indeterminate**
If stones present:	☐ single		
	☐ multiple		
	☐ largest measured: ____mm		
	☐ mobile		
	☐ non-mobile		
	☐ in fundus		
	☐ in body		
	☐ in neck		
Gallbladder wall:	☐ thickened	☐ not thickened	☐ indeterminate
	Wall thickness:_____mm		

Pericholecystic fluid:	□ present	□ absent	□ indeterminate
Sonographic Murphy's sign:	**□ present**	**□ absent**	**□ indeterminate**
Common Bile Duct:	□ normal	□ enlarged	□ indeterminate

Largest Diameter:_____mm

Biliary Sludge:	□ present	□ absent	□ indeterminate
Polyp:	□ present	□ absent	□ indeterminate
Adenomyomatosis	□ present	□ absent	□ indeterminate

Transverse gallbladder diameter: _____mm

Longitudinal gallbladder diameter: _____mm

□ other: _____

Interpretation:

□ **No significant biliary pathology identified**

□ **Cholelithiasis without sonographic evidence of cholecystitis**

□ **Cholelithiasis with sonographic evidence of cholecystitis**

□ Sonographic evidence of acalculous cholecystitis

□ Choledocholithiasis

□ Polyps

□ other: _____

Quality assurance:

Suggested Quality Assurance Grading Scale

	1	2	3	4	5
Grading Scale Definitions	No recognizable structures, no objective data can be gathered	Minimally recognizable structures but insufficient for diagnosis	Minimal criteria met for diagnosis, recognizable structures but with some technical or other flaws	Minimal criteria met for diagnosis, all structures imaged well and diagnosis easily supported	Minimal criteria met for diagnosis, all structures imaged with excellent image quality and diagnosis completely supported

Image quality   1   2   3   4   5

Accuracy of interpretation of images as presented   TP   TN   FP   FN

Accuracy of interpretation of images as compared to
gold standard (ie, CT, operative report)   TP   TN   FP   FN

Comments: _____

FOCUSED RENAL/URINARY TRACT

The elements that are **BOLDED** *represent the core emergency ACEP views, findings and interpretations for each application.*

Patient/ exam demographics:

Patient name: _____
Patient gender: ☐ M ☐ F
DOB: ___ / ___ / ___
MR#: _____
Bar Code/Patient Identifier:_____
Hospital Name:_____
Date and time of exam: ___ / ___ / ___
Exam type:
    ☐ Diagnostic
    ☐ Educational
    ☐ Procedural

Clinical category:
    ☐ Resuscitative
    ☐ Symptom based
    ☐ Therapeutic
    ☐ Unknown/ other
☐ Initial exam
☐ Repeat exam

Primary person obtaining/ interpreting images: _____
Secondary person obtaining/ interpreting images: _____
Additional person(s) obtaining/ interpreting images: _____

Indication(s) for exam:

☐ abdominal pain   ☐ dysuria
☐ flank pain   ☐ acute renal failure
☐ back pain   ☐ anuria
☐ hematuria   ☐ post-void
☐ urinary retention   ☐ educational
☐ other: _____

Views obtained:

Right kidney long axis (coronal):	☐ adequate	☐ limited	☐ not obtained
Right kidney short axis:	☐ adequate	☐ limited	☐ not obtained
Left kidney long axis (coronal):	☐ adequate	☐ limited	☐ not obtained
Left kidney short axis:	☐ adequate	☐ limited	☐ not obtained
Transverse bladder:	☐ adequate	☐ limited	☐ not obtained
Sagittal bladder:	☐ adequate	☐ limited	☐ not obtained

☐ other: _____

Findings:

Right kidney

Hydronephrosis:	☐ **present**	☐ **absent**	☐ **indeterminate**
If present:	☐ **mild**	☐ **moderate**	☐ **severe**
	☐ **present degree unspecified**		
Hydoureter:	☐ present	☐ absent	☐ indeterminate
Kidney stones:	☐ present	☐ absent	☐ indeterminate
If present:	size of largest stone: ___mm		

	stone location(s):		
	☐ parenchyma		
	☐ renal pelvis		
	☐ UPJ		
	☐ Ureter		
	☐ UVJ		
Renal Cyst:	☐ present	☐ absent	☐ indeterminate
If present:	☐ simple	☐ complex	
	Diameter_____mm		
Extra-renal Pelvis:	☐ present	☐ absent	☐ indeterminate
Duplicated Ureteral System:	☐ present	☐ absent	☐ indeterminate

☐ other: _____

Left kidney

Hydronephrosis:	**☐ present**	**☐ absent**	**☐ indeterminate**
If present:	**☐ mild**	**☐ moderate**	**☐ severe**
	☐ present degree unspecified		
Hydoureter:	☐ present	☐ absent	☐ indeterminate
Kidney stones:	☐ present	☐ absent	☐ indeterminate
If present:	size of largest stone: ___mm		
	stone location(s):		
	☐ parenchyma		
	☐ renal pelvis		
	☐ UPJ		
	☐ Ureter		
	☐ UVJ		
Renal Cyst:	☐ present	☐ absent	☐ indeterminate
If present:	☐ simple	☐ complex	
	Diameter_____mm		
Extra-renal Pelvis:	☐ present	☐ absent	☐ indeterminate
Duplicated Ureteral System:	☐ present	☐ absent	☐ indeterminate

☐ other: _____

Bladder Dimensions
width: ___mm   height: ___mm depth: ___mm
volume: _____mL
Right ureteral jet: ☐ present ☐absent ☐indeterminate ☐ not assessed
Left ureteral jet: ☐ present ☐absent ☐indeterminate ☐ not assessed
other: _____

Interpretation:

☐ No sonographic evidence of renal tract obstruction			
☐ Hydronephrosis present	**☐ left**	**☐ right**	**☐ bilateral**
☐ **mild**			
☐ **moderate**			
☐ **severe**			
☐ **present, degree not specified**			
☐ Hydroureter present	☐ left	☐ right	☐ bilateral
☐ Nephrolithiasis	☐ left	☐ right	☐ bilateral
☐ parenchyma			
☐ UPJ			
☐ UVJ			
☐ Renal Cyst	☐ left	☐ right	☐ bilateral
☐ simple			
☐ complex			

❑ **Bladder Size**   ❑ **distended**   ❑ **collapsed**   ❑ **normal**
☐ other: _____

<u>**Quality assurance:**</u>

Suggested Quality Assurance Grading Scale

	1	2	3	4	5
Grading Scale Definitions	No recognizable structures, no objective data can be gathered	Minimally recognizable structures but insufficient for diagnosis	Minimal criteria met for diagnosis, recognizable structures but with some technical or other flaws	Minimal criteria met for diagnosis, all structures imaged well and diagnosis easily supported	Minimal criteria met for diagnosis, all structures imaged with excellent image quality and diagnosis completely supported

Image quality   1   2   3   4   5
Accuracy of interpretation of images as presented   TP   TN   FP   FN
Accuracy of interpretation of images as compared to
gold standard (ie, CT, operative report)   TP   TN   FP   FN

Comments: _____

FOCUSED THORACIC

The elements that are **BOLDED** *represent the core emergency ACEP views, findings and interpretations for each application.*

Patient/ exam demographics:

Patient name: _____
Patient gender: ☐ M ☐ F
DOB: ___ / ___ / ___
MR#: _____
Bar Code/Patient Identifier:_____
Hospital Name:_____
Date and time of exam: ___ / ___ / ___
Exam type:
    ☐ Diagnostic
    ☐ Educational
    ☐ Procedural

Clinical category:
    ☐ Resuscitative
    ☐ Symptom based
    ☐ Therapeutic
    ☐ Unknown/ other
☐ Initial exam
☐ Repeat exam

Primary person obtaining/ interpreting images: _____
Secondary person obtaining/ interpreting images: _____
Additional person(s) obtaining/ interpreting images: _____

Indication(s) for exam:

☐ dyspnea	☐ hypotension
☐ chest pain	☐ blunt thoracic trauma
☐ pleurisy	☐ penetrating thoracic trauma
☐ hypoxia	☐ educational
☐ other: _____	

Views:

Right anterior/ superior thorax:	☐ **adequate**	☐ **limited**	☐ **not obtained**
Right lateral/ inferior thorax:	☐ **adequate**	☐ **limited**	☐ **not obtained**
Left anterior/ superior thorax:	☐ **adequate**	☐ **limited**	☐ **not obtained**
Left lateral/ inferior thorax:	☐ **adequate**	☐ **limited**	☐ **not obtained**

    ☐ other: _____

Findings:

Right thorax

lung sliding:	☐ **present**	☐ **absent**	☐ **indeterminate**
lung point sign:	☐ present	☐ absent	☐ indeterminate
Interstitium:			
a-lines:	☐ present	☐ absent	☐ indeterminate
b-lines:	☐ present	☐ absent	☐ indeterminate
anterior/ superior region:	☐ present (greater than 3 per view)	☐ absent	
inferior/ lateral region:	☐ present (greater than 3 per view)	☐ absent	
pleural effusion:	☐ **present**	☐ **absent**	☐ **indeterminate**
If present:	☐ **small**	☐ **large**	

	anechoic	**complex**	
lung consolidation:	☐ present	☐ absent	☐ indeterminate
air bronchograms:	☐ present	☐ absent	☐ indeterminate
	☐ other: _____		

Left thorax

lung sliding:	**present**	**absent**	**indeterminate**
lung point sign:	☐ present	☐ absent	☐ indeterminate

Interstitium:

| a-lines: | ☐ present | ☐ absent | ☐ indeterminate |
| b-lines: | ☐ present | ☐ absent | ☐ indeterminate |

anterior/ superior region: ☐ present (greater than 3 per view)   ☐ absent

inferior/ lateral region: ☐ present (greater than 3 per view)   ☐ absent

pleural effusion:	**present**	**absent**	**indeterminate**
If present:	**small**	**large**	
	anechoic	**complex**	
lung consolidation:	☐ present	☐ absent	☐ indeterminate
air bronchograms:	☐ present	☐ absent	☐ indeterminate
	☐ other: _____		

Interpretation:

☐ **No sonographic evidence of acute pulmonary disease**

| ☐ **Pneumothorax** | ☐ **left** | ☐ **right** | ☐ **bilateral** |
| ☐ **Pleural effusion** | ☐ **left** | ☐ **right** | ☐ **bilateral** |

☐ Alveolar interstitial syndrome (focal)

☐ Alveolar interstitial syndrome (diffuse)

| ☐ Lung consolidation | ☐ left | ☐ right | ☐ bilateral |

☐ other: _____

Quality assurance:

Suggested Quality Assurance Grading Scale

	1	2	3	4	5
Grading Scale Definitions	No recognizable structures, no objective data can be gathered	Minimally recognizable structures but insufficient for diagnosis	Minimal criteria met for diagnosis, recognizable structures but with some technical or other flaws	Minimal criteria met for diagnosis, all structures imaged well and diagnosis easily supported	Minimal criteria met for diagnosis, all structures imaged with excellent image quality and diagnosis completely supported

Image quality   1   2   3   4   5

Accuracy of interpretation of images as presented   TP   TN   FP   FN

Accuracy of interpretation of images as compared to
gold standard (ie, CT, operative report)   TP   TN   FP   FN

Comments: _____

FOCUSED LOWER EXTREMITY VENOUS

The elements that are **BOLDED** *represent the core emergency ACEP views, findings and interpretations for each application.*

Patient/ exam demographics:

Patient name: _____
Patient gender: ☐ M ☐ F
DOB: ___ / ___ / ___
MR#: _____
Bar Code/Patient Identifier:_____
Hospital Name:_____
Date and time of exam: ___ / ___ / ___
Exam type:
    ☐ Diagnostic
    ☐ Educational
    ☐ Procedural

Clinical category:
    ☐ Resuscitative
    ☐ Symptom based
    ☐ Therapeutic
    ☐ Unknown/ other
☐ Initial exam
☐ Repeat exam

Primary person obtaining/ interpreting images: _____
Secondary person obtaining/ interpreting images: _____
Additional person(s) obtaining/ interpreting images: _____

Indication(s) for exam:

    ☐ leg pain: ☐ left   ☐ right ☐ bilateral
    ☐ leg swelling: ☐ left   ☐ right ☐ bilateral
    ☐ leg erythema: ☐ left   ☐ right ☐ bilateral
    ☐ dyspnea
    ☐ tachypnea
    ☐ pleurisy
    ☐ educational
    ☐ other: _____

Views:

Right saphenofemoral junction:	☐ **adequate**	☐ **limited**	☐ **not obtained**
Right common femoral vein:	☐ **adequate**	☐ **limited**	☐ **not obtained**
Right femoral vein:	☐ **adequate**	☐ **limited**	☐ **not obtained**
Right popliteal vein:	☐ **adequate**	☐ **limited**	☐ **not obtained**
Right popliteal trifurcation:	☐ **adequate**	☐ **limited**	☐ **not obtained**
Left saphenofemoral junction:	☐ **adequate**	☐ **limited**	☐ **not obtained**
Left common femoral vein:	☐ **adequate**	☐ **limited**	☐ **not obtained**
Left femoral vein:	☐ **adequate**	☐ **limited**	☐ **not obtained**
Left popliteal vein:	☐ **adequate**	☐ **limited**	☐ **not obtained**
Left popliteal trifurcation:	☐ **adequate**	☐ **limited**	☐ **not obtained**

☐ other: _____

Findings:

Right leg

     Saphenofemoral junction: ❏ compressible ❏ NOT compressible ❏ indeterminate
     Common femoral vein: ❏ compressible ❏ NOT compressible ❏ indeterminate
     Femoral vein: ❏ compressible ❏ NOT compressible ❏ indeterminate
     Popliteal vein: ❏ compressible ❏ NOT compressible ❏ indeterminate
     Popliteal trifurcation: ❏ compressible ❏ NOT compressible ❏ indeterminate
     ❏ other: _____

Left leg

     Saphenofemoral junction: ❏ compressible ❏ NOT compressible ❏ indeterminate
     Common femoral vein: ❏ compressible ❏ NOT compressible ❏ indeterminate
     Femoral vein: ❏ compressible ❏ NOT compressible ❏ indeterminate
     Popliteal vein: ❏ compressible ❏ NOT compressible ❏ indeterminate
     Popliteal trifurcation: ❏ compressible ❏ NOT compressible ❏ indeterminate
     ❏ other: _____

Interpretation:

     ❏ no sonographic evidence of deep vein thrombosis
     ❏ DVT present
         Location(s):

❏ R saphenofemoral junction	❏ L saphenofemoral junction
❏ R CFV	❏ L CFV
❏ R FV	❏ L FV
❏ R popliteal	❏ L popliteal
❏ R popliteal trifurcation	❏ L popliteal trifurcation

     ❏ indeterminate for DVT
     ❏ other: _____

Quality assurance:

Suggested Quality Assurance Grading Scale

	1	2	3	4	5
Grading Scale Definitions	No recognizable structures, no objective data can be gathered	Minimally recognizable structures but insufficient for diagnosis	Minimal criteria met for diagnosis, recognizable structures but with some technical or other flaws	Minimal criteria met for diagnosis, all structures imaged well and diagnosis easily supported	Minimal criteria met for diagnosis, all structures imaged with excellent image quality and diagnosis completely supported

Image quality   1   2   3   4   5
Accuracy of interpretation of images as presented   TP   TN   FP   FN
Accuracy of interpretation of images as compared to
gold standard (ie, CT, operative report)   TP   TN   FP   FN

     Comments: _____

FOCUSED CARDIAC ULTRASOUND

The elements that are **BOLDED** *represent the core emergency ACEP views, findings and interpretations for each application.*

Patient/ exam demographics:

Patient name: _____
Patient gender: □ M □ F
DOB: ___ / ___ / ___
MR#: _____
Bar Code/Patient Identifier:_____
Hospital Name:_____
Date and time of exam: ___ / ___ / ___
Exam type:
    □ Diagnostic
    □ Educational
    □ Procedural

Clinical category:
    □ Resuscitative
    □ Symptom based
    □ Therapeutic
    □ Unknown/ other
□ Initial exam
□ Repeat exam

Primary person obtaining/ interpreting images: _____
Secondary person obtaining/ interpreting images: _____
Additional person(s) obtaining/ interpreting images: _____

Indication(s) for exam:

    □ cardiac arrest   □ chest wall injury
    □ hypotension   □ dyspnea
    □ shock   □ syncope
    □ chest pain   □ tachypnea
    □ shortness of breath   □ fever
    □ tachycardia   □ educational
    □ palpitations
    □ other: _____

Views:

Subxiphoid (4 chamber):	□ adequate	□ limited	□ not obtained
Parasternal long axis:	□ adequate	□ limited	□ not obtained
Parasternal short axis:	□ adequate	□ limited	□ not obtained
Subxiphoid (long axis, IVC view):	□ adequate	□ limited	□ not obtained
Apical four-chamber:	□ adequate	□ limited	□ not obtained
	□ other: _____		

Findings:

Pericardial effusion: □ present   □ absent □ indeterminate size
    if present   □ small   □ moderate □ large □ present size not specified
        Evidence of tamponade   □ **IVC plethoric**
                                   □ **R atrial collapse**
                                   □ **R ventricular collapse**
                                   □ **Excessive mitral inflow variation**

Global Ventricular Function: ❏ hyperdynamic   ❏ normal
                                   ❏ reduced   ❏ severely reduced
                                   ❏ asystole   ❏ indeterminate
Right Ventricular Size: ❏ normal   ❏ dilated   ❏ indeterminate
              Signs of RV strain   ❏ RV hypokinesis
                                              ❏ Paradoxical septal motion
                                              ❏ McConnell's Sign
                                              ❏ Tricuspid regurgitation
                                                      Max velocity: ___m/s
                                              ❏ RV hypertrophy
Thoracic aorta: ❏ present   ❏ absent   ❏ indeterminate
                             Aortic root: ____mm
                             Thoracic aorta diameter: _____mm
IVC: ❏ normal   ❏ dilated   ❏ collapsed   ❏ indeterminate
                             Maximum diameter: ___mm
                             Minimum diameter: ___mm
                             Collapse: ❏ >50%   ❏ <50%
       other: _____

Interpretation:
❏ **No sonographic evidence of significant cardiac dysfunction**
❏ **No sonographic evidence of significant pericardial effusion**
❏ **Pericardial effusion**
        ❏ **small**   ❏ **moderate**   ❏ **large**
        ❏ **present size not specified**
❏ **Pericardial effusion with evidence of pericardial tamponade**
❏ **Global ventricular function:**
        ❏ **hyperdynamic**   ❏ **normal**
        ❏ **reduced**   ❏ **severely reduced**
❏ **No cardiac activity/ Cardiac standstill**
❏ **No sonographic evidence of RV size dilation**
❏ **RV dilation**
❏ **No sonographic evidence of volume depletion**
❏ **Sonographic findings suggestive of volume depletion**
❏ **Dilated IVC**
❏ No evidence of sonographic aortic root dilation
❏ Dilated Aortic Root
❏ other: _____

Quality assurance:

Suggested Quality Assurance Grading Scale

	1	2	3	4	5
Grading Scale Definitions	No recognizable structures, no objective data can be gathered	Minimally recognizable structures but insufficient for diagnosis	Minimal criteria met for diagnosis, recognizable structures but with some technical or other flaws	Minimal criteria met for diagnosis, all structures imaged well and diagnosis easily supported	Minimal criteria met for diagnosis, all structures imaged with excellent image quality and diagnosis completely supported

Image quality	1	2	3	4	5				

Image quality   1   2   3   4   5

Accuracy of interpretation of images as presented   TP   TN   FP   FN

Accuracy of interpretation of images as compared to
gold standard (ie, CT, operative report)   TP   TN   FP   FN

    Comments: _____

SOFT TISSUE/MUSCULOSKELETAL

The elements that are **BOLDED** *represent the core emergency ACEP views, findings and interpretations for each application.*

Patient/ exam demographics:

Patient name: _____
Patient gender: ☐ M ☐ F
DOB: ___ / ___ / ___
MR#: _____
Bar Code/Patient Identifier:_____
Hospital Name:_____
Date and time of exam: ___ / ___ / ___
Exam type:
   ☐ Diagnostic
   ☐ Educational
   ☐ Procedural

Clinical category:
   ☐ Resuscitative
   ☐ Symptom based
   ☐ Therapeutic
   ☐ Unknown/ other
☐ Initial exam
☐ Repeat exam

Primary person obtaining/ interpreting images: _____
Secondary person obtaining/ interpreting images: _____
Additional person(s) obtaining/ interpreting images: _____

Indication(s) for exam:

☐ Swelling	☐ Mass	☐ Decreased Range of Motion
☐ Redness	☐ Fever	☐ Deformity
☐ Pain	☐ Foreign Body	☐ Educational
☐ other: _____		

Views:

Skin and subcutaneous tissue:	**☐ adequate**	**☐ limited**	**☐ not obtained**
Muscle:	☐ adequate	☐ limited	☐ not obtained
Tendon:	☐ adequate	☐ limited	☐ not obtained
Joint:	☐ adequate	☐ limited	☐ not obtained
Bone:	☐ adequate	☐ limited	☐ not obtained
	☐ other: _____		

Findings:

Skin and subcutaneous tissue:

Tissue thickness	☐ normal	☐ thickened	☐ indeterminate
	Thickness _____mm		
Tissue Echogenicity	☐ normal	☐ increased	☐ indeterminate
Cobblestoning	**☐ normal**	**☐ increased**	**☐ indeterminate**
Subcutaneous Collection	**☐ present**	**☐ absent**	**☐ indeterminate**
If present	Diameter _____mm		

Muscle:

Appearance	☐ normal	☐ irregular	☐ indeterminate
Echogenicity	☐ normal	☐ increased	☐ indeterminate

	Collection	☐ present	☐ absent	☐ indeterminate

Tendon:

	Appearance	☐ normal	☐ irregular	☐ indeterminate
	Defect	☐ present	☐ absent	☐ indeterminate

Joint: ☐ fluid ☐ no fluid ☐ indeterminate

Bone:

	Cortex Appearance	☐ normal	☐ irregular	☐ indeterminate
	If irregular	☐ aligned	☐ angulated/misaligned	
		☐ other: _____		

Interpretation:
☐ **No sonographic evidence of soft tissue abnormality**
☐ No sonographic evidence of musculoskeletal abnormality
☐ **Cellulitis**   ☐ **location:**_____
☐ **Abscess**   ☐ **location:**_____
☐ Joint Effusion   ☐ location:_____
☐ Tendon Injury   ☐ complete   ☐ partial   ☐ indeterminate
☐ Fractured Bone   ☐ location:_____
☐ other: _____

Quality assurance:

Suggested Quality Assurance Grading Scale

	1	2	3	4	5
Grading Scale Definitions	No recognizable structures, no objective data can be gathered	Minimally recognizable structures but insufficient for diagnosis	Minimal criteria met for diagnosis, recognizable structures but with some technical or other flaws	Minimal criteria met for diagnosis, all structures imaged well and diagnosis easily supported	Minimal criteria met for diagnosis, all structures imaged with excellent image quality and diagnosis completely supported

Image quality   1   2   3   4   5

Accuracy of interpretation of images as presented   TP   TN   FP   FN

Accuracy of interpretation of images as compared to
gold standard (ie, CT, operative report)   TP   TN   FP   FN

Comments: _____

OCULAR

*The elements that are **BOLDED** represent the core emergency ACEP views, findings and interpretations for each application.*

Patient/exam demographics:

Patient name: _____
Patient gender: ☐ M ☐ F
DOB: ___ / ___ / ___
MR#: _____
Bar Code/Patient Identifier: _____
Hospital Name: _____
Date and time of exam: ___ / ___ / ___
Exam type:
    ☐ Diagnostic
    ☐ Educational
    ☐ Procedural

Clinical category:
    ☐ Resuscitative
    ☐ Symptom based
    ☐ Therapeutic
    ☐ Unknown/ other
☐ Initial exam
☐ Repeat exam

Primary person obtaining/ interpreting images: _____
Secondary person obtaining/ interpreting images: _____
Additional person(s) obtaining/ interpreting images: _____

Indication(s) for exam:

☐ eye pain   ☐ head injury
☐ eye/orbital trauma   ☐ suspected foreign body
☐ vision change   ☐ headache
☐ visual loss   ☐ educational
☐ other: _____

Views:

Right eye transverse:	☐ **adequate**	☐ **limited**	☐ **not obtained**
Right eye longitudinal:	☐ **adequate**	☐ **limited**	☐ **not obtained**
Left eye transverse:	☐ **adequate**	☐ **limited**	☐ **not obtained**
Left eye longitudinal:	☐ **adequate**	☐ **limited**	☐ **not obtained**
	☐ other: _____		

Findings:

Right eye

Retinal contour:	☐ **normal**	☐ **abnormal/ detached**	☐ **indeterminate**
Lens:	☐ normally located	☐ dislodged	☐ indeterminate
Vitreous body:	☐ **anechoic**	☐ **hyperechoic density**	☐ **indeterminate**
Optic nerve sheath:	☐ enlarged	☐ normal	☐ indeterminate
ONSD: ____ mm			
☐ other: _____			

Left eye

Retinal contour:	☐ **normal**	☐ **abnormal/ detached**	☐ **indeterminate**

Lens: □ normally located □ dislodged   □ indeterminate
Vitreous body: ⊐ **anechoic**   ⊐ **hyperechoic density** ⊐ **indeterminate**
Optic nerve sheath: □ enlarged   □ normal   □ indeterminate
                              ONSD: ____mm
                         □ other: _____

Interpretation:

⊐ **No acute abnormalities identified**
⊐ **Retinal Detachment**   ⊐ **left**   ⊐ **right**   ⊐ **bilateral**
□ Lens dislocation   □ left   □ right   □ bilateral
⊐ **Vitreous Hemorrhage**   ⊐ **left**   ⊐ **right**   ⊐ **bilateral**
□ Intraocular Foreign body   □ left   □ right   □ bilateral
□ Increased ONSD   □ left   □ right   □ bilateral
□ other: _____

Quality assurance:

Suggested Quality Assurance Grading Scale

	1	2	3	4	5
Grading Scale Definitions	No recognizable structures, no objective data can be gathered	Minimally recognizable structures but insufficient for diagnosis	Minimal criteria met for diagnosis, recognizable structures but with some technical or other flaws	Minimal criteria met for diagnosis, all structures imaged well and diagnosis easily supported	Minimal criteria met for diagnosis, all structures imaged with excellent image quality and diagnosis completely supported

Image quality   1   2   3   4   5
Accuracy of interpretation of images as presented   TP   TN   FP   FN
Accuracy of interpretation of images as compared to
gold standard (ie, CT, operative report)   TP   TN   FP   FN

Comments: _____

Essential Machine Features

EMERGENCY ULTRASOUND:
Essential Machine Features
Updated for 2014

Mark Byrne MD
Chair, Industry Relations Subcommittee
Emergency Ultrasound Section
American College of Emergency Physicians

© Springer International Publishing AG 2018   587
V. S. Tayal et al. (eds.), *Ultrasound Program Management*,
https://doi.org/10.1007/978-3-319-63143-1

1. **COMPACT & EASILY MOBILE**
   - Fits into patient rooms, limited spaces
   - Width and depth kept to a minimum
   - Wheels are high quality, multi-directional
   - Light weight, easy maneuverability
   - Most ED applications best served by a compact cart-based system
   - Storage options (e.g. for extra gel, cleaning agents, probe covers, angiocaths, etc.)

2. **IMAGE QUALITY & VERSATILITY**
   - 2-D image quality is essential
   - Maximize in difficult/obese patients
   - Capabilities for multiple applications
     - General/abdominal (wide footprint curvilinear probe)
     - Cardiac (phased array probe)
     - Vascular, soft tissue, procedural (high frequency linear probe)
     - Pelvic, obstetrical (endocavitary/transvaginal probe)
   - Midline mark on linear, curvilinear probes to facilitate procedural applications
   - Multiple probe ports (minimum 3, preferably 4), easy switching between transducers
   - Multiple holders to accommodate 3-4 probes, gel bottle(s), and barcode scanner
   - Large, bright screen, broad viewing angles
   - Monitor easily articulates in all directions
   - Needle localization/guidance technologies highly desirable

3. **EASE-OF-USE & SIMPLIFICATION**
   - Quick boot-up time (including "cold boot")
   - Battery powered sleep mode
   - Maximal battery life (at least 2-3 hours battery powered scanning)
   - Rapid battery recharging
   - Reminders (visual and auditory) when battery level low

   - Simplified control panel, essential functions highlighted

- On/Off	- Zoom
- Start/End exam	- Freeze
- Exam type	- Measure
- Depth	- Calculations
- Gain	- Still image
- Optimize	- Video

   - Control panel should be backlit, with large buttons and large print
   - Physical knobs/dials preferable for functions such as depth, gain
   - Sealed control panel surface for easy cleaning
   - Keyboard best if sealed (not easily penetrated by liquids) or pull-out
   - Should be as intuitive as possible (users of varying skill levels)
   - Retain ability to pull up more advanced features
   - Touch screen panel on cart (not monitor) well-suited for this purpose
     - Allow for maximal customization (i.e. which functions to include/exclude)
     - Default to basic functions, with option to access more advanced modes
   - Touch panels must be responsive (do not lag) and reliable, continue to function despite exposure to gel, bodily fluids

- Start exam screen fields
  - Patient name
  - Medical record number
  - Accession number
  - Examiner name(s) (two fields to allow for trainee/supervisor)
  - Probe selection
  - Exam type preset

4. DURABILITY & SERVICE

- ED is a harsh environment, demands 24/7 uptime
- Machine, probes, cords need to be rugged
  - Probes may be dropped onto the ground
  - Probe cords, power cords may be run over by the machine wheels
  - Probes, machine may be exposed to bodily fluids (blood, pus, etc.)
- Machine cord management commonly under-appreciated
- Probe cords must be durable (protected), cart designed to minimize cords tangling or being run over by machine wheels
- Probe holders should be stable, strong, easily cleaned
- Power cord ideally retractable, otherwise easily stowed and should not originate from bottom of cart, which promotes tangling in cart wheels

- Service needs to be prompt and accessible 24/7
  - Need availability beyond Monday-Friday 9am-5pm business hours
  - ED required to be in full operation nights, weekends, and holidays
- Affordable service plan options, either included plan (5 years) or contract paid yearly
- Commonly broken parts should be separate (modular) and easily replaceable
- Ability to export and import machine system settings (i.e. for loaner machines in case primary machine is out of service for repairs)
- Software failures (freezes, reboots) unacceptable

5. IMAGE ARCHIVAL & WORKFLOW

- Record as still images and cine loops to internal storage
- Internal storage capacity upgradeable (not fixed in size)
- DICOM capabilities should be standard on all machines
- Widely used export formats for still images (JPEG) and cine loops (MOV, AVI, MP4)
- Export options should include USB, CD/DVD, and (less commonly) thermal print
- Integrated Wi-Fi capabilities essential for all future machines models
- Wi-Fi adapter housed within a secured location on machine cart (not attached externally)
- Support for all IEEE 802.11 standards, security protocols used in healthcare IT

- Workflow should be designed using standardized, non-proprietary formats
- Front-end workflow: getting information into the machine (i.e. patient information, sonographer name(s), exam type, indication for scan)
- Optimize front-end workflow via barcode scanners, DICOM modality worklists
- Separate diagnostic studies from those performed for educational purposes
- Ultrasound interpretation ("worksheets") filled out directly on machines
- Worksheets should include indication, views, findings, interpretation based on ACEP Standard Reporting Guidelines, but essential that they are fully user customizable

- Back-end workflow: getting information out of the machine (i.e. transfer ultrasound images and interpretations to the PACS and EMR)
- Ideal workflow to obtain images and document findings directly on the machine, then wireless transfer of ultrasound images and report from machine to the PACS and EMR

6. FUTURE INNOVATIONS
- Wireless probe technologies highly desirable for the ED setting
- Consider incorporation of basic controls (e.g. image capture, depth, gain) onto the ultrasound probe
- Ability to pull up teaching images (standard views, probe placement, pathologic images) directly on machines

Glossary

AAMC-LCME	Association of American Medical Colleges Liaison Committee on Medical Education
AAP	American Academy of Pediatrics
ABMS-MOC	American Board of Medical Specialties-Maintenance of Certification
ACCE	Advanced Critical Care Examination
ACCP	American College of Chest Physicians
Accreditation	The process of review that healthcare organizations participate in to demonstrate the ability to meet predetermined criteria and standards of accreditation established by a professional accrediting agency.
ACEP	American College of Emergency Physicians
ACGME-RRC	Accreditation Council for Graduate Medical Education—Residency Review Committee
ACGME	Accreditation Council for Graduate Medical Education (ACGME) is a private, nonprofit organization that reviews and accredits graduate medical education (residency and fellowship) programs, and the institutions that sponsor them, in the United States.
ACR	American College of Radiologists
ADT	Admissions, discharge, and transfer system serves as the framework for most hospital IT systems. It holds essential patient information including full name, date of birth, medical record, and account numbers.
ACCE	Advanced Critical Care Echocardiography (ACCE) includes both focused cardiac ultrasound and advanced applications of echocardiography.

© Springer International Publishing AG 2018
V. S. Tayal et al. (eds.), *Ultrasound Program Management*,
https://doi.org/10.1007/978-3-319-63143-1

AHRQ	Agency for Healthcare Research and Quality—organization with mission to produce evidence to make healthcare safer, higher quality, more accessible, equitable, and affordable, and to work within the U.S. Department of Health and Human Services and with other partners to make sure that the evidence is understood and used.
AIUM	American Institute of Ultrasound in Medicine
ALARA	As Low As Reasonably Achievable, used in the context of any imaging study's energy effects towards the body.
APP	Advanced Practice Provider, typically physician assistants, nurse practitioners, and nurse anesthetists.
ASE	American Society of Echocardiography
Bioeffect	Biological effects of *ultrasound* are the potential biological consequences due to the interaction between the *ultrasound* wave and the scanned tissues.
Blended learning	Instruction where a portion of the traditional face-to-face instruction is replaced by web-based online **learning.**
CCM Ultrasound	Critical Care Medicine Ultrasound
CCUE	Critical Care Ultrasound Exam
Centers for Medicare and Medicaid Services (CMS)	US federal agency which oversees Medicare, Medicaid, and Children's Health Insurance Program
CDC	Center for Disease Control, an agency of US Department of Health and Human Services that issues infection control and disease guidelines.
CMS 1500	Standard physician billing form
CMUT	Capacitive Micromachined Ultrasound Transducer
Cold boot	Starting the Ultrasound machine from no power to full power
Compact cart	Smaller ultrasound system with monitor keyboard and probe connections (usually more than one), with narrowed footprint compared to large radiology and cardiology machine.
Competency	Having the technical, cognitive, and integrative skills to perform a procedure or group of procedures.

Consultative ultrasound	Ultrasonography done in a more traditional manner with performance by sonographers and interpreted by a physician, typically, remote to the patient. Typically in radiology and cardiology, but also in obstetrics/gynecology and vascular laboratories.
Continuing education	Education outside a formal program of education, usually in a shorter time period or framework. In the context of medical education, typically short courses taken beyond residency or fellowship.
CORD	Council of Residency Directors (Emergency Medicine)
CPOE	Computerized physician order entry
CPT	Current Procedural Terminology, a coding classification used in the United States through the American Medical Association.
Credentialing	The process of gathering information regarding a physician's qualifications for appointment to the medical staff with verification of physician's qualifications, such as residency training and board certification.
Critical Care Ultrasound (CCUS)	Noncardiac ultrasound applications as well as focused cardiac ultrasound.
Current Procedural Terminology (CPT)	AMA publication on procedural codes that physicians use to identify services rendered.
CUAP	Clinical Ultrasound Accreditation Program, a POC accreditation system run by the ACEP.
CUS	Clinical Ultrasound, or ultrasound examinations done by clinicians.
Deliberate Practice	Purposeful structured goal-oriented learning, with repetitive performance of skills, coupled with rigorous skills assessment rather than simply repeated practice of skills.
Diagnosis-related group (DRG)	System used to categorize hospital inpatients based on diagnosis code for reimbursement purposes.
DICOM	Digital Imaging and Communications in Medicine, a common international standard for creating, saving, and transmitting images.
DRG	Diagnosis-Related Group
Emergency Ultrasound	Point of care ultrasound performed by emergency physicians or providers in emergency departments or emergency settings.
EMR	Electronic Medical Record

EMS	Emergency Medical Services, typically prehospital medical care in the United States.
FDA	Food and Drug Administration, an agency of the USA. Department of Health and Human Services. It has authority over medical safety of US machine and medical devices.
Fellowship	A concentrated period of medical education post-residency in specific, typically a field of knowledge, focused practice or subspecialty in medical education.
Flipped classroom	Is a model in which the typical lecture and hands-on portion of instruction in a course are reversed. Short online lectures are viewed by students before the class session, while in-class time is devoted to exercises, projects, or discussions.
FOAMed	Free Open Access Medical Education
Footprint	The area of the face of the ultrasound probe that touches the patient.
FPPE	Focused Professional Practice Evaluation—A more specific and time-limited monitoring of a practitioner's practice performance and is utilized when a provider is initially granted practice privileges, new privileges are requested for an already privileged provider or performance nonconformance involving an already privileged provider is identified.
Frequency	The repetition rate of a wave. In ultrasound, the rate of vibratory waves emitted from the US probe.
Gain	Amplification of sound
Gel	A substance made of water and other materials that facilitates by reducing resistance to sound transmission.
Global codes	Codes that either (1) cannot by definition be broken down into professional and technical components or (2) due to the practice setting in which the procedure is occurring, include both the professional and the technical components.
Hand carried	An ultrasound machine that can be carried by hand.
HHS	Health and Human Services. An American federal cabinet level agency that oversees federal health policy and is the major payor for the elderly and poor in the United States.
HIPPA	(Health Insurance Portability and Accountability Act of 1996) is United States legislation that provides data privacy and security provisions for safeguarding medical information.
HL7	Health Level 7 refers to a set of standards used in the transfer of administrative and clinical data among various healthcare software applications. It serves to enhance interoperability, giving electronic systems the ability to exchange information.
HLD	High-level disinfection

Hot boot	Also known as warm boot, starting an US machine from sleep mode, hinbernate mode, by touching a key or toggle button
IAC	Inter-Societal Accreditation Commission
I-AIM	Indication, Acquisition, Integration, and Medical Decision-Making methodology for sonologist to use
International Classification of Diseases (ICD)	Categorization system listing signs, symptoms, and diseases for billing purposes.
IEEE	Institute of Electrical and Electronics Engineers
IOM	Institute of Medicine (IOM) reports provide objective advice to decision makers and the public.
Import course	A type of CME course that occurs at the location of a specific medical group, hospital, or department. The course travels to the participants.
IT	Information Technology
LLD	Low-Level Disinfection
LMICs	Low- and Middle-Income Countries
Local coverage determinations (LCDs)	CMS description of clinical utility for a common CPT code which applies locally to providers in a particular geographic coverage area.
MCI	Mass Casualty Incident
Medicare Administrative Contractors (MAC)	Private companies hired by CMS to administer the responsibilities of Medicare Part A or B.
Medicare Physician Fee Schedule (MPFS)	Annual publication by CMS on RVUs and for varying CPT codes.
MI Mechanical Index	A measure of the potential for nonthermal ultrasound bioeffects, particularly those related to cavitation, the collapse of gas bubbles in response to the ultrasonic field.
MIPAA	The Medicare Improvements for Patients and Providers Act of 2008 (MIPPA), which was passed in July, calls for providers of advanced diagnostic imaging services (MR, CT, PET, and nuclear medicine) to be accredited in order to receive payment for the technical component of those services.

Middleware	Software with the goal of organizing and streamlining workflow in a clinical ultrasound program, also known as workflow, ultrasound management system.
Modular course	US course as part of a large meeting or conference.
Multiple Procedure Payment Reduction (MPPR)	Bundling for radiology procedures in the same family.
National coverage determination (NCD)	CMS description of clinical utility for a common CPT code which applies nationally.
NAS	Next Accreditation System, a short form for the ACGME "The Next Step in the Outcomes-Based Accreditation Project".
NEMA	National Electrical Manufacturers Association
NQF	National Quality Forum
Open course	A type of CME course which is at a fixed location but open to all.
OPPE	Ongoing Professional Practice Evaluation—A means of evaluating professional performance on an ongoing basis to monitor professional competency, identify areas for possible performance improvement by individual practitioners and obtain objective data in decisions regarding continuance of practice privileges.
OSAUS	Objective Structured Assessment of Ultrasound Skills.
OSCE	Objective structured clinical exams. A type of standardized examination using a model, usually live but can be simulated.
Output Display Standard	ODS, was developed and required to be displayed on Track 3 ultrasound systems, usually displaying important bioeffects indices.
PACS	Picture Archiving and Communication System (PACS)
PIV	Peripheral IV
POC	Point of Care
Pocket size	US machine that fits into a pocket.
POC US	Point of Care Ultrasound—Use of ultrasound by clinicians at the bedside to diagnose disease, monitor resuscitation, and guide procedures.
PPO	Preferred Provider Organization
Prehospital	Referring to activities and medical care performed prior to arriving to an established medical facility. In the United States, called Emergency Medical Services.

Principled negotiation	A strategy of negotiation to look for mutual benefit and shared interests instead of positional stances.
Privileging	The process by which the hospital determines the specific procedures that may be performed by each medical staff applicant and appointee in the hospital.
Probe	A part of the US device that is a hand-held instrument that typically holds the crystals that transform electrical voltage to sound waves via the piezoelectric effect or other technology that creates the US waves.
Professional component	Professional work involved in a procedure. With diagnostic ultrasound, the professional work is the interpretation of the images and creation of a report.
Prospective Payment System (PPS)	A method of reimbursement in which Medicare payment is made based on a predetermined, fixed amount. The payment amount for a particular service is based on the DRG.
Quality improvement	A systematic, formal approach to the analysis of practice performance and efforts to improve performance.
Radiation	Transmission of <u>energy</u> in the form of <u>waves</u> or <u>particles</u> through space or through a material medium. Often refers to ionizing radiation that uses electromagnetic radiation in plain X-rays, CT scans, fluoroscopy, and nuclear medicine.
Relative Value Scale Update Committee (RUC)	Multiply-specialty group reviews RVUs for approved CPT codes.
Relative value units (RVUs)	Measure of value used to weight physician services.
SAEM	Society of Academic Emergency Medicine
SCCM	Society of Critical Care Medicine
SCUF	Society of Clinical Ultrasound Fellowships
SDOT	Standard Direct Observation Tool
Simulator	Imitation of the operation of a real-world process or system in a device, model, computer program.
SOCCA	Society of Critical Care Anesthesiologists
Sonographer	Medical professional who performs ultrasonography. Mostly commonly refers to professional who has finished training in an Ultrasound school or finished sonographer training in an undergraduate college degree. Often anyone who performs ultrasound may be given this name.

Sonography	Noninvasive medical procedure that uses the echoes of high-frequency sound waves (ultrasound) to construct an image (sonogram) of internal organs or body structures.
Sonologist	A physician or advanced practitioner who performs, interprets, and integrates ultrasound into the clinical care of their patient.
SRLF	Société de Réanimation de Langue Française The French Intensive Care Society (FICS) is a learned society founded in 1971. Its mission is continuing medical education and post-university teaching and promotion of clinical research and assessment of hospital-based intensive care.
Sustainability	Anticipating and meeting the needs of society, both directly through actions in their local communities, and by preparing students for their future roles.
Technical component	Technical work involved in performing a procedure. With diagnostic ultrasound, the technical component covers the cost of equipment, technician salaries, image archiving, overhead, etc.
TI	Thermal Index is a ratio of the intensity of the ultrasound beam to the relative amount of energy required to raise the tissue temperature 1 °C.
TJC	The Joint Commission (formerly JACHO), an independent, not-for-profit organization that assesses hospitals for accreditation and certification to meet certain performance standards.
UBO4 Form	Medical insurance claim forms used by "facilities" to bill insurance companies for services rendered.
Ultrasonography	Use of high frequency sound waves the diagnosis, monitoring, or treatment in clinical care.
Ultrasound	Sound having an ultrasonic frequency >20,000 Hz used in medical imaging.
Ultrasound Management	The management of an ultrasound program in a department, facility, enterprise, or organization.
US workflow	See middleware also. The steps or process of US examination including patient ID, settings, performance, image capture, labeling measuring, interpretation, and reporting.
VPN	Virtual private network
Web-based	A system that reports data to the world wide web as opposed to local system or databases.
WINFOCUS	World Interactive Network for Focused Ultrasound

Index

© Springer International Publishing AG 2018
V.S. Tayal et al. (eds.), *Ultrasound Program Management*,
https://doi.org/10.1007/978-3-319-63143-1